Fluency Disorders

Fluency Disorders

Kenneth J. Logan, PhD, CCC-SLP

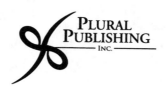

PLURAL
PUBLISHING
INC.

KH

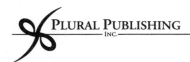

5521 Ruffin Road
San Diego, CA 92123

e-mail: info@pluralpublishing.com
Website: http://www.pluralpublishing.com

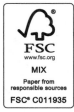

Copyright © by Plural Publishing, Inc. 2015

Typeset in 10½ × 13 Garamond by Flanagan's Publishing Services, Inc.
Printed in the United States of America by McNaughton & Gunn, Inc.

For permission to use material from this text, contact us by
Telephone: (866) 758-7251
Fax: (888) 758-7255
e-mail: permissions@pluralpublishing.com

*Every attempt has been made to contact the copyright holders for material originally
printed in another source. If any have been inadvertently overlooked, the publishers
will gladly make the necessary arrangements at the first opportunity.*

Library of Congress Cataloging-in-Publication Data

Logan, Kenneth J., author.
  Fluency disorders / Kenneth J. Logan.
      p. ; cm.
  Includes bibliographical references and index.
  ISBN 978-1-59756-407-6 (alk. paper)—ISBN 1-59756-407-9 (alk. paper)
  I. Title.
  [DNLM: 1. Speech Disorders. WL 340.2]
  RC423
  616.85'5—dc23
                                                          2014022905

7/15/15

Contents

Preface

This is an exciting era for those who have an interest in fluency disorders. For centuries—including a good portion of the 1900s—laypeople and experts alike have possessed only a marginal understanding of what causes disfluent speech and fluency disorders like stuttering and cluttering. This situation has led to misconceptions about not only the nature and treatment of fluency disorders but also the people who have such disorders. Fortunately, this situation seems to be changing.

Advances in technology and research methodologies during the past two decades have enabled researchers to examine aspects of biology, anatomy, physiology, and speech production that previously could be assessed only in a rudimentary manner, if they could be assessed at all. This has led to refinements in the understanding of speech production and to new insights into the nature of disorders such as stuttering and cluttering. With such information, researchers have created increasingly specific models about the types of deficits that are at the heart of these disorders. Substantial progress also has been made in recent years in understanding the consequences that fluency disorders have on affected individuals. Work in this area has, for example, led to a more detailed and accurate picture of how impaired fluency affects a person's psychosocial well-being, school and work experiences, and overall quality of life.

All of these advances are welcome news to speech-language pathologists. At the very least, there now is a sense of optimism that clinicians will soon have an accurate, precise answer to provide to clients who are curious about why they have difficulty speaking fluently. More broadly, these advances create hope for the development of new and more effective treatments for fluency disorders, as well as the prospect of improved societal understanding of fluency disorders and the various adverse effects that fluency disorders can have on an individual's functioning during daily activities. Of course, not everything about the study of fluency disorders is brand new. For example, there exists a host of well-established procedures for fluency assessment and a core set of behavioral treatment approaches that have been studied extensively. Even in these areas, however, researchers and clinicians are constantly refining and expanding existing clinical methods in ways that improve the reliability, validity, effectiveness, and/or efficiency of existing practices. Clearly, there is much to discuss in the arena of fluency disorders.

My purpose in writing *Fluency Disorders* was to provide readers with a comprehensive and up-to-date overview of the topics that I have outlined above. I have attempted to capture the current state of affairs in terms of our knowledge about areas such as normal aspects of speech fluency, the nature and characteristics of fluency disorders, and contemporary assessment and treatment procedures. I also have attempted to provide specific details about particular aspects of fluency assessment, caseload selection, and treatment. Such information should provide readers with a solid platform upon which they can build requisite clinical skills and develop an appreciation for the decision-making processes that underlie clinical practice.

As all authors do, I have written this book from a certain perspective. More precisely, I have approached *Fluency Disorders* from three interlocking perspectives that, when taken together, map rather neatly on to contemporary notions of evidence-based practice. The first perspective deals with research. Here, my goal was to provide readers with a comprehensive overview of what science tells us about fluency disorders. Consideration of high-quality, peer-reviewed research is critical to clinical practice, as it enables clinicians to evaluate not only the effectiveness of particular treatments but also the breadth and depth of what we understand about the nature and characteristics of particular disorders. The volume of research on fluency disorders is substantial, and it seems as if during the past century, scientists have examined virtually every variable that conceivably might pertain to fluency disorders. Rather than attempt to address *everything* that researchers have studied with respect to fluency disorders, I instead opted to focus primarily on a combination of those topics that are addressed in contemporary research on fluency disorders and those topics that were addressed in "older" research but continue to have relevance to either contemporary research or clinical practice.

The second perspective in *Fluency Disorders* deals with clinical practice. Here, my goal was to provide readers with a comprehensive overview of key practices associated with assessing and treating fluency-related behaviors. In contemporary models of evidence-based practice, clinical data provide clinicians with "internal evidence;" that is, an index of client performance in relation to particular tasks, settings, and treatment approaches. A treatment that is deemed to be highly effective at a group level may not be effective at all at an individual level, and internal evidence will help clinicians determine when this is the case. Throughout the years, several practical and conceptual problems have been identified with respect to fluency measurement. These problems can lead to imprecise and, in some instances, illogical statements about a client's functioning. For this reason, I discuss procedural approaches for fluency measurement at some length within the text. Not every detail of clinical practice can be specified, however. Thus, in other portions of the book, I present clinically relevant information in the form of general principles that are designed to provide readers with a framework to guide clinical practice.

The third perspective within *Fluency Disorders* is that of the client/patient. I can write from this perspective relatively easily by virtue of my lifelong experiences as a "person who stutters" and by having interacted with many fluency-impaired people in my roles as "fluency clinician" and "fluency researcher." Many of the examples that I offer with regard to what a client might do in a particular situation are drawn from personal experience in one of these three roles. Within the context of evidence-based practice, the client/patient perspective is just as important to consider as the *research* and *clinical practice* perspectives are.

Some clinicians I have met seem to think that one must have a fluency disorder in order to provide effective fluency treatment services to clients. This notion is simply untrue. In fact, many of the most valuable insights that I have gained about management of my stuttering have come from people who had typical fluency.

What *is* critical for effective service provision, however, is that clinicians have a solid understanding of both the research literature on fluency disorders and the client's current level of functioning, as well as a good sense of what the client with impaired fluency experiences during daily life and what he or she desires from treatment. There are many resources, including this textbook, available to learn about effective treatment approaches and evaluation of a client's functioning. Information about the client's experiences with stuttering may seem more difficult to attain but such information is readily available as well. Textbooks like this are, again, one source of information. Other sources include peer-reviewed research, internet discussion forums, conference presentations, and multimedia materials from professional organizations and self-help groups. And, of course, clinicians simply can ask clients to talk about their unique experiences.

In summary, *Fluency Disorders* is a book about research, clinical practice, and clinician and client perspectives on fluency, fluency impairment, and communication disability. It is my hope that, after reading the book, readers will have a good sense of what fluency and fluency disorders are, how fluency disorders affect people, and how speech-language pathologists can help those who have impaired fluency to function as effectively as possible in all daily activities.

Introduction

The purpose of this brief introduction is to provide readers with a sense of the basic structure and content of the book. With regard to physical organization, *Fluency Disorders* is divided into four main sections that follow a progression from normal to impaired functioning and from assessment to treatment. Each of the chapters concludes with a brief summary, which functions as an abstract of the main concepts that were presented. The terms *client* and *patient* are used in instances when the discussion focuses on clinical interactions and activities.

Section I deals with the nature of fluency: what fluent speech is, how typical speakers accomplish fluent speech, how disfluent speech arises, and what "normal fluency" is. A key point to be taken from this section is that "fluent speech" is by no means perfectly smooth. Thus, in a speaker who exhibits "typical fluency," speech is *mostly*, but not entirely, continuous, and the interruptions in fluency that do occur generally have little effect on the speaker's ability to communicate. Another key point is that fluency is more than just continuous speech. Rather, it is manifested in multiple ways, including speaking rate, rhythm, and effort; speech naturalness and talkativeness; as well as the stability of performance across situations and over time.

Section II deals mainly with the nature and characteristics of fluency disorders. The primary focus in this section is on developmental stuttering, which is the most common type of fluency disorder. Cluttering and acquired forms of fluency impairment are discussed at length in this section, as well. Also included in Section II is information about disfluency patterns observed in people who have concomitant disorders that affect language and/or cognition functioning. The disfluency patterns observed in these instances sometimes can be quite severe, but in many cases, they are relatively mild in terms of their impact on communication and, thus, are not likely to be the person's primary area of disability. Still in other cases, the disfluency patterns may be relatively mild in terms of frequency of occurrence but quite unusual in form and thus quite noticeable to listeners. The section offers discussion of the scope of fluency difficulties that exist, along with their associated etiologies and characteristics.

In Sections III and IV, the focus shifts toward practical matters associated with assessment and treatment. Section III deals with issues associated with assessing individuals who have fluency-related concerns. Topics in this section include basic assessment concepts, methods for collecting data about clients' fluency-related performance, details associated with analyzing aspects of fluency within a speech sample, as well as issues related to diagnosis, severity rating, prognosis, and clinical recommendations. Section IV deals with issues related to improving fluency functioning. The latter section begins with a detailed discussion of how to establish treatment goals, define treatment success, and select treatment approaches. The discussion then shifts toward general treatment principles. Basic properties of six general principles are outlined, and the evidence base associated with each of the principles is summarized. It is argued that a principle-based approach to intervention provides clinicians with a mechanism for integrating research-based treatments with data from clinical practice and the client's unique problem profile and treatment values. This is not a prescriptive, one-size-fits-all approach to intervention but rather one that is intended to promote individualized intervention within an evidence-based context. The focus on treatment principles also leads naturally to discussion about the *commonalities* that exist among the numerous treatment strategies that have been described in the treatment literature. As a consequence, traditional dichotomies between "fluency shaping approaches" and "stuttering modification approaches" are downplayed, while the similarities that exist across intervention approaches (e.g., regulation of speech motor movements) are emphasized.

The book concludes with an overview of the treatment literature, with particular emphasis on outcome studies conducted with speakers who stutter. Studies are organized according to the particular treatment principles that the researchers in a particular study emphasized most. Many of the treatment protocols in these studies incorporate more than one of the six treatment principles we have outlined. Still, in most of these cases, one or two treatment principles are emphasized to a much greater extent than the others. Review of these studies will provide readers with examples of how clinical scientists have implemented treatment principles within a research context. General summaries of these treatments are presented in this text. Readers are advised to consult the original sources for specific details on the implementation of a particular treatment. Summaries of the research literatures on altered auditory feedback and drug-based intervention are presented as well, so that readers will have a sense for the status of these approaches to intervention. The book ends with a brief discussion of approaches to evaluating treatment outcomes. A multidimensional framework to outcome assessment is described, wherein progress can be examined from both clinician and client perspectives and within skill-building contexts as well as real-world settings.

Acknowledgments

Although my name stands alone on the cover of this book, in reality there are many people who contributed to its content and production. These contributions range from large to small, direct to indirect, and immediate to remote. I appreciate each of them greatly.

Lori Altmann, Lisa Edmonds, Paul Fogel, Lisa LaSalle, Nancy Logan, Charlie Osborne, Iomi Patten, Jamie Reilly, Dale Williams, and several anonymous reviewers offered critical commentary and/or helpful background information on initial drafts of various chapters. Natalie Logan developed the concept for the front cover design, and she and Chris Logan helped with preliminary cross-checking of the citations and references. Aaron McEnery patiently answered all of my questions that dealt with technical issues. Linda Lombardino, Nan Bernstein Ratner, and Chris Sapienza provided valuable input when the project was at the pre-proposal stage.

Many people have played significant roles in shaping my understanding of fluency disorders, but I particularly want to acknowledge the many undergraduate, master's, and doctoral students who have passed through the Speech Fluency Lab and the *Introduction to Speech Disorders* and *Stuttering* courses at the University of Florida. There have been many times when their questions and comments have prompted me to think about fluency disorders in new ways. I also wish to acknowledge C. Woodruff (Woody) Starkweather, whose 1987 text helped me appreciate how *fluency* and *stuttering* fit together. That notion has stuck with me since I first read his book in the late 1980s, and it runs throughout this book. Special appreciation goes to Edward G. Conture for his invaluable mentorship and insights about fluency disorders at all stages of my career.

I also wish to acknowledge the production staff at Plural Publishing for their assistance and input during all phases of the project. I am particularly appreciative of the efforts put forth by Milgem (Gem) Rabinera, the primary project editor. Her ability to combine good-natured prodding with a calm demeanor and ample patience played a critical role in pushing the book to completion. I extend my gratitude to Dr. Sadanand Singh for providing the opportunity to develop this book. His energy and enthusiasm for publishing inspired me throughout the writing process. Finally, I wish to thank my family—and especially my wife, Nancy—for all of the cheerful assistance, thoughtful gestures, and unwavering support at all stages of this project.

*To those people who have difficulty speaking fluently
and the professionals who work with them.*

SECTION
I

Foundational Concepts

1

Conceptualizing Fluency

The term *fluency* has several connotations, one of which is to characterize the way in which people perform tasks that require sequenced movements. Consider, for example, the seamless twists and turns that a gymnast makes while performing a routine on the parallel bars or the sweeping finger movements that a pianist makes while playing a classical music piece. The notion of fluency has relevance in the domain of human communication as well, where one can describe the fluency with which people read, write, sign, and speak. Our primary focus in this text is on *speech fluency*; that is, the fluency that people exhibit when speaking. That said, we also touch on fluency as it pertains to other domains of communication such as oral reading.

Demonstrations of highly fluent speech are commonplace and, at times, truly impressive. Consider the carefully measured sentences of a woman who is delivering a eulogy for a lifelong friend, the rapid-fire remarks of an auctioneer who attempts to entice a roomful of bargain hunters to purchase items at a favorable price, or the fiery rhetoric of a politician who seeks the support of voters in an upcoming election. Instances of highly fluent speech are evident in many mundane activities as well—ordering a cup a coffee, for example, or scheduling a medical appointment. Indeed, fluent speech is so commonplace during daily activities that most people take very little notice of this aspect of communication. When an individual's speech fluency deviates significantly from the norm, however, it can literally turn heads. It seems as if everyone wants a glimpse of the disfluent speaker.

The word *fluency* derives from the Latin word *fluere*, which means *fluid*. Not surprisingly, the notion of fluidity figures prominently in both academic and nonacademic definitions of fluency. Dictionary definitions for fluency typically list descriptors such as *ease, effort,* and *proficiency*. These same terms appear in academic discussions of fluency, as well. Although ease, effort, and proficiency are integral to understanding the construct of fluency, there also are other aspects of fluency that warrant consideration. These issues are discussed in the next section.

Dimensions of Fluency

In one sense, descriptors such as *ease*, *effort*, and *proficiency* capture some of what is most important in speech fluency, but, in another sense, they only scratch the surface in describing the nature of speech fluency and its relationship to verbal communication. As a general rule, the study of any subject area can be enriched by the use of a conceptual framework or model. A model provides interested parties with a "roadmap" of the territory that is to be examined along with a sense for the number and types of variables that should be considered when studying the subject area (Bernstein Ratner, 2005; Friel-Patti, 1994). The use of a conceptual model also helps focus the kinds of questions that one asks about the subject area, and it leads to predictions about the kinds of answers one expects to get in response to the questions.

It is against this backdrop, that we introduce the concept of *fluency dimensions*; that is, the perspectives from which one can study fluency. As we will see, fluency is a multidimensional construct, and it is important to clarify what these dimensions are prior to discussing a comprehensive model of fluency. We begin our discussion of fluency dimensions with an overview of influential work by Fillmore (1979) and Starkweather (1987), each of whom proposed multidimensional frameworks that one can use to study fluency. Fillmore (1979) approached the concept of fluency as it pertains both to the general population and to individual differences in performance. Fillmore primarily viewed fluency competence as a reflection of a speaker's language abilities. Accordingly, his thoughts on fluency overlap to some extent with what speech-language pathologists now regard as *pragmatic*

functioning. Fillmore (1979) noted that it is important to differentiate . . . between "*how* people speak (a) language and *how well* people speak (a) language." He then went on to argue that fluency is one measure of how well people speak their language.

Fillmore (1979) proposed four dimensions through which one can measure a speaker's fluency competence:

- "The ability to talk at length with few pauses" (which we will term *talkativeness*);
- "The ability to talk in coherent, reasoned, and 'semantically dense' sentences" (which we will term *succinctness*);
- "The ability to have appropriate things to say in a wide range of contexts" (which we will term *flexibility*); and
- "The ability . . . to be creative and imaginative in . . . language use" (which we will term *creativity*).

In the following sections, we explore the relevance of Fillmore's fluency dimensions to the assessment, diagnosis, and treatment of speakers who exhibit impaired fluency.

Starkweather (1987) extended Fillmore's (1979) work by proposing additional dimensions of fluency that pertained more directly to physical aspects of speech production. Starkweather defined speech fluency as "a normal level of skill in the production of speech" (p. 12). Like Fillmore, he proposed four primary dimensions of fluency:

- *Continuity* (i.e., the connectedness of sounds, syllables, and words within a spoken message);

- *Rate* (i.e., the speed at which a spoken message is delivered);
- *Rhythm* (i.e., prosodic patterns within a spoken message); and
- *Effort* (i.e., the amount of energy a speaker expends when speaking).

Starkweather noted that continuity, rate, and rhythm are associated with aspects of speech timing, and he argued that each is subordinate to effort. In other words, utterances[1] that a listener perceives to be highly effortful are those that feature deviations in the continuity, rate, and/or rhythm of what a speaker has said.

We have flagged two additional aspects of speech production that merit consideration as fluency dimensions. One of these is *speech naturalness* (Nichols, 1966; Parrish, 1951), a construct that researchers began to study in earnest during the 1970s to 1980s. Traditionally, researchers have used naturalness as a means of evaluating the quality of speech in individuals who are attempting to manage stuttering through application of various stuttering management strategies (e.g., Ingham & Packman, 1978; Martin, Haroldson, & Triden, 1984; Runyan, Bell, & Prosek, 1990). In most studies of speech naturalness, researchers have been interested in comparing the post-treatment speech of treated individuals to that of typical speakers to determine whether the speech of the two groups sounds similar. Measures of speech naturalness have become increasingly common in studies of treatment efficacy with speakers who stutter (e.g., Riley & Ingham, 2000; Teshima, Langevin, Hagler, & Kully, 2010), and they

are recommended for use as a standard treatment outcome measure (Ingham & Riley, 1998). We suspect that naturalness, like effort, functions as a superordinate dimension of fluency and that it reflects the combined effects of other fluency dimensions, particularly those associated with continuity, rate, rhythm, and effort.

The other aspect of speech production that warrants consideration as a fluency dimension is *stability*, a construct that pertains to speech consistency (e.g., Kleinow & Smith, 2000; Smith & Goffman, 1998; Van Riper, 1971; Yaruss, 1997). Stability differs from other fluency dimensions because it reflects *repeated measurements* of speech performance; that is, how a person performs over time. Normally, the speech production system functions in a relatively stable manner. That is, a typical speaker exhibits essentially the same degree of fluency when asked to say a particular utterance 10 times in succession or when asked to speak in the same situation day after day. *Variability* is a construct that is closely associated with stability. An unstable speech system yields more variable results than a stable speech system does.

With the addition of naturalness and stability, the number of prospective fluency dimensions swells to 10. At present, we are unsure if each of the 10 fluency dimensions is equally important to advancing our understanding of fluency and fluency disorders, or if all 10 dimensions are even necessary to include in a fluency model. For now, however, we will include all of them in our working model of fluency. We present an overview of these prospective fluency dimensions (Table 1–1) and other details in

---

[1]An *utterance* is a string of words or clauses that communicates an idea and is bound by a single intonational contour (e.g., Logan & Conture, 1995, 1997; Meyers & Freeman, 1985). Utterances often are set apart by pauses, as well. An utterance can consist of a single word (e.g., *me*) or multiple words (e.g., *In the morning.*). All sentences are utterances, but not all utterances are sentences.

Table 1–1. Overview of the Primary Dimensions of Fluency

Dimension	Description
Continuity	The extent to which spoken utterances are free from unexpected or unintended interruptions that are related to errors in speech planning or execution.
Rate	The speed at linguistic information is expressed (includes the promptness with which a spoken utterance is initiated or terminated).
Rhythm	Variations in the duration of syllables (and their associated speech sound segments) during the course of a spoken utterance; prosodic patterns in utterances.
Effort	The amount of physical or mental energy used to produce an utterance. (Related issues include physiological [e.g., muscle activation] and cognitive [e.g., allocation of attention and memory] variables.)
Naturalness	The extent to which spoken utterances sound like those of typical speakers in terms of continuity, rate, rhythm, and/or effort.
Talkativeness	Overall verbal output; the ability to fill time with talk; the extent to which a speaker verbally participates in daily activities (includes issues related to verbal participation).
Communicative flexibility	The ability to generate appropriate verbal remarks across a range of communicative settings and conversational partners (includes issues related to conversational pragmatics).
Succinctness	The organization and semantic density of utterances; the ability to speak in a compact way, with minimal use of meaningless "filler."
Creativity	The ability to produce novel, clever, or distinctive utterances spontaneously during discourse (includes issues related to producing performative speech acts).
Stability	Pertains to the variability of fluency and/or speech-related movements across successive iterations of a particular utterance; the ability to say a particular utterance in the same way time after time.

the remainder of this section. We discuss interrelationships among the fluency dimensions near the end of this chapter through presentation of a working model of fluency.

Continuity

Continuity refers to the connectedness with which a person speaks. More specifically, continuity concerns the extent to which a speaker articulates the sounds within syllables, the syllables within words, and the words within utterances in a seamless, ongoing manner. In another sense, we can view continuity as the extent to which spoken utterances are free from interruption. Continuity is perhaps the most extensively researched fluency dimension, and it is a basic component of most, if not all, fluency assessment protocols. Thus, we devote a relatively large amount of space to continuity in this chapter.

Interruptions in the continuity of speech are common, even for speakers who have "normal" levels of speech fluency. As we explain below, many factors can precipitate such interruptions. However, some forms of continuity interruption are more relevant than others are to the assessment of speech fluency and to the clinical management of fluency disorders.

Nonspeech Physiological Events

Many nonspeech physiological events have the potential to trigger interruptions in speech continuity. Examples of these include the following: *breathing, sneezing, yawning, hiccupping, burping,* and *coughing.* When these events occur during the course of speech production, breaks in speech continuity are likely. Continuity interruptions that result from speech breathing are commonplace; however, continuity interruptions that result from other nonspeech physiological events are not.

Because continuity interruptions of this sort do not directly reflect a speaker's communicative competence, a clinician usually will *not* note them during a fluency assessment. Exceptions to this rule include instances in which a speech-language pathologist judges that a speaker produces such behaviors deliberately to conceal or postpone symptoms of fluency impairment. For example, a speaker who stutters may anticipate difficulty in saying an upcoming word fluently. The speaker is uncomfortable with letting other people see or hear the fluency problem and consequently delays the initiation of the word by pretending to yawn.

Prosodic Structure

The term *prosody* is a phonological concept that refers to the rhythmic and intonational properties of a spoken utterance (Kent & Read, 1992). As such, the term encompasses the temporal properties of spoken utterances, including phenomena such as segment duration, word duration, and pause duration (Ferreira, 1993, 2007; Selkirk, 1984). The classic view is that a speaker specifies the durational properties associated with individual words within a metrical plan for an utterance (see, for example, Selkirk, 1984). Speech scientists and psycholinguists regard metrical planning as a primary source of the *final syllable lengthening* phenomenon; that is, the tendency for a syllable to be longer in duration when it occurs within an utterance-final context than it is when it occurs within a nonfinal utterance context (Ferreira, 1993; Fon, Johnson, & Chen, 2011; Klatt, 1974, 1975; Snow, 1994, 1997). Others, however, have argued that the motor system contributes to word duration. For example, final syllable lengthening has been noted in normally hearing 3-month-old infants as well as in infants and preschoolers who are deaf (Nathani, Oller, & Cobo-Lewis, 2003).

Other aspects of speech that have a prosodic basis include the syllable stress and segment lengthening associated with the conveyance of certain communicative intentions. For example, a speaker can convey equivocation through vowel lengthening, as in the lengthening of the vowel [ɛ:] in the word "well" (*Well, it's complicated.*) Pausing is another aspect of prosody that is relevant to both verbal communication and the assessment of speech continuity. Speakers use pauses for a variety of purposes. Chief among these is to mark syntactic boundaries (e.g., *Our dog eats from this dish* |*pause*| *and our cat eats from that dish*). Speakers also use pauses to convey communicative intentions such as suspense (e.g., *The winner of this week's $10 million lottery drawing is* |*pause*| *<insert name here>!*) and equivocation (e.g., Speaker₁: *Does my car have a tiny dent?* Speaker₂: *Well* |*long pause*| *that depends on what you mean by 'tiny.'*

When assessing fluency, it is necessary to distinguish between those metrical events that a speaker appears to have planned and those that a speaker appears not to have planned. Usually, continuity interruptions that appear to be planned (i.e., a pause of typical duration at the end of major grammatical unit) *are not* necessary to note in a clinical fluency analysis. Alternately, clinicians typically will make note of metrical patterns that appear to be unplanned or unintended because they are likely to be symptomatic of an error or problem in speech production.

Other aspects of prosody include *fundamental frequency* (which listeners perceive as pitch) and *intensity* (which listeners perceive as loudness) (Kent & Read, 1992). Processing pitch and loudness data over time yields information about the intonation of an utterance. Although the intonation pattern of an utterance is not directly associated with its continuity, it can provide information about *speech effort*, a dimension of fluency that we will discuss shortly. A clinician might show interest, for example, when a speaker's vocal pitch changes in an atypical manner because such a pattern probably is not part of the speaker's speech production plan. Speakers who stutter sometimes produce sudden upward shifts in pitch while talking, a behavior that coincides with the release of excessively tense vocal fold adduction at the initiation of disfluent vowels.

Goal Shifts

Continuity interruptions also can occur when a speaker shifts his or her attention away from the communicative intention at hand in order to pursue another behavioral goal. The main pattern is that the speaker attends to something that he or she regards as either more interesting or important than the current message. For example, a woman might stop talking after remembering that she left a candle burning near an arrangement of dried flowers, or a man might stop talking after noticing that a spider is crawling on his arm. The goal shift results in a prompt cessation of speech—sometimes in mid-utterance. When a speaker interrupts an utterance because of a goal shift, he or she may not resume it immediately. The utterance is, in a sense, abandoned. (The speaker may revisit the general theme of the interrupted utterance later in the conversation, however.) In most cases, interruptions of this sort occur infrequently and are not indicative of fluency impairment. Nonetheless, clinicians often do note them as part of a fluency assessment, because frequent occurrence of this behavior could signal impairment in either attention or language use, or a sign of frustration in cases of severe impairment in the ability to speak fluently.

Speaking Partner Behavior

Some interruptions in speech continuity result from the behavior of a conversational partner. Physical interruption of another person's speech (e.g., a mother places her hand over the mouth of her child to prevent the child from speaking) is not common. Verbal interruption is quite common, however. The most common scenario for verbal interruption is for a conversational partner to talk at the same time as the speaker. As the partner begins to talk over the speaker, the speaker then has the option to yield the speaking turn to the conversational partner. In doing so, the speaker interrupts his or her ongoing utterance. In a sense, continuity interruptions of this sort are a special case of the "altered behavioral goals" scenario described in the previous section. That is, the speaker chooses to yield the conversational turn to the other person rather than electing to compete for talking time with the other person. Some factors that can influence a speaker's decision to yield a speaking turn include the speaker's social status relative to that of the partner and the relative importance of the partner's utterance in relation to the speaker's utterance.

Continuity interruption that occurs secondary to verbal interruption generally *is* important to note in a fluency assessment. This is because verbal interruption tends to occur more often than usual when one of the conversational participants has impaired fluency (Meyers & Freeman, 1985), and verbal interruption has the potential to exacerbate the problems of speakers who have fluency difficulties (Kelly & Conture, 1992; Millard, Nicholas, & Cook, 2008; Starkweather, Gottwald, & Halfond, 1990).

Planning Errors

Another source of speech interruption involves problems in planning what is about to be said. As will be described further in Chapter 2, speech production is a complex process that requires the generation of multiple, hierarchical representations (i.e., plans). All utterances,

even superficially simple ones, take some amount of time and multiple steps to plan. Although some utterance planning seems to take place concurrently with speaking, a portion of it also seems to take place during the pauses that are inserted within or between utterances (Ferreira, 2007). When pauses occur at major syntactic boundaries, it can be challenging to determine how much of the pause reflects aspects of utterance prosody (i.e., *planned pauses*) and how much of the pause reflects activities related to the planning of upcoming segments of the utterance (i.e., *planning pauses*). This is because both may occur within the same period of silence (Ferreira, 2007).

Continuity interruptions that appear to be associated with utterance planning usually are included only in a fluency analysis when the interruption lasts for longer than the norm or when the speaker exhibits concomitant behavior (e.g., excessive muscle tension, irregular speech breathing) that is not a customary component of utterance planning. The factors that lead a speaker to take an unusually long time to plan upcoming speech often are *covert*; that is, not outwardly observable (Postma & Kolk, 1990). Presumably, continuity interruptions that last for an unusual amount of time reflect some underlying difficulty in one or more aspect of speech planning (see Chapters 2 and 3 for more details).

Continuity interruptions also may occur if a speaker determines that the content of an ongoing utterance either is incorrect or is mismatched with a listener's needs or expectations. In such cases, the speaker must assess the portion of the utterance that was incorrect or problematic for the listener, and then alter the original utterance accordingly by re-planning the pertinent segment.

Errors in speech production also can result when something a speaker has said deviates from what he or she intended to say (see Postma & Kolk, 1990). If a speaker detects the deviation and elects to "repair" it, an interruption in continuity often occurs. In such cases, the speaker's error becomes *overt*, meaning that the incorrect portion of the utterance is apparent to both the speaker and the listener. Every speaker exhibits at least some overt errors when talking. In the general population, such errors typically are linguistically based. During fluency assessment, clinicians typically will note continuity interruptions that arise from linguistic errors. Such interruptions are of particular significance when they deviate significantly from the norm in frequency, duration, or manner. As will be discussed in Sections II and III of this text, the main objectives in a clinical setting are to determine how often such interruptions occur, how long it takes a speaker to resolve them, and what it is that the speaker has corrected.

Motor Control Problems

Motor control problems constitute another potential source for continuity interruption. As will be discussed in Chapter 2, the execution of speech movements is a multifaceted process that seems to require both "feedback" and "feedforward" mechanisms. Some speakers may report *movement initiation difficulties*; that is, instances in which they know precisely what they want to say and how they want to say it but are temporarily unable to initiate the speech-related movements that are needed to execute the utterance. Continuity interruptions of this sort are common among speakers who have impaired flu-

ency. Thus, a clinician typically *will* note them during a fluency assessment.

Continuity Interruptions Versus Disfluency

As we noted in the previous section, not all interruptions in speech continuity are indicative of fluency-related communication problems. For instance, some continuity interruptions result from general physiological phenomena that are unrelated to speech production; others are planned features of the speaker's utterance; and others are rooted in errors or delays in speech planning or production. This leads to the question of whether one needs to record *all* instances of continuity interruption—regardless of their source—when describing a speaker's fluency. As we have suggested in the previous sections, the answer to this question largely depends on an examiner's objectives for assessment and the level of behavioral detail that the examiner deems necessary to record.

The relationship between continuity interruption and disfluency is summarized in Table 1–2. In most cases, it is necessary to note only those continuity interruptions that reflect *disfluency*, which we define here as *interruptions in the execution of a speech plan that arise from either (a) errors in the speech planning and execution process or (b) partner-based behaviors such as verbal interruption that impede a speaker's ability to execute an utterance completely* (see Postma & Kolk, 1990). In this view, disfluency constitutes a subcategory of continuity interruptions. We then can divide the subcategory of disfluency further into: (1) disfluencies that originate with the speaker and (2) disflu-

Table 1–2. Sources of Interruption in Speech Continuity and Their Relevance to Disfluency

Source	Example[a]	Relevance to Fluency Disorders
General physiological event	*The alligators are-* [speaker yawns] *lounging in the sun.*	Relevant only if produced deliberately to conceal or delay genuine symptoms of fluency impairment.
Prosodic structure	*And the winner of grand prize is . . . ticket number 237!*	Relevant only when prosodic pattern is significantly different from what is normal for the communication context.
Goal shift	*Yeah, it's really-* [Speaker shifts attention to something other than the utterance, which triggers the moment of interruption.]	Relevant only if produced deliberately to conceal or delay symptoms of fluency impairment.
Speaking partner actions	Speaker: *I want-* Partner: Hey, look at that!	Relevant. Documentation of partner-based interruptions yields information about conversational dynamics, a speaker's access to conversational participation, and the effect of interruption upon a speaker's subsequent fluency performance.
Repair of planning error	*The ǀsmails-ǀ snails smell bad.*	Relevant. The speaker interrupts speech to alter an overt error (i.e., *smails*).
Motor-based problems	*ǀseveral abortive attempts at phonationǀ I'm at Green Lake.*	Relevant. The speaker experiences difficulty in producing the sequence of articulatory movements that correspond to the utterance (i.e., *I'm at Green Lake*).

[a]Utterances with continuity interruptions are shown in italics. Hyphens indicate the moment at which continuity is interrupted. Ellipsis indicates a lengthy, silent pause.

encies that originate with the conversational partner.

Many fluency assessment protocols call for documenting the frequency, type, and/or duration of disfluencies that originate with the speaker. Sources for disfluency that originate with the speaker include the following:

- Delays in the retrieval of utterance-related information,

- Errors in the accuracy or appropriateness of the information that is retrieved,
- Errors in the assembly of the information that is retrieved, and
- Errors in the execution of planned utterances.

Continuity breaks that arise from events that are unrelated either to speech planning or execution (e.g., burps, hiccups, yawns, breathing) or events that appear to be an intended part of an utterance (e.g., pauses associated with speech prosody) are not documented unless a clinician judges that a speaker uses them deliberately to conceal or postpone the onset of an anticipated disfluency.

Disfluency Versus Dysfluency

Even casual readers of the fluency disorders literature will likely note the use of the alternate spellings *dis*fluency versus *dys*fluency. Both spellings appear commonly in journals and textbooks, with individual authors preferring one form to the other. Quesal (1988) noted that the prefix *dis-* refers to the absence or lack of something (in this case, fluency), whereas the prefix *dys-* refers to something that is abnormal in nature. On this basis, he argued that *disfluency* is the preferred spelling for assessment of speech continuity because of its utility in describing the fluency interruptions of both unimpaired speakers and impaired speakers without having to make assumptions about the underlying nature of specific interruptions. Bernstein Ratner (1988) countered that the distinction between the *dis* and *dys* has largely been lost in contemporary American English; thus, it is acceptable to use either spelling. We prefer the spelling *disfluency*, largely for the reasons that Quesal noted and will use it throughout the text except when quoting an author who has used the alternate spelling.

Rate

Rate is another of the fluency dimensions Starkweather (1987) identified. In a general sense, the term *rate* refers to the speed at which a speaker conveys information during speech (Logan, Byrd, Mazzocchi, & Gillam, 2011). There are two general approaches to measuring speaking rate. The first approach, which variably has been termed *articulation rate, articulatory rate*, and *articulatory speaking rate*, is computed using stretches of speech that are free from interruptions in continuity. Some researchers have based articulation rate analyses on a unit called a *run*, which they define as some minimum number of consecutive syllables (e.g., four or five) that a speaker produces without a break in continuity. Thus, a run can constitute either an entire utterance (see Example 1–1 below) or a portion of an utterance (see the underlined segment within Example 1–2 below).

Example 1–1: *The storm dumped 12 inches of rain in our county.*

Example 1–2: *The |s- s-| storm dumped 12 inches of rain in our county.*

As we will explain further in Section II, articulation rate is computed by dividing the total number of syllables sampled across all fluent utterances (or runs) by the total amount of time taken to articulate all of the fluent utterances (or runs). Speech-language pathologists usually base articulation rate on assessment of a preset number of utterances or runs (e.g., 10 or 20) that they select randomly from some larger speech sample. Analysis of these selected samples will presumably yield an accurate estimate of a speaker's customary articulation rate. Because articulation rate is based on perceptibly fluent stretches of speech, it is essentially a measure of how rapidly a speaker talks at times when the speech production system is functioning optimally. It appears that adult speakers attain increases in articulation rate by increasing the amount of *coarticulatory overlap* across adjacent speech sound segments rather than simply increasing the velocity of articulatory movements (Gay, 1978; Gay, Ushijima, Hirose, & Cooper, 1974). Coarticulation refers to the extent to which the articulatory movements for one speech sound segment carry over into the production of an adjacent speech sound segment (Nicolosi, Harryman, & Kresheck, 1989).

A second measurement approach, *speech rate* involves the analysis of both fluent *and* disfluent utterances. When assessing speech rate, an examiner elicits a series of utterances from a speaker and then randomly selects a subset (e.g., 10 or 20) of those utterances for analysis. The number of syllables (or words) within each utterance is tallied and then summed across all sampled utterances. (Excluded in the tally are any syllables [or words] that are associated with disfluent segments of speech.) The total number of syllables (or words) in the sample then is divided by the time spent speaking during all of the utterances, including time spent during disfluent segments of an utterance.

Because the syllables within disfluent segments are included within utterance timings but not within the counts of how much speech has been spoken, speech rate almost always will be slower than articulation rate. Similarly, a highly disfluent speaker usually will have a much slower speech rate than a speaker who is mildly disfluent. This is because speech disfluency consumes time that a speaker might otherwise have devoted to productive communication (i.e., fluent speech). Speech-language pathologists can use speech rate to quantify how a speaker's disfluency characteristics change over

time. A speaker who exhibits a decrease in the number and the duration of disfluencies over time generally will exhibit an increase in speech rate. We illustrate the effect of disfluency on rate measures in Table 1–3.

The expected articulation and speech rate values for a speaker vary according to variables such as the type of task the speaker is performing, the speaker's familiarity with the speaking topic, and the type of communicative intention that the speaker is conveying. In general, listeners tend to view the use of a brisk speech rate favorably. For instance, speech rate values correlate positively with ratings of a speaker's competence, intelligence, and truthfulness (Apple, Streeter, & Krauss, 1979; Brown, Giles, & Thakerar, 1985; Smith, Brown, Strong, & Rencher, 1975). Nonetheless, listeners do not always view rapid speech favorably. For example, listeners tend to rate speakers who use a moderate speech rate as being more benevolent than those who use a rapid speech rate (Smith et al., 1975). Starkweather (1987) noted that the habitual speech rate used by a speaker tends to fall toward the upper end of his or her rate range. In other words, people tend to talk about as fast as they are able to talk, without compromising the intelligibility or accuracy of their spoken message.

A third way to view rate is in terms of how promptly a speaker can initiate an utterance following a cue to begin speaking. Researchers use terms such as *speech reaction time* and *speech initiation time* to refer to this behavior. A similar measure is *laryngeal reaction time*, which encompasses initiation times for nonspeech vocalizations such as throat clearing. As we will explain in Section II, speakers who stutter tend to have longer speech initiation times than speakers who do

Table 1–3. Example of Differences Between Articulation Rate and Speech Rate in Fluent and Disfluent Utterances

Line	Spoken Utterance	# of Syllables	Speaking Time (in seconds)	Articulation Rate (syll/s)	Speech Rate (syll/s)
1	*We went kayaking at Cedar Key last weekend.*	12	2.8	4.3	4.3
2	*We saw |ma- ma-| <u>manatees in the bay near the refuge</u>.*	12 in utt, 10 in run	3.4 in utt, 2.1 in run	4.2 in run	3.5 in utt
3	*The |um| manatees swam |be- be-| beside |our-| our little kayaks.*	12	3.9	NA	3.1
4	*We |um| hoped to |um| see some |um| dolphins, but |um| they were |um| elsewhere.*	12	5.2	NA	2.3

Note. Underlined text indicates a "run" of five or more continuous syllables within a disfluent utterance. *Utt* = utterance, *syll* = syllable, *NA* = not applicable. Articulation rate cannot be computed for lines 3 and 4 because neither utterance contains five consecutive syllables that are uninterrupted by disfluency. Disfluent speech is excluded from tallies of the number of syllables within an utterance. Note that the speech rates for utterances 2, 3, and 4 (the disfluent utterances) are slower than that for utterance 1, even though the core utterance on each of these lines contains 12 syllables. The disfluencies in utterances 2, 3, and 4 take time to produce. Consequently, speech rate is slower in these utterances than in utterance 1.

not stutter—even during utterances that listeners perceive to be fluent. Speakers who stutter also report that they tend to produce disfluencies more often within speaking contexts that obligate prompt initiation of speech (e.g., saying "hello" after answering a phone call). Thus, issues related to utterance initiation rate have clinical relevance, as well.

Rhythm

Rhythm is an aspect of prosody and, as such, it includes variations in syllable, segment, and pause duration throughout the course of an utterance. Rhythm is regarded as a *suprasegmental* aspect of speech because its effects are realized across syllables, words, phrases, and sentences (Bauman-Waengler, 2012). Some authors use the term *tempo* instead of or in addition to rhythm to capture the notion of rate as well as rhythm. The rhythm of an utterance differs from its *intonation*, with the latter referring to the pitch and stress patterns that transpire over the course of an utterance (Kent & Read, 1992).

Multiword utterances are comprised of consecutive syllables, some of which are *stressed* and some of which are not. In English, the distribution of stressed syllables is uneven, meaning that the number of unstressed syllables occurring between stressed syllables is variable (Huggins, 1972). Thus, speech rhythms are not fixed in the same sense that musical rhythms are. A speaker can express the same utterance via a variety of rhythmic patterns (Kent & Read, 1992). Such variations may affect the meaning that the speaker conveys (e.g., *YOU want that?* versus *You WANT that?* versus *You want THAT?*). Of course, in clinical settings, the primary focus is on instances wherein a speaker alters speech rhythm in an unplanned or unintended way, such as during disfluency or a stress assignment error (e.g., *parachute* → paraCHUTE). Disfluency can markedly disrupt speech rhythm, particularly when it occurs frequently.

Effort

The next fluency dimension to be discussed is effort. In the context of speech production, a clinician can examine effort from either a mental or physical standpoint (Starkweather, 1987). *Mental effort* refers to the amount of thought or attention a speaker expends while talking, whereas *physical effort* refers to the amount of muscular exertion a speaker expends while talking (Hoit, Lansing, & Perona, 2007). Although researchers probably understand the physical characteristics of speech production better than the mental characteristics of speech production, both areas have received considerable attention in research throughout the years. Also, as technological advances allow for increasingly precise inquiry into the neurophysiological correlates of various cognitive processes, the relationships between objective measures of neural and muscular activity and subjective perceptions of mental and physical activity have become better understood (e.g., Schmidt, Lebreton, Cléry-Melin, Daunizeau, & Pessiglione, 2012).

The physical properties of speech sounds are well documented. One widely used objective index of physical effort during speech sound production is *intraoral air pressure*. A variety of studies have been conducted to examine differences in intraoral air pressure values across age levels, sound classes, linguistic contexts, and articulation rates (e.g., Klatt, 1974; Oller, 1973; Prosek & House, 1975; Subtelny, Worth, & Sakuda, 1966; Umeda, 1977).

Subglottal and *intraoral air pressures* have been used as an index of effort, as well (e.g., Hixon, 1973; Prosek & House, 1975). Prosek and House reported a significant linear relationship between the amount of intraoral air pressure that is present during speech production and a speaker's perception of speaking effort. In other words, greater intraoral pressure corresponds with greater perceived effort. Other physical indices of speaking effort include electrodermal activity, peripheral blood flow, oxygen saturation levels, blood pressure, and heart rate (Craig et al., 1996; Hoit, Lansing, & Perona, 2007; van Lieshout, Starkweather, Hulstijn, & Peters, 1995; Weber & Smith, 1990). Studies of cerebral blood flow patterns via neuroimaging have provided insight into the involvement of various neural centers in assorted cognitive and motor processes (e.g., Ingham et al., 2004).

The relationship between mental effort and speech production tasks has been examined as well. Methods for documenting mental effort include the use of multipoint rating scales, adjective listing, and narrative description (e.g., Hoit et al., 2007; Ingham, Warner, Byrd, & Cotton, 2006). Clinicians may use such methods with an eye toward determining whether a speaker feels that he or she needs to exert conscious management or attention to speech production. Research in nonspeech domains such as ball throwing reveals that use of consciously mediated control strategies (i.e., mental effort) for activities that ordinarily are executed in an automatic manner leads to greater variability in joint coordination as well as changes in movement dynamics and timing (Higuchi, 2000).

Naturalness

Another dimension of fluency that has clinical relevance is *naturalness*. Researchers often use the construct of naturalness in conjunction with fluency treatment protocols that require the regulation of articulation rate. Although many speakers who stutter produce fewer disfluencies through application of rate regulation strategies, it is possible for the resulting speech patterns to sound "mechanical" (i.e., unnatural) when compared to the speech of speakers who do not stutter (e.g., Ingham, Gow, & Costello, 1985; Onslow & Ingham, 1987). Speakers who stutter can improve speech naturalness using feedback from a clinician about their current naturalness levels (e.g., Ingham, Martin, Haroldson, Onslow, & Leney, 1985). In past research studies, raters have not received a precise definition for naturalness; thus, the assumption is that a listener will know a natural utterance when he or she hears one. To some extent, this appears to be the case, as individual naturalness ratings have proven to be quite reliable (Martin et al., 1984).

Research findings suggest that ratings for speech naturalness correlate strongly with both speech rate and disfluency frequency (Logan, Roberts, Pretto, & Morey, 2002; Martin & Haroldson, 1992). However, naturalness ratings for disfluent speech samples are affected by whether speech is presented to raters via an audio-only or audio-visual format (Martin & Haroldson, 1992). As expected, seeing a person speak disfluently yields less favorable naturalness ratings than merely hearing the person speak disfluently. Thus, there may be other factors that contribute to naturalness ratings in addition to rate and disfluency. In Figure 1–1, we illustrate the extent to which a speaker's articulation rate can predict the naturalness ratings that he or she receives from listeners. As shown in the figure, adult raters' perceptions of speech naturalness are strongly tied to the speakers' articulation rates.

Based on findings from Logan et al. (2002), one might wonder whether deviations in virtually any aspect dimension of fluency would be sufficient to affect a rater's perceptions of naturalness. This hypothesis awaits investigation. Given current findings, however, it would not be surprising to find that naturalness ratings correlate strongly with fluency dimensions such as effort and rhythm in addition to rate and continuity.

Talkativeness

According to Fillmore (1979), an essential component of fluency is "the ability to fill time with talk." Although Fillmore did not use the label *talkativeness*, the term seems appropriate for this fluency dimension as it fits his criterion for talking at length, and it is consistent with terminology used by researchers who specialize in studying issues related to verbal output and participation (e.g., Leaper & Ayres, 2007; Leaper & Smith, 2004). Given the many communicative functions that speakers convey through talking, talkativeness

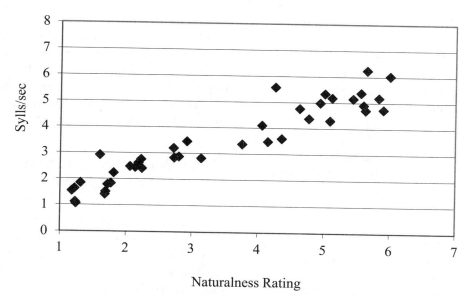

Figure 1–1. A scatterplot showing the relationship between speech rate and speech naturalness. The speech rate data were obtained from 40 typical adults who participated in an experiment wherein they practiced various techniques for slowing speech rate. The naturalness ratings were obtained from a separate group of 39 typical adults who listened to audio recordings of the sentences and then rated them using a 7-point speech naturalness scale. The correlation coefficient for the two variables was .95, which indicates that an utterance's speech rate is a strong predictor of its associated naturalness rating. Reprinted with permission from "Speaking Slowly: Effects of Four Self-Guided Training Approaches on Adults' Speech Rate and Naturalness," by K. J. Logan, R. R. Roberts, A. P. Pretto, and M. J. Morey, 2002, *American Journal of Speech-Language Pathology, 11,* pp. 163–174.

carries many advantages. Of course, the amount of verbal output a speaker produces does not necessarily correspond with how effectively he or she communicates. Thus, in clinical settings, it is imperative to weigh a speaker's verbal output against the extent to which it meets the needs and expectations of conversational partners as well as the speaker's personal communication goals.

The tension that exists between verbal output and verbal economy is reflected in Grice's (1975) widely cited *conversational maxims*. Grice's maxims pertain to the quantity, quality, relevance, and manner of what a speaker says.

- The *maxim of quantity* states that conversational contributions should be as informative as possible but not be overly informative. In other words, it is generally desirable for a speaker to say only what is necessary and avoid superfluous or excessive detail. We address this concept in greater detail below, under the headings of "verbal output and participation" and "succinctness."

- The *maxim of relation* calls for conversational contributions to be relevant. Inclusion of irrelevant details in a conversation can boost overall verbal output, but it risks diminishing the overall quality of communication. We address this concept in greater detail below, under the heading of "succinctness."

- The *maxim of manner* is similar to the maxim of quantity, in that it stipulates a speaker should seek to be as clear, brief, and orderly as possible. We address this concept below, under the headings of "succinctness" and "situational flexibility."

- The *maxim of quality* states that conversational contributions should be truthful. In other words, speakers should avoid saying things that are patently false or that cannot be corroborated. Of the four maxims, this one seems to have the least relevance to speech fluency; thus, we will not discuss it further, other than to say that speakers who stutter sometimes express concern that listeners will mistake their disfluent speech for instances of lying or deception (Bloodstein & Bernstein Ratner, 2008).

Determination of what constitutes excessive, irrelevant, or disorderly speech is not easily accomplished, and standards for acceptable performance in these areas seem to vary across cultures (Norris, 1995; Tulviste, Mizera, De Geer, & Tryggvason, 2003). For instance, in studies of mealtime conversations, American and Swedish teenagers talk more than Estonian teenagers do, and Swedish teenagers use a greater proportion of behavioral directives than American and Estonian teenagers do (Tulviste, Mizera, & De Geer, 2006). In addition, there are contextual scenarios such as conversational storytelling and comic routines wherein speakers intentionally violate conversational maxims in ways that make speech performance highly effective or entertaining. Consequently, one should apply these maxims cautiously within clinical settings.

Verbal Output and Participation

Researchers often define talkativeness in terms of verbal output. Several measures of verbal output have been reported: (1) the number of syllables, words, or utterances a speaker produces during an interaction; (2) the number of syllables or words a speaker produces per unit of time; (3) the average number of syllables or words a speaker produces per utterance; and (4) the total amount of time a speaker spends talking.

Talkativeness also relates to the notions of *participation* and *participation restriction*, aspects of verbal output that figure prominently into assessments of communicative functioning (World Health Organization, 2001). Within the sphere of verbal communication, participation pertains to matters such as the number and variety of social contexts in which a speaker makes verbal contributions as well as to the depth and breadth of a speaker's contribution during specific situations. The notion of participation restriction pertains to the absence or lack of participation in ways that limit or hinder a person's ability to function within the context of daily activities. Thus, the basic goal when measuring verbal output and participation is to capture how much talking a person does in various situations. We present additional details about the clinical assessment of verbal output in Section II of this text.

Selective mutism is a disorder that offers an unambiguous example of the functional limitations that arise when one consistently does not to talk in one or more contexts (Giddan, Ross, Sechler, & Becker, 1997; Harris, 1996). In this case, an individual's absence of speech in specific situations is unrelated to his or her language competence or background knowledge for a topic, and it can interfere markedly with social interactions as well as educational and occupational achievement. Selective mutism may coincide with social phobia and fear of social embarrassment (Giddan et al., 1997). Although selective mutism is not a fluency disorder, per se, it nonetheless involves behaviors that are relevant to fluency: verbal output and verbal participation. Participation restrictions also occur—albeit less dramatically—in developmental stuttering. In this case, a speaker's embarrassment over speech disfluency and concerns about how listeners will react to speech disfluency may lead the person to avoid talking in certain situations or to say as little as possible when talking.

Succinctness

Another dimension of fluency that Fillmore (1979) noted is the ability to speak in logically organized and semantically dense sentences such that ideas are expressed in "a compact and careful way." Thus, a speaker who is skilled in this dimension of fluency may communicate in eight words what another speaker takes 15 words to communicate. We use the term *succinctness* as a label for this dimension of fluency because it is con-

sistent with Fillmore's description and it captures Grice's (1975) maxims of quantity and manner, as well.

Fillmore (1979) conjectured that one's ability to speak succinctly is associated with his or her general linguistic aptitude and background knowledge for a particular topic. Succinctness also might be associated with the amount of experience that a speaker has with conveying a particular story, concept, procedure, and so forth to others. In this view, the succinctness of a message should improve over time, as the speaker rehearses content or practices information delivery.

Other terms that are relevant to the notion of succinctness are *coherence* and *circumlocution*. The term *coherence* refers to a speaker's ability to present information in a logical, unified manner. In clinical settings, clinicians assess coherence by examining a person's topic maintenance skills. Coherence deficits are found in an assortment of disorders that affect functioning in cognition or language. These include the following: developmental language impairment (Bliss & McCabe, 2008; Ketelaars, Hermans, Cuperus, Jansonius, & Verhoeven, 2011); dementia (Dijkstra, Bourgeois, Allen, & Burgio, 2004); aphasia (Rogalski, Altmann, Plummer-D'Amato, Behrman, & Marsiske, 2010); and cluttering (St. Louis, Myers, Faragasso, Townsend, & Gallaher, 2004; van Zaalen-op't Hof, Wijnen, & DeJonckere, 2009). In such cases, succinctness of message delivery is reduced or lost, as the speaker strays toward topics that have, at best, only marginal relevance to the focal topic.

Within the context of fluency disorders, the term *circumlocution* is used to describe instances in which a speaker inserts semantically acceptable but communicatively unnecessary words into an utterance. Some speakers who stutter use circumlocution to cope with the expectation of being unable to produce the motor movements associated with upcoming syllables. We present an example of circumlocution below.

> Example 1–3: *Uncle Alston returns tonight.* (Intended or preferred utterance.)

> Example 1–4: *My mom's baby brother returns tonight.* (Utterance with circumlocution.)

An utterance like the one in Example 1–4 might occur when a speaker expects disfluency on the word *Alston* and reacts to it by substituting alternate and less precise words (e.g., *my mom's baby* brother) or by inserting additional, unnecessary words prior to it (e.g., *Dear sweet old Uncle Alston*). Thus, circumlocution leads to avoidance or postponement of key words within an utterance. Circumlocution is rarely a highly reliable strategy for coping with the anticipated disfluency of developmental stuttering and, by filling speech with imprecise or unnecessary words, the speaker often creates more communication problems than he or she solves by avoiding or delaying the key word.

As noted above, problems with coherence, circumlocution, and lack of succinct expression occur in conjunction with various types of language impairment. These problems also are seen in *cluttering*, a disorder that often features evidence of impairment in both speech and language (see Section II for additional details). Speakers who consistently and substantially exceed the verbal output requirements that are customary within a particular situation or who consistently report information that is irrelevant often are labeled as having a pragmatically based communication impairment (Douglas, 2010; Meilijson, Kasher, & Elizur, 2004; Philofsky, Fidler, & Hepburn, 2007). Thus, it is functional to be talkative but dysfunctional to be so talkative that others become annoyed, distracted, confused, or disinterested.

Communicative Flexibility

Another of the fluency dimensions that Fillmore (1979) proposed pertains to a speaker's ability to generate appropriate verbal remarks across a range of social or communicative situations. According to Fillmore, a person who is fluent in this way talks easily with both friends and strangers and manages to find the "right thing to say" during situations that leave other speakers fumbling for words. Examples of such situations include consoling someone who is in distress and delivering unpleasant feedback to someone. We use the term *communicative flexibility* to describe this dimension of fluency and place it under the heading of talkativeness.

Of course, clinical intervention programs will not transform every person who has impaired fluency into a comforting confidant or the "life of the party." Although the latter attributes often are valued and are consistent with the notion of fluency as it pertains to the general population, the primary aim in clinical settings is to help a speaker establish functional communication skills. Thus, in this text, we view the notion of communicative flexibility in a broader sense than Fillmore did (1979). That is, we regard it as the ability to use speech to accomplish a variety of communicative purposes—the ability for a speaker to say *something* (though not necessarily the "right" or "best" thing) across a range of communicative contexts. Many people who have impaired fluency find this type of social fluency challenging to attain.

Fey (1986) developed a system for classifying the functional characteristics of particular utterances within a conversation. The analysis is rooted in Searle's (1975) concept of the speech act. With Fey's speech act analysis, each conversational utterance is described in terms of the communicative function that the speaker accomplishes by uttering it. With the system, a clinician can describe the functional characteristics of each conversational utterance a speaker produces in two ways: (1) the role that the utterance assumes in relation to the previous utterance (i.e., its *utterance-level* function) and (2) the role the utterance assumes in relation to the topic structure of the ongoing conversation (i.e., its *discourse-level* function). Within a given conversation, the utterances that a speaker produces typically will accomplish a range of communicative functions. The main categories of Fey's speech act analysis are diagrammed in Figure 1–2. Clinicians can use the categories shown in the figure to describe the communicative function associated with each of the utterances that a speaker says and, in doing so, discover the types of communicative functions that are conveyed most and least often. Analysis of *utterance function* has relevance to speech fluency in that impaired speakers often report that certain types of speech acts (e.g., *responding to a request for clarification*) are more difficult to say fluently

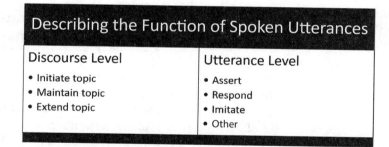

Describing the Function of Spoken Utterances	
Discourse Level	**Utterance Level**
• Initiate topic • Maintain topic • Extend topic	• Assert • Respond • Imitate • Other

Figure 1–2. Utterance-level and discourse-level categories within Fey's (1986) speech act analysis. A clinician can use the analysis to describe the function of clients' conversational utterances in relation to the function of a preceding utterance (utterance-level analysis) and the topic structure of the overall conversation (discourse-level analysis). At the discourse level, an utterance can initiate a topic, maintain a topic, or extend a topic. At the utterance level, conversational utterances function in one of four general ways: (1) as an assertion (e.g., to make a request, statement, comment, disagreement), (2) as a response (i.e., to respond to another person's request for information, action, attention, and so forth), (3) as an imitation (i.e., to repeat an utterance that another person has just said), or (4) other.

than other types of speech acts (Bloodstein & Bernstein Ratner, 2008).

Creativity

A fourth dimension of fluency that Fillmore (1979) identified pertains to the spontaneous expression of ideas in novel, clever, or distinctive ways during discourse. As Fillmore noted, speakers who are highly proficient in this dimension of fluency not only are able to express ideas clearly in a variety of settings but also do so in a way that is pleasing, entertaining, or amusing to others. Although Fillmore did not specifically use the term *communicative creativity* as a label for this fluency dimension, it fits his description well. Examples of communicative creativity include the abilities to generate puns, jokes, alliterations, or metaphors spontaneously during conversation. Together, they constitute a specific form of talkativeness.

For many people with impaired fluency, the ability to talk in the creative way that Fillmore (1979) described might be regarded as "icing on the cake;" that is, something beyond what is necessary for functional communication. Thus, a clinician normally would not designate creative verbal expression as a high priority within a treatment plan for a person with impaired fluency. On the other hand, performative speech acts such as joke telling are integral to social interaction and are valued as an aspect of communication. People who stutter commonly report that it is challenging to speak fluently within time-constrained speaking contexts such as joke telling (Manning, 2010). One main challenge with telling jokes is that the speaker's frequent disruptions in speech continuity interfere with the timing that

is integral in conveying humor. Although creative communication is unlikely to receive substantial attention in a treatment program, certain aspects of it may warrant inclusion in specific treatment plans.

Stability

The term *stability* refers to consistency of performance. The notion of stability is relevant to fluency dimensions such as continuity, rate, rhythm, effort, naturalness, and talkativeness. In general, speakers with disordered fluency perform less consistently than speakers with normal fluency do in both speech and nonspeech tasks that require sequential movements (Kleinow & Smith, 2000; Olander, Smith, & Zelaznik, 2010; Smits-Bandstra & De Nil, 2007, 2009; Yaruss, 1997).

Within-Task and Between-Task Perspectives

The construct of stability can be studied from both *within-task* and *between-task* perspectives. The within-task perspective refers to the extent to which a speaker performs in a similar manner when asked to perform the same task repeatedly (e.g., reading a paragraph aloud five times in succession). Each attempt at the task is called a *trial*, and a researcher compares the speaker's fluency performance across the trials. The speaker usually completes a series of trials in rapid succession. This approach provides information about a variety of issues including whether a speaker's disfluency frequency, speech rate, and/or motor coordination change as a function of practice.

In contrast, the between-task perspective deals with the extent to which a speaker performs in a similar manner across different types of speaking tasks. For example, one might compare a speaker's performance during a sentence production task, a reading task, and a conversational task. In this way, one can answer questions such as whether a speaker's disfluency frequency or speech rate changes as a function of the activity or task they perform. Both perspectives are important to consider in order to obtain a complete understanding of a person's fluency functioning.

Score Dispersion

The concept of *variability* is closely associated with stability. Variability is a statistical concept. One can quantify it by computing the *standard deviation* of a data set. The standard deviation is a statistic that captures the manner in which data points (e.g., the individual trials during a series of consecutive trials) disperse around the mean score for the data set. The more variable a speaker's performance is on a task, the larger the standard deviation value for that task will be. In general, speakers who stutter will show greater variability on most fluency-related measures than speakers who do not stutter will. The behavioral patterns that characterize both groups are illustrated in Figure 1–3.

Another statistical term that relates to variability is *range*, which is the difference between the minimum and maximum scores in a data set. A speaker who is more stable at performing a particular task will have a smaller score range for the task than a speaker whose performance is less stable.

Measures of Central Tendency

Measures of dispersion are viewed in relation to measures of central tendency, particularly the *mean* (i.e., the sum of all scores divided by the number of scores that were summed). A common approach used by researchers is to compare speakers with disordered fluency and speakers with typical fluency in terms of their means scores on a particular variable. In this comparison, the researchers are primarily interested in determining whether the means for the two groups differ significantly from each other when score variability for each group is taken into account.

A Working Model of Fluency

In Figure 1–4, we present a working model of fluency. The model constitutes our attempt to explain how the various fluency dimensions that we have discussed in this chapter fit together.

As shown in the model, rate and continuity are considered overlapping concepts. That is, speech rate is predictably linked with the number of disfluencies a person produces. A speaker who frequently is disfluent usually will have a relatively slow speech rate because disfluencies consume time that otherwise would be spent in productive speech.

In the model, continuity and rate are embedded within rhythm. This is because both disfluency frequency and rate contribute to a listener's perceptions about the rhythm of speech (Logan et al., 2002; Martin et al., 1984). However, rhythm is more than just these two facets of speech production. For instance, disfluency duration (i.e., the amount of time disfluencies

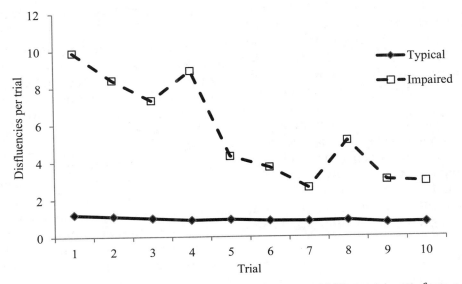

Figure 1–3. An example of the type of data one would expect to see from a speaker with typical fluency (Typical) and a speaker with impaired fluency (Impaired) during a story generation task that involves 10 consecutive trials. The speaker with typical fluency produces a mean of 0.91 disfluencies per trial, with a standard deviation (*SD*) of 0.15. Thus, about 68% of the 10 disfluency scores for the typical speaker fall within 0.15 points of the mean score. The line graph for the typical speaker is nearly straight and has very little slope, a pattern that indicates stable performance. In contrast, the mean number of disfluencies per trial for the impaired speaker is 5.61 (*SD* = 2.76). The *SD* statistic for the impaired speaker indicates that the disfluency scores disperse much more widely about the mean than the scores for the typical speaker do. That is, about 68% of the 10 disfluency scores for the impaired speaker fall within 2.76 points of the mean score. The line graph for the impaired speaker shows much more fluctuation across trials than the line graph for the typical speaker, a pattern that also is indicative of unstable performance and consistent with the speaker's relatively high standard deviation statistic.

last) can affect speech rhythm, as can prosodic features such as pause duration.

Effort is presented broadly to include both mental and physical aspects of the construct. In Figure 1–4, effort is a reflection of speech continuity, rate, and rhythm. Thus, speakers who exhibit deficits or marked differences in these dimensions of fluency would likely be perceived as speaking in an effortful manner (see, for example, Ingham et al., 2009). Effort,

in turn, is embedded within naturalness. Thus, within the scope of the model, atypical performance in rate, rhythm, continuity, and/or effort would be likely to result in the perception that speech production is unnatural (Hodgman & Logan, 2013).

We positioned talkativeness in the outermost ring of the model and use the term in a broad sense to capture the following concepts:

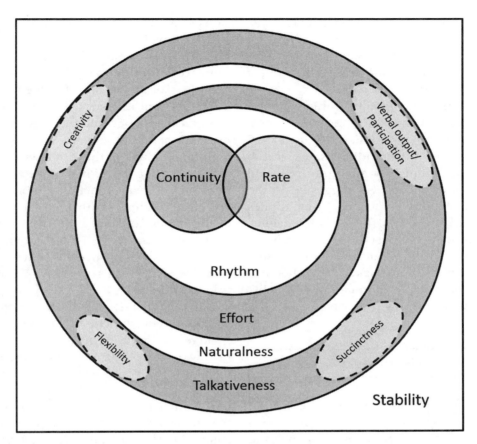

Figure 1–4. A working model of speech fluency. Solid lines enclose the primary fluency dimensions; dashed lines enclose secondary fluency dimensions. Each dimension either overlaps with or embeds within other fluency dimensions. Verbal output, creativity, flexibility, and succinctness are aspects of talkativeness. Stability is a way of characterizing the other fluency dimensions (e.g., rate stability, effort stability) and can be determined only after conducting repeated observations of a person's speech.

- The amount of speech a person produces at a particular time (verbal output);
- The extent to which a person engages or participates in the various interpersonal activities encountered during daily life (participation);
- The appropriateness of verbal output for a particular activity (succinctness);

- The range of communicative functions that are accomplished verbally (flexibility); and
- The ability to express ideas in novel, clever, entertaining, or distinctive ways (creativity).

The location of talkativeness within the model implies that speakers are most apt to exhibit a typical degree of talkativeness when they are proficient at other dimensions of fluency, namely continuity, rate, rhythm, effort, and naturalness. Of course, other factors, such as a person's temperament, may influence talkativeness characteristics in a person.

We present stability within a square that lies beyond the concentric rings. We do this to symbolize the idea that, unlike other fluency dimensions, stability is determined by analyzing repeated samples of speech. As suggested in the model, stability is a concept that applies to all of the other fluency dimensions. Assessments of speech fluency are likely to be most valid when based on repeated observations of a speaker. Only then can one gain an appreciation for how variable a speaker's fluency performance is.

Summary

Fluency is a multidimensional construct that is based on both physical speech production (i.e., speech articulation) and abstract message formulation (i.e., cognitive processing, linguistic planning). Accordingly, there are many potential sources for fluency difficulty during the speech production process. In this chapter, we have outlined seven primary dimensions of fluency, along with four other concepts that we regard as special cases or subcategories of certain primary fluency dimensions. One can conceive of the fluency dimensions as vantage points or perspectives from which to study fluency. Largely, the fluency dimensions are interrelated. For example, speech continuity is associated with speech rate, rhythm, naturalness, and perhaps with effort as well. We have assembled these dimen-

sions into a working model of fluency, to which we will return throughout the text. The model is useful as an organizational framework for discussing the characteristics associated with specific fluency disorders as well as issues that are related to clinical practice such as assessment, prevention, and treatment. Although it is tempting to think of these fluency dimensions as reflecting either "speech functions" or "language functions," it probably is more accurate to say that most, if not all, of the dimensions are reflective of *communicative functions*. To the extent that is so, the analysis of speech fluency offers an index of a person's overall communicative functioning.

In the remainder of this textbook, we explore fluency functioning in relation to a range of clinical populations. We focus mainly on issues related to disordered fluency, a topic which we discuss against the backdrop of typical fluency functioning. A final point that bears mention is that speech fluency has relevance to the study of both communication *differences* and *modalities* of communication. For instance, one benchmark for distinguishing between native and nonnative speakers of a language is the fluency with which they speak. Fluency also is used as a primary measure of a person's competence with skills such as oral reading and sign language use. We briefly explore these topics as well, later in the text. Before doing these things, however, we first turn our attention to several other fundamental topics: the speech production process (Chapter 2), the nature of disfluency (Chapter 3), and characteristics of normal fluency performance (Chapter 4). All are key foundational concepts that inform the clinical management of fluency disorders.

2

Fluency and Speech Production

In this chapter, we discuss some basic properties of speech production and explore how they relate to speech fluency. In doing so, we examine general features of speech production models as well as specific speech production processes involved in language formulation and speech articulation. It is our purpose to provide readers with an overview of the structural and functional bases of fluent speech production, as well as an appreciation for the number of things a speaker must "get right" in order to speak fluently.

Most people possess only a limited understanding of how fluently they communicate and even less understanding of how they attain fluent communication. Ordinarily, when speaking, it seems as if one only has to open his or her mouth and a stream of words springs forth. One might interpret the relative ease with which most people talk as evidence that the process of fluent speech production is simple and straightforward. This is not the case, however, as even the casual remarks a person says result from a series of neurophysiological events that he or she must perform accurately and integrate precisely

if fluency is to occur. It is perhaps surprising that fluency impairment is as uncommon as it is.

Speech production has been a subject of longstanding interest to physicians, speech-language pathologists, psycholinguists, neuropsychologists, and related professionals (Schuell, Jenkins, & Jiminez-Pabon, 1964). During the 1800s, researchers such as Paul Broca and Carl Wernicke managed to link unique patterns of speech impairment to lesions within specific regions of the nervous system and, in doing so, they deduced the functions of those regions. Understanding of the speech production process and its neuroanatomical correlates progressed steadily during the early-to-mid 1900s through scientific experiments with animals and study of people with brain injury (Schuell et al., 1964). In the years since then, the development of increasingly sophisticated computer-based tools for describing, measuring, and modeling neuroanatomical structures and neurophysiological events has resulted in a markedly more accurate and detailed description of speech production and, with it, speech fluency.

Nonetheless, there still are many details of the speech production process that require additional investigation before we can regard them as well understood.

Models of Speech Production

Numerous speech production models have been presented in recent decades (e.g., Bock & Levelt, 1994; Dell, 1986; Fromkin, 1971; Garrett, 1975, 1984; Levelt, 1989; Levelt, Roelofs, & Meyer, 1999). The authors of these models typically depict the speech production process as a series of stages or levels within which specific aspects of an utterance are developed or represented. The basic components of three well-studied models of speech production appear in Table 2–1. As can be seen, the models appear generally similar in terms of the number and types of components included within them. In the remainder of this section, we discuss some of the primary features that these models share, as well as the evidence base for the existence of components contained within them.

Basic Components of Speech Production

In a sense, the representational levels within contemporary speech production models constitute the necessary ingredients for the production of a spoken utterance. As shown in Table 2–1, speech production generally is agreed to begin with a semantic (i.e., meaning-based) representation of a communicative goal. At this

Table 2–1. Representational Levels Associated with Three Speech Production Models

	Model		
	Fromkin (1971)	**Dell (1986)**	**Levelt, Roelofs, & Meyer (1999)**
Level or Type of Representation	Meaning representation	Semantic (Meaning) representation	Conceptualization (Meaning)
	Syntactic specification of lexical items	Syntactic processing for lexical items	Syntactic specification of lexical items
	Intonation contour for syntactic frame		
	Content words fit to syntactic frame	Morphological processing	Morphological encoding
	Morphological specification		
	Phoneme specification	Phonological processing	Phonological encoding
	Phonological rules that fit phonemes with context		Phonetic encoding
	Articulation	Articulation	Articulation

point, the speaker identifies a message that he or she wishes to convey to others. This message has been labeled variously by authors as a *proposition* (Fromkin, 1971), an *intention* (Garrett, 1984), and a *lexical concept* (Levelt et al., 1999). The message (i.e. proposition, intention, lexical concept) is essentially a preverbal representation, rooted in thought, visual imagery, emotion, or feeling (Bock & Levelt, 1994)—forms that are not readily understandable to other people. Consequently, the speaker must translate the preverbal message into a language-based code that can be understood by other people who use the same language codes.

Although the speech production models presented in Table 2–1 share a number of similarities, they differ in several ways as well. For instance, Fromkin's (1971) model is oriented toward capturing the properties of sentence production whereas later models (Dell, 1986; Levelt et al., 1999) are more closely oriented toward lexical access and word production. The models also differ with regard to the assumptions the authors (cf. Dell, 1986; Levelt et al., 1999; Roelofs, 2000) make about issues such as the following:

- The extent to which certain linguistic representations are stored in memory (versus being constructed on an "as needed" basis),
- The extent to which processing across levels of linguistic representation occurs in serial fashion (versus simultaneously),
- The extent to which linguistic formulation occurs in a unidirectional (e.g., morphology $\rightarrow$ phonology) versus a bidirectional (e.g., morphology $\leftrightarrow$ phonology) manner.

In any case, as shown in Table 2–1, it is widely agreed that language formulation is multidimensional, such that it consists of distinct syntactic, morphologic, and phonologic representations. *Syntax* pertains to the grammatical roles of specific words and the language-specific rules for word ordering in phrases, clauses, and sentences (Zukowski, 2013). As such, the syntactic representation creates or implies a structural form for the soon-to-be spoken utterance. Some researchers (e.g., Shattuck-Hufnagel, 1979) have likened this structural form to a *frame* or to *slots*, into which message-relevant lexical items subsequently can be inserted. The frames are recognizable as the familiar units of syntax; that is, the *phrase*, the *clause*, and the *sentence*. A syntactic phrase is a word or a string of words that fulfills a specific grammatical function within an utterance, such as *subject, object, verb,* and *adverb*. A clause is a syntactic unit that is organized around a verb phrase: All grammatically complete sentences contain at least one clause.

Syntactic units have a hierarchical structure, such that phrases nest within clauses, and clauses nest within sentences. In sentences that contain more than one clause, it is common for one of the clauses to fulfill a grammatical function as well. In such cases, one clause is regarded as being *subordinate* to another superordinate clause within the utterance. In Figure 2–1, for example, the subordinate clause *after he had eaten lunch* functions as an adverb by providing information about *when* the repair occurred.

Morphology deals with the structural aspects of words, particularly meaning units within words. Linguists commonly distinguish between *free* and *bound* morphemes. Free morphemes can stand alone to convey meaning. Bound morphemes are

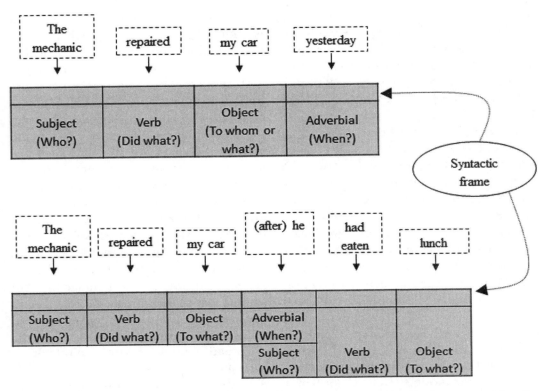

Figure 2–1. Examples of simple and complex sentences. A syntactic frame provides the speaker with a mechanism for linking message-relevant lexical items (*dashed boxes*) with their corresponding positional slots and their grammatical functions in the emerging utterance. The top sentence is *simple* because it contains a single verb phrase and, therefore, one clause. The bottom sentence is *complex* because it contains two verb phrases and, therefore, two clauses. Also, the second clause in the bottom sentence (*after he had eaten lunch*) is subordinate to the first clause (*the mechanic repaired my car*) because it functions as an adverb in the overall sentence. In other words, the subordinate clause modifies the verb *repaired* in the first clause clause by specifying *when* the repair took place.

affixed to free morphemes. Examples of bound morphemes in English include the plural -*s* marker, the past tense -*ed* marker and the present progressive verb marker -*ing*. Bound morphemes are meaningful only when attached to a free morpheme. The particular affixes that a speaker selects for a lexical item are determined by the syntax of an utterance and a word's grammatical function within the utterance.

One common approach to quantifying the structural complexity of preschool-er's spoken language is to compute the mean number of morphemes per utterance within a speech sample (i.e., Mean Length of Utterance (MLU); Miller, 1981). The more morphemes an utterance contains, the more complex it is. The effect of morphological complexity on speech fluency of conversational utterance has been assessed in a number of research studies involving children who stutter (e.g., Lattermann, Shenker, & Thordardottir, 2005; Ntourou, Conture, & Lipsey, 2011; Watkins, Yairi, & Ambrose, 1999; Zackheim & Conture, 2003), and the general finding has been that the likelihood of disfluency increases as the number of morphemes in an utterance increases.

Phonology

Phonology deals with the sound system of a language as well as sound-based features such as stress and intonation (Gleason, 2013). The phonological system functions as an interface between the language system and the motor (articulatory) system. At the phonologic level, the speaker creates a sound-based representation of a lexical item. This representation includes the phonemes that correspond with the selected lexical items and their positional location within syllables.

Phoneme assignment gives rise to *phonetic specification,* wherein the speaker specifies the speech sounds that will be spoken. With the phonetic realization in place, the speaker possesses a rough blueprint for how to say the utterance. The phonetic plan will be modified further based on proprioceptive and kinesthetic input during the articulation stage.

Sources of Evidence

There are several lines of evidence to support the existence of representational stages such as the ones shown in Table 2–1. As noted earlier, researchers gained initial insights into the component processes of speech production through studies of people who presented with lesions, diseases, developmental disorders, and so forth that affect the nervous system. The effects of injury and illness often are diffuse, however. This complicates the researcher's task of isolating

the presenting symptoms to a specific anatomical location or neural subsystem. Consequently, researchers have turned to a host of additional research methodologies, most of which allow for more precise control over extraneous variables.

Speech Error Analysis

Speech errors occur when the spoken form of an utterance deviates in one or more ways from its intended form. The errors are nonsystematic in nature, meaning that they occur less often and less reliably than, say, the phonological simplification patterns (e.g., "cluster reduction") or morphological overgeneralizations that preschoolers commonly produce.

Speech errors usually are rooted in language processing. Examples include errors in syntactic formulation (e.g., *If I was done to that . . . If that was done to me . . .* (Stemberger, 1982); lexical selection (e.g., *My uncle- uh, grandfather will be joining us.*); and phonological planning (e.g., *The pig bancakes- uh, big pancakes . . .*). Much of the data on speech errors comes from the study of typical speakers during everyday situations (e.g., Boomer & Laver, 1973; Stemberger, 1989). More recently, however, researchers (e.g., Dell & Warker, 2007) have studied speech errors that they induce within laboratory settings using stimuli that increase the likelihood of error occurrence.

With speech errors, speakers show evidence of *dissociation* in linguistic formulation. In other words, the speaker formulates some aspects of the utterance correctly and others incorrectly. For instance, in the *pancake* example above, the speaker demonstrates syntactic correctness through construction of a well-formed noun phrase (*Determiner + Adjective + Noun*). The speaker shows evidence of morphological correctness as well, by correctly affixing the plural marker to the noun, rather than to the adjective. The utterance even contains all of the necessary speech sounds. The speaker's error involves the assignment of those speech sounds to their correct positional order within the utterance (i.e., the /b/ and /p/ exchange). The fact that the speaker detects and then repairs this error suggests the existence of a representation of how the phrase *should sound* and the presence of a checking mechanism in which the spoken form of the phrase is compared with an internal representation of the phrase. Because the speaker has detected and corrected this error, it appears that the speech monitoring system functions properly, as well. Dissociations such as this support the idea that word ordering (i.e., syntax) and plural marker specifications are separate processes from phoneme positioning.

Chronometry and Response Latencies

Chronometry is another method that researchers use to identify the components of speech production (Levelt, 2001). In psycholinguistic research, chronometry involves the study of the time course within which particular language-related events unfold. The approach is rooted in concepts associated with *spreading activation theory* (described in the next section), and it is used extensively in research. The broad goal is to examine the time course associated with the production of various target responses. One of the primary dependent variables in chronometric experiments is the research participant's *response latency* (e.g., the amount of time that has elapsed between the introduction of a stimulus and initia-

tion of the participant's response to that stimulus). A researcher presents stimuli under various experimental conditions and then examines how the participant's response latencies vary.

One common experimental manipulation in this type of research is to present a second stimulus either before or at the same time as the presentation of the target stimulus. The researcher then examines the effect of this competing stimulus on the latency of the participant's response to the primary stimulus and uses the results of the analysis to make inferences about the structure and function of the speech production system. For example, Schriefers, Meyer, and Levelt (1990) found that semantic distracters (e.g., the word *goat* paired with the target word *sheep*) affected naming speed only when presented before the presentation of the picture that they asked participants to name. In contrast, phonologic distracters (e.g., the word *sheet* paired with the target word *sheep*) affected naming speed only when presented concurrently with or shortly after the presentation of a picture of a sheep. Experiments of this sort incorporate what researchers refer to as a *priming paradigm*. That is, the researcher seeks to identify the types of information that facilitate (i.e., prime) response initiation as well as those that impede or interfere with it, along with the time at which such facilitative or interference effects occur. In the Schriefers et al. (1990) study, the results suggest that semantic processing occurs prior to phonologic processing during the time course of word preparation.

Anderson and Conture (2004) used response initiation data to make inferences about children's syntactic processing during sentence production. The researchers presented line drawings to children who stuttered and children who did not stutter. The children were instructed to describe the sentences using simple declarative sentences (e.g., *The man is walking the dog.*). In one condition, the children produced the sentences without having the syntactic form of the sentence primed. Interestingly, in this condition, the children who stuttered exhibited slower speech initiation times than the nonstuttering children did. The speech initiation times for the two groups were comparable, however, in another condition wherein the syntactic form of the target sentence was primed through presentation of another simple declarative sentence. (For example, the sentence *The boy is kicking the ball* was presented just before the target sentence *The man is walking the dog.*). Based on the improved speech initiation times that children who stuttered attained when the syntax for the response target was primed, Anderson and Conture concluded that children who stutter might present a deficit or weakness in syntactic formulation.

Connectionist and Neuro-Computational Models

A third approach that researchers use when attempting to determine the architecture of the speech production system involves computer-based simulations. Examples of such simulations include the WEAVER++ model (Levelt et al., 1999; Roelofs, 2000) and the DIVA/GODIVA models (Bohland, Bullock, & Guenther, 2009; Guenther, 1995, 2006).[1] The computer models are organized around discrete information units (i.e., *nodes*), which are analogous to neurons or neuron assemblies that store information in memory.

The nodes connect to one another to create a network through which information can be stored, exchanged, and integrated. In recent years, researchers have used such computer models to test hypotheses about how the speech production system functions under certain conditions. They then compare results of such experiments against neuroimaging data that they collect for the same tasks in order to match specific types of information processing to specific neuroanatomical regions (e.g., Bohland et al., 2009; Indefrey & Levelt, 2004).

Spreading activation is a fundamental property of connectionist/computational models. The notion of spreading activation theory is rooted in a model developed by Quillian (1967), which primarily dealt with the problem of computer-based speech recognition. Collins and Loftus (1975) extended Quillian's work to model basic properties of lexical (word-based) representation. Both models feature interconnected nodes that form a network. In the Collins and Loftus model (Figure 2–2), the lengths of the lines that connect the nodes represent the "closeness" or semantic relatedness of the concepts. When one node activates, other linked nodes activate as well, via spreading activation. In Figure 2–2, activation of *car*, for example, would spread to *truck, street*, and *vehicle* as well as other nodes. Activation then would spread to whatever nodes connect to the secondary nodes.

The link between *car* and *truck* would be stronger than, say, the links between *car* and *ambulance* or *car* and *house*, because of the relative difference in semantic similarity across the paired concepts. Another important principle of spreading activation is that the strength of the

---

[1]WEAVER is an acronym for *Word-form Encoding by Activation and Verification*; DIVA is an acronym for *Directions into Velocities of Articulators*, while GODIVA is the *Gradient Order* version of DIVA.

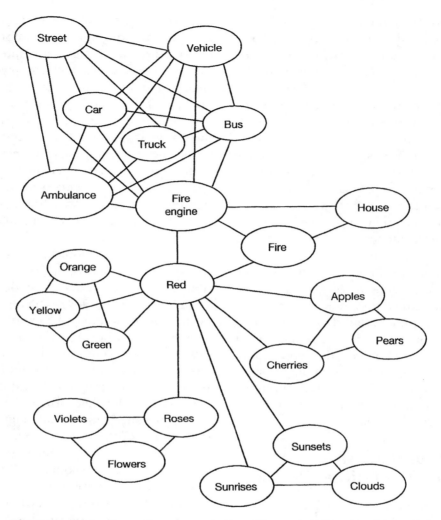

Figure 2–2. A schematic representation of how conceptual information is stored in human memory from Collins and Loftus (1975). In the model, similar concepts are highly interconnected, but dissimilar concepts are not. The length of a connecting line represents the strength or degree of relatedness between concepts. According to spreading activation principles, when a node activates, energy spreads from that node throughout the network. The strength of the spreading activation decreases as the distance between nodes increases. From "A Spreading Activation Theory of Semantic Processing," by A. M. Collins and E. F. Loftus, 1975, *Psychological Review, 82,* pp. 407–428. Reprinted with permission.

activation diminishes as the (conceptual) distance from a node increases. Thus, if a speaker activates the node for *car*, that activation would spread very weakly, if at all, to semantically distant nodes such as *roses* and *cherries*. The notions of network interconnectivity and spreading activation have been used to explain certain types of speech errors (Dell, 1986) and they have been argued to have relevance to speech fluency as well (Postma & Kolk, 1991, 1993).

In more contemporary models (e.g., Bohland et al., 2009; Dell, 1986; Levelt et al., 1999; Roelofs, 2000), spreading activation is said to occur across processing levels. Thus, nodes at the semantic level connect with nodes at the syntactic level, which in turn connect with nodes at the morphological-phonological level (Levelt et al., 1999) and have the potential to influence one another.

Other Sources of Evidence

Researchers have used a variety of other research methodologies in addition to the approaches described above to make inferences about structure and time course of speech production processing. Examples of such methodologies include the following: analysis of eye movements via eye tracking technology; analysis of cortical and subcortical electrical activity via electrophysiological measures; and analysis of blood flow activity within both the cortex of the brain and subcortical structures via hemodynamic imaging. In subsequent chapters, we touch on the use of these methodologies in the study of fluency-impaired speakers.

Primary Stages of Speech Production

Levelt and colleagues (e.g., Bock & Levelt, 1994; Levelt, 1989, 2001; Levelt, Roelofs, & Meyer, 1999; Roelofs, 1997, 2000, 2003; Roelofs & Meyer, 1998) have been

engaged in a large and long-term research program that has been designed to model the process of speech production.[2] The speech production model from Levelt (1989) is in Figure 2–3.

The model includes many components, several of which overlap with the ones that we outlined under the Levelt et al. model in Table 2–1. For now, we will focus on three processing stages within the model shown in Figure 2–3: the *Conceptualizer*, the *Formulator*, and the *Articulator*.

- The Conceptualizer is that part of the speech production process wherein the speaker develops a semantically based concept or intention to express.
- The Formulator is that part of the process wherein the speaker assembles linguistic codes that translate a concept into a form that is recognizable to others. The formulation stage encompasses several familiar aspects of language form; namely *syntax, morphology,* and *phonology*.
- The Articulator is that part of the speech production process where a person plans and then executes a sequence of movements that correspond to the linguistic representation. In this way, the speaker can convert linguistic representations into acoustic output (i.e., speech).

As is evident from Figure 2–3, word preparation models include stages of representation: conceptual preparation leads to specification of word function and

---

[2]Research teams have conducted numerous studies to test these concepts at laboratories in Nijmegen, a city in the Netherlands. Thus, the model sometimes is called "the Nijmegen model."

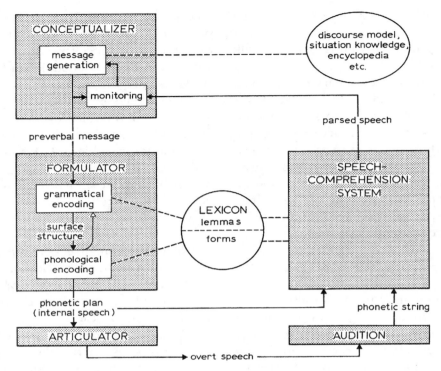

Figure 2–3. Speech production model proposed by Levelt (1989). The boxes represent processing components and the circled areas represent informational stores. Five primary processing mechanisms are included in the model. Three of these (Conceptualizer, Formulator, and Articulator) figure prominently in message generation and production. The Audition and Speech Comprehension Systems are particularly relevant to monitoring message development and message output. From Levelt, Willem J. M., *Speaking: From Intention to Articulation*, figure 1.1, page 9, © 1989 Massachusetts Institute of Technology, by permission of The MIT Press.

form, which in turn leads to the planning of relevant motor movements, and the eventual execution of those motor movements in the form of speech articulation. In the following sections, we discuss the processes of conceptualization, formulation, and articulation in more detail. We return to concepts associated with the Nijmegen model and other relevant models in several of the following chapters, particularly those models that address fluency impairment.

Conceptualizing a Message

As discussed above, speech production begins with *conceptualization*. At this stage, the speaker establishes the essential meanings that he or she wishes to convey to others. Conceptualization entails the act of mapping an *intention* that one wants to express to corresponding *lexical concepts*. The speaker subsequently will transform lexical concepts into corresponding morphologic, phonologic, phonetic, articulatory, and acoustic representations during the *formulation* and *articulation* stages (see below).

Lexical Concepts

Conceptualization essentially is a *preverbal* processing state (Levelt, 1989). The speaker's goal is to mold a preverbal intention into appropriate *lexical concepts* (Levelt et al., 1999). A lexical concept is a semantically based representation of the speaker's intention. Following the principles of spreading activation, when a speaker attempts to realize a communicative goal such as "*label the object in this picture*," he or she must select an appropriate lexical concept from a field of other potentially relevant lexical concepts (see Figure 2–2).

Levelt et al. (1999) give an example of how conceptual networks function: When a researcher presents a participant with a picture of a four-legged animal that has a mane, hooves, and a long tail and wears a saddle, several lexical concepts activate simultaneously. <*Horse*> will be one of them, but <*animal*>, <*mare*>, <*colt*>, and other such concepts will likely activate, as well. Factors that affect the lexical concept that a speaker ultimately selects include the characteristics of the pictured object itself as well as the speaker's ability to engage in *perspective taking*, which is an aspect of social cognition wherein the speaker assesses what type of concept a particular situation calls for (Crystal & Varley, 1998).

With perspective taking, the speaker must evaluate the status of the ongoing conversation. That is, the speaker must consider what he and the other conversationalists have said thus far, determine the degree of specificity or formality that is appropriate in the situation, and determine the amount of background information the audience needs (Crystal & Varley, 1998; Levelt, 1989; Levelt et al., 1999). The act of conceptualizing typically is not problematic for speakers, especially when a speaker and conversational partner are well acquainted. Still, there are times when even highly proficient speakers fumble with conceptualization. For example, a person might hesitate while attempting to generate an intention in a situation that calls for consoling a friend over the loss of a loved one. At such times, speech becomes disfluent.

Intentions and Memory

Intentions are rooted in the ideas and thoughts that one has. Ideas and thoughts are based on one's stored knowledge of the world. In the so-called *multiple memory systems* view, knowledge is represented across several memory systems, which can be broadly divided into whether they involve declarative memory or not (Neath & Surprenant, 2003; Tulving, 1983).

Declarative Memory

Neath and Surprenant (2003) describe declarative memory as knowledge that can be consciously described and is open to conscious awareness. They list three subtypes of memory under the heading of declarative memory: *episodic memory*, *semantic memory*, and *working memory*.

Episodic memory pertains to personal, autobiographical, and event-based knowledge, including the ways in which specific events relate to one another in time.

Semantic memory is conceptual in nature and, thus, a foundation for one's lexical concepts. The term *object knowledge* refers to information that pertains to particular objects (e.g., *Mom, Earth*) and object classes (e.g., people, planets). Traditionally, researchers viewed lexical concepts as packages of bundled information known as *semantic features* (see Bloom & Lahey, 1978, for a discussion of this approach). In this view, a lexical concept consists of a core set of attributes or qualities that are unique to that concept. For example, the word *tree* might include semantic features like [wood], [tall], [bark], [leaves], and [roots]. Some of the features for *tree* (e.g., [roots]) are shared with *flower* and *tooth* as well.

Levelt et al. (1999) argued against a feature-based type of representation, however, noting that speakers rarely, if ever, substitute superordinate concepts (e.g., *animal*) for subordinate concepts (e.g., *horse*) when naming objects. Levelt et al. also noted that words with a complex array of semantic features are no harder for people to access than words with simple feature sets. Based on these observations, Levelt et al. argue that lexical concepts behave more like "undivided wholes." Also included under semantic knowledge are the notions of *relational memory* (e.g., knowing how one entity relates to another) and *spatial memory* (e.g., spatial relations among objects).

Neath and Surprenant (2003) characterize *working memory* as a subtype of declarative memory. Following Baddeley (1992), they describe working memory as a form of immediate memory that incorporates a central mechanism for directing one's attention (i.e., an *executive* function) and several so-called *slave systems* that are specialized for tasks such as phonological processing and visual-spatial processing.

Nondeclarative Storage

Declarative memory typically is contrasted with *procedural memory*, which is a nondeclarative type of storage (Crystal & Varley, 1998). Neath and Surprenant (2003) indicate that *procedural memory* encompasses knowledge that pertains to knowing how to do something. It is an implicit form of knowledge, which means that it is based on previous experiences for which the individual lacks conscious awareness. Examples include specific motor skills and cognitive skills. Neath and Surprenant list *perceptual representation* as a second type of nondeclarative memory. Subtypes of perceptual representation include visual word forms and auditory word forms.

Utterance Functions

Spoken utterances can be viewed from both semantic and pragmatic perspectives. From a semantic perspective, one can examine the meaning conveyed in an utterance. From a pragmatic perspective, one can examine the functional role that a particular utterance assumes within a conversation. As noted in Chapter 1, Fey (1986) described a system for classifying the functional roles of conversational utterances. His system extended the work of others (e.g., Dore, 1974; Searle, 1975) who had studied functional uses of language through a process called *speech act analysis*. With this approach, a clinician describes utterances in two ways: (1) in terms of how they function in relation to the immediately preceding utterance (an *utterance-level analysis*); and (2) in terms of how they function in relation to the conversational topic (a *discourse-level analysis*). Also noted in Chapter 1, fluency impairment may cause speakers to restrict the range of communicative functions that they express.

Utterance-Level Functions

Fey (1986) identifies four utterance-level categories: (1) assertive acts, (2) responsive acts, (3) imitative acts, and (4) other acts.

- *Assertive acts* are unsolicited speech acts. In other words, these are utterances that the speaker produces without being obligated to do so by the communicative actions of another person. Fey further specifies assertive acts into the following four subtypes: *statements* (remarks pertaining to one's internal feelings, thoughts, or beliefs); *comments* (remarks pertaining to objects, events, and activities external to the speaker); *disagreements* (comments or statements that deny or negate a previously made assertion); and *requestives* (remarks that are intended to solicit information or actions from another person). *Performative* acts consist of utterances that involve joking, teasing, protesting, or warning (e.g., *Look out!*). Performative acts tend to be rhetorical in nature. As such, a verbal response is not obligated or expected from a conversational partner.
- *Responsive acts* are solicited by requests that another person has made. They can be further specified, as well, based on what a conversational partner has asked a speaker to do. Subtypes of responsive acts include *responses*

to requests *for* (a) *information*, (b) *clarification*, (c) *attention*, and (d) *action*. As such, speakers produce responsive acts following either a question (e.g., *What is your name?*) or a command (e.g., *Tell me about the movie.*) that a conversational partner poses.

- *Imitative acts* are a verbatim copy of an utterance that another person has just said. Imitative acts usually are produced much less often than assertive and responsive acts. Neither imitative acts nor performative speech acts advance a conversation in the way other assertive and responsive acts do.

Discourse-Level Functions

At the *discourse level* of analysis, utterances can be described in terms of how they relate to the unfolding conversation. From this perspective, an utterance can fulfill one of three roles during conversation: initiate a topic, maintain a topic, or extend a topic.

- *Topic initiation* occurs when an utterance is not preceded by another utterance (i.e., it is the first utterance in a conversation) or when the semantic theme of an utterance is unrelated to the semantic theme found in previously spoken utterances during a conversation.
- *Topic maintenance* occurs when a speaker produces an utterance that relates to the ongoing topic but does not add substantive semantic information to it (e.g., a child answers "yep" or "mhmm" when asked if he wants an ice cream cone).

- *Topic extension* occurs when a speaker's utterance adds semantic details to an established topic or moves an existing topic in a new, but semantically relevant, direction.

As with utterance-level functions, fluency impairment may cause speakers to restrict the range of discourse-level functions that they express. For example, a speaker who stutters may decide to limit his or her conversational contributions to verbal remarks that merely maintain a conversation. In such instances, the speaker assumes a very passive role in communication.

Conceptualization and Fluency

Analysis of the utterance functions that a speaker produces has relevance to fluency disorders.

It yields information about patterns of conversational *participation,* such as whether the person uses mostly responsive acts—a pattern that indicates the person "speaks only when spoken to." It also provides insight into the pragmatic contexts within which speech is most disfluent. With regard to the latter point, some communicative intentions (e.g., assertive acts) often are more linguistically complicated than others (e.g., responsive acts) to accomplish and thus are more prone to disfluency (Logan, 2003a; Weiss & Zebrowski, 1992).

Formulation

Formulation entails the process of converting lexical concepts or messages into a linguistic representation that others are likely to comprehend. *Language* is "a code

whereby ideas about the world are represented through a conventional system of arbitrary signals for communication" (Bloom & Lahey, 1978, p. 4). *Speech*, in contrast, is a mode of expressing linguistic codes; that is, it is the physical realization of linguistic symbols. It is common for authors who write about fluency disorders to use the term *speech fluency* when discussing a speaker's performance. Although use of this term implies a narrow interest in articulation, it is understood that one cannot have speech fluency without also having linguistic fluency. Linguists and other professionals who are interested in language study the structural aspects of language from three distinct perspectives: *syntax*, *morphology*, and *phonology* (Bloom & Lahey, 1978).

Lemma Activation and Syntactic Specification

According to Levelt et al. (1999), selection of a lexical concept at the conceptualization stage of word production leads to *lexical selection*, wherein the speaker selects the *lemma* (Kempen, 1977, 1978) that corresponds to the lexical concept. The lemma contains an address or label for a lexical item, along with its associated syntactic role. Also included within the lemma is information about the syntactic environment within which the lexical item occurs. For example, the lemma for an action-related meaning not only indicates that the lexical item fits into the grammatical class called a *verb*, but also it specifies whether the lexical item is obligated to be followed by an object (e.g., the verb *want* obligates the use of a direct object: *I want <u>coffee</u>.*).

Also represented in the lemma are *diacritical parameters*: the kinds of morphological affixes that are associated with the lexical item. This allows for specification of how the speaker will realize a particular word within a particular syntactic environment. For example, the lemma for the verb *jump* will specify the type of affixes that are necessary when the speaker produces *jump* in the present tense or the past tense, in the first, second, or third person, and so forth.

Morphological and Phonological Encoding

In Levelt's (2001) model, activation of the lemma leads to specification of the morpho-phonemic form of a word. As noted in the previous section, the morphological form of a lexical item is specified within its lemma. It includes a base morpheme and any diacritics (i.e., *bound* morphemes) associated with it. The values of a diacritic for a particular lemma are derived from the speaker's communicative intention and conceptual goals for the utterance (e.g., <*I am commenting about an event that occurred in the past*>). Also included in the word form representation is information about the prosodic (stress) patterns within both the lexical item and its broader syntactic environment (Ferreira, 1993).

Word form specification leads to *phonological encoding*. Figure 2–4 includes the phonological encoding framework from Levelt (2001). As shown, phonological encoding for the word *horses* begins with the retrieval of the phonemes that are associated with each of the morphemes in the word. Levelt (1989, 2001) terms this retrieval process *the phonological spell-out*. So, for *horses*, the speaker retrieves the phonemes /h/, /ɔ/, /r/, /s/, /ɪ/, and /z/. At this point in Levelt's model, the speaker retrieves information about the syllable position that the phonemes assume, as well.

Syllable Structure

Syllables are phonological units that are organized around vowels. In English, vowels may be preceded or followed by one or more consonants. It is widely held that, for most languages, syllable representations are hierarchical (Ball, Müller, & Rutter, 2010).[3] That is, some parts of the syllable are nested within other parts. Support for this view comes from studies of non-systematic speech errors or "slips of the tongue" as well as language manipulation activities such as rhyming and alliteration. These data suggest that syllables consist of two main nodes: the *onset* and the *rime*. The rime, in turn, consists of two sub-components: the *nucleus* (also called the *peak*) and the *coda*. In models of speech production (e.g., Shattuck-Hufnagel, 1979), the onset, nucleus, and coda are commonly viewed as positional slots for the sound segments (i.e., "the filler") within a syllable. The speaker's use of an organizational frame of this sort presumably minimizes the occurrence of sound sequencing errors (e.g., "bat" → "tab") in speech (Berg, 1998), and it promotes efficiency in speech articulation by allowing for the coarticulation of articulatory gestures (Fowler, 2007). See Figure 2–5 for an illustration of a syllable frame.

As noted above, a syllable is organized around a nucleus, which is a *sonorous* speech sound. Sonority refers to the degree of vocal tract openness associated with a phoneme. From a distinctive feature

---

[3]Berg and Abd-El-Jawad (1996) present data from Arabic, which suggest that syllable structure representation within that language is linear in nature; that is, based largely on tri-consonantal roots that serve as word frames (e.g., $C_1\_\ C_2\_\ C_3\_$) and strong phonotactic constraints against repetition of identical sounds within a word boundary.

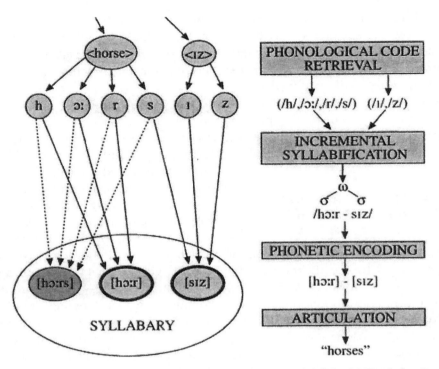

Figure 2–4. The portion of the WEAVER++ model (Levelt, Roelofs, & Meyer, 1999; Roelofs, 2000) that deals with word form development. The developing word is *horses*. Nodes containing the word's morphological structure (top level) link with associated phonemes. Phoneme selection leads to determination of the word's syllable structure. In this case, the syllable boundaries do not match the morpheme boundaries so that the speaker can accommodate the maximization of (syllable) onset rule. At the phonetic encoding level, the speaker selects syllables from a syllable store (i.e., syllabary), based on the syllabification process performed earlier. From *Spoken Word Production: A Theory of Lexical Access*, by W. J. M. Levelt, 2001. *Proceedings of the National Academy of Sciences* [PNAS], *98*, 13464–13471. Copyright (2001) National Academy of Sciences, USA. Reprinted with permission.

perspective, every vowel sound is [+sonorant]. Some consonants (in English, /m/, /n/, and /l/), can function as syllabic nuclei in certain phonetic contexts (e.g., the /m/ in *rhythm*). For a sound or sound sequence to be considered a syllable, the nucleus slot must be filled with a sonorant sound. For example, the vowel /o/ can stand alone as a syllable, but the nonsonorous consonant /f/ cannot.

Sound Sequencing

The onset serves as a placeholder for consonant sounds that precede the nucleus of a syllable (e.g., *no*, *snow*).[4] In English,

---

[4]The notion of positional slots during phonological encoding is not universally accepted, however, and some speech production models make no assumptions about their existence (cf. Dell, Juliano, & Govindjee, 1993).

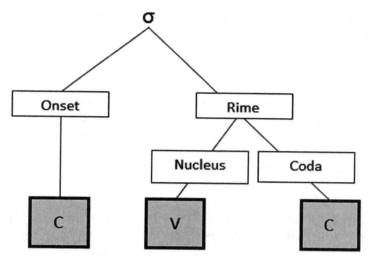

Figure 2–5. Hierarchical model of syllable (σ) structure. Syllable representation is thought to have a hierarchical, right-branching structure. The *onset* serves as a placeholder for syllable-initial consonants (C). The rime consists of the *nucleus* (also called the *peak*) and the *coda*. The nucleus is a placeholder for sonorous sounds—usually vowels (V). The coda is a placeholder for post-vocalic consonants within the syllable. In English, onsets can contain 0 to 3 consonants and codas can contain 0 to 4 consonants.

it is permissible for the onset slot to be unfilled (e.g., *on, eat*).

The coda follows the vowel. Like the onset, it may be filled (e.g., *cat, bad*) or unfilled (e.g., *go_, he_*) in English. Each language has phonotactic rules that specify the types of consonant configurations that are permissible in the onset and coda slots. In English, clusters of more than one consonant are permissible in both the syllable onset and coda. English onsets may contain between 0 to 3 consonants; English codas may contain between 0 to 4 consonants (Berg, 1998).

When the onset or coda features more than one consonant, sequential ordering is determined largely by sonority (Berg, 1998; Gierut, 1999). The ordering hierarchy, from most to least sonorous, is as follows: glides, liquids, nasals, fricatives, affricates, and stops (Berg, 1998). Thus, the most sonorous consonants are positioned closest to the syllable nucleus and the least sonorous consonants are positioned furthest from the nucleus. In a two-segment consonant cluster such as *bl*, the more sonorous of the two phonemes (/l/) is positioned closer to the vowel than the less sonorous sound (/b/). Codas follow the same principle. In the cluster *nd* (as in the word *band*), /n/ is more sonorous than /d/; consequently, it is positioned closer to the vowel than /d/.

The sonority principle accounts for phoneme sequencing patterns within most English consonant cluster forms. The general rule is violated, however, during some /s/ clusters. For example, within syllables such as *stay* and *skill*, a stop consonant lies closer to the vowel than the /s/, even though fricatives are more sonorous than stops. This situation leads some researchers (e.g., Gierut, 1999; Selkirk, 1984) to speculate that, at least in this context, /s/ is represented as an "adjunct" or "appendage" to the syllable.

Sonority effects exist within clusters that span syllable boundaries within words as well. Berg (1998) reported that in most English words that feature "cross-syllable" clusters, the constituent sounds are phonologically dissimilar and ordered in decreasing sonority. The most common clusters of this type feature either a *nasal + stop* sequence as in *.hin.der* or a *nasal + fricative* sequence as in *.mon.ster.* Berg suggested that this patterning of sounds reduces the occurrence of sound sequencing errors.

Syllabification

In Levelt's (1989) model, the phonological spellout leads to the specification of a word's syllabic structure (see *incremental syllabification* in Figure 2–4). For one-syllable words like *cat* or *cats,* this process is straightforward. For multisyllable words like *horses,* however, syllabification may result in reformulating syllable boundaries in ways that differ from those found in the word's morphemic representation. This is illustrated in Figure 2–4, wherein a consonant that occupies the coda position in the word's base morpheme (*horse)* is reassigned to the (empty) onset position of the syllable that corresponds with the plural marker, *-iz.* The resyllabification is performed through a processing strategy that maximizes the number of consonants that occur within the onset position of noninitial syllables in a word (Levelt, 1989; Selkirk, 1984). Resyllabification enhances the ease with which words are pronounced. Levelt et al. (1999) illustrate how a word such as *escorting* is much

easier to pronounce when the speaker relocates morpheme-final /t/ in *escort* to the onset of the following syllable. In its original position, the /t/ is unreleased. Use of a "word-final" /t/ in what ends up as a word-medial position makes for cumbersome (and, arguably, *disfluent*) articulation. Relocation of the /t/ to the onset of the morpheme *-ing* allows the /t/ to be released and aspirated within the word.

According to Selkirk (1984), if the phonotactic rules of a language allow a syllable to lead off with a particular consonant or string of consonants, then the resyllabification process will take place. The main rule is that the onset of a syllable will capture as many consonants as the phonotactic rules of the language allow. In the case of the word *mushroom,* for example, the syllable boundaries are marked *.mu.shroom,* rather than *.mush.room.*

Levelt (2001) cites experimental evidence that suggests word syllabification occurs during word formulation, rather than being stored in a fixed form. When the syllabification process is complete, the speaker has formulated a *phonological word.* We discuss phonological words further in the following section on prosodic representation.

Prosodic Encoding

Prosody is a phonological construct that pertains to the metrical and intonation properties of a spoken utterance (Ferreira, 2007; Kent & Read, 1992; Levelt, 1989; Selkirk, 1984; Wheeldon, 2000). Included within the domain of *metrical phonology* are the stress patterns, segment durations, pause locations, and pause durations that characterize an utterance—aspects of production that a listener perceives as the *rhythm* or *metrical properties* of connected speech (Kent & Read, 1992). Research data suggest that speakers construct *prosodic plans*, in which they specify the metrical and intonation patterns to be used in an utterance (Ferreira, 2007; Wheeldon, 2000).

Researchers hypothesize that prosodic representations have a hierarchical structure. The units nested within this hierarchy are as follows: *syllables, feet, phonological words, phonological phrases, intonational phrases,* and *utterances* (Selkirk, 1984, Levelt, 1989; Wheeldon, 2000). In other words, syllables combine to form feet, feet combine to form phonological words, phonological words combine to form phonological phrases, and so on. An utterance's syntactic structure influences its prosodic structure. Evidence for hierarchical representation of prosody comes, in part, from cross-language analyses of certain phonological rules (see Nespor & Vogel, 1986, for more detail) and analysis of the metrical patterns that occur with certain types of speech errors and phonologically based word manipulations such as rhyming and alliteration (Ball et al., 2010). Data from studies of the pause locations and pause durations that occur during various types of syntactic constructions (e.g., Ferreira, 1993) provide a third leg of evidence for hierarchical prosodic representation. Although the phonologic system is a primary source of input for the prosodic system, other factors (e.g., the attitude or emotion that a speaker wishes to convey) affect aspects of prosody such as articulation rate and pause patterns, as well (Levelt, 1989).

Syllables and Feet in Metrical Phonology

In English, stressed syllables generally are louder, longer, and have greater pitch movement than unstressed syllables (Ball et al., 2010). In contemporary clinical practice, procedures involved in the analysis and description of stress patterns are commonly based on principles from *metrical phonology* (Goldsmith, 1990; Liberman & Prince, 1977). Within the framework of metrical phonology, the degree of stress for a particular syllable is determined through analysis of the stress characteristics of surrounding syllables. For example, in the two-syllable word *table,* the first syllable carries more stress than the second syllable. Thus, the first syllable is designated as "strong" (*s*), the second syllable as "weak" (*w*), and the stress pattern for the word is "strong-weak" (*sw*). In English, most two-syllable words are characterized by either a "strong-weak" stress pattern or a "weak-strong" stress pattern, and most multisyllable words in English feature *alternating stress* (i.e., *swsw, wsws*).

In metrical phonology, syllables fall into one of three stress categories: *unstressed* (weak)*, secondary stress,* and *primary stress.* Ball et al. (2010) use the term *secondary stress* to describe a syllable that carries more stress than at least one other syllable within a word but has less stress than another syllable within that word. They use the term *primary stress* in reference to a syllable that carries the most stress within a word (Example 2–1). Only one syllable per word can carry primary stress. In Example 2–1, lowercase characters indicate secondary stress and weak stress (*s* and *w,* respectively) and the uppercase *S* indicates primary stress.

Example 2–1

a. Graduation: [.græ.dʒu.eɪ.ʃən.] = *swSw*

b. Velocity: [.və.lɑ. sɪ. tɨ.] = *wSws*

Syllables within words fit into higher-order units called *feet*. A foot is a span of two syllables that differ in stress. In Example 2–2, the foot boundaries for the words from Example 2–1 are marked with parentheses. Each foot consists of one strong syllable and one weak syllable.

Example 2–2

a. Graduation: (græ. dʒu) (eɪ.ʃən)

b. Velocity: (ə.lɑ) (sə.tɨ)

In *graduation*, the third syllable (and thus the second foot) bears primary stress. Thus, the second foot within *graduation* is strong in relation to the first foot. In *velocity*, the second syllable (and thus the first foot) bears primary stress. Consequently, the first foot is strong in relation to the second foot. Word stress patterns often are modeled using tree diagrams like those shown in Figure 2–6.

In English, several factors influence stress assignment. One such factor involves the segmental characteristics of the rime (Ball et al., 2010). That is, weak syllables are considered "light" from a segmental standpoint because the rime consists of a short vowel (e.g., /ɪ/, /ɛ/, /ə/) and one consonant. The rimes in strong syllables, however, are "heavy" from a segmental standpoint; that is, they have one of the following: (a) a short vowel and two or more consonants or (b) a long vowel such as /i/, /e/, or /u/ or a diphthong in combination with zero or more consonants.

Phonological Words

Phonological words consist of the phonemes associated with a lexical item, organized in terms of syllable position and the stress pattern associated with those syllables (Selkirk, 1984; Wheeldon, 2000). Each phonological word is comprised of a smaller metrical unit, the foot (Selkirk, 1984; Wheeldon, 2000). Some phonological words consist of a single stressed foot, while others consist of both a stressed foot and an unstressed foot (Ball et al., 2010). The notion of a phonological word differs from the traditional sense of a word. For instance, Ball et al. (2010) explain that a word string like *black + bird* can be regarded as one phonological word when it is used as a compound noun to refer to a certain species (e.g., *Blackbirds are common throughout Europe.*). In that case, the component syllables follow a clear *strong-weak* stress pattern. When the word string is used to refer to the color of an unspecified bird species, however (e.g., *An unusual black bird visited the feeder today*), both *black* and *bird* are stressed and regarded as separate phonological words.

Function words such as determiners, conjunctions, and auxiliary verbs can combine with lexical words to form distinct phonological words as well (Selkirk, 1984; Wheeldon, 2000). Levelt (1989) gives the example of *I've*, in which an unstressed function word (*have*) is reduced such that it no longer has a sonority peak (i.e., *have* → [v]). Because [v] is no longer a syllable, it attaches to the preceding word to form the phonological word [aɪv]. Cases in which a reduced word joins with a preceding word are termed *enclitization*. In English, enclitic forms often include pronouns, auxiliary verbs, or verb particles (see Example 2–3A–D, below). *Proclitic* forms are possible as well (Ball et al., 2010). In this case, a reduced function word merges with a following word to make a single phonological word (see Example 2–3E–G).

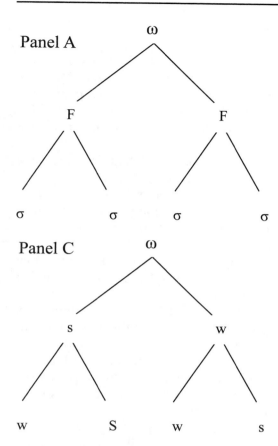

Panel A

Panel B

Panel C

Figure 2–6. Metrical trees are useful for describing the prosodic structure of *phonological words* (ω). **A.** The hierarchical nature of prosodic units is illustrated. As shown, a phonological word (*top tier*) is composed of feet (F, *middle tier*) which, in turn, are composed of syllables (σ, *bottom tier*). **B.** The metrical tree represents the stress characteristics for a phonological word (ω) like *graduation*, wherein primary stress falls on the third syllable (i.e., the left branch of the second foot) and secondary stress falls on the first syllable (i.e., the left branch of the first foot). **C.** For a phonological word like *velocity*, primary stress falls on the second syllable (i.e., the right branch of the first foot) and secondary stress falls on the fourth syllable (i.e., the right branch of the second foot). In four-syllable words like these, the foot that carries primary word stress is designated as *strong* (s), and the foot that carries secondary word stress is designated as *weak* (w).

Example 2–3

a. *get him* → [gɛdm̩]

b. *want to* → [wɑnə]

c. *I am* → [aɪm]

d. *Tess will* → [tɛsl̩]

e. *you want* → [jəwɑnt]

f. *and go* → [ŋgo]

g. *an apple* →[ənæpl̩]

From a phonological perspective, it seems that function words often behave as affixes to lexical words (Au-Yeung, Howell, & Pilgrim, 1998). Selkirk (1984) described a straightforward method for setting phonological word boundaries: *attach weak (de-stressed) monosyllable function words to the lexical words with which they are semantically associated.* With this approach, weak auxiliary verbs attach to full verbs (e.g., *can take* → [kn̩teɪk], weak prepositions attach to noun complements (e.g., *for Jeff* → [fɚ.dʒɛf], and so forth. However, when a function word bears primary stress (e.g., MY red coat) or is located at the end of a phrase boundary (e.g., *I mean the cookies we ran out OF*), it becomes a distinct phonological word.

Phonological Phrases

The *phonological phrase* is superordinate to the phonological word. As such, it is comprised of one or more phonological words (Selkirk, 1984). Within each phonological phrase, one syllable bears primary stress. Phonological phrase boundaries often overlap with syntactic phrase boundaries (Ferreira, 1993). When an utterance consists of a single syntactic phrase (e.g., a noun phrase like *the dog*), the boundaries for the phonological word, the phonological phrase, and the *intonation phrase* (described below) are the same. Levelt et al. (2001) argue that the phonological phrase is the basic unit of phonetic planning. If so, this may explain how speakers who stutter can "sense" that they are likely to stutter on an upcoming syllable. In this view, the speaker has planned a string of syllables for articulation but detects a problem or weakness within the plan.

Intonation Phrases

The *intonation phrase* is the largest prosodic unit over which an intonation contour applies (Selkirk, 1984). Intonation phrases are comprised of phonological phrases and are organized around one strong syllable, which represents the focus of the prosodic unit. Wheeldon (2000) noted that sentence constituents such as tag questions (*That horse is fast, isn't he?*) and parenthetical remarks always are marked as discrete intonation phrases within their respective sentences.

Utterances

The *utterance* is the largest unit in the prosodic hierarchy (Wheeldon, 2000). An utterance can be either a grammatically complete sentence or some other string of words that lacks a verb but nonetheless communicates a coherent idea. The process of ellipsis (i.e., deleting redundant or shared information) often results in utterances that lack a verb. For example, when asked what color the sky is, most people reply by saying "blue." In this case, the speaker deletes the shared information (*the sky is*). Either way the speaker says it (*blue, the sky is blue*), it is regarded as an utterance.

In Figure 2–7, a longer utterance is presented to illustrate the hierarchal relationships among levels of prosodic representation. The prosodic form in the figure is consistent with the model of prosody that Selkirk (1984) and Ferreira (1993) have described.

Phonetic Encoding

Phonological encoding gives rise to a *phonetic plan*, which includes information about the types of articulatory movements that are necessary to say a word (see the lower sections of Figures 2–3 and 2–4). The phonetic plan consists of the *syllable programs* that go with the phonological words that a speaker intends to say (Cholin, 2008). In an analysis of English and Dutch speakers, Schiller, Meyer, Baayen, and Levelt (1996) found that the 500 most frequent syllable forms in each language accounted for 80 to 85% of all syllable tokens used by adult speakers in everyday speech. Based on this and other observations, Schiller et al. suggested that the most frequently used syllables within a

Utterance				
Intonational Phrase		Intonational Phrase		
PPhr	PPhr	PPhr	PPhr	
ω	ω	ω	ω	ω
Ed	*said*	*my* | *Dad*	*won*	*a* | *CAR*

Figure 2–7. Levels of prosodic representation within a complex utterance (Utt). From a syntactic perspective, the sentence contains two clauses; from a prosodic perspective, it contains two intonational phrases. Phonological words (ω) embed within phonological phrases (PPhr), which in turn embed within intonational phrases (IPhr). Syllables (not shown in this figure) embed within phonological words (see Figure 2–6) and carry stress. If the word *car* carried primary stress for the entire utterance, the right-branching IPhr in the utterance would be strong relative to the left-branching one, and within the right-branching IPhr, the right-branching PPhr would be strong relative to the left-branching PPhr.

language are stored as ready-to-use programs in what they termed a *mental syllabary*. They also suggested that speakers assemble low-frequency syllables on an as-needed basis during speech planning. Their model for syllable production is based on results from speech-initiation time research during various experimental contexts (Cholin, Schiller, & Levelt, 2004) and the observation that priming of syllabic information, especially syllable onsets, facilitates speech-initiation times for low-frequency syllables more so than for high-frequency syllables (Cholin & Levelt, 2009).

In older models of speech production, researchers tended to regard the phonetic plan as a set of relatively detailed instructions for articulatory movements. Over time, however, researchers have come to view the phonetic plan in a minimalist sense; that is, as a specification of only the most basic actions a speaker must undertake to accomplish a particular articulatory goal. In the latter view, the phonetic plan is a *context-independent* representation. Some authors (e.g., Browman & Goldstein, 1990, 1992; Fowler, 2007; Goldstein & Fowler, 2003) have likened the form of a phonetic plan to that of a multi-tiered musical notation, which they term a *gestural score*. Instead of representing treble and bass notes, the gestural score specifies the spatial/dimensional configuration of the vocal tract during the course of prosodic units as long as a phonological phrase. The notion of a gestural score is rooted in a branch of phonology called *articulatory phonology* (Bauman-Waengler, 2012).

In Figure 2–8, we present an example from Goldstein and Fowler (2003) that illustrates the gestural score for the word *team*. As shown in the figure, the gestural score essentially is a plot of the location and degree of vocal tract constrictions the speaker must realize during the time course of the syllable. The key articulatory structures involved in vocal tract constriction are the *velum, lips, tongue body, tongue tip,* and *larynx*. The actions of these articulators are represented on specific tiers, a configuration that allows movements in different parts of the speech articulation system to overlap in time (e.g., lip constriction can occur at the same time as tongue raising). Speech sound segments routinely assume the characteristics of surrounding sounds —a process known as *coarticulation*. The

"team"

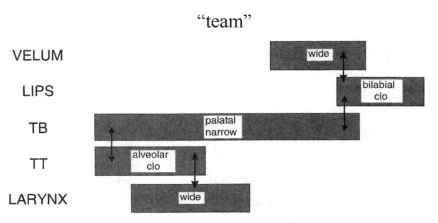

Figure 2–8. According to principles of articulatory phonology, speakers organize articulatory movements for syllables using a spatiotemporal representation called a *gestural score*. A schematization of a gestural score for the word *team* is shown in this figure. Each of the rows represents a speech-related structure (e.g., *TB* = tongue body, *TT* = tongue blade). The shaded bars indicate the activity of each speech-related structure during the course of the one-syllable word. The label within each bar indicates the specified goal for the organ (e.g., for the tongue tip, the goal is closure of the vocal tract at the alveolar ridge; for the lips, the goal is bilabial closure). The arrows indicate gestures that are "critically coordinated" and the thickness of the arrow represents the strength of the coordinative bonding between the gestures. From L. Goldstein and C. A. Fowler, *Articulatory Phonology: A Phonology for Public Language Use.* In Phonetics and Phonology in Language Comprehension and Production, N. O. Schiller & A. S. Meyer (Eds.); Mouton de Gruyter; 2003, New York, NY, p. 165. Courtesy of Mouton de Gruyter.

multitiered framework of the *gestural score* accounts for coarticulation by showing how speech sounds can overlap in time through the coordinated actions of articulators (Hixon, Weismer, & Hoit, 2008).

It is hypothesized that the gestural score specifies only the *task invariant* goals needed to produce a speech gesture (Browman & Goldstein, 1990, 1992; Fowler, 2003; Goldstein & Fowler, 2003). This means that the gestural score is a general plan, rather than an all-encompassing blueprint of which muscles will contract and the force with which they will contract. The generality of the plan affords the flexibility that a speaker needs to produce articulatory gestures in a variety of contexts, such as when attempting to say *bat*

while holding a pen in one's mouth. To reiterate, a gestural score is a statement of *what* must happen but not necessarily *how* it must happen.

According to Goldstein and Fowler (2003), a gestural score like the one shown in Figure 2–8 is specified further through actions of the peripheral articulatory system. Modifications of this sort are necessary to account for unanticipated or atypical articulatory conditions. These *task dynamic* parameters specify, among other things, context-specific movement properties such as *muscle stiffness*, which affects movement duration and velocity, and *damping*, which affects articulator behavior at the time an articulator nears a place of articulation. Although the exact mechanisms that control peripheral articulatory adjustments currently are being debated, the notion that speakers utilize a multilevel, spatiotemporal plan as a platform for articulation has gained growing acceptance among speech scientists.

Neural Correlates of Word Formulation

During the past century, researchers have shown great interest in localizing the processes of speech production to specific neuroanatomical regions of the central nervous system. Advancements in neuroimaging technology and the use of increasingly refined experimental tasks have aided these efforts greatly. Indefrey and Levelt (2004) conducted a meta-analysis of 82 studies in which researchers used neuroimaging technology to identify the neural regions associated with specific speech production processes. Through the meta-analysis, they isolated a number of regions that are reliably active during speech production. These areas include portions of the frontal lobe, the temporal lobe, the thalamus, and the cerebellum. In a follow-up to this research, Indefrey (2007) reached several tentative conclusions regarding the neural correlates of various word production stages (Table 2–2). As shown, the seemingly

Table 2–2. Brain Regions Associated with Stages of Speech Production (Based on Indefrey, 2007)

Component	Activated Region(s)	
	General	**Specific**
Conceptual planning above the sentence level	Frontal lobe	Left middle frontal gyrus, left angular gyrus; anterior region of left medial frontal gyrus; precuneus
Syntactic encoding during sentence production	Frontal lobe	Posterior region of the left inferior frontal gyrus (Brodmann's areas 44, 45)
Lemma selection	Temporal lobe	Mid-region of the left middle temporal gyrus
Word form retrieval (morpho-phonological code)	Temporal lobe	Posterior region of the left temporal lobe (middle and superior temporal gyri)
Phonological encoding/ syllabification	Frontal lobe	Posterior region of left inferior frontal gyrus (Broca's area [Brodmann's area 44] and the adjacent [posterior] cortex [Brodmann's area 6])
Phonetic encoding and articulation	Frontal lobe, Thalamus, Cerebellum	Left precentral gyrus; left thalamus; cerebellum (supplementary motor area?; left anterior insula?)
Internal self-monitoring	Temporal lobe	Mid-region of the right superior temporal gyrus; mid- to anterior regions of left superior temporal gyrus
External self-monitoring	Temporal lobe	Left and right superior temporal gyri

simple act of word production involves widespread neural activation.

Indefrey and Levelt (2004) also analyzed reaction time data from numerous picture-naming studies to map the time course for the various stages of word production (Table 2–3). As shown, word encoding involves four main stages: conceptual preparation, lemma retrieval, word form encoding, and phonetic encoding. Indefrey and Levelt estimated that the time spent in syllabification varies according to the number of phonemes within a word, with speakers appearing to take about 25 ms per phoneme. Thus, the value shown in Table 2–3 (125 ms) would correspond to a word that contains 5 phonemes. The time spent in phonetic encoding would vary depending on whether the motor plans for syllables had to be created on the fly (as seems to be the case for infrequently used syllables) or retrieved from a mental syllabary (as seems to be the case for frequently used syllables). Presumably, one would see deviations in the time course of these stages if a speaker exhibited impairment in one or more aspects of word form encoding.

Formulation and Fluency

The multistage nature of word formulation presents many possible mechanisms for breakdown in speech fluency. Levelt (2001) notes that one key "fault line" in the process occurs at the boundary between a selected lexical item and selection of its corresponding phonological code. When speakers encounter difficulty at this point in the word production process, it results in the familiar "tip of the tongue" state: The speaker has selected the meaning and syntactic form of what he or she wishes to convey but is unable to match that information with its associated sound form.

Other components of the production process are potentially vulnerable to impairment. In their neuropsycholinguistic theory of stuttering, Perkins, Kent, and Curlee (1991) hypothesized that stuttered speech is symptomatic of impairment in the phonological encoding system. In their theory, stuttered speech can arise when a speaker is unable to integrate the phonemic segments that comprise a target word or phrase with their corresponding temporal (prosodic) frame. They pro-

Table 2–3. Estimated Time Windows for Successive Operations in Spoken Word Encoding

Operation	Duration (ms)
Conceptual preparation (from picture onset to selecting the target concept)	175
Lemma retrieval	75
Form encoding:	
Phonological code retrieval	80
Syllabification	125
Phonetic encoding (till initiation of articulation)	145
Total	600

Source: Reprinted from *Cognition, 92,* P. Indefrey & W. J. M. Levelt, The Spatial and Temporal Signatures of Word Production Components, pp. 101–144. Copyright (2004), with permission from Elsevier.

posed that the integration problem arises from impairment in either the ability to construct the temporal frames or the ability to execute the segmental spellout. The mismatch in the availability of information (i.e., either the phonemes are selected, but the timing frame is not yet constructed or vice versa) leads to fluency disruption of the sort seen in stuttered speech.

Wingate (1988), in contrast, hypothesized that stuttered speech is symptomatic of impairment in syllable planning. He proposed that speakers who stutter have difficulty in retrieving the syllable rime. When the speaker retrieves a syllable onset but lags in the retrieval of the syllable rime, part-word repetitions (e.g., *b- b-back*) and sound prolongations (e.g., *wwwwe*) result. People who stutter tend to produce these types of fluency interruptions more often than they produce other types of fluency interruptions. We will return to these and other theories of disfluent speech in subsequent chapters.

Articulation

Creation of the phonetic plan leads to motor planning and the act of speech articulation. Articulation entails the physical movement of numerous speech-related structures. The function of these movements is to create an acoustic representation of the speaker's intention. In some respects, speech articulation is a well-understood process. For example, researchers have identified the various muscles, cartilages, and peripheral nerves associated with speech articulation, as well as their respective actions and functions in speech production. They have described the biomechanical characteristics of the speech breathing and phona-

tion systems in depth, as well. There are, however, aspects of speech articulation that researchers understand only partially. Most of the murkier aspects of articulation fall under the domain of *speech motor control*. There are two topics of long-standing debate in this area:

- *The nature of speech motor plans*: How much detail does a speech motor plan contain? What type of information does it contain? How are speech motor plans organized, stored, and executed?
- *The nature of articulatory targets*: Which type of target is the speaker aiming for when articulating? Is the speaker aiming toward an acoustic target or a sensory target?

Several key concepts that pertain to articulation and the nature of speech motor control are discussed in the remainder of this section.

Articulatory Subsystems

In academic texts, the speech articulation system is commonly divided into three main parts: the *respiratory* system, the *laryngeal* system, and the *supralaryngeal* system. The basis for these divisions is both anatomical and functional. The supralaryngeal system, in turn, can be divided into the *pharyngeal, lingual, velar, mandibular*, and *labial* subsystems (Behrman, 2007; Borden & Harris, 1984; Gracco, 1990). See Figure 2–9 for an illustration of each subsystem and brief descriptions of their functions in speech production.

Kent (2004) reviewed the biomechanical and histological properties of

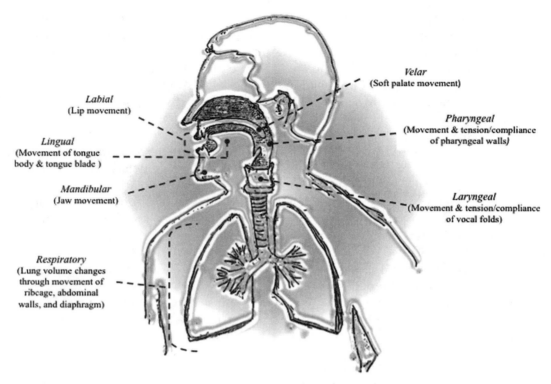

Figure 2–9. Subsystems of speech articulation. The *respiratory system* powers speech by pushing air through the vocal tract. It includes the lungs, ribs, trachea, and muscles of the chest wall and abdominal wall. During speech, the *laryngeal* system regulates expiratory airflow and generates phonation. It includes the larynx and various extrinsic muscles that anchor the larynx in the neck. Superior to the larynx is the pharyngeal subsystem, which plays a role in the resonance and articulation of speech. The remaining subsystems (the lingual, velar, mandibular, and labial) are associated with articulation. Their movement alters the dimensions of the vocal tract, which is critical for the production of speech sounds.

the craniofacial and laryngeal muscles and concluded that the speech motor system differs in several ways from other motor systems. He noted that speech production is characterized by fast, precise, and often long-lasting movements, and that the muscles of the speech production system are specialized to produce such movements. The muscles of the larynx, for example, are capable of contracting for long periods of time, meaning that they resist fatigue, and they shorten at twice the speed of limb muscles, a property that facilitates airway protection and the ability to articulate rapidly.

Kent (2004) also noted the remarkable diversity of muscle types within the speech production system. There are muscles that control joint movement; muscles that control sphincter actions at the lips, pharynx, and velopharynx; muscles such as those within the larynx that are capable of vibratory and valving actions; and muscles that inflate and deflate the lungs. There also is the tongue, an organ that is capable of *hydrostatic* (i.e., fluid-like) movement. He also noted the degree to which speech production muscles are *polymorphic* (i.e., composed of multiple types of muscle fiber). The heterogeneous fiber compositions of muscles associated with mandibular movement, for example, allow for a range of contraction speeds instead of only a basic "all or nothing" response.

The various subsystems of the speech production mechanism are reviewed briefly in the remainder of this section. Readers who need a more thorough discussion of this topic should consult contemporary sources on speech and voice science (e.g., Behrman, 2007; Hixon et al., 2008; Sapienza & Ruddy, 2009).

Respiratory System and Speech Breathing

The respiratory system creates the air movement that is necessary for the production of speech sounds. Without substantial air movement, speech sound production is not possible. Speech breathing consists of cycles: a cycle equals one inhalation plus one exhalation. During speech breathing, the inspiratory phase occupies about 10% of the total time in a cycle, and the expiratory phase occupies the remaining 90% of the time (Kent & Read, 1992). This pattern of brief inhalations and extended exhalations allows a speaker to produce relatively many syllables on one breath, and it is markedly different from that observed during quiet breathing, wherein the inspiratory and expiratory phases are more similar; that is, roughly 40% inspiration and 60% expiration (Kent & Read, 1992).

Inspiration is accomplished by increasing the volume of the thoracic cavity and, with it, the lungs. Expansion of the thoracic cavity is accomplished by

expanding the chest wall upward and outward and by lowering the floor of the thorax through contraction of the diaphragm, the large muscle that comprises the floor of the chest cavity. These actions create an increase in lung volume, which in turn drops air pressure within the lungs below atmospheric pressure. Air molecules then flow into the lungs until the pressure imbalance equalizes.

During quiet breathing, exhalation essentially is a passive process. The speaker relaxes the inspiratory muscles, after which gravity and the elastic properties of the chest wall structures result in a return of the chest cavity dimensions to resting level. Muscles activation patterns during the expiratory phase of speech breathing are different, however. One main difference is that muscles that are ordinarily active during the inspiration phase of both quiet and speech breathing now are active during portions of expiration phase, as well. The activation of these muscles during expiration counteracts the natural tendency of the chest wall to recoil to its resting state rapidly. As such, expiration of air occurs much more gradually than it ordinarily would. The diaphragm—which typically is inactive during the expiration phase of quiet breathing—is active during the initial stages of speech exhalation, as well, for the same reason.

During the mid-to-late phases of a spoken utterance, the muscles that expand the chest wall deactivate and other muscles of the rib cage wall begin to contract. Actions of the latter muscles actively compress the thoracic cavity. In this way, the exhalation phase continues well beyond the point at which it normally would cease in quiet breathing. This enables a speaker to increase the number of syllables spoken per exhalation. Muscles of the abdominal wall are active throughout the course of an extended utterance, as well. Activation of these muscles appears to make speech exhalation more precisely controlled than it otherwise would be (Hixon et al., 2008).

The Laryngeal System

During speech production, the *larynx* acts as a valve to regulate the rate at which air flows through the vocal tract. In addition, the larynx functions as the source of *phonation* during speech production. Phonation is a physiological process whereby the energy of moving air is transformed into acoustic energy (Nicolosi, Harryman, & Kresheck, 1989). The larynx consists of a cartilaginous frame and several paired *intrinsic muscles*. The primary cartilages of the larynx include the *thyroid*, the *cricoid*, and the (two) *arytenoids*. In addition to providing structural integrity to this segment of the airway, the cartilages serve as origin and insertion points for the intrinsic laryngeal muscles involved in phonation.

The valving action of the larynx is accomplished primarily through movement of the right and left *thyroarytenoid* muscles (Sapienza & Ruddy, 2009). The vocal folds can be positioned via contraction of several other intrinsic laryngeal muscles along a continuum ranging from fully *abducted* (both vocal folds are maximally spread from the airway midline) to fully *adducted* (the right and left vocal folds make contact at the airway midline). When the vocal folds are properly approximated and tensed, and exhaled air pushes against them with sufficient force and in a sustained manner, they begin to vibrate in a quasi-periodic manner. Vocal fold vibration essentially chops the exhaled airstream into a series of brief sound bursts that subsequently are resonated in the vocal tract and perceived as voice. When a speaker adducts the vocal folds tightly, the force of the eggressive airstream may be insufficient to initiate or sustain vocal fold vibration. At such times, phonation ceases. The issue of tightly adducted vocal folds arises in some speakers who stutter and is associated with breaks in speech fluency.

The Pharyngeal System

The pharynx is a tube-like portion of the vocal tract with three identifiable regions: the larynopharynx, the oropharynx, and the nasopharynx. During speech production, the pharynx primarily acts as a resonating chamber; however, portions of it, particularly the oropharynx, are involved in the articulation of some speech sounds (Hixon et al., 2008).

A speaker can alter the dimensions and cross-sectional configurations of the pharynx (i.e., its *lumen*) through contraction of the primary pharyngeal muscles and can move the pharynx itself in different directions through the contraction of other muscles in the neck region. The actions of the *tongue, velum, sternothyroid* muscle, and the *mandible* can affect the dimensions of the pharynx, as well.

The Lingual System

The main structure in the *lingual system* is the tongue, which is comprised of four intrinsic muscles and four extrinsic muscles. The tongue also contains fibrous, elastic connective tissue, which forms an encapsulating framework that defines tongue shape and augments the effects of muscle contraction during speech (Hixon et al., 2008). The intrinsic tongue muscles alter the shape of the tongue and thus are integral to the production of many consonants. The extrinsic tongue muscles primarily affect tongue body positioning and thus are particularly relevant to vowel production (Hixon et al., 2008). The intrinsic and extrinsic tongue muscles function in a complementary manner during speech production. In this view, speech essentially is a stream of vowels (which result primarily from extrinsic tongue muscle movement) on which consonants (which result primarily from intrinsic tongue muscle movement) are superimposed (Levelt, 1989).

The Labial System

The labial system consists of 14 muscles. The *orbicularis oris* muscle lies within the lips and thus rings the mouth opening. It includes both intrinsic and extrinsic components. The remaining 13 muscles insert in or near the lips. The contractions of these muscles allow for a multitude of configurations in lip positioning and mouth opening.

The Mandibular System

The *mandible* (i.e., lower jaw) is capable of an array of directional movements (Hixon et al., 2008). Examples include the following: lowering, elevation, side-to-side movement, and forward-to-backward movement. During speech, movement of the mandible affects the degree of mouth opening and, consequently, tongue height in relation to the palate. Movements of this sort are integral to the production of vowels and consonants.

The Velar System

The velum is the primary structure in the velar system. It constitutes the "soft" region of the palate and, at rest, resembles a curtain that arcs across the posterior of the oral cavity (Hixon et al., 2008). The uvula, a pendulum-like structure, extends from the velum. During the articulation of most speech sounds, the vocal tract is configured in a tube-like manner, extending from the superior face of the vocal folds through the pharynx into the oral cavity. For some speech sounds such as /m/, /n/, and /ŋ/, however, the oral cavity is coupled with the nasal cavity at the velopharyngeal port. When this happens, the nasal cavity serves as an additional chamber for resonance.

The palatal muscles function more like facial muscles than like limb muscles in that some muscles in the system (e.g., palatopharyngeus, uvulus) are capable of rapid movements, and others (e.g., palatal levator, palatal tensor muscles) are specialized for slow, continuous contractions (Kent, 2004). Hixon et al. (2008) noted that there is considerable variability, both within and across speakers, in the attainment of velopharyngeal closure. Multiple gestural configurations are possible and can involve either movements of a single structure (i.e., elevation of the velum alone, inward movement of the lateral pharyngeal walls alone), combinations of those movements, or combinations of those movements in conjunction with forward (anterior) movement of the posterior pharyngeal wall. In other words, there are many ways to attain velopharyngeal closure.

The Nature of Speech Motor Control

In this section, several basic characteristics of the speech motor system are reviewed. Fluent speech depends on efficient, well-timed, and error-free functioning in this arena.

Staged Production

Similar to the process of word preparation, speech articulation unfolds in stages
or phases. Levelt (1989) outlined the following four-phase progression. Evidence
for this progression comes from various
chronometric experiments.

- *Planning phase*, wherein phonetic
  (motor) plans are constructed. As
  noted previously, these plans seem
  to specify only general aspects of
  a movement sequence such as
  where and when vocal constrictions
  must occur. A plan can be as long
  as a phonological phrase and as
  short as a single stressed syllable
  (i.e., a foot).
- *Motor plan retrieval phase*, wherein
  the speaker retrieves motor plans
  from memory. During sentence
  production, motor planning
  overlaps with motor execution.
  That is, while people are speaking,
  they are simultaneously planning
  what they will say next. This
  means that motor plans must be
  buffered in memory so that they
  will be ready for retrieval when
  the speaker completes whatever
  is being said now. Because motor
  plans are relatively short—they
  typically span only a few syllables
  —a speaker might need to retrieve
  several plans during the course of
  saying a long sentence.
- *Unpacking phase*, wherein the
  selected motor plans are "opened"
  and "read." In this phase, the
  speaker, in a sense, scans the
  contents of the plan to access
  the specific utterance-specific
  instructions for movement.

- *Execution phase*, wherein neural
  commands travel to the appropriate
  muscles or muscle groups to
  yield articulatory movement. The
  execution phase is not the "end
  of the story" when it comes to
  motor control, however, as speech
  movements undergo further
  updating through a peripheral
  feedback system (Behrman, 2007;
  Guenther, 2006; Kröger, Birkholz,
  Lowit, & Neuschaefer-Rube, 2010).
  The latter process enables the
  speaker to address unexpected
  or unusual circumstances in the
  vocal tract that may force the
  speaker to pursue unique gestural
  configurations in order to attain
  the articulatory goals for the
  utterance.

Synergistic Movements

Earlier in this chapter, we alluded to the
many muscles that are involved in speech
production. It is natural to think that each
of the muscles operates autonomously
during speech production. If this were
the case, the speech plans that one would
need to construct would become quite
complex. In fact, the plans would likely
be so complex that the planning time and
storage space needed to manage them
would be incompatible with the notion
of fluent speech (Levelt, 1989). The need
for a speaker to direct the many muscles
within the speech production system creates a scenario that authors have termed
the "degrees of freedom" problem (Behrman, 2007). The crux of the problem is
this: What kind of system is able to attain
coordinative control over so many muscles, many of which have the potential to
contract in many different ways?

Findings from studies of speech motor control have shed light on the degrees of freedom problem. It appears that speech muscles do not adhere to an "every muscle for itself" organizational pattern. Rather, the movements of functionally related muscles are inextricably linked to one another. This organizational property is termed *synergism*. The concept of synergy refers to the cooperative or collaborative actions of muscles for the achievement of a particular outcome such as the production of a speech sound or a syllable (Behrman, 2007). Put another way, speech muscles seem to operate as a functional unit—a single, coordinative structure in which *vocal tract configuration* is the basic functional unit of speech articulation (Ackermann & Riecker, 2010; Fowler, 2007; Gracco, 1990). Therefore, rather than having to control a plethora of structures, the speaker needs to control only one primary structure—the vocal tract (Behrman, 2007; Fowler, 2007; Gracco, 1990).[5]

In the synergistic view, the adjustment of one articulator leads to adjustments in all of the other articulators that are functionally associated with it. For example, the speech-related movements of the upper lip, lower lip, and jaw have been shown to be functionally intertwined during the production of bilabial sounds, as are the movements of the lower lip and the larynx during production of [f] (see Gracco, 1990; Levelt, 1989; Fowler, 2007). More generally, the movements of the orofacial system have been shown to be tightly coupled with those of the laryngeal and respiratory systems (McClean & Tasko, 2002), and the production of stressed syllables leads to adjustments in *all* portions of the vocal tract—not only in one or two articulators (Gracco, 1990).

The synergistic nature of muscle movement within the speech production system has led to the view that sound and syllable production is a matter of learning an assortment of *vocal tract configurations* that are specific to the phoneme and syllable shape inventories of a language. For instance, Goldstein and Fowler (2003) argue that "phonological knowledge" reflects a speaker's ability to learn specific vocal tract configurations and the ways in which one vocal tract configuration relates to another. This view contrasts with the traditional linguistic notion of phonological knowledge as consisting of bundles of abstract distinctive features.

Data from studies of motor movements suggest that muscle synergisms are task specific. Thus, the synergisms that underlie speech sound production differ from those that underlie chewing and swallowing—even though the tasks incorporate the same muscles (Bunton, 2008; Wilson, Green, Yunusova, & Moore, 2008). For this reason, one would expect nonspeech oral motor exercises to have little facilitative effect on a person's ability to produce speech-based gestures. Indeed, this seems to be the case. For example, research with children who exhibit delayed speech sound development shows that treatments based on speech-based movement patterns lead to significantly better speech production outcomes than treatments that are based on nonspeech oral motor exercises (Forrest & Iuzzini, 2008).

---

[5]An alternate view is that the speaker needs to control only a few subregions, each of which features synergistic patterning of its constituent muscles (Gracco, 1990).

Motor Equivalence

A second general characteristic of the speech motor system is *motor equivalence,* which is the ability to accomplish a particular articulatory objective via more than one movement pattern. Consider, for example, articulation of /p/. In the word *peace*, a speaker typically produces the sound by approximating the upper and lower lips in a symmetrical, spread manner. In the word *push,* however, it is produced with a rounded or pursed lip posture. The articulatory movements for the two tokens of the sound differ due to the effects of phonetic context: one features spread lips and the other features pursed lips. Nonetheless, the two gestural postures have an equivalent result: production of a bilabial plosive that listeners recognize as /p/.

The notion of motor planning has relevance to the concept of motor equivalence. As noted at the start of this section, in older models of speech production, phonetic plans were assumed to be highly specific (for a review, see Borden & Harris, 1984). Over time, this view became less attractive because of the sheer number of plans one would need to compile in order to cover all possible phonetic permutations and because of the motor system's well-demonstrated ability to adapt immediately to unexpected or novel intrusions (i.e., *perturbations*).

Returning to the production of /p/, imagine a speaker who attempts to say *peace* and *push* while holding a carrot between the left molars. In this scenario, the mandible deviates markedly toward the left during production of the sound. The lips swing in that direction too. Although the semipursed articulatory posture in the carrot-holding context is awkward to make, speakers are able to plan the posture instantly and without instruction. Furthermore, the new, awkward posture allows for lip closure around the carrot and, hence, the ability to say the target sound. Thus, phonetic plans seem to include information about where vocal tract constrictions must occur (in this case, at the lips) and the articulatory subsystem(s) involved in creating the constriction (in this case, the lips and mandible). However, the phonetic plans apparently do not specify exactly how each of the muscles within the subsystem(s) must contract to accomplish the articulatory goal. Instead, the speech motor control system is able to utilize sensory feedback to determine the current state of the articulators and then compute a context-specific plan that leads to attainment of the general phonetic goal.

The Nature of Articulatory Targets

People construct plans in order to reach goals. Researchers who study speech production and speech motor control have long debated the nature of the articulatory targets or goals that a person aims for when speaking. The two most commonly mentioned possibilities are acoustic/auditory targets and sensorimotor targets. The essential question is this: When a speaker is articulating, is he or she aiming for a certain sound or a certain feel?

Some authorities have proposed an auditory frame of reference for articulation (e.g., Kent, 1984; Stevens, 1972). They have argued that the speaker aims for a certain acoustic result. In this view, the acoustic target includes the spectral characteristics that a listener would need to have in order to perceive a particular phoneme or syllable. Because phonemic boundaries are not strictly limited, a speaker would aim for an "acoustic space" rather than a narrowly specified acoustic goal. On the somatosensory side, several models have been proposed.

- One view is that a speaker aims for *proprioceptive* targets. That is, speakers use the alpha-gamma loop to monitor muscle spindle activity, and contraction ceases when a target length within a muscle spindle is realized (Behrman, 2007; Levelt, 1989).
- An alternative view comes from the so-called "mass-spring theory" (e.g., Fowler & Turvey, 1980). The idea here is that a speaker monitors the lengths of agonist and antagonist muscles through the muscle spindle system. Muscles move toward a target length, which is realized when agonist and antagonist reach a resting position and are at equilibrium.
- Other forms of orosensory feedback have been hypothesized as components of the speaker's target. These include tactile feedback from mechoreceptors as well as feedback from pressure sensors in the oral cavity and pharynx (Behrman, 2007; Levelt, 1989).

As we discuss later, contemporary models of speech motor control hypothesized that speakers pursue multiple frames of reference when executing an utterance.

The Role of Feedback in Motor Control

After a speaker constructs a phonetic plan, he or she enacts it through the articulatory system. Enactment of the plan leads to *context-dependent* modifications to the general phonetic plan. As noted above, such modifications are based on data from the auditory, somatosensory, and motor systems and the use of *feedforward* and *feedback* pathways (Guenther, 2006). The feedforward component entails the enactment of a motor plan (i.e., gestural score) that corresponds to a phonetic goal. The feedback component entails an evaluation of whether motor plan enactment results in attainment of the phonetic goal. When novel or unexpected articulatory conditions are encountered (such as the carrot-in-the-mouth scenario described in the previous section), a speaker also uses sensory data to create compensatory movements that adjust the motor plan.

Models of Speech Motor Control

Many speech motor production and control models have been proposed throughout the years. In this section, we discuss several of them. The first models we review are grouped under the heading of "Early Models." The review of such models is by no means exhaustive. The main goal is to offer a sense of the kinds of approaches that researchers have proposed. Later in this section, we review two contemporary models: the DIVA model and the ACT model. The latter models incorporate some key concepts from early models and add other novel concepts. As such, they demonstrate how explanations of speech motor control have evolved over time.

Early Models

Borden and Harris (1984) reviewed several of the models that were under consideration in the early 1980s. In this section, we summarize their descriptions of models from that era.

- The *multiple conversion model:* Liberman and colleagues (Liberman, Cooper, Shankweiler, & Studdert-Kennedy, 1967) proposed that speakers do not directly convert phoneme representations into speech gestures; rather, their phoneme representations are modified progressively through the influence of surrounding phonemes and the neuromotor, myomotor, and articulatory rules that control speech production. They proposed that, through this process, a static phonemic representation blends or "smears" with those of surrounding phonemes to yield articulatory overlap between sounds in connected speech.
- *Target-based models:* During the late 1960s to early 1970s, several authors emphasized the notion of speech-related *targets* within speech production models. A target essentially is a reference point that the speaker aims to match or approximate. Borden and Harris (1984) summarized the various forms that a target could assume. Possible forms included the following: auditory/ acoustic, proprioceptive, tactile, or multidimensional representations such as spatial and auditory. Some of these forms continue to be mentioned in contemporary models of speech production.

The DIVA Model

More recently, Guenther and colleagues (Bohland, Bullock, & Guenther, 2009; Ghosh, Tourville, & Guenther, 2008; Guenther, 2003, 2006) described a computer-based model of the speech articulation system. The model, named *Directions into Velocities of Articulators* (DIVA), seeks to capture the mechanisms associated with both the production of learned speech sounds and the process of speech sound development.[6]

The DIVA model includes two main subsystems: *feedforward control* and *feedback control*. In the model, speech production begins with the activation of "cells" within a *speech sound map*, which corresponds to the left frontal operculum (Broca's area) in the human brain. The speech sound map links with the model's "motor cortex" by feedforward and feedback connections. The feedforward commands are of the sort found in a gestural score (see Browman & Goldstein, 1990). When the model operates in the feedforward mode, motor commands from the speech sound map are projected to the motor cortex both directly and indirectly. The indirect projections are routed through the cerebellum, which plays a role in integrating information about the current state of the vocal tract state and, in doing so, facilitates the timing of feedforward commands.

According to Guenther (2006), people develop gestural scores over time through a "tuning" procedure that begins during babbling and utilizes auditory and somatosensory feedback. Following repeated experiences with sound produc-

---

[6]Within the context of the DIVA model, a speech sound is defined as a sound, syllable, or a word, as each can be mapped with a single motor plan.

tion, auditory targets for specific speech gestures such as sounds and syllables emerge. Connections between the motor and auditory regions of the model make it possible for cells in the speech sound map to activate when a person perceives sounds and when a person produces sounds. It also means that the representation in the speech sound map includes information about the auditory target region for the sound.

In the DIVA model, the auditory targets for speech sounds are conceived as *regions* rather than as narrowly specified acoustic events. In this way, an auditory target can accommodate the subtle variations in speech sound realization that arise through coarticulation, rate variation, prosodic effects, and so forth, as well as variations that arise externally through the introduction of physical perturbations to the speech articulatory system. In the DIVA model, an infant who is learning to talk relies on auditory feedback extensively during sound production and, over time, the auditory feedback leads to refinement of motor representations. In the model, somatosensory targets, which consist of the tactile and proprioceptive sensations associated with a sound's production, emerge through experience with sound production, as well. Eventually, the representations that emerge within a speech sound map are specified well enough to allow a speaker to say speech sounds accurately without having to rely on auditory feedback. At this point, the speaker is using what are termed *feedforward commands*. When a speaker operates in this mode, speech articulation unfolds in a largely automatized manner.

When a speech sound is produced, information about the expected auditory feedback is sent to the auditory cortex and is stored in an auditory error map. The representation in the auditory error map is compared against the speaker's actual outcome, which is represented in the auditory state map. If the two representations differ, cells in the auditory error map activate and corrective motor commands are relayed back to the motor cortex. Similarly, during speech sound production, information about the actual somatosensory state associated with a sound, which is represented in the somatosensory state map, is compared with the expected outcome, which is represented in the somatosensory error map. If the two representations differ, cells in the auditory error map activate and corrective commands are relayed to the motor cortex to alter the velocity and/or positioning of speech movements.

The ACT Model

Kröger et al. (2010) described an action-based neurocomputational (ACT) model of speech articulation. Like the DIVA model, the ACT model is a computer-based simulation of the speech production process. The ACT model differs from the DIVA model in several ways. For example, it places a greater emphasis on the roles of sensorimotor feedback and articulatory gestures during speech. Hence, those parts of the model are a bit more elaborate than they are in the DIVA model, as evidenced by the many representational "maps" that are included in the ACT model. In addition, the ACT model features separate mechanisms for processing frequently used and infrequently used articulatory gestures. One main difference is that plans for frequently used articulatory gestures are stored in memory, and thus are "ready-made." In contrast, plans for infrequently used articulatory gestures are constructed on an "as needed" basis. In this way, the ACT model attempts to simulate the details of the normal syllable planning process (Kröger et al., 2010). Like the DIVA model, the ACT model incorporates the notion of feedforward and feedback components. It also posits the existence of "maps" that contain representations of the distinct sensory and motor "pieces" that comprise a particular articulatory gesture. The maps correspond to unique neural processing centers in the human nervous system.

The primary representational maps within the DIVA and ACT models are summarized in Table 2–4. As shown, both models propose that speech articulation requires the representation and integration of multiple forms of information. A complete discussion of these models is beyond

Table 2–4. A Comparison of Processing Maps in the DIVA Model (Guenther, 2006; Guenther, Ghosh, & Tourville, 2006) and the ACT Model of Speech Articulation (Kröger, Birkholz, Lowit, & Neuschaefer-Rube, 2010)

DIVA Model		ACT Model	
Map	**Characteristics**	**Map**	**Characteristics**
Speech sound map	Phoneme, syllable, and word representations akin to gestural scores	Phonemic map	Representations of phonemes and frequent syllables
Articulatory velocity and position map	Analogous to primary motor cortex; receives input from speech sound map and auditory and proprioceptive regions	Phonetic map	Representation of the sensory states associated with phonemes and syllables
Auditory state map	Expected or allowable auditory "regions" for target speech sounds	Motor plan map	Invariant vocal tract actions associated with particular syllables
Auditory error map	Compares expected and actual auditory features of speech sound; generates corrective motor feedback, if needed	Primary motor map	Three-dimensional model of the vocal tract
Somatosensory state map	Expected tactile and proprioceptive sensations for a speech sound (i.e., phoneme, syllable, word)	Articulatory state map	Specifies the location of one articulator relative to another at a particular point in time
Somatosensory error map	Compares expected and actual somatosensory features of sound; generates corrective motor feedback, if needed	Somatosensory map	Representations of proprioceptive and tactile states during the course of a movement.
		Auditory state map	Representations of speech sound formant structures

the scope of this chapter, but the information presented in Table 2–4 gives some sense of the type of neural processing that is thought to be required to meet even very basic articulatory goals such as sound and syllable production. Neuro-computational models such as the ACT and the DIVA are useful in that they point toward potential ways in which the speech articulation process can break down. Possible points of impairment include the ability to create stored representations, the ability to access stored representations, and the ability to integrate one type of representation with another. Problems such as these presumably can lead to errors in accuracy or precision of articulatory movements and perhaps to difficulties in speech fluency, as well. Computer-based models of the speech production process offer a potentially useful tool for systematically testing the effects of various types of impairment on speech output.

Neural Correlates of Speech Motor Control

Earlier in this chapter, we identified several key cortical structures involved with neurolinguistic processing. In this section, we focus on the neuroanatomical correlates of events in the late stages of speech production, particularly those that involve phonetic processing.

Guenther (2006) attempted to validate several aspects of the DIVA model by comparing the model's structure and performance to neuroimaging data that were collected from adults during specially designed speech production tasks. Through this research, he found links between the various processing modules of the DIVA model and actual neuroanatomical structures. For instance:

- The DIVA's *speech sound map* corresponds to the left frontal operculum;
- The DIVA's *articulatory velocity* and *position maps* correspond to the motor cortex;
- The DIVA's *auditory error map* and *auditory state map* correspond to the superior temporal cortex;
- The DIVA's *somatosensory error map* and *somatosensory state map* correspond to the inferior parietal cortex.

Analysis of neuroimaging data has led to other insights about the relationships between speech production processing and neural processing regions. For example, Indefrey and Levelt (2004) conducted a meta-analysis of dozens of neuroimaging studies in which researchers had studied aspects of phonological encoding, phonetic encoding, and speech articulation. The meta-analysis revealed the following findings:

- An association between the intra-sylvian cortex and phonological code retrieval;
- An association between Broca's area and phonological word development (in particular, the syllabification of phonological words); and
- An association between speech motor control and the cortical region that is bound by the pre- and post-central sulci, including the Sylvian fissure.

Other authors have sought to identify the specific neural regions that are associated with motor planning and motor execution. In this regard, Riecker et al. (2005) examined neural activation patterns in adult speakers during a syllable repetition. Results of their analysis suggested the existence of two motor-related loops that are integral to speech production.

- *A premotor loop.* The first loop consists of the supplemental motor area (SMA), the inferior frontal gyrus, the anterior insula, and the superior cerebellum. In their research, activation occurred earlier in these structures than it did in other neural regions that were active at some point during the task. On this basis, Riecker et al. (2005) concluded that these structures are involved with premotor tasks such as movement preparation and movement initiation.

- *A motor execution loop.* In Riecker et al.'s research, a second cluster of neural regions was active only during later stages of the task. This cluster included the following areas: the sensorimotor cortex, the thalamus, the basal ganglia, and the inferior cerebellum. On this basis, Riecker et al. concluded that these areas are involved with motor execution. Involvement of the basal ganglia in motor execution is not surprising, as other researchers have noted its role in the timing of sequenced articulatory movements, in the development of newly learned movement sequences, and in the disruption in the continuity of articulatory movements (Smits-Bandstra & De Nil, 2007). It is well known that fluctuations in levels of the neurotransmitter dopamine affect cell functioning within the basal ganglia. Such fluctuations have been linked to a loss in the specificity of movement direction and to slowness in the initiation of sequenced movements (Smits-

Bandstra & De Nil, 2007). Thus, speech motor control seems to unfold in stages and specific neural processing regions regulate or control specific aspects of the overall task.

Speech Motor Production and Fluency

The production of speech movements seems to be a multifaceted process. In the current view, the plans that drive speech articulation are not highly detailed. Instead, they seem to include only the most basic targets that the speaker must realize in order to accomplish a functional goal like saying a sound or a syllable. Data from speech error research support the idea that articulatory plans can be as long as a phonological phrase, which is a prosodic unit that consists of a lexical word plus any of its associated function words. It is thought that the finer details of a movement are not specified until the speaker is in the act of saying an utterance. This allows the speaker to fine-tune the basic motor plan so that it fits the circumstances of the current utterance.

The precise nature of the speaker's articulatory target still is under study. Older models favored explanations that centered on one type of target, for instance, an acoustic goal or a proprioceptive goal. In contemporary models, scientists allow for the possibility that speakers have access to multiple, interconnected production "maps" or neural centers that represent information about the articulatory, acoustic, and somatosensory properties of the target sound. Speakers access information from these maps, as needed, depending on the circumstances present in a particular utterance. The syllable has emerged as a basic unit of speech production. It is thought that speakers store the articulatory plans for a language's most common syllables.

Issues related to the planning and control of motor movements assume a prominent role in contemporary models of fluency disorders. There are several potential ways in which problems in the speech motor arena could result in impaired fluency. Disfluency, for example, could reflect impairment in the ability to construct or store the gestural scores associated with specific syllables or, perhaps, impairment in the ability to compile syllable-level motor programs into sequences that form phonological phrases. It also is conceivable that a speaker might have well-formed gestural scores but is unable to specify those gestural scores when articulating due to faulty integration of sensory feedback from the tactile, proprioceptive, or auditory domains.

Disturbances in rate are likely to have a motoric basis, as rate-related behavior has been associated with the activities of both the basal ganglia and the cerebellum, neural centers that are integral to motor control. Motor-based explanations for stuttering have some intuitive appeal because they fit well with the report from speakers who stutter of "knowing what to say but being unable to say it," and they match with the most common treatment approaches for the disorder. That said, research also has uncovered evidence of deficits in cognitive and language mechanisms among some people with impaired fluency (see Chapter 6). Thus, it may be that speakers who have impaired fluency have deficits across multiple parts of the speech production system. The latter issue is discussed in more depth within the following chapters on fluency disorders (Chapters 5–8).

Summary

To understand fluency impairment, a clinician must have a basic understanding of how people speak. In this chapter, we discussed some basic properties of speech production and outlined several speech production models. In each model, the act of speaking is said to commence with the selection of a specific meaning or concept that the speaker intends to express. The speaker then converts the intention into appropriate linguistic codes and corresponding motor plans that allow for message-specific articulatory movements.

Language formulation is a multilayered process. Using Levelt's (1989) model and its derivatives as a basis, we saw that linguistic formulation entails the assignment of a lemma—a syntactic representation—to a lexical concept. Following lemma selection, the corresponding morphologic and phonologic structures of a word are formulated. During the latter process, the speaker accesses each of the requisite phonemes in the word and assembles them into the proper sequence and, in doing so, creates pronounceable syllables. The syllables are specified further in terms of their metrical properties. This results in the development of a phonetic plan, which functions as a blueprint—similar to a musical score—for the types of vocal tract configurations that the speaker must realize in order to convey the word to other people. The multilayered nature of speech production implies that there are several potential paths to fluency disruption. The common view is that disfluency can arise wherever there is slowness, inaccuracy, or imprecision in message conceptualization or formulation. From this perspective, fluency is an index of the extent to which the entire speech production process is functioning normally.

Much of the early scientific data on speech production came from case studies of people with lesions or neurological diseases that affected speech-language centers of the brain. In recent decades, researchers have markedly advanced the understanding of speech production through systematic laboratory experiments that have provided evidence for the existence of the various components of speech production. The use of computer-based simulations to model speech production processes has become more common and increasingly sophisticated. Computer-based modeling provides researchers with the potential to examine a wide range of speech production questions efficiently, noninvasively, and in considerable depth.

Although understanding of syntactic, morpho-phonologic, and phonetic processing has improved exponentially during the last 50 years, there still is much work left for researchers to do. One of the more vexing problems that researchers have faced involves the modeling of motor planning and control mechanisms. Contemporary models seem to converge on the idea that the vocal tract behaves as a single, functionally related, coordinative structure during speech. How speakers develop these coordinative patterns requires additional research. Current thinking is that infants' prelinguistic vocalizations play a role in "tuning" the functional organization of the vocal tract musculature and, with it, the eventual creation of stored motor plans that correspond to the sounds, syllables, and words in a language.

Data from neuroimaging studies show that even the most basic speech vocalizations involve widespread neural activation at both the cortical and subcortical levels (Ackermann & Riecker, 2010; Guenther, 2006). Incremental changes in articulatory complexity—for example, progressing from the vowel [ɑ] to the CV combination [pɑ]—result in even greater neural activation (Bohland et al., 2009; Ghosh et al., 2008). Given the many components that are involved in speech production, it perhaps is surprising that the prevalence of fluency disorders is as low as it is. For most people, the speech production system operates smoothly, accurately, and efficiently.

As noted, fluency disorders are understood best when they are examined within the context of data on normal speech production. The multistage model of speech production presented in this chapter provides a starting point for explaining problems in fluency. In the context of such a model, there are several plausible routes to speech disfluency. Some possibilities include the following: poorly developed or unstable representations of linguistic or motoric information; slowness or interference during the selection or retrieval of stored representations; breakdown in the ability to integrate one representation with another; and weakness in the ability to evaluate or update the progress of a developing plan or an ongoing motor movement. On this basis, we see that fluency problems are rooted in neurophysiological events. As such, a clinician's approach to conceptualizing fluency problems needs to go much deeper than the intuitive hypotheses (e.g., "he got nervous," "he's thinking about it too much") that sometimes are used to explain fluency disorders.

3

Conceptualizing Disfluency

Clinical descriptions of fluency performance usually are rooted in an analysis of disfluency. Instances of disfluency often are described in terms of what the speaker *does* while being disfluent (Williams, Darley, & Spriestersbach, 1978). On the surface, disfluency description might seem to be a relatively straightforward process. In practice, however, it can be a challenging undertaking. Indeed, clinical authorities have noted several problems and pitfalls with regard to the identification, quantification, and labeling of disfluency (Cordes, 2000; Einarsdóttir & Ingham, 2005; Logan, 2009; Smith & Kelly, 1997). The main goal of this chapter is to help the reader develop a thorough understanding of disfluency: its structure, origins, and variations. Such information is critical if one hopes to measure speech continuity accurately and interpret disfluent speech patterns in a conceptually sound manner.

Defining Disfluency

Disfluency is essentially a place within an utterance where speech production is disrupted due to a problem in either speech planning or execution. Such disruptions are unintended. Consequently, the speech that occurs during disfluent segments of an utterance is superfluous or extraneous to its ideal or intended form (Onslow, Gardner, Bryant, Stuckings, & Knight, 1992). A primary goal in the clinical analysis of disfluency is to separate those portions of a spoken utterance that *are* intended or desired (i.e., the "fluent" parts) from those that *are not* (i.e., the "disfluent" parts). Upon doing so, a clinician then can begin to describe disfluency in terms of its frequency and manner.

The task of identifying points of disfluency within a spoken utterance usually is straightforward. This is because speakers often provide listeners with easy-to-recognize signs that a problem in speech production has occurred. Examples of behaviors that are symptomatic of disfluency include the following:

- An atypically long break in utterance continuity;
- A break in continuity that occurs at an unusual location with the utterance;

- A rhythmic pattern that is unusual or unexpected within the context of the utterance;
- Evidence of excessive physical effort during speech sound production;
- Production of meaningless sounds or vocalizations;
- Phonologically or morphologically malformed words or unintended words that the speaker subsequently corrects; and
- Repeating portions of an utterance for reasons other than emphasis.

The disfluencies that speakers produce often contain more than one of the behaviors listed above. Other behavioral markers of disfluency exist, as well.

Isolating Disfluent Segments

Several disfluent utterances are presented in Table 3–1. In the utterances, vertical lines are used to separate disfluent segments from the productive words that constitute the fluent portions of the utterance. Descriptive detail is presented about each of the disfluencies as well.

The term *core utterance* refers to the portion of a spoken utterance that remains after all disfluent segments are removed. As such, the core constitutes the "fluent

Table 3–1. Examples of Disfluency Within a Transcript of Spoken Utterances

Line	Transcribed Utterance[a]	Target Utterance[b]	Descriptive Detail
1	The- | *1 s silence* | weather is cool.	The weather is cool.	Unusually long and unusually located continuity break.
2	It- |may$_1$| may$_2$ get even cooler.	It may get even cooler.	Break in continuity after *may$_1$* followed by a restart of the word (i.e., *may$_2$*).
3	It |r-| rains most afternoons.	It rains most afternoons.	Break in continuity during production of *rain*, which is followed by a restart of the word.
4	Uncle |Joe's-| Jim's knees hurt.	Uncle Jim's knees hurt.	Unintended word, which subsequently is revised.
5	A storm is- |uh| expected later.	A storm is expected later.	Meaningless vocalization inserted into continuity break.
6	|D|o we have an umbrella?	Do we have an umbrella?	Excessive physical effort on [d] (not coded in transcript).
7	|LLLL|et's buy one now.	Let's buy one now.	Excessive duration of the [l] segment.
8	This one looks |choo| cheap.	This one looks cheap.	Phonological error, which subsequently is revised.

[a]Boundaries of disfluent segments are marked with vertical lines; *s* = second; hyphens indicate a break in utterance continuity that is not part of the planned utterance.

[b]The term *target utterance* corresponds to the intended or core form of the utterance and it shows how the utterance would have sounded without disfluency.

portion" of an utterance. In utterances that contain no disfluent segments (i.e., *fluent utterances*), the core utterance consists of whatever words the speaker has said. In utterances that contain disfluent segments, however, the core utterance is essentially the way in which the utterance would have sounded had the speaker not produced any disfluency (see Table 3–1). One can think of a core utterance as the speaker's linguistic target. Therefore, the terms *core utterance* and *target utterance* will be used interchangeably throughout the text.

In speakers with typical fluency, it is reasonable to assume that the core utterance is equivalent to the speaker's *intended utterance*. With speakers who have impaired fluency, this assumption is more tenuous, however. For example, impaired speakers may report that they sometimes abandon the words they intend to say when they anticipate that they will say those words disfluently. Speakers report that, at such times, they stealthily substitute words that they *can say* for the words they *would like to say*. Consequently, the words that they actually speak fail to fully reflect their intended wording. An example of this follows:

Example 3–1:

(intended utterance) *You did a superb job.*

(spoken utterance) *You did a wonderful job.*

In this case, the speaker substituted the word *wonderful* for the intended word *superb* and said the substituted word without overt signs of disfluency. Thus, to a listener, the spoken utterance sounds "fluent." However, to the speaker, it feels "disfluent" because the act of executing a word substitution effectively interrupted production of the intended utterance. In cases like this, there is no way for the listener to know that word substitution has occurred without asking the speaker about it directly. Thus, although it may be appropriate to equate the concept of a "core utterance" with that of an "intended utterance" for much of what a speaker says, this association may not hold true for everything a speaker says.

The Structure of Disfluency

Speech disfluencies most commonly are classified using descriptive labels. However, the labels that are used in contemporary clinical practice provide only a limited view of what a speaker does during disfluency. Therefore, it is useful to consider the underlying structure of disfluency. Levelt (1983) presented a useful framework for examining the structure of disfluency. He used the framework mainly to analyze disfluencies that resulted from the correction of overt speech errors (e.g., misnamed objects). In this chapter, we have extended Levelt's framework to analyze the structure of other categories of disfluency.

We discuss four concepts, each from Levelt's (1983) framework, with regard to disfluency structure: the *reparandum*, the *moment of interruption,* the *editing phase*, and the *repair phase*.[1] The concepts

---

[1]Levelt (1983) included a fifth component, the *original utterance*, in his structural analysis, which we will not discuss at length in this chapter. The term refers to whatever a speaker has said in an utterance up to the point of an interruption in speech continuity. An example of an original utterance appears in Figure 3—1.

are illustrated briefly in Figure 3–1, and they are explained in greater detail in the remainder of this section.

In Figure 3–1, we see an example from Levelt (1983) of an utterance within which the speaker has made a word choice error (the use of "left" rather than "pink"), which is then corrected. The speaker continues to talk for three syllables beyond the erroneous word (the latter is termed the "reparandum" in Levelt's system). The editing phase follows the error and is characterized by the interjection *uh* and silence (as indicated by the ellipsis). The speaker then repairs the error.

The Reparandum

Levelt (1983) used the term *reparandum* to refer to the portion of an utterance that features the error or problem that the speaker attempts to repair. As such, the reparandum is the trigger for disfluency. Sometimes the reparandum is *overt* (Postma, Kolk, & Povel, 1990). This means that the error that triggers disfluency is spoken aloud such that the speaker and the listener can hear it. As noted, an example of an overt error is shown in Figure 3–1. Overt errors assume a variety of forms, including those that involve word order, word pronunciation, and word stress. If a speaker detects an overt error *and* then elects to correct it, the overt error becomes a reparandum (see Figure 3–1). If the speaker does not detect the overt error or detects it but decides to ignore it, the error simply remains an error.

At other times, the reparandum is *covert* in nature (Postma et al., 1990). Covert errors are, by definition, hidden.

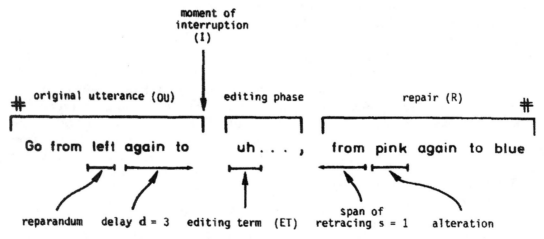

Figure 3–1. The structural components of an instance of disfluency as described by Levelt (1983). In this figure, disfluency is triggered by an error (the *reparandum*) in the execution of an intended utterance (the speaker says "left" instead of "pink"). Utterance articulation is interrupted two words (and three syllables) after the incorrect word (the *delay*). After interrupting speech, the speaker enters the *editing phase*, during which a plan is formulated to correct the reparandum. The speaker interjects "uh" while editing. The repair phase consists of the speaker's attempt to correct the error. During the repair phase, the speaker retraces to the word before the reparandum in the original utterance and then resumes speech to correct the reparandum. From "Monitoring and Self-Repair in Speech" by W. J. M. Levelt, 1983, *Cognition, 41,* pp. 41–104. Reprinted with permission.

Thus, neither the listener nor the speaker hears the covert error in the speech signal. Presumably, covert errors are located within portions of an utterance that the speaker has planned but has not yet spoken. Upon detecting the impending error, the speaker may do one of the following: (1) stop the ongoing utterance and, in doing so, create disfluency; or (2) ignore the detected error and, in doing so, incorporate the error into the utterance. Covert error detection is such that the speaker may sense something is wrong with an upcoming segment of the utterance but be unable to describe what the problem is.

The Moment of Interruption

Levelt (1983) described the *moment of interruption* as the point at which a speaker stops an ongoing utterance due to the detection of an error. The stoppage in speech informs the listener that the speaker has detected an error or problem in speech production. Levelt notes that the point of interruption is not linguistically constrained, which means that a speaker may stop an utterance at any point: in mid-word, after a word (as in Figure 3–1), after a phrase, and so on. The positional relationship between the moment of interruption and the reparandum varies. When the reparandum is based on an overt speech error, the moment of interruption can occur within the reparandum itself; immediately following the reparandum; or at some later point in the utterance (as in Figure 3–1). However, the general rule is that once a speaker has detected an overt speech error, he or she will not talk much beyond the error before interrupting the utterance. Indeed, studies of typical adult speakers show that the average latency

for utterance interruption following overt word choice errors is about 200 ms (i.e., two-tenths of a second; Levelt, 1983). In the example shown in Figure 3–1, the speaker interrupts the utterance three syllables beyond the incorrect syllable.

In the case of covert speech errors, the relationship between the location of the moment of interruption and the reparandum is less clear. As noted, covert errors often are positioned within portions of an utterance that the speaker has planned but has not yet spoken. Thus, with covert errors, the moment of interruption can occur just before the reparandum, within the reparandum, or one or two words in advance. Several examples of covert errors are shown in Examples 3–5 through 3–8 below, in the section on covert repair.

The Editing Phase

Levelt (1983) describes the *editing phase* as the stage of disfluency that follows the moment of interruption. Here, the speaker presumably constructs a plan for resolving the error that triggered the moment of interruption. The editing phase usually is characterized by silence and/or production of one or more *editing terms*. Common editing terms in American English include nonword vocalizations such as *um* or *uh* (see Figure 3–1) or other types of "filler" such as *like* and *well*. Many authors refer to editing terms of this sort as *interjections* (Logan, 2009; Williams et al., 1978). The concept of an editing term is a bit broader than this, however, in that it also includes *personal asides* and *editorial comments*, remarks that are directed as much toward the speaker as they are toward the listener. Examples of the latter are indicated by the italicized words in the Examples 3–2 and 3–3, where the errors are underlined, the editing terms are italicized, and pauses are denoted by ellipses.

> Example 3–2: You need to buy the <u>big</u> . . . *oh no, wait,* the little one.

> Example 3–3: It looks like a <u>back</u> . . . <u>back</u> . . . *that's easy for you to say!* . . . black backpack.

The Repair Phase

In Levelt's (1983) analysis of disfluency structure, the *repair phase* of disfluency follows the editing phase, and it consists of the speaker's attempt to correct the overt or covert error (i.e., the reparandum). In Figure 3–1, the speaker successfully repairs the reparandum on the first attempt by saying the word *pink* correctly. However, Levelt noted that the term *repair* does not necessarily mean a speaker's attempt to fix an error has been successful. For instance, speakers sometimes "repair" words that were not obviously incorrect in the original utterance, and sometimes the repairs they construct are incorrect. In other cases, the speaker's attempt at repairing the error will be unsuccessful and lead to either repetition of the original error or to new errors. In the latter cases, the speaker then may commence additional repairs in an effort to reestablish the original communicative intention. Often, the additional attempts to repair the utterance result in the same segment of speech being repeated over and over (e.g., *w- w- w- why*).

Overt Repairs

Overt repairs are those in which the speaker's repair alters something that already has been said. Repairs usually are accomplished by changing, adding, or deleting words or portions of words in the part of the utterance that already has been spoken (see Examples 3–2 and 3–3 above and Figure 3–1). Speakers also may alter the prosodic characteristics of what has been previously said. With overt errors, the reparandum is available to both the speaker and the listener. In such cases, the repair usually involves retracing to some previously spoken point in the utterance and then restarting the utterance. When a speaker retraces to a point before the reparandum, he or she will end up repeating portions of the original utterance (see the word *the* in Example 3–2, above) and, in doing so, create a disfluency type that many authorities term "repetition."

Sometimes, retraces will extend to the start of the syntactic phrase that contains the reparandum. This process is illustrated in Example 3–2 above, where the speaker retraced to the beginning of the noun phrase in which the reparandum (i.e., *big*) was located. When the reparandum is located near the start of an utterance, the speaker's repair may result in a retrace to the beginning of the utterance. Alternately, in Example 3–4 below, the speaker retraces only to the beginning of the reparandum. In this example, none of the words from the original utterance are repeated verbatim during the repair. The intended word (*black*) is simply inserted after the reparandum, *back*.

> Example 3–4: It looks like a *back*-black bear.

Covert Repairs

With covert repairs, the location of the reparandum is unknown and is likely to exist in a portion of the utterance that has been planned but not yet spoken. This is illustrated in Examples 3–5 to 3–8 below, wherein the speaker interrupts the utterance even though there was nothing obviously wrong with it up through the point of interruption. Covert repairs can commence either from the point of interruption (see *ack hole* in Example 3–5 and *black hole* in Example 3–6 below), at the start of the word that immediately precedes the moment of interruption (see *black hole* in Example 3–7 below), or at some earlier point within the original utterance (see *like a black hole* in Example 3–8 below). Note that in Example 3–8, the onset of the covert repair coincides with the start of the syntactic phrase within which the moment of interruption occurs. In covert repairs that feature retracing (see Examples 3–7 and 3–8), the speaker repeats portions of the original utterance verbatim; that is, without changing, add-

ing, or deleting morphemes. This is in contrast to overt repairs, wherein some portions of the original utterance may be repeated, but other portions are altered (see Example 3–2).

Example 3–5: It looks like a bla-*ack hole*.

Example 3–6: It looks like a- . . . *black hole*.

Example 3–7: It looks like a bla-*black hole*.

Example 3–8: It looks like a bla-*like a black hole*.

In Figure 3–2, we illustrate the structural aspects of covert repair further. In

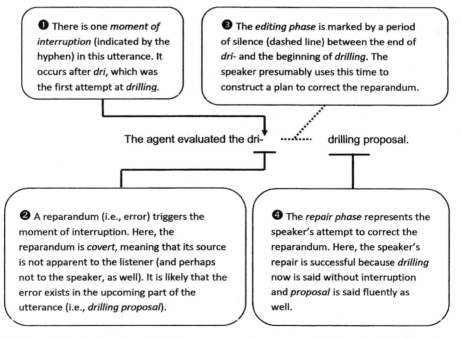

Figure 3–2. Extension of disfluency structure concepts to a stutter-like disfluency. In this case, the utterance is interrupted in mid-word, prior to the error point (see Boxes 1 and 2). The editing phase consists of silence (see Box 3), after which the speaker commences a repair by restarting the previously interrupted word. The repair is successful, as shown by the absence of continuity interruption in the second attempt at saying *drilling*.

this case, the disfluency results in the repetition of a part of a word. Disfluency of this sort is common in the speech of many speakers who stutter but relatively uncommon in the speech of speakers with typical fluency.

Labeling Disfluency

When assessing breaks in speech continuity, clinicians typically attempt to determine how often speech is interrupted as well as what the speaker does when speech is interrupted. This has led to the development of disfluency-labeling systems. Throughout the years, numerous disfluency-labeling systems have been presented (e.g., Conture, 2001; Gregory, 2003; Dollaghan & Campbell, 1992; Hieke, 1981; Johnson 1961; Loban, 1976; MacLachlan & Chapman, 1988; MacWhinney & Osser, 1977; Teesson, Packman, & Onslow, 2003; Yairi & Ambrose, 1999).

In Table 3–2, we illustrate the breadth of terminology that exists across labeling systems. As shown, the labeling approaches vary widely in content and scope. Though the specific terminology varies across labeling systems, it is apparent that most of the approaches shown in Table 3–2 include terms for capturing repeated speech, unusual silence, and error correction. Many of the labels are transparent; that is, they describe what the speaker does during disfluency. Not all disfluency-labeling terms are equally transparent, however. For instance, Loban (1976) used the term *maze* as a synonym for the term *disfluency*, particularly those that are based on linguistic errors. Others (e.g., Miller, Chapman, & Nockerts, 1998) have followed suit. To our way of

thinking, a maze is something that is convoluted, complex, or difficult to emerge from. As illustrated in the previous section on disfluency structure, however, continuity interruptions often are quite simple in form. For this reason, we suggest avoiding use of the term *maze* as a generic descriptor for disfluency. If the term is to be used at all, it perhaps is best reserved for instances of disfluency that involve multiple and varied unsuccessful attempts to repair an overt or covert error.

As shown in Table 3–2, the labeling systems also vary in specificity. For instance, some systems have relatively few labels (e.g., Hieke, 1981), while others have many (e.g., Johnson & Associates, 1959; MacWhinney & Osser, 1977). Several labeling systems distinguish between repetitions that involve part of a word or an entire word, and some systems further specify whether the repeated unit is a monosyllabic or polysyllabic word (e.g., see Williams et al., 1978, Table 3–3).

Many of these disfluency labeling systems were developed for use within clinical or experimental research. It seems likely that the differences in specificity across labeling systems reflect the different purposes and needs of the researchers. Unimpaired speakers typically do not produce much disfluency, and the disfluency they do produce tends to assume a fairly restricted range of forms. Thus, when the research is focused on unimpaired fluency (e.g., Hieke, 1981), there may not be a need for more than a few descriptors. Impaired speakers tend to produce more disfluency, and the disfluency they produce is more variable in form. Thus, when the research focus involves impaired speakers, researchers are more apt to have a need for using systems that include many descriptors (e.g., John-

Table 3-2. Examples of Terminology Variations in Disfluency Labeling Systems

Disfluent Utterance[a]	Labeling System			
	Johnson & Associates (1959)	Kowal, O'Connell, & Sabin (1975)	MacWhinney & Osser (1977)	Hieke (1981)
The dog- |silence, without assuming posture for |b|| barked	N/A	Unfilled pause	Unfilled pause	N/A
The dog- |you know| barked	N/A	Parenthetical remark	Filled pause	N/A
The dog- |um| barked	Interjection	Filled pause	Filled pause	
The d|ooo|g barked	Sound prolongation	N/A	Drawl	
The do- |silently hold vowel posture| og barked	Broken word	N/A	N/A	
The |d-| dog barked	Sound and syllable repetition		Initial segment phonological repetition	Stall
|The d-| The dog barked	Sound and syllable repetition	Repeat	Word-included phonological repetition	
|The-| The dog barked	Word repetition		Word repetition	
|The dog-| The dog barked	Phrase repetition		Several word repetition	
|The dog-| . . . Hey, I'm hungry	Incomplete phrase	False start	Sentence incompletion	Abandoned utterance
|The cat-| The dog barked	Revision		Retraced false start	
The |bog-| dog barked			Phonological correction	Repair

Note. N/A = not applicable (i.e., this type of disfluency was not included in the disfluency labeling system).

[a]Disfluency boundaries are marked with vertical lines. A single dash within a disfluency boundary indicates the moment of interruption. Three consecutive typed letters (e.g., mmm) within a disfluency boundary indicate that a speech sound is produced for an excessive length of time. Ellipsis denotes a period of silence.

Table 3–3. Disfluency Labels Described by Williams, Darley, & Spriestersbach (1978)

Disfluency Type	Description	Example[a]
Interjections	Extraneous sounds (e.g., *uh, er, hmm*), words (e.g., *well, like*), and phrases (e.g., *you know*).	Jack- |*um*| fell off the *like* bicycle.
Part-word repetitions	Repetition of syllables or speech sounds within a word.	Jack |*f-*| fell off the |*b-*| bicycle.
Whole-word repetitions	Repetition of entire words (monosyllable or polysyllable), excluding words that are repeated for emphasis.	|*Jack-*| Jack fell off the bicycle.
Phrase repetitions	Repetition of consecutive words.	|*Jack fell-*| Jack fell off the bicycle.
Revisions	The content or grammatical form of what has been said is modified.	Jack |*falled-*| fell off the bicycle.
Incomplete phrases	Instances in which an utterance is started but not completed (with no evidence of attempt at revision or repetition).	Jack fe-
Broken words	Cessation of speech sound production within a word boundary that disrupts rhythm and interferes with the "smooth flow of speech"	*Ja-* |*silently hold vowel posture*| *ack* fell off the bicycle.
Prolonged sounds	"Unduly prolonged phonemes" or parts of words. (May be accompanied by unusual effort, tension, or strain.)	*J*|*aaa*|*ck* fell off the bicycle.
Dysrhythmic phonation	Phonation that "disturbs or distorts the . . . normal rhythm of speech." May feature excessive tensing. May be attributable to sound prolongation or usual timing, improper stress, or "other speaking-behavior infelicity" incompatible with fluent speech.	{*J*}*ack* fell off the bicycle.
Tension pause	Barely audible sounds associated with speech breathing or muscle tightening that precede a word.	Jack fell off the |*abortive vocalizations of schwa vowel*| bicycle.

[a]Disfluent segments are italicized. Parentheses indicate excessive physical tension.

Note. Williams et al. (1978) stated that disfluencies that assume a form such as \|*we um-*\| *we are going* . . . , are tabulated as having two instances of disfluency. In this textbook, we identify disfluency boundaries by referring to points of interruption within the speaker's target utterance. In the case of \|*we um-*\| *we are going* . . . , the point of interruption lies between *we* and *are*. Thus, the interjection *um* occurs during the editing phase that is associated with the speaker's attempt to repair the covert error that led to the interruption between *we* and *are*. Consequently, the segment of speech is scored as having one point of disfluency.

son & Associates, 1959). The main point is that disfluency-labeling systems are flexible and can be adapted as needed to meet research or clinical needs. If the goal is to measure changes in a speaker's disfluency behavior over time, however, it is important to use a fixed labeling system so that comparable comparisons can be made at each observation point.

Many of the labeling systems currently used by speech-language pathologists for the study of fluency disorders derive from the work of Johnson and Associates (1959) or subsequent revisions to that work by Williams et al. (1978). Although the disfluency labels utilized in these systems are oriented toward capturing the common symptoms of stuttered speech, they also are applicable for use with describing disfluency in unimpaired speakers, nonnative speakers of a language, and speakers from other clinical populations. They also are appropriate for use in situations in which normally functioning and disordered speakers are compared.

The disfluency labels from Williams, Silverman, and Kools (1968) are shown in Table 3–3. This labeling system expanded on Johnson and Associates's (1959) system. Many contemporary sources (e.g., Conture, 2001; Logan & Conture, 1995, 1997; Pellowski & Conture, 2002; Yairi & Ambrose, 1999; Yairi & Seery, 2011) discuss disfluency-labeling systems that are similar to the one in Table 3–3.

The structural properties associated with the most common disfluency types from the Williams et al. (1978) system are analyzed in Table 3–4 using Levelt's (1983) disfluency structure framework. When the disfluency labels are analyzed in this way, we see that the labels for revision and repetitions are oriented toward the type of repair strategy a speaker uses. In both cases, the repair strategy involves retracing to some earlier point in the utterance. In contrast, the labels for pausing, prolonging, and interjecting are oriented toward what the speaker does during the editing phase of disfluency. With prolongation, the editing phase is marked by the length-

ening of a sound segment. With pausing, it is marked by relatively lengthy silence and with interjecting, it is marked by the use of semantically unproductive syllables such as *um* (and probably silence as well). It is unclear how or why disfluency labeling evolved in this way. Perhaps, the various labels capture the phase of a disfluency that is most salient to a listener.

In the remainder of this section, we present a detailed discussion of the most commonly used disfluency labels in contemporary writing on fluency disorders.

Revising

In this section, we discuss basic characteristics associated with disfluency that involves revision.

Description

The term *revision* refers to disfluency that features the repair of something that a speaker has just said. Revision is the only disfluency type of those mentioned in Table 3–4 in which an overt error occurs in the original utterance. Some authors (e.g., MacWhinney & Osser, 1977; Naremore & Dever, 1975) appear to use the term *false start* as a synonym for revision. We prefer the term *revision* because it avoids the suggestion that this type of disfluency is restricted to the onset of an utterance.

It is possible to confuse revision with *elaboration*. The main difference between the two concepts is that revision involves a change in the form or content of what the speaker has just said. Elaboration involves leaving whatever has just been said intact, but expanding it with additional information that clarifies or enriches meaning. As such, elaboration often involves parenthetical remarks. The elaborated content

Table 3–4. Structural Characteristics of Common Disfluency Types

Disfluency Label	Spoken Utterance	Original Utterance (Before Interruption)	Error Detection Phase			Repair Phase	
			Reparandum (Error)	Moment of Interruption	Editing Phase	Repair Type	Repair
REV	*After school- um work, we'll leave.*	*After school*	*school*	Follows reparandum (*school*)	Silence after "school" + *um*	Overt	Retrace to start of reparandum, alter reparandum.
PWR	*After w- work, we'll leave.*	*After w-*	*work*⁺	Prior to reparandum	Silence after moment of interruption	Covert	Retrace to start of word that is interrupted, restart from there.
WWR	*After work- work, we'll leave.*	*After work*	*we'll*⁺	Prior to reparandum	Silence after "work"	Covert	Retrace to start of word before the interruption, restart from there.
PhR/MWR	*After work- after work, we'll leave.*	*After work*	*we'll*⁺	Prior to reparandum	Silence after "work"	Covert	Retrace to onset of the syntactic phrase that precedes the interruption, restart from there.
PRO	*After wwwork, we'll leave.*	*After w*	*work*⁺	Prior to reparandum	Lengthening of [w]	Covert	Resumption of "work" following [w].
INT	*After work- um we'll leave.*	*After work*	*we'll*⁺	Prior to reparandum	Silence following "work," plus semantically empty filler	Covert	Resumption of utterance at point of interruption.
PAU	*After work |silence| we'll leave.*	*After work*	*we'll*⁺	Prior to reparandum	Silence after "work"	Covert	Resumption of utterance after editing, beginning with *we'll.*

Note. REV: Revision; *PWR:* Part-word repetition; *WWR:* Whole-word repetition; *PhR:* Phrase repetition (also termed multiword repetition [MWR]); *PRO:* Prolonged speech sound; *INT:* Interjection; *PAU:* Pause. Superscript ⁺ indicates that the reparandum could be some part of the utterance *after* the word indicated in the column.

often is delivered within the context of a new clause. This is in contrast to revision, wherein the repair usually occurs within the clause that contains the error. Elaboration typically occurs when a speaker determines that a listener requires additional information about an ongoing utterance. In such cases, it is an indicator of pragmatic competence.

We illustrate the difference between revision and elaboration further in Examples 3–9 and 3–10 below:

> Example 3–9: *I gave the coupon to Andrea, I mean Allison. (Andrea is revised to Allison)*

> Example 3–10: *I gave the coupon— the one that gets you 50% off—to Celia. (coupon is elaborated)*

Structural Aspects of Revision

- *Moment of interruption:* With revision, the moment of interruption usually occurs in close proximity to the overt error. In some cases, it occurs while the reparandum is being spoken and in other cases, it occurs either immediately after the reparandum is spoken (as in Example 3–9 above) or a word or two after the reparandum (as in Figure 3–1).
- *Editing phase:* The editing phase of a revision usually is characterized by either silence or the production of an editing term (e.g., *um*). In some revisions (see Example 3–9), the speaker produces an editorial comment as well.
- *Repair phase:* The repair associated with a revision involves a retrace to some earlier point in the original utterance. This may be either to

the start of reparandum (as in Example 3–9) or to some point in the original utterance prior to the reparandum. In either case, the repair will lead to an alteration of the original utterance. It is possible for a speaker to detect an error but then choose to leave it unrepaired. In such cases, the speaker can do one of the following: (1) continue speaking without interruption or (2) interrupt the utterance briefly and resume speaking from the point of interruption.

Several examples of revision are shown in Table 3–5. As indicated there, the linguistic errors that trigger revision can assume a variety of forms and encompass all facets of language.

Revision and Fluency Impairment

Revision can be symptomatic of fluency impairment if it occurs more frequently than normal or if instances of revision routinely last for an unusual length of time.

Abandoning Utterances

In this section, we discuss basic characteristics associated with abandoned utterances.

Description

In an *abandoned utterance*, the speaker stops an utterance before its completion and makes no immediate attempt to complete it. Speakers abandon utterances for a variety of reasons, some of which include the following: (a) shifting attention to an

Table 3–5. Examples of Linguistic Errors That Can Trigger Revision

Error Type	Example
Phonologic error	The |Cand-| <u>Grand</u> Canyon is beautiful in March.
Lexical error	|Jane-, *I mean*| <u>Joan</u> plans to run with us in the race.
Morphological error	The |boy were-| <u>boys</u> were going fishing.
Pragmatic (appropriateness) error	We'll ride with that |dude- *uh*| <u>teacher</u>.
Syntactic error	|Bob pushed Bi-, *no wait* . . . | <u>Bill pushed Bob</u>.

Note. Each linguistic error (i.e., reparandum) and any accompanying editing terms are set apart by vertical lines. Speech within the vertical lines is regarded as disfluent. Revisions (i.e., error repairs) are underlined.

activity other than talking; (b) forgetting the intention that was being conveyed; (c) deciding that the content of the utterance is inappropriate or uninteresting for the listener; and (d) being thwarted from speaking by external events such as environmental noise or another person's speech.

An abandoned utterance sometimes is confused with a revision. The two types of disfluency are contrasted in the examples below.

Example 3–11: *Today, it was* \|*unsue-*\| *unseasonably cool.* (Error is revised, utterance is completed)

Example 3–12: \|*He was-*\| *They never ride the bus.* (Error is revised, utterance is completed)

Example 3–13: *Today, it . . .* (Utterance is interrupted and is not completed)

Example 3–11 is a clear case of revision because the speaker corrects an overt error. In Example 3–12, the eventual utterance *they never ride the bus* possibly is a revision of the speaker's original intention, which never was fully expressed but began with *he was.* Example 3–13 clearly

differs from the previous two examples in that the person interrupts speech in mid-utterance but never resumes it.

Williams et al. (1978) used the term *incomplete phrase* as a label for utterances that are abandoned. We prefer the term *abandoned utterance* because the speech unit that the speaker discontinues is not always a phrase. Rather, it can be any linguistic unit that is less than a complete utterance (e.g., a sound, a syllable, a phrase, two phrases, a phrase and half, a clause, etc.). Some authors (e.g., Brookshire & Nicholas, 1995) have used the term *false start* as global term to capture both revision and abandonment. In this text, we will distinguish between the two concepts because the effects that each has on communication can be quite different.

Structural Aspects of Abandoned Utterances

- *Moment of interruption:* In abandoned utterances, a moment of interruption occurs after the speaker has produced some portion of an utterance.
- *Editing phase:* In some abandoned utterances, the moment of interruption is followed by an

editing term (e.g., saying *um*). However, in many abandoned utterances, there is no evidence of an editing phase. Rather the utterance is simply discontinued after the moment of interruption.

- *Repair phase:* There is no evidence of a repair phase in an abandoned utterance. This is the main difference between abandonment and all other types of disfluency.

Abandoned Utterances and Fluency Impairment

Most clinical assessments of speech are based on dyadic (i.e., two person) exchanges, and it is our experience that, within such settings, utterance abandonment is a rare occurrence and unlikely to be a primary symptom of fluency impairment. Still, abandoned utterances are worthwhile to document because they can provide information about the communication environment within which a speaker participates and, possibly, a speaker's reaction to fluency impairment. For example, in cases where a person abandons utterances frequently due to interruptions from others, a clinician might direct treatment goals toward the speaking partners rather than toward the speaker. In cases where abandoned utterances occur in the absence of interruption from another speaker, a clinician then might evaluate whether the behavior indicates that a speaker has "given up" on verbal communication due to fluency-related difficulties.

Pausing

In this section, we discuss basic characteristics associated with disfluency that involves pausing.

Description

The term *pause* refers to a period of silence during the course of speech production. Such silence can occur either (a) within a single utterance or (b) between consecutive utterances within a narrative or a conversation. In the professional literature, researchers have differentiated between periods of silence that pertain to articulatory processes and periods of silence that pertain to linguistic processes. The notion of pausing is more closely associated with silence that pertains to linguistic processes. Still, in the present section, we will briefly discuss periods of silence that arise for articulatory reasons because of their relevance to the study of disfluency.

Most periods of silence that are articulatory in nature are associated with the stop-closure phase of stop and affricate consonants. Stop-closure intervals are readily identifiable on spectrographic images of speech. During this phase of consonant articulation, the vocal tract is completely sealed, a configuration that results in a blocking (stopping) of egressive airflow and a temporary cessation of sound (Hixon, Weismer, & Hoit, 2008). Byrd (1993) examined the stop-closure characteristics of 630 speakers during connected speech. This approach allowed for the study of stop-closure across an assortment of phonetic contexts. The average closure duration was 59 ms for voiceless stop consonants and 56 ms for voiced stop consonants. Closure durations were shortest for alveolar stops (~52.5 ms) and longest for labial stops (~66.5 ms). Other researchers (e.g., Stathopoulos & Weismer, 1983) have reported slightly longer stop-closure durations, particularly for voiceless stops, in studies that featured relatively small sample sizes and tasks that featured sets of target words within standard carrier phrases. No matter what the context, it is uncommon for stop-closure durations to exceed 100 ms (Hixon et al., 2008). Because stop-closure is articulatory in nature, it typically is not included in discussions of pausing. Nonetheless, if the stop-closure duration of a particular consonant is unusually long, it can be relevant to the identification of speech disfluency and thus warrant clinical consideration. We discuss this issue later in this section, under the heading of sound prolongation.

Within utterances, periods of silence are commonly observed at linguistic boundaries such as those between phonological words and prosodic phrases (Ferreira, 1993). In contexts such as narration and conversation, periods of silence also are routinely observed between the boundaries of consecutive sentences (Kelly & Conture, 1992). Silence at these locations is termed a pause. Most within-utterance pauses are thought to reflect the effects of linguistic planning and/or prosodic marking (Ferreira, 1993). Based on experimental evidence, the average duration for within-utterance pauses is anywhere from 20 ms to 100 ms, depending on the location of the pause in relation to the prosodic structure of the utterance and the temporal characteristics of the final word in a phrase or clause (Ferreira, 1993, 2007). Overall, there seems to be general agreement that most of the pauses that reflect cognitive-linguistic processing fall into the range of 50 to 250 ms (Deputy, Nakasone & Tosi, 1982; Hieke, Kowal, & O'Connell, 1983; Robb, Maclagan, & Chen, 2004; Rochester, 1973; Schönpflug, 2008).

This leads to the question of which pauses should be counted as disfluency. The most basic question is whether one should count *all* of the pauses that speaker produces or only those pauses that are atypical and, thus, perhaps indicative of impaired fluency. When the analysis is

focused on a speaker with suspected or actual fluency impairment, speech-language pathologists usually adopt the latter approach; that is, they analyze only pauses that are atypical.

A pause can be atypical in terms of either its duration (i.e., it lasts much longer than average) or its location (i.e., it occurs in a place where typical speakers rarely pause). At present, there is not a standard definition for how long a pause must be in order to be regarded as atypical. In studies of speakers who stutter, many researchers have considered pauses that exceed 250 ms as instances of disfluency (Logan, Byrd, Mazzocchi, & Gillam, 2011; Walker & Archibald, 2006; Walker, Archibald, Cherniak, & Fish, 1992; Yaruss, 1997). Such an approach fits reasonably well with data on the duration of linguistically based pauses that typical speakers produce. Pauses that exceed 250 ms in length are longer than most pauses that involve linguistic planning and/or prosodic marking and, as such, are suggestive of problems or errors in sentence formulation.

Example 3–14 illustrates the impact that one's definition for pause identification can have on the number of pauses that are identified in a speech sample. Imagine that a clinician set the threshold for pause identification at 250 ms for this sentence.

Example 3–14: *I want │Silence = 270 ms│ this one │Silence = 82 ms│ but not that one.*

Using the 250 ms criterion, the clinician would label the first silent period as a pause because its duration exceeds 250 ms, but the second period of silence would be ignored because its duration is less than 250 ms. Note that neither of the silent periods would be labeled as a pause if the clinician had set the threshold for pause identification to 333 ms. Thus, using the 333 ms criterion, the sentence in Example 3–14 would be considered fluent. Some researchers have set much higher thresholds for determining which pauses should be regarded as disfluent. For example, in Sturm and Seery's (2007) study with children, the threshold was set at 2000 ms, an approach that would likely eliminate most within-utterance pauses from consideration as disfluency.

As noted, another approach to pause identification is to consider *where* a period of silence occurs within an utterance. With this approach, a clinician labels silence that occurs in unexpected or atypical locations as disfluency as a pause, regardless of its duration. The sentence in Example 3–15 features a silent break in the middle of the word *telephoning*.

> Example 3–15: *I am tele-* |*Silence = 75 ms*| *phoning the salesman for an explanation.*

Because this silent break occurs in a highly unusual location, and it does not appear to be associated with either the prosodic structure of the utterance or sentence planning, it would be labeled as an instance of disfluency—despite its relatively short duration.

Structural Aspects of Pausing

Pauses can occur before the start of an utterance or within the boundary of an utterance. In an utterance-internal context, pauses are structured as follows:

- *Moment of interruption*: During a pause, the speaker usually interrupts the ongoing utterance at word boundaries, particularly those that coincide with phrase or clause boundaries. Examples of each are shown below:
  - After dinner- |pause|, Chris walks the dog. (pause at phrase boundary)
  - After he eats dinner- |pause| Chris walks the dog. (pause at clause boundary)

  Pauses routinely occur between sentence boundaries, as well:
  - Chris eats dinner. |pause| Then, he walks the dog. (pause at utterance boundary)

- *Editing phase*: The editing phase of a pause is characterized by silence. If the length of the editing phase exceeds some predetermined threshold (e.g., 250 ms), the pause is regarded as an instance of disfluency. Ideally, the threshold for deciding if a pause will be included in a disfluency analysis should be based on normative data from typical speakers, as opposed to being set arbitrarily.

- *Repair phase*: Pauses that fit the criteria for disfluency presumably are associated with covert errors that arise from difficulties in utterance planning and information retrieval. The repair phase commences with the resumption of speech from the original point of interruption. Thus, the speaker will not repeat or revise any portion of the utterance that preceded the moment of interruption.

Speakers are sometimes able to identify the nature of the problem that triggers a pause. One common trigger for pausing is the speaker's temporary inability to retrieve linguistic codes that are associated with a lexical concept. In such cases, the pause continues until the speaker resolves the formulation problem.

Pausing and Fluency Impairment

Pauses can be symptomatic of fluency impairment when a speaker produces them unusually often, when a speaker produces them in unusual locations, or when instances of pausing last for an unusual length of time. Because utterance planning and information retrieval are typical aspects of speech production, pause identification is not always consistent with the idea of disfluency, a term that implies the presence of speech production errors. In the approach outlined here, short pauses that are positioned at expected locations within an utterance are presumed to reflect ordinary or typical speech production processes. Unusually long pauses, in contrast, are considered to be a sign of disrupted or atypical speech production processes. The threshold that one uses for defining "unusually long" will influence the number of disfluencies that a clinician identifies within a speech sample.

Interjecting

In this section, we discuss basic characteristics associated with disfluency that involves interjection.

Description

Interjection is a form of disfluency that is characterized by the presence of semantically unproductive vocalizations. Examples of such vocalizations include *uh, um, mmm,* and *er.* A clinician may even judge

throat clearing as evidence of interjection if it occurs consistently, appears unrelated to signs of airway discomfort, and coincides with linguistic contexts that are associated with linguistic planning. The *uhs* and *ums* that permeate daily speech occur during the editing phase of disfluency. Hence, they are referred to as *editing terms.* Some authors use the term *filled pause* as a synonym for interjection because the speaker is inserting a vocalization into what is essentially a between-word period of silence. Although editing terms such as *um* and *uh* do not carry lexical meaning, they do serve as a signal to listeners that the speaker is actively editing an utterance and intends to resume speaking shortly. As such, editing terms act as a device for holding conversational turns, and they reduce the likelihood that the conversational partner will interrupt the speaker (Norrick, 2009).

Words such as *like* and *well* and expressions such as *you know, hold on,* and *let's see* sometimes function as editing terms, as well. In such instances, they can be considered as interjections. In Example 3–16 below, the italicized words are considered interjections (and, hence, disfluencies) because one could delete them from the utterance and still communicate exactly the same idea. In this example, the terms are equivalent to *uh* and *um* in that they are extraneous to the core utterance and, as such, do not alter the meaning of what has been said.

Example 3–16: Evan was hoping to get *you know* invited to *like* the football camp.

Of course not all instances of *like, well,* and *you know* are considered interjections. For instance, *like* functions as a comparative in Example 3–17 below, *well* functions as an adverb in Example 3–18, and *you know* functions as the subject and verb, respectively, in Example 3–19. Thus, in these contexts, the words are integral to the structure and meaning of the respective sentences and are not regarded as signs of disfluency.

> Example 3–17: The car was *like* a rocket, speeding around the track.

> Example 3–18: George used to play the accordion *well*.

> Example 3–19: *You know* that we will be leaving at 6 a.m. tomorrow.

Likewise, not all instances of non-lexical editing terms are symptomatic of disfluency. That is, speakers occasionally use interjections like *um* intentionally to signal equivocation, disagreement, or sarcasm (Norrick, 2009) or to mark another person's utterance as flawed (Lange, 2008). An instance of intentional use of *um* to signal disagreement is presented in Example 3–20.

> Example 3–20

> Speaker₁: I can't wait for the breakfast. I've heard Patrick is a terrific cook.

> Speaker₂: *Ummm* . . .

> Speaker₁: He's not terrific?

> Speaker₂: That would be correct.

Intentional use of editing terms is not common in everyday discourse; thus, most of the *um*s and *uh*s that a clinician encounters will be evidence of disfluency.

A speaker may be able to describe the nature of the problem or error that precipitates an interjection. As with pausing, a commonly reported trigger for interjection is the temporary inability to retrieve linguistic codes that are associated with an intended utterance. Some authors argue that pausing and interjecting are functional behaviors because they afford the speaker extra time for utterance planning or programming (Hieke, 1981; Starkweather, 1987). In this view, the time spent in interjecting prevents the speaker from making a more substantial formulation error that would end up taking him or her much longer to repair.

Structural Aspects of Interjection

From a structural standpoint, interjections are nearly identical to pauses.

- *Moment of interruption*: During an interjection, the ongoing utterance is most apt to be interrupted between word boundaries, particularly those that coincide with phrase, clause, or utterance boundaries. (See the pause examples in the preceding section.)
- *Editing phase*: The editing phase of an interjection is characterized by the use of one or more editing term, which may be surrounded by silence. In some instances of interjection, the silence may be long enough to meet the criterion for pause identification. Traditionally, disfluencies of this sort have been nonetheless classified as interjections. One certainly could make a case, however, that such instances of disfluency deserve a unique classification label.
- *Repair phase*: Interjections are associated with covert errors. The repair phase of interjection

commences with the resumption of speech (i.e., after the editing term).

Interjection and Fluency Impairment

Clinicians who are new to fluency assessment seem prone to draw the mistaken conclusion that *um* or other editing terms are not exemplars of disfluency because "everybody says *um*." This line of reasoning is, of course, faulty and is akin to saying that "*2 + 2 = 6* is not an addition error because everybody makes addition errors sometimes." Unless there is clear evidence that the speaker is using an interjection intentionally, editing terms like *uh* and *um* are always treated as evidence of disfluency. The main goal of fluency assessment is to describe what a speaker *does*. Each time a speaker says *um* or *uh,* the examiner should make note of it. Determining whether the speaker's verbal behavior is "normal" or "abnormal" is accomplished by comparing the frequency and manner of the speaker's interjecting against that of the general population. Thus, a woman who produces 2 interjections per 100 words during a story-telling task most likely will be judged as interjecting in a normal way because most adults produce interjections at a similar frequency during story telling. In contrast, a speaker who produces 40 interjections per 100 words during the same task will be judged as "atypical" because very few speakers produce interjections so frequently. A speaker who routinely produces strings of consecutive interjections (e.g., *He um, um, um, um, um doesn't like to eat lobster*) would be regarded as atypical as well, because most people use only one editing term per disfluency.

To reiterate, a main goal in fluency assessment is to record what one observes. Interpretation of what one has observed comes later. As with revisions and pauses, interjections can be symptomatic of fluency impairment when a speaker produces them too often, for an excessive amount of time, or in unusual locations.

Repeating

Repetition involves the act of saying the same word or series of words in the same way, for reasons other than emphasis. Several subcategories of repetition have been identified in the fluency disorders literature. The most common of these are part-word repetition, whole-word repetition, and phrase repetition. We discuss each of these subcategories below.

Part-Word Repetition

With part-word repetition, the speaker interrupts ongoing speech in mid-word and then retraces to the beginning of the interrupted word, at which point speech is resumed. In doing so, the speaker repeats, verbatim, the part of the interrupted word that has just been previously spoken. An example of a part-word repetition follows:

Example 3–21: *Our dog Riley |l-| loves to chase squirrels.*

Some authors (Conture, 2001, Williams et al., 1978) use the term *sound/ syllable* repetition when referring to a disfluency that is structured in this manner. Others (MacWhinney & Osser, 1977) have termed it *phonologic repetition*. Both terms are similar to the term part-word repetition in that they indicate that something shorter than a complete word is being repeated.

Part-word repetitions are infrequent in the speech of typical speakers, but they occur relatively often in the speech of many speakers who stutter. Part-word repetition presumably reflects the speaker's attempt to repair a covert error. When asked about the location of the problem or error that triggered the part-word repetition, speakers who stutter frequently report that it lies within the upcoming segments of the interrupted word. In Example 3–21 above, this would be the speech sounds that follow /l/ in the word "loves." In this view, the speaker is not "having trouble saying 'l' sound," per se. Rather, the speaker will report knowing what needs to be said (in this case, the word "loves") and even how it should be said but has difficulty in executing the necessary articulatory movements in a way that seamlessly connects the sounds within the word.

A structural variant of the part-word repetition occurs when the speaker interrupts speech in the midst of a word and then retraces to some point *before* the interrupted word in the original utterance. In such instances, the repair usually commences at the first word within the syntactic phrase that contains the interrupted word. This is illustrated in Example 3–22.

Example 3–22: |*In the m-*| *In the morning, we went fishing.*

The form of the disfluency in Example 3–22 resembles both a part-word repetition and a phrase repetition (described below). Disfluent instances like the one in Example 3–22 have received scant attention in the speech-language pathology literature. To our knowledge, there is no widely accepted label for the phenomenon. It is unclear why a speaker sometimes would begin the disfluency repair by retracing to the onset of the interrupted word and, at other times, do so by retracing to the start of the syntactic phrase that contains the interrupted word. In either

case, mid-word interruption of speech is not common among typical speakers. Thus, if a speaker produces disfluencies like those in Example 3–22 several times per 100 words during the course of a speech sample, it could be an indication of fluency impairment.

Whole-Word Repetition

The structure of *whole-word repetition* is very similar to that of part-word repetitions. The only difference is that the moment of interruption in a whole-word repetition occurs *after* completion of the word that subsequently is repeated during the repair phase (e.g., *at- at night*). As with part-word repetition, the reparandum is covert. When clinicians ask speakers to identify the location of the problem that triggers word repetition, the speaker often mentions some upcoming portion of the utterance—often it will be the word that immediately follows the point of interruption.

With whole-word repetition, the editing phase usually consists of a pause. The speaker then commences the repair phase by retracing to the onset of the word that immediately precedes the moment of interruption and restarts the utterance from that point. In doing so, the speaker repeats the word that was spoken immediately before the moment of interruption.

When identifying instances of whole-word repetition, the clinician should consider the possibility that the speaker's repetition is intentional. In Example 3–23, for instance, it is plausible that the intensifier *very* is repeated for emphasis.

Example 3–23: *Her dog was very, very thirsty.*

In cases like this, information about fluency dimensions such as rate, rhythm, prosody, effort, and naturalness can be used to judge whether the word is repeated intentionally.

Phrase (Multiword) Repetition

Another form of repetition mentioned in many disfluency classification systems is *phrase repetition*. With this form of disfluency, the speaker interrupts speech after completing a word and, after editing, initiates the repair by retracing two or more words before the point of interruption. This is illustrated in Example 3–24, where the speaker initiated the repair three words before the point of interruption.

> Example 3–24: *Yesterday |the two teachers-| the two teachers went out for breakfast.*

Often, the repair commences at the onset of the syntactic phrase that contains the moment of interruption (as in Example 3–24). Also common are instances wherein the speaker's repair involves a retrace to the onset of the utterance, as shown in Example 3–25.

> Example 3–25: *|Ralph is planning-| Ralph is planning to change jobs next year.*

In Example 3–25, the moment of interruption occurs following the verb phrase (*is planning*), but the repair commences at the onset of the noun phrase that precedes the verb phrase (*Ralph*). In this case, the label "phrase repetition" is inaccurate from a syntactic standpoint because more than one phrase is repeated. For this reason, we prefer the term *multiword repetition* as a label for repetitions of this kind.

Repetition and Fluency Impairment

Repetition in any form can be symptomatic of fluency impairment if a speaker produces it at a frequency greater than what typically is observed in the general population or when a speaker routinely requires more than one attempt to repair the covert error (e.g., |*w- w- w-*|*wait*; |*In the morning- In the morning- In the morning-| we'll leave*). When typical speakers produce repetition, the moment of interruption is more likely to occur at a word boundary than it is within a word boundary. Thus, it also is unusual for a typical speaker to produce part-word repetition at a greater frequency than either word or multiword repetition.

Prolonging and Blocking

Some instances of disfluency are characterized by fixed articulatory postures, wherein the production of particular speech sounds appears to be "frozen," "locked," or "stuck." This results in specific consonant or vowel sounds being produced for an unusually long duration. In speakers who exhibit impaired fluency, sound prolongation may be accompanied by excessive physical tension in the speech-related musculature. The presence of excessive physical effort, especially muscle tremor, can be used to discriminate instances of disfluency from instances of intentional sound prolongation as in phrases like "noooo waaaay." Clinicians sometimes specify sound prolongations further by indicating whether they are audible or inaudible (Conture, 2001). Some authors (e.g., Ambrose & Yairi, 1999; Williams et al., 1978) use the term *disrhythmic phonation* to include disfluency that features prolonged and/or unusually tense speech sounds.

Audible Sound Prolongation

As suggested by its name, both the speaker and the listener can hear an *audible sound prolongation.* We represent audible sound prolongation in the examples below using a sequence of three consecutive letter characters. (See the "m" and "e" in the words *most* and *when,* respectively, below). In each of these examples, the prolonged sound is separated from the remainder of the utterance by vertical lines.

Example 3–26: *|MMM|ost of the students have graduated.*

Example 3–27: *Wh|eee|n is the shuttle leaving for Orlando?*

Audible sound prolongation most often is observed on vowels, continuant consonants (fricatives, liquids, glides), and nasal consonants—speech sounds that can be naturally lengthened due to the absence of complete vocal tract obstruction during articulation. In our experience, audible prolongation is less apt to occur in conjunction with stop-plosive and affricate sounds, as these consonant classes naturally feature complete blockage of airflow in the oral cavity (and perhaps at the glottis, as well) along with closure of the velopharyngeal port. Thus, the articulatory configurations for these sound classes do not foster audible segment lengthening. If audible prolongation does occur on stop-plosive or affricate sounds, it will likely result from a lengthening of the release phase. For stop-plosives, this will be realized as lengthened aspiration, as represented by the multiple superscript *h* symbols in Example 3–28.

Example 3–28: Zeke was |p^{hhh}|acking the camping gear.

With affricates, audible prolongation can be realized through lengthening of the [ʃ] or [ʒ] posture during the production of /tʃ/ and /dʒ/, respectively. Speakers sometimes abruptly close the glottis while prolonging a sound. This leads to silence, which results in the disfluency sounding like a part-word repetition when speech resumes. This is illustrated in the example below.

Example 3–29: *The green |aaa-*[closed glottis]aaa*|apples were very tart.*

Some authors (e.g., Williams et al., 1978) refer to the latter type of disfluency as a "broken word." However, a similar pattern can occur during word-initial consonant production as well. In such cases, the clinician may find it difficult to decide whether to label the disfluency as a form of repetition or prolongation.

Inaudible Sound Prolongation

During *inaudible sound prolongation,* the speaker assumes the articulatory posture associated with a particular speech sound and attempts to speak but, while doing so, does not produce audible sound. If inaudible sound prolongation is observed, it often is in conjunction with production of stop-plosives and affricates—sounds that feature complete obstruction in the vocal tract. Inaudible sound prolongation also tends to coincide with vowel initiation, wherein the vocal folds may be adducted tightly, a configuration that results in an absence of phonation and a sensation of heightened air pressure in the thoracic cavity. Inaudible sound prolongation is difficult to represent using orthographic characters. In this text, we do so by noting the speech sound the speaker is attempting to say and then by following it with a series of consecutive hyphens. In Example 3–30, the partitioned disfluency represents a case where the speaker silently holds the articulatory posture for [p] for an unusual length of time. Some authors (e.g., Gillam, Logan, & Pearson, 2009; Guitar, 2006) use the term *block* to label this type of disfluency.

Example 3–30: |*P- - -*|*eter is driving to Maine this weekend.*

Structural Aspects of Sound Prolongation

As noted, the essential feature of prolongation is that the speaker lengthens a speech sound or its posture inappropriately but then eventually moves into the next speech sound. With audible prolongation, the utterance is not interrupted by silence, as is the case with other disfluency types. The lengthened segment still is a form of continuity interruption, however, because (a) the speaker takes longer than intended to get from one sound to another within the utterance, and/or (b) the speaker attempts to move from one sound to another within an utterance but temporarily is unable to do so. Sometime during the course of the lengthened sound, the speaker presumably enters the editing phase, which then leads to a resolution of problem that triggered the disfluency. After that, the repair phase commences, as the speaker transitions from the prolonged sound to the sound that follows it. Inaudible prolongation, in contrast, features a silent editing phase. Unlike a pause, however, the speaker continues to hold the articulatory posture

that was present at the moment of interruption. The repair phase commences when the speaker transitions from the held or blocked sound to the sound that follows it.

Both audible and inaudible sound prolongations are associated with covert errors. The reparandum lies beyond the lengthened sound, in an upcoming portion of the planned utterance. Thus, when prolonging a speech sound, a speaker is not having difficulty "on" the prolonged sound, per se, but rather has difficulty connecting the articulatory posture of the prolonged sound with the articulatory posture(s) of the following sound(s).

Sound prolongation is potentially more challenging to identify than other types of disfluency. This is because identification of this disfluency type depends on judgments about the temporal characteristics of sound segments. Recall that, in disfluency analysis, pause identification is customarily accomplished through the application of a somewhat arbitrary temporal criterion (e.g., "silence longer than 250 ms between word boundaries is regarded as disfluency"). Fixed temporal criteria cannot be applied to the labeling of sound prolongation, however, because speech sounds have inherently different durations and, in normal speech production, the duration of any particular sound segment varies with its context, as well.

According to Kent and Read (1992) several factors affect segment duration. These include the following: (1) the position of a word within an utterance; (2) whether a word is stressed or not; (3) whether a particular word conveys new or old information within the discourse setting; (4) whether a speech sound occurs as part of a consonant cluster or not; and (5) whether a speech sound occurs in the initial or final position of a word.

The functional role of an utterance also can affect segment duration, as well. Consider, for example, performative speech acts like those produced by a sports announcer after a player scores a key goal in a soccer match, i.e., *Scoooooooooooorrrrre!* In this context, the extreme segment lengthening is intentional and welcomed by listeners—at least those listeners who root for the scoring team! Other less dramatic examples of this phenomenon occur in everyday speech. Think, for example, of a person who expresses incredulity by saying the phrase "No way!" (e.g., [nːoːːwːeːː]). Because these instances of segment prolongation are done intentionally, they are not regarded as exemplars of disfluency.

Jones, Logan, and Shrivastav (2005) conducted a study of the effects of articulation rate and consonant type on prolongation identification. A panel of judges listened to computer-generated sentences in which both the duration of target sounds and background articulation rate within the sentence stimuli were systematically varied. Stimuli were presented in a stepwise manner, similar to the method used when determining pure-tone thresholds during a hearing assessment. This method made it possible to determine a judge's temporal threshold for prolongation identification. Analysis of group data showed that the judges considered a target speech sound to be "prolonged" when the presented duration exceeded the original (i.e., "customary") duration of a segment by about 38%. Thus, a speech sound that originally lasted 20 ms long was perceived as "prolonged" when it was lengthened to about 28 ms (i.e., 20 × 1.38 = 28). It was determined that the articulation rate within the surrounding sentence affected prolongation identification as well. That is, within the context of a relatively slow articulation rate, the observed durations of speech sounds that listeners judged as "prolonged" were longer than they were when the same speech sounds occurred in the context of a relatively fast articulation rate.

In clinical settings, identification of sound prolongation is quite straightforward when the affected segment shows evidence of extreme lengthening and is even more so when the lengthened segment is accompanied by excessive articulatory effort. For example, virtually all listeners will agree that a tense 4-second-long sound is an example of disfluency because there are no circumstances under which a speech sound will be produced in that manner. A prolonged sound segment—even one with relatively short duration—is likely to be labeled as disfluent when accompanied by observable muscle tremor. (In the latter context, a speech sound may appear to be "blocked" without necessarily sounding "prolonged.") However, reliable prolongation identification can become more challenging when a speech sound only slightly exceeds a typical duration and lacks signs of obviously excessive muscle tension.

Prolongation and Fluency Impairment

As with other types of disfluency, prolongation can be symptomatic of fluency impairment when it occurs more frequently than what is observed in the general population, when the prolongation is of unusually long duration, and/or when excessive physical effort accompanies the production of the sound segment. Prolongation is uncommon among speakers with typical fluency. Thus, the observed frequency for prolongation can be relatively low in an absolute sense (e.g., 1 or

2 per 100 syllables) and still be indicative of impaired fluency (see Chapter 4 for further discussion of prolongation frequency in the general population).

Variations in Disfluency Form

Thus far, most of the disfluency examples we have presented have featured a prototypical structure. In natural settings, however, disfluency forms sometimes are quite different from the classic forms that are noted in textbooks and research reports. This creates challenges for clinicians who are attempting to label disfluent speech. We suspect that the lack of an agreed-upon method for dealing with these nonstandard disfluency forms contributes to the relatively low reliability found in studies of clinicians' disfluency labeling (Cordes, 2000; also see Einarsdóttir & Ingham, 2005).

Variations in the Editing Phase

The editing phase for revision and repetition typically is characterized by silence: The speaker interrupts an ongoing utterance, pauses, and then retraces to some previous point within the original utterance to either repeat verbatim what has been said before (repetition) or alter what has been said before (revision). Revision and repetition do not always assume this classic form, however.

Use of Editing Terms During Revision and Repetition

A variation of the classic revision and repetition forms is for the speaker to pro-duce an editing term during the editing phase. Contrasts between the two forms of editing during revision are shown in Examples 3–31 and 3–32 below.

> Example 3–31: |*Charles-*| *Roberto filed the report with the agent.* (Classic form)

> Example 3–32: |*Charles- um*| *Roberto filed the report with the agent.* (Variation)

Contrasts between the two forms of editing during repetition are shown in Examples 3–33 and 3–34 below.

> Example 3–33: |*Ro-*| *Roberto filed the report with the agent.* (Classic form)

> Example 3–34: |*Ro- um*| *Roberto filed the report with the agent.* (Variation)

Examples 3–31 and 3–33 feature classic forms of revision and part-word repetition, respectively: The editing phase for each of the disfluencies is marked by silence. Examples 3–32 and 3–34, in contrast, feature the editing term *um* during the editing phase. In some approaches to disfluency analysis (e.g., Miller et al., 1998), the utterances in Examples 3–32 and 3–34 are coded as containing *two* disfluencies; that is, the editing term *um* is counted as the second disfluency within each utterance. When the structure of the disfluencies in Examples 3–32 and 3–34 are analyzed, however, we see that, in both cases, continuity is interrupted only once and it is interrupted in the same place. We also see that the disfluencies have the same general structure as the disfluencies in utterances in Examples 3–31 and 3–33; that is, a moment of interruption, an editing phase, and a repair phase. Furthermore, in Examples 3–31 and 3–32, the revisions are organized around the same reparandum: the speech error *Charles*. Likewise, there is nothing in the structure of Examples 3–33 and 3–34 to suggest that the covert problems that trigger the repetitions differ across the utterances. On this basis, we conclude that each of the four utterances should be regarded as containing one instance of disfluency.

Wingate (1984a) examined patterns of interjecting in typical adults and adults who stuttered and found that 13 of the 20 participants in the stuttering group produced editing terms such as "um" during the course of repetition disfluencies; however, none of the 20 adults with typical fluency did. This suggests that there is value in noting structural deviations in the form of disfluency.

Use of Multiple Editing Terms During Revision, Repetition, or Interjection

Another variation of the classic forms of disfluency is for a speaker to produce more than one editing term during the editing phase of revision, repetition, or interjection. This is illustrated in Examples 3–35, 3–36, and 3–37 below.

> Example 3–35: $|$*Charles- um um um* $|$ *Roberto filed the report with the agent.*

> Example 3–36: $|$*Ro- um um um* $|$ *Roberto filed the report with the agent.*

> Example 3–37: *Roberto* $|$*um um um* $|$ *filed the report with the agent.*

In Examples 3–35 and 3–36, the general structure of the disfluency is similar to that of a classic revision and part-word repetition, respectively: a moment of inter-

ruption, an editing phase, and a repair phase. The multiple interjections are indicative of a longer-than-typical editing phase, which suggests that the error that triggered the moment of interruption is taking longer than usual to resolve. The same conclusion applies for Example 3–37, wherein the speaker requires more time than usual to construct a repair for the covert error that triggered the interruption between "Roberto" and "filed." We consider utterances like these to have one instance of disfluency because there is only one place where the continuity of the core or target utterance is interrupted.

Variations in the Repair Phase

The repair is the final phase of disfluency. Onset of the repair phase is a signal that the speaker is attempting to implement a "fix" for the problem that triggered disfluency and, in doing so, complete the intended utterance. Most of the examples of disfluency given in this chapter thus far have featured successful repair of the reparandum on the first attempt. Repair patterns of this sort are the norm for speakers with typical fluency skills. Speakers with impaired fluency, however, are not always so successful. Consequently, the repair phase may need to be initiated two or more times before the reparandum is successfully resolved. Examples 3–38 and 3–39 illustrate instances of disfluency in which the speaker initiates the repair phase more than once to successfully address a covert error.

> Example 3–38: *The* $\lfloor fl_0$- fl_1- $\lfloor flights_2$ *to San Juan are less expensive in May.*

> Example 3–39: *The flights to* $\lfloor San_0$- San_1- $\lfloor San_2$ *Juan are less expensive in May.*

In Example 3–38, the speaker interrupts the ongoing utterance at fl_0. The speaker's first attempt at repairing the covert error (i.e., fl_1) is unsuccessful, as indicated by the moment of interruption immediately after it. After additional editing (i.e., the silence that follows fl_1), the speaker attempts a second repair (i.e., $flights_2$), which is successful, as indicated by the speaker's ability to advance the target utterance beyond the original point of interruption. Example 3–39 features the same general structure as Example 3–38, but in this case, the multiple repair attempts occur within the context of whole-word repetition.

In Examples 3–38 and 3–39, each of the utterances contains one *multiple-iteration repetition* (each repair attempt is termed an *iteration*). Each of the multiple-iteration repetitions is regarded as one instance of disfluency, because there is one point of continuity interruption and the speaker's repair attempts are aimed at resolving it.

Some authors describe multiple-iteration repetitions in terms of the number of extra *repetition units* they contain. The notion of a repetition unit refers to an abortive attempt at the production of syllable; thus, it differs slightly from the notion of a repair. Both instances of disfluency in the examples above are regarded as having two repetition units (i.e., fl_0 and fl_1 in Example 3–38; San_0 and San_1 in Example 3–39). In clinical settings, one may encounter instances wherein a speaker with impaired fluency routinely produces multiple repetition units during disfluency.

Nested Errors

A third variation in disfluency form involves the *nesting* of errors; that is, an instance in which one fluency-related error embeds within another. An example of this situation is provided in Figure 3–3, where the speaker produces a part-word repetition within a portion of the original utterance that is subsequently revised. There is no straightforward way to label a fluency disruption like this using traditional disfluency-classification systems. It is plausible that the part-word repetition and revision are related events. If so, a situation like this might warrant the use of a unique term, one that captures the unique structure of what has transpired. At present, there is no such term in wide use in the clinical literature. The term *maze* is a possibility but offers only a very general description of what the speaker does.

Repetition of Word- and Utterance-Final Segments

Repetition of Word-Final Sounds During Utterance-Internal Words

In nearly all instances of repetition, a speaker commences the repair phase at the *beginning* of some previously initiated word. All of the examples of part- and whole-word repetition given thus far in this chapter feature this form. On rare occasions, however, speakers repeat either a syllable *rime* (e.g., *white -ite, -ite*) or *coda* (e.g., *red -d -d*) located within a word that just has been spoken. So, rather than retracing to the beginning of a previously spoken word, the speaker retraces to a medial position with a previously spoken word and commences the repair from there. Terms such as *word-final repetition* (when a syllable rime is repeated) and *final consonant repetition* (when a syllable coda is repeated) have been used to describe repetitions of this

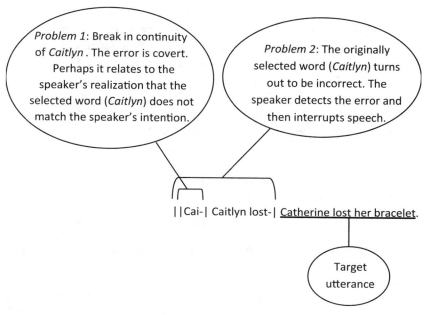

Figure 3–3. An example of an instance where one fluency problem (repair of a covert error during the word *Caitlyn*) nests within another fluency problem (a word selection error that is subsequently repaired). The part-word repetition occurs in a segment of speech that the speaker ultimately edits out of the target utterance. The interruption in utterance continuity occurs prior to production of the first word in the target utterance (i.e., *Catherine*). Traditional disfluency classification systems do not clearly capture this type of disfluency. This increases the likelihood that clinicians will label the disfluent speech in different ways and thus reduce the reliability of clinical data.

sort (Lebrun & Van Borsel, 1990; Mowrer, 1987; Stansfield, 1995). These repetitions share properties of both whole- and part-word repetition. That is, like whole-word repetition, the moment of interruption occurs at a word boundary, and like a part-word repetition, the repair phrase results in only a portion of a previously spoken word being repeated.

The contrast between final segment repetitions and typical forms of repetition is illustrated in Examples 3–40 to 3–43.

Example 3–40: *L|et's-| et's ask him where we can get coffee.*

Example 3–41: *Let's a|sk-| sk him where we can get coffee.*

Example 3–42: *Let's |ask-| ask him where we can get coffee.*

Example 3–43: *Let's |a-| ask him where we can get coffee.*

In Example 3–40, the speaker initiates the repair phase at the start of the previously spoken rime (i.e., *et's*) and in Example 3–41 at the start of the previously spoken coda. Examples 3–42 and 3–43, in contrast, show the standard forms of whole- and part-word repetition, wherein the repair commences at the *start* of a previously spoken word. Several case studies have been published in academic journals concerning individuals who exhibit disfluency patterns that include these atypical repetitions (e.g., Cosyns, Mortier, Corthals, Janssens, & Van Borsel, 2010; McAllister & Kingston, 2005; Mowrer, 1987; Lebrun & Van Borsel, 1990; Stribling, Rae, & Dickerson, 2007). These studies are discussed further in Chapter 9. In cases of final-position repetition, it is unclear whether the reiterations merely reflect individual differences in the repair strategies for certain types of covert errors or, instead, whether they reflect the presence of some unique impairment that leads to unique covert errors which, in turn, require a unique form of repair.

Repetition of Utterance-Final Elements

Another structural variant of disfluency that is observed occasionally involves repetition of utterance-final elements. In this case, the repeated unit can be either sublexical (e.g., an utterance-final coda or rime) or something more substantial (e.g., an utterance final word or phrase, or the entire utterance itself). Repetition of utterance-final words and phrases is associated with a condition known as *palilalia,* a pattern of speech production that is associated with basal ganglia dysfunction (Duffy, 1995). In palilalic speech, repetitions may feature multiple iterations, which increase progressively in rate and decrease progressively in loudness (Kent & LaPointe, 1982). An example of palilalic speech follows:

> Example 3–44: *I like to swim |like to swim- like to swim- like to swim- like to swim |.*

Because the repeated speech occurs *after* successful completion of the core utterance, it is plausible that this type of disfluency is symptomatic of perseveration. In other words, it appears that the speaker does not "shut off" a completed utterance. This pattern contrasts with the other forms of repetition presented in this chapter, wherein the repeated speech reflects a restart strategy that allows for resumption of an incomplete utterance. Additional information about palilalia is presented in Chapter 9.

Limitations of Disfluency-Labeling Systems

As suggested throughout this chapter, there are several limitations associated with contemporary disfluency-labeling systems and their use in describing fluency-related performance. In this section, these limitations are discussed in greater detail.

Lack of Standard Terminology

As shown in Table 3–2, many terms have been used to describe disfluency-related behaviors. In some cases, multiple terms exist to describe essentially the same behavioral phenomenon. The lack of standard terminology for disfluency labeling can potentially impede communication between clinicians, particularly when terms are either undefined or defined only minimally.

Lack of Comprehensive Terminology

As demonstrated in previous sections of this chapter, the surface form of disfluency can vary widely and traditional disfluency-labeling systems are not comprehensive enough to capture these variations adequately. Thus, it appears that new approaches to disfluency labeling are needed, particularly for analyses of disordered fluency. The challenge is to create a system of labels that is, at once, practical, comprehensive, and sufficiently descriptive. It is possible that the path toward a more satisfactory disfluency-labeling system may involve the use of fewer and less specific descriptors. We discuss this concept in Section III in conjunction with the topic of disfluency analysis.

Inconsistent Relationship Between Labels and Structure

The labeling terms that are most widely used today seem to be oriented toward describing the most salient features of disfluency. However, the descriptive labels are inconsistent with respect to how they correspond to the structural aspects of disfluency. For example, the terms *pause* and *interjection* describe what a speaker does during the editing phase of disfluency, the terms *part-word repetition, whole-word repetition, phrase repetition*, and *revision* describe what a speaker does during the repair phase of disfluency, and the term *prolongation* describes what a speaker does during the editing phase and perhaps the repair phase as well. The effects of this inconsistency on clinical practice are unclear, but we suspect that it contributes to the less-than-satisfactory reliability that often is reported for disfluency measurement. This problem is illustrated in the following example.

Example 3–45: *Natalie |will- uh| will fly to Athens next week.*

In Example 3–45, the speaker produces a repeated word along with the interjection *uh*. As noted earlier in the

chapter, some authors (i.e., Miller et al., 1998) would code the utterance as containing two disfluencies: a word repetition *and* an interjection. When the structure of the disfluency is analyzed, however, we see that the editing term *uh* (which constitutes the second disfluency in Miller et al.'s approach) occurs during the editing phase that follows the moment of interruption associated with the repetition of *will*. Thus, instead of simply pausing after *will$_1$*, as a speaker usually would do, this speaker inserts an editing term along with some silence into the editing phase. The key point is that the *um* and the repeated word *will* are associated with the same fluency challenge—repairing the covert error that leads to the break in continuity between the words *will* and *fly*. Thus, in this utterance, it appears that there is one primary problem to be solved: how to advance the intended utterance beyond the word *will*. Consequently, there is one instance of disfluency. The act of disfluency analysis might be accomplished more easily and with better reliability and validity when it is approached in this way; that is, by first attempting to identify the number and nature of the speaker's fluency challenges within a target utterance (e.g., difficulty in moving from a syllable onset to a syllable rime or from one word to the next) and *then* describing what the speaker does at each phase of disfluency while attempting to resolve the difficulty. This possibility awaits scientific investigation.

Reliance on Listener-Based Analyses

Traditionally, disfluency analysis is conducted from a listener's perspective. A clinician listens to a sample of speech and attempts to determine when, where, and how interruptions in continuity have occurred. This approach is inherently limited because it considers neither the speaker's perspective on fluency nor other dimensions of fluency.

In Figure 3–4, we present an example of an utterance that, from a listener's perspective, is free of continuity interruptions and thus is judged as "fluent." Upon further examination, however, we see that the speaker perceived this utterance to require excessive effort to produce. Consequently, the speaker perceived the utterance as "disfluent," or at least as something less than "normal" fluency. Mismatches between a speaker's and a listener's evaluation of utterance fluency occur routinely in the context of clinical interactions that involve people who stutter. Clinicians must be alert to this possibility during assessment and treatment activities.

Summary

In this chapter, we reviewed the types of disfluency that speakers commonly produce. We discussed structural aspects of common disfluency types, noting the characteristics of their interruption points, editing phases, and repair phases. We noted that disfluency tends to assume a limited number of forms and that, in

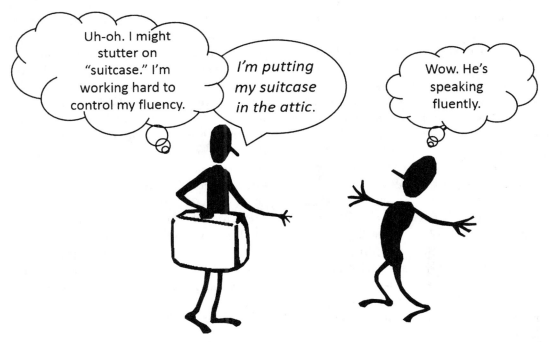

Figure 3–4. In clinical settings, clinicians typically rely on analysis of acoustic signals to evaluate speech fluency. This figure illustrates the limitations associated with this approach. In this example, the listener judges the speaker's utterance to be "fluent" because it is free from interruptions in continuity. The speaker, however, perceives the utterance differently. That is, the speaker anticipates disfluency on the word "suitcase" and exerts considerable effort at monitoring speech production in order to produce the utterance without overt interruption in continuity.

most instances, disfluency is a symptom of problems in the speech production process. The nature of the speech production problem that underlies an instance of disfluency is sometimes apparent to both the listener and speaker, but at other times, it is apparent only to the speaker, and at other times, to neither person.

Speakers often detect the overt speech errors they make and, upon doing so, correct them through a revision process that results in disfluency. Overt speech errors often arise under one of two scenarios: (1) inappropriate code selection (i.e., choosing linguistic codes that are incompatible with the utterance intention) and (2) inappropriate code ordering (i.e., the selected code is part of the intended utterance; however, it is located in the wrong position within the utterance).

Many of the classic disfluency types share structural similarities. For example, part-word repetition, whole-word repetition, and revision all involve a retrace to an earlier portion of an utterance that the speaker already has produced. The extent of retracing often is minimal—in many instances only to the onset of the word that immediately precedes the point of utterance interruption. This pattern increases communicative efficiency because it limits the duration of disfluency. In some instances, however, the speaker's retrace will extend further back into the utterance, which results in the repetition of several words that the speaker already has said and a longer disfluency. In the latter scenario, the speaker's repair for the disfluency is likely to coincide with the start of either a phrase or a clause.

With many disfluencies, the nature of the problem that triggers disfluency is hidden or covert. In some instances, the speaker may be able to describe the nature of the error; however, at other times, the exact nature of the error is unknown. Theoretically, covert errors can reflect problems in either speech planning or speech execution. Often, it is not possible to identify what triggers certain instances of disfluency or even to make a general statement about whether it is a language problem or a motor problem.

Numerous classification systems for disfluency have been presented in the linguistics and speech-language pathology literatures. Classification systems that are used with unimpaired speakers tend to contain far fewer categories than those that are used with impaired speakers. This reflects the fact that impaired speakers tend to produce a wider variety of disfluency types than unimpaired speakers do. Nonetheless, there is considerable overlap between groups in the types of disfluency they produce. The structural aspects of common disfluency types and their relationship to fluency impairment were discussed in detail.

The chapter concluded with a discussion of the limitations associated with contemporary disfluency-labeling systems. Among the problems noted was the lack of a universal method for describing disfluent segments that feature forms other than those in the classic disfluency categories. Limitations such as this can adversely affect the reliability and validity of clinical measures of disfluency. Disfluency is a dynamic process; hence, the disfluency description system that one uses may need to be dynamic as well. That is, a clinician may need to adapt existing classification systems when necessary in order to describe the disfluency characteristics of a particular patient accurately. Clinicians who possess a rich understanding of the nature of disfluency will be in a good position to do this.

4

Speech Fluency in Typical Speakers

In this chapter, we discuss the topic of normal fluency performance. The term *normal* has a statistical connotation, one that deals with the probability or likelihood that an event will occur. Normal events are those that are commonplace, expected, or observed in a majority of people. Abnormal events, in contrast, are uncommon, unexpected, or observed in a small number of people. The main area of focus in this chapter is on the type of fluency performance that most people exhibit and the point at which the boundary of typical fluency ends and atypical fluency begins. Our discussion of normal fluency performance is organized around the fluency model that was introduced in Chapter 1. The typical features of fluency performance are described in relation to each of the various dimensions of fluency. Ultimately, the determination of "normal fluency" requires the synthesis of clinical data from across these fluency dimensions. This allows a clinician to create a comprehensive appraisal of a speaker's fluency performance.

Defining Normal Performance

Qualitative Versus Quantitative Perspectives

A clinician can evaluate the normalcy of a speaker's fluency from both a *qualitative* and a *quantitative* perspective. The qualitative perspective entails description of the *types* of fluency-related behaviors a speaker produces. Some behaviors appear in many speakers and thus are expected or typical. Other behaviors appear in very few speakers and thus are unexpected or atypical. Individuals who exhibit "normal fluency" mainly produce typical fluency behaviors. Speakers with atypical or impaired fluency, in contrast, are apt to produce a wider range of fluency behaviors, including ones that are seldom, if ever, observed in the general population.

Analysis of the kinds of fluency behaviors a speaker produces tells only half of the story, though. For this reason, it also is important to adopt a *quantitative perspective* when interpreting fluency performance. From this perspective, a clinician attempts to describe variables such as disfluency frequency, disfluency duration, speech rate, and so forth, in numerical terms. With a quantitative analysis, the variable nature of fluency quickly becomes apparent. That is, some speakers will perform at the upper end of the fluency performance continuum while others will perform at the lower end. Most, however, will perform somewhere between these extremes. The primary focus in this chapter is on this "middle" segment of the fluency performance continuum.

Type Versus Manner of Behavior

As noted above, the identification of normal fluency involves consideration of both qualitative and quantitative data. The interplay between these perspectives is illustrated in Figure 4–1.

The behavioral patterns that correspond most directly to atypical or impaired fluency are those in the second row. These include the following scenarios:

- Producing typical behavior in an atypical manner. For example, saying "um" (typical), at a markedly greater frequency than other people (atypical).
- Producing atypical behavior in an atypical manner. For example, producing a physically tense sound prolongation (atypical) with a duration that is markedly longer than that of most people, including those with impaired fluency (atypical).

The notion of normal fluency, in contrast, is most consistent with the scenario presented in cell 1:

- Producing typical behavior in a typical manner. For example, revising speech (typical) at a frequency that is similar to most people in the general population (typical).

The scenario presented in cell 2—producing atypical behavior in a typical way—is less straightforward to interpret. Most often, it is compatible with the notion of normal fluency, such as when a speaker produces sound prolongation (atypical) at a frequency that is similar to or less than most people in the general population (typical). Such a scenario would suggest that the sound prolongation is an inconsequential feature in the person's speech profile. Some behaviors, however, are so unusual that their mere occurrence, even once, in a speech sample is sufficient to trigger concern about a person's fluency. Consider for example, a speaker who silently repeats the articulatory movements associated with the final few words of an utterance that he had just spoken aloud. Such a behavior is highly unusual, even among people with fluency disorders such as stuttering and cluttering. Therefore, the typical frequency for this type of repetition is essentially zero in the general population and close to zero in disordered populations.

Performance Variability

Fluency performance is inherently variable: a speaker exhibits one level of performance during one situation and another during some other situation.

Type of behavior produced

	Typical	Atypical
Typical	**1** Typical behavior produced in a typical manner	**2** Atypical behavior produced in a typical manner
Atypical	**3** Typical behavior produced in an atypical manner	**4** Atypical behavior produced in an atypical manner

Manner in which behavior is produced

Figure 4–1. The normalcy of fluency performance can be viewed in terms of the types of behaviors a person produces and the manner in which he or she produces them. The notion of "normal fluency" is most consistent with the performance profile shown in cell 1 (speakers who produce typical behavior in a typical way). Cells 3 and 4, in contrast, represent performance profiles that are consistent with the notion of "atypical" or "abnormal" fluency. Although the performance profile described in cell 2 generally is indicative of normal performance, there are scenarios in which it could represent atypical performance, such as when the atypical behavior consists of something that most disordered speakers never produce.

Thus, the notion of "normal" in speech fluency is inextricably bound to performance variability and the tasks a speaker performs. To define normal performance *for a particular task*, one must consider the pattern of fluency that most people would exhibit when performing that task. To define normal performance *for a particular person*, one must consider the patterns of fluency that most people would exhibit both over time and across a wide range of tasks.

Researchers have identified many factors that are associated with fluency variability. Included among them are the following: (1) the linguistic complexity of what is said; (2) time constraints that affect the speaker's ability to obtain or maintain a speaking turn; (3) environmental stimuli that compete with a speaker's attempts to talk; and (4) the speaker's level of concern for how listeners evaluate what he or she says.

Obviously, it is not normal for a speaker to exhibit wild fluctuations in fluency performance over time or across speaking tasks. In general, speakers with "normal fluency" show much less *within-subject variability* in fluency performance than speakers with atypical fluency do (Kleinow & Smith, 2000; Yaruss, 1997). That is, they perform at a similar level of proficiency when they do the same task repeatedly, and they perform at a similar level of proficiency across the various activities of daily living. Speakers with typical fluency also show much less *between-subject variability*. That is, people who fit into the category of "normal fluency" perform similarly to one another. Alternately, people who fall into the category of *disordered fluency* exhibit fluency performance that differs markedly from that of most speakers.

Continuity in Typical Speakers

One way to consider the notion of normalcy in speech fluency is through analysis of speech continuity. As discussed in Chapter 1, the term *continuity* refers to the connectedness of speech movements during utterance production. To measure continuity, clinicians typically describe the number and nature of disfluencies a speaker produces. Disfluency involves a break in the continuity of an utterance, and it is an intrinsic feature of speech production. All speakers, even gifted orators, are disfluent sometimes. Thus, the main issue to consider is not whether a speaker has produced disfluency but whether the

speaker's *pattern of disfluency* is similar to the pattern that most speakers in the population exhibit.

Disfluency Frequency

When one attempts to define "normal fluency," a fundamental matter to consider is the frequency with which most speakers produce disfluency. Disfluency is an unintended or undesired part of an utterance. In general, whatever a speaker says within the boundaries of disfluency is extraneous to his or her communicative intention. This concept is illustrated in Example 4–1, wherein a speaker repeats the name *Sasha* as well as the consonant sequence /st/. Both of the repeated units occur within the context of repairing covert errors. The speaker's first attempts at *Sasha* and *stood* are marked as disfluent, as indicated by the vertical lines, because the speaker has not advanced the intended utterance to the words that follow these segments.

Example 4–1: |Sasha-|Sasha
|st-|stood by her brother.

When computing disfluency frequency, a clinician must locate where continuity interruption occurs within an utterance. In Example 4–1, there are two points of continuity interruption: one between *Sasha* and *stood* and another between the onset and rime of *stood*. After the points of interruption are located, the clinician tallies them throughout the speech sample and then tallies the total number of *words* or *syllables* in target utterances throughout the sample. The word or syllable tally enables the clinician to report disfluency frequency in reference to the number of linguistic units produced in the speech sample. The clinician can compute a speaker's overall disfluency frequency using the following formula:

- *(number of continuity interruptions/ number of target words [or syllables])*100*[1]

This formula yields a disfluency metric that adjusts for sample size: the *number of disfluencies per 100 words* (or *syllables*). For example, if a speaker produces 34 disfluencies during a 457-word speech sample, it translates into an adjusted disfluency frequency of 7.44 disfluencies per 100 words (i.e., (34/457)*100. This approach allows a clinician to make direct comparisons of disfluency frequency data across speech samples of varying lengths.

By averaging disfluency frequency scores across many speakers, one can obtain estimates of the average frequency of disfluency within the general population and the extent to which disfluency frequency varies across speakers. Score variation is commonly reported via a statistic called the *standard deviation (SD)*. With this approach, one can define the bounds of normal fluency performance. Thus, for disfluency frequency, the normal range would be defined as follows: disfluency frequency scores that fall within ±1 *SD* of the mean disfluency frequency score.

Disfluency Frequency During Childhood

In the speech-language pathology literature, much of the data on disfluency frequency comes from comparisons between children who stutter and children who do not stutter. In most of these studies, speech sample elicitation takes place in laboratory settings during conversational or narrational tasks. The children in these studies typically interact with either a parent or an adult researcher. In most studies, the sample sizes range from 200- to 500-words in length.

In Table 4–1, we summarize research findings from nine studies that report data on children's disfluency frequency during conversation. We have sorted the findings from top to bottom within the table according to participant age. As can be seen, the average participant age ranges from 2;5 (29 months) to 10;7 (127 months). In three of the studies (DeJoy & Gregory, 1985; Logan, Byrd, Mazzocchi, & Gillam, 2011; Wexler, 1982), the researchers report data for more than one age level. Most of the researchers report data for children who are less than six years old. Upon scanning Table 4–1, it is apparent that the disfluency frequency values vary substantially across studies, particularly for those studies that reported data for preschool children.

Most likely, several factors contribute to the variations in disfluency frequency values. One factor is methodological differences across the studies. For example, DeJoy and Gregory (1985) and Logan et al. (2011) both included pauses in their disfluency frequency computations, but other researchers did not. In the Logan et al. study, pauses constituted an average of 44% of all disfluencies among typical children. If the authors had not counted pauses, the disfluency frequency value for their total cohort (shown on the second-to-last row in Table 4–1) would have decreased from 8.89 disfluencies per 100 syllables to 5.01 disfluencies per 100 syllables. Thus, when pauses are excluded, the Logan et al. data

---

[1]Note that this formula does not account for the *types* of disfluency that a speaker produces (e.g., *interjections, repetitions*). The focus is, instead, on whether *any form* of disfluency has occurred.

Table 4–1. Disfluency Frequency Characteristics of Children With Typical Fluency During Conversational Tasks

Source	Participants			Disfluency Frequency			
	n^a	M age[b]	Age Range	M	SD	± 1 SD	Reference Unit
Yairi (1981)	33	29	24 to 33	6.49	5.04	1.45 to 11.53	Per 100 words
Wexler (1982)[c]	12	30	26 to 33	14.56	5.71	8.85 to 20.27	Per 100 words
Ambrose & Yairi (1999)	54	39	24 to 60	5.66	1.56	4.11 to 7.22	Per 100 syllables
DeJoy & Gregory (1985)	30	42	39 to 45	11.40	4.68	6.72 to 16.08	Per 100 words
Natke et al. (2006)	24	43	26 to 62	3.75	0.91	2.84 to 4.66	Per 100 words
Pellowski & Conture (2002)	36	46	36 to 59	2.60	1.80	0.80 to 4.40	Per 100 words
Logan & Conture (1997)	14	52	38 to 67	4.04	1.91	2.13 to 5.95	Per 100 syllables
Wexler (1982)[c]	12	54	50 to 59	9.10	3.16	5.95 to12.26	Per 100 words
DeJoy & Gregory (1985)	30	60	57 to 63	9.30	3.31	5.99 to 12.61	Per 100 words
Yairi & Clifton (1972)	15	66	61 to 71	7.65	2.60	5.05 to 10.25	Per 100 words
Wexler (1982)[c]	12	77	73 to 81	9.08	4.08	5.00 to 13.16	Per 100 words
Logan et al. (2011)[d]	17	82	66 to 91	9.57	3.59	5.98 to 13.16	Per 100 syllables
Logan et al. (2011)[e]	34	98	66 to 127	8.89	3.34	5.55 to 12.23	Per 100 syllables
Logan et al. (2011)[f]	17	114	96 to 127	8.20	3.03	5.17 to 11.12	Per 100 syllables

Note. Frequency values are totals, i.e., combined across all types of disfluency.

[a] Number of participants per age cohort or in the entire study.

[b] Ages reported in months; Age 3;0 = 36 months; 5;0 = 60 months; 7;0 = 84 months; 9;0 = 96 months; 11;0 = 132 months.

[c] All participants were male.

[d] Data in this row are from the younger children in the study (*M* age = 6;10) and include pauses.

[e] Data in this row are from all children in the study (*M* age = 8;2) and include pauses.

[f] Data in this row are from the older children in the study (*M* age = 9;6) and include pauses.

are in a range that is consistent with data from other studies (e.g., Logan & Conture, 1997; Ambrose & Yairi, 1999).

A second methodological issue pertains to how atypically structured disfluencies were counted. Most authors of the studies in Table 4–1 did not specify how they scored atypically structured disfluencies. DeJoy and Gregory (1985) were an exception in this regard. Based on information presented in their method section, it appears that an utterance like the following one was scored as having two disfluencies: |*He um*| *he was ready to go* (i.e., a word repetition and an interjection). Under the disfluency analysis method that Logan et al. (2011) used, which is consistent with the method described in this text, the utterance above would have only one instance of disfluency (the continuity interruption between the words *he* and *was*). Assuming that all other aspects of disfluency measurement were the same, this means that disfluency frequency values in the DeJoy and Gregory study were apt to be somewhat higher than those in the Logan et al. study.

The reference metric for disfluency frequency varied across studies in Table 4–1, as well: In some studies, researchers reported disfluency frequency *per 100 words* and, in others, *per 100 syllables*. Because the number of syllables within a speech sample is almost always greater than the number of words, the disfluency frequency values for the "per 100 syllables" studies are somewhat lower than they would be if the computations had been based on words. Sample size differences across the studies also may account for some of the variability in the estimates of disfluency frequency. With small participant samples (e.g., 10 to 20 people), extreme scores from one or two participants have a greater impact on the

sample mean than they do in large samples. This might partially explain why the Wexler (1982) study (*n* = 12) reported a mean disfluency frequency for 30-month-old children that was more than twice as high than the ones reported by either Yairi (1981) or Ambrose and Yairi (1999). The latter studies featured many more participants than the Wexler study did.

Despite the many methodological differences across the studies, several general patterns emerge with regard to what constitutes normal disfluency frequency in children. These include the following:

- The average disfluency frequency for the six studies that used a word-based reference was 6.96 disfluencies per 100 words.
- The average disfluency frequency for the three studies that used a syllable-based reference was 6.20 disfluencies per 100 syllables. Thus, the disfluency frequency for these studies was about 11% lower when it was referenced to syllables rather than words. This is roughly consistent with research on the number of syllables per word in children's speech, i.e., 1.13 syllables per word in Dyson (1988); 1.15 in Yaruss (2000); and 1.18 in Flipsen (2006).
- In studies of children who were five years old or younger, the reported disfluency frequencies ranged from 2.60 to 14.56 disfluencies per 100 words. However, the three studies with the largest sample sizes (Ambrose & Yairi, 1999; Pellowski & Conture, 2002; Yairi, 1981) reported frequencies that were toward the low end of this range (5.66, 2.60, and 5.04, respectively).

- In studies of school-aged children, the reported disfluency frequencies are more consistent, with two studies (DeJoy & Gregory, 1985; Wexler, 1982) reporting mean frequencies of approximately 9 disfluencies per 100 words and one study (Logan et al., 2011) reporting a mean frequency of approximately 9 disfluencies per 100 syllables.

- The upper limit of the normal range for school-aged children's disfluency frequency is approximately 10 to 13 total disfluencies per 100 words. The disfluency frequency value varies depending on whether pauses are counted as a disfluency type or not.

- Estimates of the upper limit of the normal range for preschool-aged children's disfluency frequency are less precise. Among the studies listed in Table 4–1, values range from as low as 4.40 disfluencies per 100 words (Pellowski & Conture, 2002) to as high as 20.27 disfluencies per 100 words (Wexler, 1982). The Ambrose and Yairi (1999) study had the largest sample size of those listed in Table 4–1. The upper bound of the normal range in that study was 7.22 total disfluencies per 100 syllables.

Based on this brief review, it is apparent that total disfluency frequency offers only a general understanding of fluency normalcy. For this reason, it is important to consider other dimensions of fluency when making decisions about whether a client's performance is normal. Although speakers with fluency impairment generally produce more total disfluencies than speakers with typical fluency do, it is possible for some people with fluency impair-

ment to have disfluency frequencies that are comparable to, or even lower than, those of typical speakers. Thus, as others (e.g., Adams, 1977; Pindzola & White, 1986; Van Riper, 1982) have noted, it always is advisable to weigh many types of fluency data (e.g., disfluency frequency, disfluency types, speech rhythm, effort, naturalness) when making decisions about fluency normalcy.

Disfluency Frequency During Adulthood

Several researchers have reported data on adults' disfluency frequency. We report findings from three such studies in Table 4–2. As shown in the table, the reported mean values range from about 4 to 7 disfluencies per 100 syllables and they are slightly lower than the disfluency frequency values reported for school-aged children. As is the case with children, the majority of disfluencies in normally functioning adults consist of interjections and revisions (and pauses, if pauses are included in the analysis). For example, Logan, Haj Tas, and Metcalf (2002) reported that 77% of the disfluencies that the typical adults in their study produced were either interjections or revisions. In contrast, only 23% of the adults' disfluencies consisted of repetitions or sound prolongations.

Of note, none of the data reported in Table 4–2 are from spontaneous conversation. That said, the data are based on tasks that are relatively challenging, including referential communication, public speaking presentation, and personal narratives. Thus, these results are likely to approximate the types of conversational demands that adults encounter and, consequently, offer a reasonable approximation of conversational disfluency.

Adulthood often spans five decades or more. Thus, it is reasonable to ask

Table 4–2. Disfluency Frequencies for Adult Speakers as Reported in Three Studies

Source	Participants	Task	Sample Size	Disfluency Frequency	
				M	**Reference Unit**
Bortfeld et al. (2001)	YA	Referential speaking	32	5.55	Per 100 words
	MA		32	5.68	Per 100 words
	OA		32	6.65	Per 100 words
	All groups		96	5.97	Per 100 words
Goberman et al. (2011)	YA_M	Public speaking	9	5.07	Per 100 syllables
	YA_F		7	3.72	Per 100 syllables
Logan et al. (2002)	YA	Personal Narratives	10	6.92	Per 100 syllables

Note. YA = young adult; *MA* = middle-aged adult; *OA* = older adult; *M* = male; *F* = female.

whether the characteristics of "normal fluency" during the early part of adulthood differ from those of late adulthood. Research findings suggest that there are subtle differences across this segment of the lifespan. For example, in one study, older adults (*M* age = 67 years) produced more disfluency than either young or middle-aged adults, with most of the effect attributable to an increase in interjection frequency (Bortfeld, Leon, Bloom, Schober, & Brennan, 2001). The researchers hypothesized that increased interjection frequency among older adults is associated with decreased efficiency in lexical retrieval in the later stages of life.

Types of Disfluency

In the preceding section, we discussed data on disfluency frequency for typical (i.e., nonimpaired) speakers. As we noted, disfluency frequency data, alone,

may be insufficient for deciding whether a speaker exhibits a normal pattern of fluency. For this reason, researchers and clinicians routinely report information about the frequency with which a speaker produces various *types* of disfluency, as well.

Much of the data in the speech-language pathology literature that pertain to disfluency types come from comparisons of children who stutter with children who do not stutter. In many of these studies, the researchers have used either Johnson and Associates's (1959) disfluency classification system or a disfluency classification system that derives from it. Consequently, the labeling terms for disfluency are similar across authors, but they do vary somewhat. Broadly speaking, the disfluency categories that are commonly included in these classification systems include the following: *repetitions* (e.g., part-word, whole-word, and multiword); *prolonged sounds* (with or without audible phonation); *interjections*; and *revisions*.[2]

---

[2]Pauses are not included in many disfluency-labeling systems. This may be due to the need to use instrumentation in order to measure pause duration precisely; however, there also is the practical difficulty of determining how long a pause must be before it is a valid indicator of fluency difficulty.

Several findings have emerged with regard to the types of disfluency that typical speakers produce. Among them are the following:

- *Typical speakers produce a variety of disfluency types, including ones that speakers with fluency impairment produce.*

A typical fluency profile includes a variety of disfluency types: repetitions, interjections, revisions, pauses, and even occasional sound prolongations. Thus, in many cases, analysis of disfluency type, alone, will not enable a clinician to distinguish an impaired speaker from a normally fluent speaker (Adams, 1977; Pindzola & White, 1986). We illustrate this concept in Figure 4–2 by summarizing some data that we derived from two studies: Ambrose and Yairi (1999) and Johnson and Associates (1959). Both studies featured two groups: children who stuttered and typi-

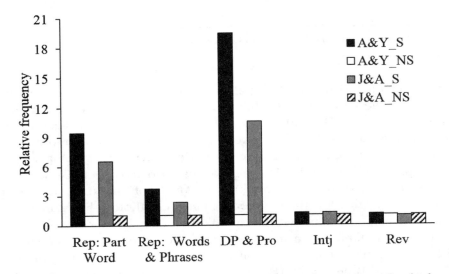

Figure 4–2. A bar graph illustrating the relative frequency with which children who stutter produce various types of disfluency relative to nonstuttering children. Data for the figure were derived from two studies to compute ratios that compared the two groups. Ambrose and Yairi ([A&Y], 1999) reported on 90 preschool-aged children who stuttered (S) and 54 age-matched nonstuttering children (NS), while Johnson & Associates ([J&A], 1959) reported on 89 children who stuttered and 68 nonstuttering children. In the figure, values for the two nonstuttering groups are held constant at 1. In this way, one can see how many times more often children who stutter produce certain types of disfluency. The findings from the two studies were similar. Differences between the groups were apparent on disfluency types involving repetition and prolongation. In these categories, children who stutter produced between 2.3 and 19.4 times as many disfluencies as the nonstuttering children, depending on the study and disfluency type. *Note:* Disfluency data in the Ambrose and Yairi study are per 100 syllables; data in the Johnson & Associates study are per 100 words. Data from some disfluency categories in the original studies were collapsed to permit comparisons.

cally fluent children. Precise comparisons between the two studies are challenging because of differences in disfluency terminology and measurement units (Ambrose and Yairi reported disfluencies per 100 syllables, while Johnson and Associates reported disfluencies per 100 words). Nonetheless, it is possible to get a sense of how the two groups of children compare in terms of the types of disfluency they produce. Note in Figure 4–2 that, in both studies, the nonstuttering group produced the same types of disfluency as the stuttering group. (The two groups did differ markedly in the *frequency* with which they produced certain types of disfluency, however. We discuss the latter point in more detail below.).

- *Typical speakers produce fewer total disfluencies than speakers with impaired fluency do.*

In a typical fluency profile, the total number of disfluencies a speaker produces usually will be consistent with the data reported in Table 4–1. In contrast, most speakers with impaired fluency produce disfluency excessively; that is, the total number of disfluencies produced will significantly exceed the values shown in Table 4–1. In the Ambrose and Yairi (1999) study, for instance, children who did not stutter produced an average of 5.66 disfluencies per 100 syllables. This frequency stands in stark contrast to the data for the children who stutter, who produced an average of 15.79 disfluencies per 100 syllables—nearly three times the frequency for typical children. Johnson and Associates (1959) reported a similar, though somewhat less dramatic difference, between their two groups. Thus, although speakers with typical fluency tend to produce the same types of disflu-

ency as speakers with impaired fluency, the two groups differ in the amount of disfluency they produce.

- *Typical speakers produce certain types of disfluency more often than other types.*

When disfluency frequency is broken down by type of disfluency, it is apparent that typical speakers mainly produce interjections and revisions. Many researchers have reported this pattern (e.g., Ambrose & Yairi, 1999; Bortfeld et al., 2001; Johnson & Associates, 1959; Logan & Conture, 1997; Pellowski & Conture, 2002; Yairi, 1981). Although speakers with typical fluency occasionally produce part-word repetitions and sound prolongations, the observed frequencies for these disfluency types tend to be quite low. In the Ambrose and Yairi (1999) study with preschool-aged children, for example, the children who did not stutter produced 0.56 part-word repetitions per 100 syllables (i.e., a frequency of about once every 200 syllables) and 0.09 disrhythmic phonations (a disfluency category that includes sound prolongation) every 100 syllables, which converts to a frequency of about once every 1000 syllables. Whole-word and multiword repetitions followed a similar pattern in that study as well. Therefore, while producing repetitions and prolongations was not, in itself, atypical in these studies, producing these types of disfluency more than about once or twice per 100 syllables is atypical.

In Figure 4–2, we illustrate the disfluency frequency differences between typical children and children who stutter in another way. That is, in Figure 4–2, the disfluency data are presented in ratio form. This approach allows us to determine how many times more often the children who stuttered produced certain types of disfluency in comparison to the nonstuttering children. In Figure 4–2, the bars for the nonstuttering children are held constant at one. This allows us to make statements like, "For every one part-word repetition nonstuttering children produce, children who stutter produce *x* part-word repetitions." If the heights of the bars for a particular disfluency type are roughly equal, it means that the two groups produced that disfluency type at a similar frequency. This is the case for the interjection and revision categories in Figure 4–2. If the bar heights differ markedly, however, it of course means that one group produces the disfluency type more or less often than the other.

Note in Figure 4–2 that the bars for some disfluency types (most notably "disrhythmic phonation and prolongation" (DP&Pro) are markedly different between the two groups. In the Ambrose and Yairi (1999) study, children who stuttered produced about 19 times as many disfluencies that involved disrhythmic phonation as the nonstuttering children did. In the study by Johnson and Associates, the children who stuttered produced this disfluency types about 10 times more often than the nonstuttering children did. Differences for the repetition categories are not as dramatic but children who stutter still clearly produced these disfluency types much more often than the nonstuttering children do, e.g., about 7 to 10 times as many part-word repetitions across the two studies.

The "frequency-by-disfluency type" approach to interpreting fluency performance is illustrated further in Figure 4–3, where a disfluency profile for a hypothetical normally functioning child is presented. The total frequency of disflu-

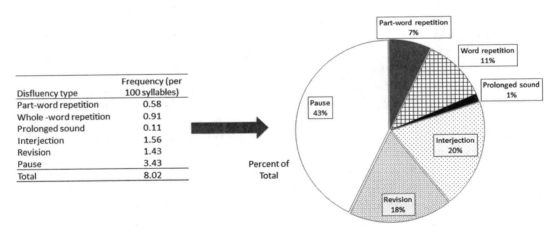

Disfluency type	Frequency (per 100 syllables)
Part-word repetition	0.58
Whole -word repetition	0.91
Prolonged sound	0.11
Interjection	1.56
Revision	1.43
Pause	3.43
Total	8.02

Figure 4–3. Example of a disfluency profile from a hypothetical child with normally developing fluency. The child's overall frequency of disfluency (8.02 disfluencies per 100 syllables) is consistent with disfluency frequency data from studies of conversational speech in normally developing children. If pauses are excluded from the analysis, the total frequency drops below 5 per 100 syllables. The frequencies for repetitions and sound prolongations are very low, as would be expected. Interjections, revisions, and pauses constitute 81% of the total disfluency frequency and, together, are produced at a frequency of 6.43 per 100 syllables. Repetitions and sound prolongations, in contrast, constitute only 19% of the total and, together, are produced at a frequency of 1.60 per 100 syllables.

ency is relatively low (about 8 per 100 syllables) and is consistent with findings from studies of disfluency frequency in children with typical fluency. The child produces most, but not all, types of disfluency. The child did not produce any sound prolongations. This is not surprising, however, given that this disfluency type seldom is produced in the general population. Revisions and interjections constitute the majority of the child's disfluency (66% in this case), a pattern which also is consistent with research on the disfluency frequency of children with typical fluency (Yairi, 1997).

- *Any type of disfluency can be symptomatic of fluency impairment.*

In recent years, some researchers have adopted the practice of regarding interjections and revisions as "normal disfluencies." This practice can be conceptually problematic. That is, although it is true that typical speakers normally produce these disfluency types at a higher frequency than other types of disfluency, it is not the case that these disfluency types are never symptomatic of fluency impairment. In other words, none of the disfluency categories in Johnson and Associates's (1959) typology or its many derivatives are inherently normal. One can only define the normalcy of interjections, revisions, and other types of disfluency in reference to data on their frequency of production. If interjections and revisions are produced excessively, it is appropriate

to regard those disfluency types as symptoms of fluency impairment. In addition, it is possible for a speaker to present with a fluency impairment in which the primary symptoms are excessive production of interjections and revisions.[3]

We illustrate this point further with a fictitious example of a preschool-aged boy who produced 7.75 interjections per 100 syllables during a conversational interaction. Imagine that we then compared the child's performance to Ambrose and Yairi's (1999) data, wherein children in the control (i.e., nonstuttering) group produced an average of 2.08 interjections per 100 syllables ($SD = 1.89$). Upon doing so, we see that the child's interjection frequency is 3.0 standard deviations above what is typical for preschool-aged children (i.e., $[(7.75-2.08)/1.89] = 3.0$). This means that nearly all preschoolers in the general population have an interjection frequency that is lower than the child's frequency. In this case, there is nothing "normal" about the way the child produces interjections.

Context Effects

Breaks in speech continuity are not random occurrences. Rather, at the sentence level, their occurrence is influenced by linguistic context and, at the discourse level, by a host of other factors including the physical setting and audience/speaking partner behavior. In this section, we focus primarily on sentence-level factors that affect disfluency.

---

[3]In clinical reporting writing, it is critical to avoid equating the term "normal disfluency" with disfluency types such as interjection, revision, and pausing because this practice can result in nonsequiturs such as the following: "The client's fluency disorder is characterized by normal disfluency." A more accurate explanation of clinical data might read as follows: "The client's speech fluency is characterized by excessive production of interjections. Although this disfluency type is common in the general population, the speaker produces it at a frequency that is significantly greater than normal."

Location of Disfluency Within Utterances

Among speakers with typical fluency, disfluency is more likely to occur at some positions in conversational utterances than others. Many instances of children's disfluency coincide with the *onset* of major syntactic units such as utterances, sentences, and clauses (Logan, 2009; Wijnen, 1990). The effect is relatively strong. For example, Logan and LaSalle (1999) reported that 82% of the conversational disfluencies produced by typical preschoolers in their study (*M* age = 4;4) occurred in conjunction with either utterance or clause initiation. In a longitudinal case study of a two-year-old boy, Wijnen (1990) reported that 44% of the child's repetitions occurred in the sentence-initial context.

The distribution of disfluency within an utterance varies with disfluency type, however, Interjections, for example, are likely to occur in grammatical contexts that differ from those for revisions or repetitions (Bortfeld et al., 2001). The distribution of pauses seems similar to that for interjections (Kowal, O'Connell, & Sabin, 1975; Logan et al., 2011); that is, both disfluency types can occur within phrases, prior to phrases, or prior to clauses.

Examples of onset-located disfluency include the following:

Example 4–2: |Af-| After breakfast.

In this example, the speaker's moment of interruption occurs within the boundary of the first word within a two-word utterance. The speaker restarts the utterance and, upon doing so, successfully advances the utterance beyond the original point of interruption.

Example 4–3: |The Bronc-| The Patriots just signed a new quarterback.

In this example, the speaker interrupts the utterance prior to completing the subject noun phrase. The speaker then revises the subject noun phrase to convey a different meaning.

Example 4–4: |um-| I'm not sure.

In this example, the speaker produces an interjection prior to the target utterance. Here, the disfluency seems to afford the speaker additional time to prepare the utterance.

Example 4–5: I do not mind flying$_{(Clause1)}$, |if the-| if the fares drop a bit$_{(Clause2)}$.

In Example 4–5, the disfluency occurs in mid-utterance, but the moment of interruption still is associated with the onset of a major syntactic unit. In this case, the moment of interruption occurs prior to the head noun of the subject noun phrase that introduces the second clause.

Researchers who have studied disfluency location in speakers who stutter (e.g., Brown, 1945; Silverman & Williams, 1967; Williams, Silverman, & Kools, 1968) have linked disfluency occurrence to other linguistic factors, as well, including word shape, word stress, and word grammatical class.

Syntactic Characteristics of Disfluent Utterances

Many researchers have examined the effect of syntactic complexity on speech fluency. In research settings, researchers have defined syntactic complexity based on either (a) the number of syntactic units produced within a sentence (e.g., Gaines, Runyan, & Meyers, 1991; Logan & Conture, 1995, 1997; Logan & LaSalle, 1999; Yaruss, 1999) or (b) developmental data pertaining to the age-of-emergence for syntactic forms within an utterance (Gordon & Luper; 1989; Gordon, Luper, & Peterson, 1986; Logan & Conture, 1995). Examples of the kinds of sentences that researchers regard as having relatively simple and relatively complex syntax appear in Table 4–3.

Counting syntactic phrases is a straightforward way to characterize sentence complexity (see rows 1 and 2 in Table 4–3). Logan and Conture (1997) compared the number of syntactic constituents within children's fluent and disfluent conversational utterances. To control for potential phonological complexity effects, they matched the fluent and disfluent utterances on the number of syllables they contained. Upon doing so, they found that disfluent utterances contained significantly more syntactic phrases than the fluent utterances did. This suggests that the syntactic form of an utterance affects fluency independently of its phonological form. In a related study, Logan and LaSalle (1999) found that the number of syntactic phrases in an utterance affected the structural form

Table 4–3. Examples of Sentences That Vary in Syntactic Complexity

Complexity Definition	Relative Complexity	Examples[a]	Syntactic Form
Number of syntactic phrases per utterance	Low	*On this spaceship.*	A 4-syllable utterance containing one syntactic phrase.
	High	*(He) (has) (a jet).*	A 4-syllable utterance containing three syntactic phrases.
Age-of-acquisition	Low	*The dog found the bone.*	Simple active affirmative declarative
	Low to Mid	*The dog didn't find the bone.*	Negative
	Mid	*The man gave the dog a bone.*	Dative
	Mid	*The dog found the man with the treats.*	Prepositional phrase
	Mid to High	*The man was bitten by the dog.*	Passive
	Mid to High	*The car belongs to the man who drives fast.*	Right embedded relative clause
	High	*The bike that was stolen belongs to the boy.*	Left embedded relative clause
	High	*The dog licked the man after eating the food that was on the floor.*	Adjunct clause

Note. Age-of-acquisition rankings based on Bernstein Ratner & Sih (1987).
[a]Parentheses indicate boundaries for syntactic phrases.

of disfluency. That is, utterances with the most syntactic constituents tended to contain disfluencies that had a complex or atypical structure; utterances with an intermediate number of syntactic constituents tended to contain disfluencies that had a simple or typical structure; and utterances with the fewest syntactic constituents tended to be spoken fluently. Zackheim and Conture (2003) also adopted a quantitative approach to define the complexity of utterance form. They examined the number of morphemes per utterance and found that it too affected the likelihood of disfluency in an utterance.

Several researchers have used a developmental-ranking approach to define syntactic complexity (see the lower half of Table 4–2). For example, Bernstein Ratner and Sih (1987) developed a syntactic complexity hierarchy that was based on previously published data regarding the ages at which various syntactic forms normally emerge in children's speech. Eight children with typical fluency and eight children who stuttered imitated 70 sentences: 7 sentences at each of 10 complexity levels. The researchers reported that the complexity ranking for a given sentence type was strongly predictive of whether the sentence contained disfluency and, if it did, the number of disfluencies the sentence contained. In the study, phonologic complexity (defined by the number of syllables per utterance) also predicted the children's disfluencies, but less powerfully than syntactic complexity did. Many other researchers (e.g., Gordon & Luper, 1989; Gordon, Luper, & Peterson, 1986; Pearl & Bernthal, 1980; Prelock & Panagos, 1989; Silverman & Bernstein Ratner, 1997) have reported significant effects for syntactic complexity on both children's and adolescent's disfluency frequency using sentence imitation tasks. In

young nonstuttering children, utterances that feature passive voice (e.g., *The man was bitten by the dog*) are particularly prone to being spoken disfluently (Gordon & Luper, 1989; Gordon et al., 1986).

Findings from other research studies have led to speculation that syntactic complexity may have less impact on speech fluency after mid-childhood or adolescence (Gordon et al. 1986; Logan, 2001; Silverman & Bernstein Ratner, 1997). For example, Logan (2001) compared the syntactic structures of fluent and disfluent conversational utterances produced by adolescent and adult speakers and found no difference in the number syntactic phrases within the utterances. In that study, there also was no difference in disfluency frequency during a sentence production task that featured four levels of syntactic complexity. More recently, however, Tsiamtsiouris and Cairns (2013) reexamined this issue with adult speakers. They developed a sentence production task that featured more complicated syntactic forms than those used in previous studies. With this approach, both typical speakers and speakers who stuttered were more disfluent when producing the most syntactically complex sentences. Thus, syntax may affect fluency beyond childhood if the structure of a sentence is sufficiently complex.

Disfluency Variations Across Speaking Tasks

In speakers with impaired fluency, disfluency frequency can vary markedly across speaking tasks (Byrd, Logan, & Gillam, 2012; Johnson, Karrass, Conture, & Walden, 2009; Yaruss, 1997). Speakers with typical fluency certainly can exhibit fluctuations in disfluency frequency across tasks, as well. However, their fluctuations usually are smaller in magnitude than those of impaired speakers. For example, in two recent studies (Byrd et al., 2012; Johnson et al., 2009), children who stuttered produced significantly different levels of disfluency during narration than they did during conversation. Typical children, in contrast, exhibited similar levels of disfluency across the two tasks.

What about adult speakers? Bortfeld et al. (2001) examined the effects of speaking role, partner familiarity, and speaking topic abstractness on speech fluency in young, middle-aged, and older adults. The researchers elicited speech samples during a referential communication task in which paired participants assumed the roles of "director" and "matcher." In the director role, a participant verbally directed his or her partner, the "matcher," to position 12 unique pictures into a spatial configuration that matched the director's configuration. Neither person could see the other person's pictures during the activity. The participants produced significantly more disfluency in the director role than they did in the matcher role, and they produced more disfluency when describing pictures of abstract objects than they did when describing pictures of children. Speaking role affected disfluency frequency more than any other variable in the study—disfluency increased from 4.93 disfluencies in the matcher role to 7.00 disfluencies per 100 words in the director role, a 42% jump. Topic abstractness resulted in an increase from 5.55 to 6.37 disfluencies per 100 words, a 15% jump. Partner familiarity had no effect on disfluency frequency. The older adults produced more disfluency than the middle-aged and young adults did during the experiment. Thus, multiple factors—in this case, communicative task and age—can influence disfluency frequency at once; however, it

is important to remember that, with non-disordered speakers, even relatively challenging tasks and relatively advanced age will only increase disfluency frequency so much. For instance, in Bortfeld et al.'s study, the highest disfluency frequency values were only about 7 per 100 words, an amount that when compared to disordered speakers still is minimal.

Many people express anxiety when asked to speak in public. On this basis, one might expect that speakers with typical fluency would experience relatively high levels of disfluency when delivering a speech to a large audience. Data from Goberman, Hughes, and Haydock (2011) failed to support this hypothesis, however. In their study, college-age adults' disfluency frequency was comparable to disfluency frequencies reported in other studies for adults who were engaged in other speaking tasks. Speakers' self-ratings of their overall fluency performance during public speaking often were less favorable than the ratings that they received from their audience, however. The researchers found that two aspects of disfluency (interjection frequency, percent of time pausing) correlated positively with the amount of apprehension and anxiety the speakers reported during their public speaking presentation. As expected, the presenters' disfluency frequency improved over time; that is, disfluency rates were lower during a second public speaking presentation than they were during an initial presentation. Preparation also seemed to facilitate fluency, as participants who reported spending the most time rehearsing their presentation spent the least amount of time pausing when presenting the material to an audience.

Rehearsal also seems to facilitate fluency during sentence imitation and oral reading. Williams, Silverman, and Kools

(1968) examined rehearsal effects in a study with typically developing elementary school-aged children. The children showed an average reduction in disfluency frequency of 19% during their second attempt at saying the target responses and a 27% reduction on their third attempt. Rehearsal effects were most prominent among children who began the study with a relatively high frequency of disfluency. Children who began with relatively low disfluency frequencies showed less proportional improvement with practice, as they essentially had relatively little room for improvement.

Disfluency in Young Children

Several researchers have studied children's fluency performance during the first three years of life. The birth-to-three period is an intriguing part of the lifespan in which to explore fluency performance, as it captures the period in which children show significant growth in their lexicon and in their use of linguistic forms associated with syntax, morphology, and phonology.

Yairi (1981) examined the fluency of 33 children, ranging in age from 24 to 33 months, during tasks that incorporated play and picture discussion. He found, as have many other subsequent researchers, that the children's disfluency scores skewed in a positive direction:

- Many children (39% of total) produced between 0 to 4 disfluencies per 100 words;
- Many other children (39% of total) produced between 5 to 9 disfluencies per 100 words;
- Some children (18% of total) produced between 10 to 14 disfluencies per 100 words; and

- Only one child (3% of total) produced more than 15 disfluencies per 100 words.

On this basis, Yairi (1981) concluded that two-year-old children's fluency skills are highly variable, but most children tend to cluster toward the "low" end of the disfluency frequency continuum. In contrast to findings from studies of older children, more than 80% of the youngsters in Yairi's (1981) study produced no repetitions of polysyllable words and more than half of the youngsters produced no revisions. The observed frequencies for part-word repetition and monosyllable whole-word repetitions were low in absolute terms (the median frequencies for the disfluency types were 0.90 and 1.00 per 100 words). Slightly more than half of the children produced prolonged sounds or sounds that featured excessive physical tension, and the median frequencies for these disfluency types were quite low as well: 0.20 per 100 words for each.

In a follow-up study, Yairi (1982) reported on longitudinal changes in the two-year-old children's disfluency during the course of about one year. Repeated measurement of the children revealed considerable variability in their performance over time. Five of the 33 children (15% of total) showed at least *four times* as much disfluency at their most disfluent observation session as they did at their least disfluent observation session. Another 18 children (55% of total) showed between 2 to 4 times as much disfluency during their most disfluent observation as they did during their least disfluent observation. Interestingly, the youngest participants at the time of the first observation showed an incremental increase in disfluency during the course of the study. Their disfluency increased from 3.67 disfluencies per 100 words at age 25 months to 6.90 disfluencies per 100 words at age 37 months—an almost two-fold increase. In contrast, the oldest participants at the time of the first observation showed an incremental decrease in disfluency during the course of the study (disfluency decreased from 8.43 disfluencies per 100 words at age 33 months to 4.26 disfluencies per 100 words at age 41 months—about half as much disfluency). This pattern suggests that, among typically developing children, disfluency frequency seems to peak between the ages of two and three and then declines as children move past age three.

Much of the change in disfluency for the younger subgroup of children in Yairi's (1982) study stemmed from increases in the frequency of revisions, monosyllable word repetitions, and phrase repetitions. In contrast, much of the change in disfluency for the older subgroup of children stemmed from decreases in the frequency of part-word and monosyllable word repetitions, interjections, and revisions. Sound prolongations (included under the term *disrhythmic phonation* in the study) and physically tense disfluencies decreased as well; however, these disfluency types constituted a very small proportion of overall disfluency at all stages of the study. Thus, the significance of the decline in the frequency of the latter disfluency types is unclear. Of note, even at times when the children were most disfluent, their average disfluency frequency values remained well below 10 disfluencies per 100 words. Thus, although the children's disfluency varied, in nearly all cases, it never increased to such an extent that it occurred more than about 10 or 12 times per 100 words.

Colburn and Mysak (1982a) reported on the relationship between children's disfluency and their language development using a longitudinal case study method with four preschoolers. Observation sessions for the study began when each of the children produced between 1.0 and 1.75 morphemes per utterance and ended when the children produced utterances that averaged 3.0 morphemes. Thus, the study captured fluency performance as the children progressed from one word, uninflected utterances into multiword utterances, some of which featured bound morphemes. In some respects, the four youngsters displayed remarkably divergent developmental pathways—two of them showed an increase in disfluency frequency during the course of the study, one child's disfluency frequency remained relatively constant, and the other child showed a decrease in disfluency frequency. The authors ranked disfluency types based on their frequency of occurrence at each MLU stage. Unlike data from Yairi (1981), the children produced phrase (multiword) repetition and word repetitions most commonly. Revision/incomplete phrase was the third-ranked category at MLU stages II, III, and IV. Interestingly, part-word repetition was the third-ranked disfluency type for 3 of the 4 children at stage I, and interjection often was ranked last or next-to-last across all four stages. The authors did not report disfluency frequency on a "per 100 words" basis, however. Thus, it is not possible to make precise comparisons between this study and others.

In a companion paper, Colburn and Mysak (1982b) examined the relationship between disfluency and the syntactic/semantic relations expressed within particular utterances. Results showed that all four children produced substantially more disfluency when expressing action-related utterances ("Daddy throw ball") than they did when expressing either state-related utterances ("that big ball") or locative-related utterances (i.e., "ball in box"). The authors concluded that disfluency seemed to correspond with the child's emerging mastery of a syntactic/semantic form and their attempts to practice its use.

Wijnen (1990) also conducted a longitudinal case study of a 2-year-old boy, and his results generally were consistent with those of previous studies with young children. Wijnen commenced data collection when the boy was just under age 2;4 and ended when he was just under age 3;0. During that time, the child's utterance length increased from 1.98 to 2.73 morphemes per utterance, which corresponds roughly to Stage II of Brown's (1973) morphological stages. Consistent with others' findings, the boy produced revisions and repetitions more often than other types of disfluency, and disfluency frequency varied noticeably over time. Changes in the child's disfluency frequency during two-word utterances unfolded as follows:

- Age 27 to 28 months:
  3.2 disfluencies per 100 words;
- Age 29 to 31 months:
  4.2 disfluencies per 100 words;
- Age 32 to 33 months:
  6.9 disfluencies per 100 words; and
- Age 34 to 36 months:
  2.0 disfluencies per 100 words.

Consistent with other reports, the youngster exhibited a sharp increase in disfluency that coincided with the emergence of syntactic sentence frames, which then was followed by a sharp decrease in disfluency frequency. Although the rise and fall in disfluency frequency for this child occurred earlier than it did for group data reported in Yairi's (1981, 1982) studies, the amount of variation was similar.

Interestingly, at the time of peak disfluency (age 32 to 33 months), most of the child's fluent utterances occurred within the following well-practiced syntactic frame: Pronoun + Verb + *Other word*. In contrast, the child's disfluency most often occurred during utterances that lacked true syntactic frames. These findings illustrate how syntax can trigger disfluency while it is developing, but also stabilize fluency once it is well established.

Disfluency Structure

As indicated in Chapter 3, each of the primary disfluency types features a prototypical or idealized structure. Within any given category of disfluency, many of the disfluencies that speakers with normal fluency produce adhere to that structure, while many of the disfluencies that speakers with impaired fluency produce do not. In this section, we briefly review each component of disfluency, discussing its typical manifestation and some atypical variations.

Moment of Interruption

The moment of interruption in a disfluency typically occurs at a word boundary. In other words, the speaker waits until a word is completed before interrupting articulation. An example of this pattern follows:

> Example 4–6: Mrs. Brugger could not find |the-| the Troutdale exit.

Less commonly, a speaker will interrupt a word *within* a word boundary. In the following example, the speaker interrupts the articulation of *find* after saying the onset consonant, and later interrupts the articulation of *Troutdale* mid-way through the first syllable.

> Example 4–7: Mrs. Brugger could not |f-|find the |Trou-|Troutdale exit.

Even less often, a speaker will interrupt a vowel prior to completing it and then resume it.[4] When speech resumes, it does so at the point of interruption. An example of this pattern follows, wherein the speaker interrupts phonation of the vowel [o] while continuing to hold the articulatory posture for the sound during the interruption. The speaker then resumes the sound.

> Example 4–8: Kate dro|---|ove into the rest area.

Editing Phase

From a structural standpoint, the editing phase of disfluency usually consists of a period of silence or both silence and the use of an editing term such as *um*. One atypical variation of these forms is the use of multiple editing terms during the course of a single editing phase. Two examples of this follow. In both cases, the speaker uses three editing terms per editing phase:

> Example 4–9: Greg went |um uh um| windsurfing near Hood River.

> Example 4–10: Andrea went |um um um| hiking in Yosemite National Park.

In the preceding examples, the editing phases are likely to be atypical in their duration because it takes longer to say three editing terms than one. The editing phases in the examples above suggest that the speaker is taking longer than usual to construct a suitable repair for the error that has triggered disfluency or, perhaps, the repair is constructed, but the speaker has difficulty initiating it. At present, there is no objective assessment that allows for determining which of these possibilities occurs at particular time.

Repair Phase

Researchers have used the terms *iteration* and *repetition unit* to refer to a speaker's attempt(s) at repairing errors that trigger disfluency. Normally functioning speakers usually require only one restart to repair the underlying problem. Examples of some typical repair attempts follow. In each of three disfluencies, the reparandum is repaired on the second attempt.

> Example 4–11: |Ju-|Justin joined the police department |last-|last month.

> Example 4–12: |His-|His brother is an English teacher.

Less commonly, a speaker will take two or more attempts to repair an error, as in the following example, where four restarts are used to move past the point of interruption.

> Example 4–13: Javier finished the |wa- wa- wa- wa-|water color painting yesterday.

Speakers usually will commence the repair at the start of the word that is closest

---

[4]In disfluency classification systems, this pattern is sometimes termed a *broken word*.

to the point of interruption. This approach leads to whole-word repetition or part-word repetition. If the speaker retraces further back in the original utterance, two or more words are repeated and multi-word (i.e., "phrase" repetition) results. Typical speakers produce multiword repetitions infrequently. The reasons that determine how far back in an utterance a speaker will retrace when attempting a repair are unclear. Perhaps word repetitions are more common than multiword repetitions because they take less time to execute and thus are less intrusive on communication.

Rate in Typical Speakers

Speaking rate can be assessed in several ways: measuring the maximum rate of repetition for syllable production (i.e., diadochokinesis); measuring how quickly a person initiates speech in response to some external signal; measuring the extent to which a speaker coarticulates consonants and vowels during syllable production; and measuring the number of linguistic units a person speaks per unit of time. We review rate performance data for tasks such as these in this section.

Articulation Rate

Articulation rate is defined as the number linguistic units—usually syllables or words—that a speaker produces per unit of time during fluent stretches of speech (Logan et al., 2011). Articulation rate is a measure of how quickly a speaker transmits information when speech continuity is uninterrupted. Computation of articulation rate is based on perceptibly fluent

speech units, preferably whole utterances or intonation phrases that consist of three or more syllables.

Articulation Rate in Meaningful Speech

Researchers have examined the articulation rate performance of children using tasks such as sentence generation, conversation, narration, and picture description. Data from studies of typical three- and four-year-old children (Hall, Amir, & Yairi, 1999; Walker & Archibald, 2006; Walker, Archibald, Cherniak, & Fish, 1992) put conversational and narrational articulation rates at approximately 3.6 to 3.9 syllables per second (syll/s), with standard deviations at approximately 0.6 syll/s. (These rates translate into a range of roughly 215 to 235 syllables per minute.)

Among five-year-old children, the research findings are less consistent. For example, Walker et al. (1992) reported an articulation rate of 4.3 syll/s for a narration task, compared to Walker and Archibald (2006) who reported 3.2 syll/s during narration, and Hall et al. (1999) who reported 3.9 syll/s during conversation. In each of the latter studies, standard deviations for articulation rate were approximately 0.6 to 0.7 syll/s. It is likely that differences in research methodology across the studies account for a substantial portion of the rate variation. It also is possible that maturational factors come into play, as others (e.g., Logan et al., 2011; Sturm & Seery, 2007) have reported age-related increases in articulation rate across the elementary school years.

Among school-aged children, articulation rate data vary across studies. Logan et al. (2011) reported articulation rates for older (*M* age = 9;6) and younger (*M* age = 6;10) subgroups of typical school-aged children using speech samples that they elicited from the Modeled Sentences, Structured Conversation, and Narration tasks on the *Test of Childhood Stuttering* (Gillam, Logan, & Pearson, 2009). Selected data from that study and the study by Sturm and Seery (2007), who elicited conversational and narrational speech samples from 7-, 9- and 11-year-old typical children, appear in Table 4–4.

In the Logan et al. (2011) study, the articulation rates for the older subgroup of children were significantly faster than the articulation rates of the younger subgroup of children during all three tasks they studied. In addition, the articulation rates were faster for both age groups during a sentence production task than they were during either conversation or narration. In the Sturm and Seery (2007) study, 9-year-old children had faster articulation rates than 7-year-old children; however, there was no difference in articulation rates of 9- and 11-year old children, a pattern that suggests articulation rate may "level off" at that age. Sturm and Seery also examined the effect of narrative elic-

itation approaches on articulation rate. They found that narration of a wordless picture book yielded faster articulation rates than either fictional story retelling or personal accounts of daily school routines. Such findings underscore the effect that a communicative task can have on articulation rate performance.

Less often, researchers have reported articulation rate in terms of phones per second. Hall et al. (1999) conducted a longitudinal study of preschoolers' speaking rates. Typical children and children who stutter were assessed at ages 3, 4, and 5 years. The typical children spoke at a rate between 11.5 and 12.0 phones per second during the course of the study. The phones per second measure differentiated the speaker groups; that is, the typical children produced more phones per second than the children who stutter did. In this case, the authors speculated that the rate difference might have been a by-product of differences between the groups in phonological development.

Not surprisingly, adults' articulation rates seem to be faster than children's,

Table 4–4. Mean Articulation Rates (and Standard Deviations) for School-Aged Children During Conversation and Narration

	Articulation Rate					
Task	**Early Elementary Years**[a]			**Late Elementary Years**[b]		
Conversation	*M*	*SD*	*±1 SD*	*M*	*SD*	*±1 SD*
Logan et al. (2011)	3.54	0.53	3.01–4.07	3.99	0.63	3.36–4.62
Sturm & Seery (2007)	4.45	0.51	3.94–4.96	5.58	0.63	4.95–6.21
Narration	*M*	*SD*	*±1 SD*	*M*	*SD*	*±1 SD*
Logan et al. (2011)	3.87	0.42	3.45–4.29	3.95	0.49	3.46–4.44
Sturm & Seery (2007)	4.51	0.56	3.95–5.07	5.27	0.70	4.57–5.97

[a]Average age for participants was approximately 7;0.
[b]Average age for participants was approximately 9;6.

with several researchers (e.g., Crystal & House, 1990; Tsao & Weismer, 1997) reporting values of about 5.0 syll/s (i.e., 300 syllables per minute). Robb, Maclagan, and Chen (2004) compared the articulation rates of American English and New Zealand English adults during oral readings. New Zealand English speakers used a significantly faster articulation rate (about 5.71 syll/s; 343 syll/min) than American English speakers (about 5.27 syll/s; 316 syll/min). Robb and colleagues proposed that vowel characteristics of the two English dialects might account for some of this difference, as vowel height tends to be higher in New Zealand English than it is in America English and high vowels generally have a shorter duration than low vowels.

Kelly and Conture (1992) examined mothers' articulation rates during interactions with their typically developing preschool-age children in a play-based conversational setting. The mean articulation rate for the mothers (M = 4.71 syll/s, SD = 0.48) was similar to, but slightly slower than, rates reported for adults during oral reading. This may reflect differences in language formulation demands between the tasks. It also may reflect parents' attempts to attune their articulation rates to those of their children. Support for this view comes from the observation that mothers of children who stuttered used an even slower articulation rate (M = 4.17 syll/s, SD = 0.74) than the mothers of typically developing children when interacting with their children.

Some researchers have compared the characteristics of "fast" and "slow" talkers. For instance, Tsao and Weismer (1997) identified the 15 fastest and the 15 slowest speakers from a cohort of 100 adults who had read a passage aloud at their habitual and maximum rates. Speakers with the slowest overall speaking rates exhibited a habitual articulation rate of 4.54 syll/s and a maximum articulation rate of 5.77 syll/s. In contrast, speakers with the fastest overall speaking rates exhibited a habitual articulation rate of 5.82 syll/s and a maximum articulation rate of 7.31 syll/s. The extent of articulation rate increase from habitual to maximum conditions was proportionally similar for the slow (+27%) and fast (+26%) speakers, which supports the long-held view that speakers tend to talk at articulation rates that are near the upper limits of their capacity (see Starkweather, 1987).

In the Tsao and Weismer (1997) study, a speaker's habitual articulation rate accounted for about 70% of the variance in his or her maximum articulation rate, with the strongest relationships existing for male speakers and for fast speakers. Tsao and Weismer (1997) argued that their results supported a neuromuscular basis for articulation rate; however, they acknowledged that sociolinguistic factors likely play a role as well. In the neuromuscular view of rate control, speakers use a central "clock" or time pattern generator to control speech (Tsao, Weismer, & Iqbal, 2006). The neural clock also may regulate other types of movements, including manual ones (Franz, Zelaznik, & Smith, 1992). In contrast, peripheral muscular characteristics such as tongue strength appear to play little role in determining articulation rate (Neel & Palmer, 2012).

Articulation Rate in the Context of Diadochokinesis

Several researchers have examined articulation rate within the context of oral diadochokinesis (see, for example, Fletcher, 1972; Yaruss & Logan, 2002). With diadochokinetic (DDK) assessment, the speaker repeats one-, two-, or three-syllable targets as rapidly as possible. Usually, nonsense targets are used: "puh," "tuh," and "kuh" are common monosyllable targets; "puh-tuh-kuh" is a common three-syllable target. Presumably, the DDK task measures maximum speech motor performance in a way that controls for language formulation effects such as those associated with lexical retrieval and morpho-phonologic encoding (Tiffany, 1980). Typically, speakers must repeat the target as quickly as possible either for a predetermined number of times (e.g., 10 times consecutively) or predetermined length of time (e.g., 10 seconds).

Robbins and Klee (1987) found that the maximum repetition rates for both one- and three-syllable targets increased throughout the preschool years. For example, production of the syllable "puh" increased from 3.70 syll/s in the 2;6 to 2;11 age interval to 5.51 syll/s in the 6;6 to 6;11 age interval. A similar increase in rate was noted during that age span for production of "tuh," that is, 3.70 syll/s at 2;6 to 2;11 and 5.37 syll/s at 6;6 to 6;11. Likewise, articulation rate during production of the tri-syllable target "puh-tuh-kuh" increased between the 2;6 to 2;11 age interval (*M* articulation rate = 3.00

syll/s) and the 6;6 to 6;11 age interval (*M* articulation rate = 5.16 syll/s).

Yaruss and Logan (2002) reported articulation rate data for production of "puh-tuh-kuh" in 15 typical children who ranged in age from 3;2 to 7;4 (*M* age = 4;9). In the study, the children's production rate was somewhat slower (i.e., 3.57 syll/s; *SD* = .69) than the average for all participants in the Robbins and Klee study (i.e., 4.23 syll/s, *SD* = .79). The source for this difference is unclear.

Fletcher (1972) conducted perhaps the most extensive study of diadochokinesis in school-aged children. He reported maximum repetition rates for nine target responses, on a year-by-year basis, for children who ranged from 6 to 14 years of age. In Fletcher's study the articulation rates for CV targets increased by 45% to 50% during the eight-year span and, for the tri-syllable target "puh-tuh-kuh," it increased by more than 80%. Thus, maturation appears to influence articulation rate performance during the DDK task.

A summary of DDK data from three studies is shown in Table 4–5. As shown, the articulation rates increase with age in each of the studies; however, across the

Table 4–5. Maximum Repetition Rates for "Puh-Tuh-Kuh" From Age 4 to 12 Years

Researcher	Age 4	Age 6	Age 8	Age 10	Age 12
Robbins & Klee (1987)[a]	1.38	1.54			
Yaruss & Logan (2002)[b]	1.00	1.30			
Fletcher (1972)[c]		0.97	1.20	1.41	1.56

Note. Data are reported as iterations per second.

[a] Reported data are averages for participant subgroups that ranged from 3;0 to 4;11 (Age 4) and 5;0 to 6;11 (Age 6).

[b] Reported data are averages for participants who ranged from 3;2 to 4;1 (Age 4) and 4;10 to 7;4 (Age 6)

[c] Reported data at each age are based on a 12-month span (e.g. Age 6 = 6;0 to 6;11). Data were originally reported in seconds per iteration and were converted to iterations per second for this table.

studies, the articulation rates are not particularly consistent. This may be due to differences in elicitation methods across the studies as well as the relatively large variability that exists across children at any age interval when performing the DDK task (Robbins & Klee, 1987).

Speech Rate

Speech rate is defined as the number of linguistic units (usually syllables or words) that a speaker produces per unit of time during randomly selected utterances (Logan et al., 2011). Because utterances are randomly selected from a speech sample, speech rate statistics usually are based on both fluent and disfluent utterances. Thus, speech rate yields information about how quickly a speaker typically transmits information. Speakers who exhibit frequent and/or long disfluencies usually will exhibit slower speech rates than speakers who exhibit infrequent

and/or brief continuity interruptions. Logan et al. (2011) reported that the combined effects of disfluency frequency and sentence length accounted for 70% of the variance in school-aged children's speech rates and that disfluency frequency was a much stronger predictor of speech rate than age was. Ingham and Riley (1998) argued that speech rate should be a standard clinical measure in the assessment of speakers who stutter.

In Table 4–6, we present data from two studies (Logan et al., 2011; Sturm & Seery, 2007) that examined speech rate in typically developing children during conversation and narration. As shown, the mean speech rates reported in the two studies were similar. For both tasks in both studies, speech rate increased only modestly between the ages of 7 and 11 years and it peaked at an average of roughly 2.8 to 2.9 syll/s.

Interestingly, in a study of preschool-aged children, Kelly and Conture (1992) reported speech rates for nonstuttering

Table 4–6. Mean Speech Rates (and Standard Deviations) in Syllables per Second for School-Aged Children During Conversation and Narration

	Speech Rate					
Task	**Early Elementary Years**[a]			**Late Elementary Years**[b]		
Conversation	**M**	**SD**	**±1 SD**	**M**	**SD**	**±1 SD**
Logan et al. (2011)	2.58	0.37	2.21–2.95	2.88	0.67	2.21–3.55
Sturm & Seery (2007)	2.41	0.38	2.02–2.79	2.70	0.29	2.41–2.99
Narration	**M**	**SD**	**±1 SD**	**M**	**SD**	**±1 SD**
Logan et al. (2011)	2.72	0.67	2.05–3.39	2.89	0.57	2.32–3.46
Sturm & Seery (2007)	2.42	0.35	2.07–2.77	2.87	0.36	2.52–3.23

Note. Sturm and Seery originally reported speech rates in syllables per minute. Values in this table were converted into syll/s.

[a] Average age for participants was approximately 7;0.

[b] Average age for participants was approximately 9;6.

children that were actually faster (*M* = 2.95 syll/s; *SD* = 0.31) than those shown in Table 4–6 for school-aged children. This underscores how variable speech rate can be as well as the extent to which disfluency frequency and other task-bound factors can affect it.

Several researchers have reported on the speech rates of typical adults. Robb et al. (2004) summarized findings from several studies and estimated that the average speech rate for adults is about 3.33 syll/s (200 syll/min) during conversation and 4.33 syll/s (260 syll/min) during oral reading. These speech rates are notably faster than the speech rates reported for children (see Table 4–6), which may reflect maturation of the speech motor system and/or the language formulation system in the years between childhood and adulthood. Robb et al. (2004) reported oral reading speech rates for the adults in their study that were similar to speech rates from previous studies: about 4.2 syll/s (250 syll/min) for a group of American English speakers and about 4.66 syll/s (280 syll/min) for New Zealand English speakers.

Rhythm in Typical Speakers

Rhythm is an aspect of prosody, manifested through utterance properties such as segment, syllable, and word duration, syllable and word stress, pause frequency, and pause duration (Ferreira, 1993; Kent & Read, 1992; Selkirk, 1984). The construct of rhythm has received less emphasis than either continuity or rate in the fluency disorders literature. In fluent utterances, speech rhythm seems to be set at

the stage of prosodic encoding (Ferreira, 1993; Levelt et al., 1999; Selkirk, 1984). Articulation rate factors into the rhythm of an utterance as well. A current hypothesis is that a central neural timing mechanism regulates a speaker's articulation rate and, in doing so, sets a speaker's habitual rate (Tsao et al., 2006).

Disfluency can adversely affect the rhythm of an utterance. For instance, listeners are likely to rate a highly disfluent speaker as having less rhythmic speech than a minimally disfluent speaker has. Other aspects of disfluency can potentially affect perceptions of speech rhythmicity as well. These include *disfluency duration* and *disfluency structure*. We discuss these variables as they pertain to speech rhythm in this section.

Disfluency Duration

Length of Repetitions and Prolongations

Researchers and clinicians often measure disfluency duration in milliseconds or seconds.[5] In the fluency disorders literature, the data usually come from comparisons between typical speakers and speakers who stutter. Consequently, researchers often focus on timing only disfluency forms that are most characteristic of stuttered speech; namely part- and whole-word repetitions and sound prolongations.

In Table 4–7, we summarize findings from several studies of disfluency duration in typically developing children. A primary limitation of these data is that typical children, by definition, produce repetitions and prolongations infrequently.

---

[5]A millisecond (ms) is 1/1000 of a second. Thus, 100 ms = 1/10 second; 600 ms = 6/10 second; and 1000 ms = 1 second.

Table 4–7. Mean Durations (and Standard Deviations) for Children's Disfluencies During Conversation

Study	Age	Disfluency Type(s)	Disfluency Duration			Adjusted M
			M	**SD**	**±1 SD**	
Throneburg & Yairi (1994)[a]	Preschool	PWR (1)	0.89	0.28	0.61–1.17	0.70
		MWR (1)	1.02	0.22	0.80–1.24	0.80
		MWR (2)	2.02	0.65	1.37–2.67	1.76
Kelly & Conture (1992)	Preschool	MWR, PWR, Pro, BW	0.65	0.20	0.45–0.85	N/A
Zebrowski (1991)[b]	Preschool	PWR	0.52	0.25	0.27–0.77	N/A
		Pro	0.40	0.23	0.17–0.63[c]	N/A

Note. Duration is reported in seconds; Adjusted means represent disfluency duration after removal of the time spent in producing the fluent repair. *PWR* = part-word repetition; *MWR* = monosyllable word repetition; *Pro* = sound prolongation; *BW* = broken word. (1) = one repair attempt; (2) = two repair attempts. *N/A* = not applicable.

[a] Duration values from this study include the fluent repair of the disfluency. Means reflect the average of each participant's average.

[b] Mean reflects the average of all disfluencies across the group.

[c] Because prolongations involve instances when a sound's duration substantially exceeds its typical duration, it is unlikely that listeners would judge sounds as short as 0.17 seconds to be disfluent unless behavior such as excessive physical tension was present.

Consequently, researchers often base their mean duration values on analysis of only a few disfluencies per child. In fact, some typical children may not produce such disfluencies at all and, consequently, cannot contribute to the analysis.

Length of Pauses

Pause behavior is another disfluency-related construct that varies significantly with both communicative task and communicative purpose. For example, adults' pause frequency is greater in tasks that involve event description than it is in tasks that involve event summarization (Goldman-Eisler, 1963). Schönpflug (2008) reported that elementary-school-aged children paused longer (*M* duration = 2.22 s) when asked to provide a verbatim recount of a story than when asked to provide the gist of the story (*M* duration = 1.57 s). Children who showed high accuracy for story recall in the gist condition exhibited an increase in pause frequency but a decrease in pause length. The children produced fewer pauses when asked to retell the gist of the story one week after originally hearing it than they did immediately after it for the first time. The author attributed the decrease in pause frequency to the children's consolidation of story-related information. Based on these data, it is clear that many factors contribute to pause duration. Included among them are the amount of linguistic detail that a task calls for and the manner in which information is stored in memory.

Many researchers have discussed the significance of pause length in relation to speech production processes. A common view is that pause duration provides clues about the source of silence during an utterance (Deputy, Nakasone, & Tosi, 1982; Goldman-Eisler, 1963; Hieke, Kowal, & O'Connell, 1983; Robb, Maclagan, & Chen, 2004). Deputy et al., for example, proposed a three-part framework for interpreting pause origin:

- Pauses shorter than 50 ms reflect articulatory processes (e.g., the closure phase of stop consonants like/t/);
- Pauses in the 50 to 250 ms range are "mixed," meaning that they reflect either psycholinguistic or articulatory processes; and
- Pauses in the 250 to 3000 ms range most likely reflect psycholinguistic processes.

Ferreira (1993) conducted a series of experiments through which she accurately predicted pause duration through analysis of a sentence's prosodic structure. Pauses that occurred at intonational phrase boundaries (IPhr) such as the one shown in Example 4–14 below were significantly longer than pauses that occurred at phonological word (PWd) boundaries such as the one between *Riley* and *always* below.

Example 4–14: Riley$_{(PWd)}$ always barks$_{(IPhr)}$ whenever another dog walks by our house.

Ferreira (1993) demonstrated that pause duration also is sensitive to word duration. In the study, pause duration increased when the length of the word preceding the pause was short. Conversely, pause duration decreased when the length of the word preceding the pause was long. Thus, the pause following a phrase that ended with a long word like *green* was shorter than the pause following a phrase that ended in a short word like *black*. (The duration of *green* is inherently longer than that of *black* because of vowel differences between the words). The main pattern of Ferreira's findings went like this:

- At a phonological word boundary, pause duration was about 20 ms if a long word preceded the pause and about 50 ms if a short word preceded the boundary;
- At an intonational phrase boundary, pause duration was about 50 ms if a long word preceded the pause and about 90 ms if a short word preceded the boundary.

Of note, the average durations for pauses at phonological word boundaries were shorter than those at intonational phrase boundaries (about 35 ms versus 70 ms, respectively). Also of note: the linguistically mediated pauses in Ferreira's (1993) experiments were well below the 250 ms criterion that researchers often use to differentiate "typical pause duration" from "lengthy pause duration." This lends support to the practice of using pause duration values such as 250 ms (and certainly 333 ms) as thresholds for the identification of unusually long pauses.

Repair Attempts and Repetition Units

A second approach to measuring disfluency duration involves counting the number of attempts a speaker needs to repair a speech production error. One can analyze repair attempts within either revisions or repetitions. In the fluency disorders literature, the study of repair attempts usually occurs within the context of comparisons between typically developing children and children who stutter. Hence, researchers often have analyzed only those repetition types that best differentiate the two groups (i.e., part- and whole-word repetitions).

The part-word repetition in Example 4–15, below, features three total attempts at saying the word *propane,* the first two of which are unsuccessful.

> Example 4–15: The *pro- pro-* propane tank is empty.

Researchers have used three methods to quantify this phenomenon. The first is to count the total number of attempts at the word, which in this case is three. The second is to count the number of unsuccessful attempts (see italics in Example 4–15), which in this case is two. The third method follows from Levelt (1983) and involves counting the number of *repair attempts*, which in this case also is two (i.e., the successful attempt and the unsuccessful attempt immediately before it). With all three methods, one would sum the counts across multiple repetitions and then report the average as *iterations per disfluency* (method 1), *repetition units per disfluency* (method 2), or *repair attempts per disfluency* (method 3). Despite the quantitative and conceptual differences across the methods, they each yield a similar sense of repetition length.

Data from studies with typically developing children show that they seldom require more than one attempt to repair a disfluency that results in repetition. Hence, a disfluency like that in Example 4–15 would be uncommon in the speech of a typically developing speaker. Yairi and Ambrose (2005) reported data from 52 typically developing children who participated in the University of Illinois Stuttering Research Program and found that they produced an average of 1.13 repetition units ($SD = 0.16$) during their part- and whole-word repetitions. Others (Ambrose & Yairi, 1999; Johnson & Associates, 1959; Zebrowski, 1991) have reported similar values.

Temporal Structure of Repetitions

Another facet of rhythm involves the temporal structure of repetitions. To get a sense of the rhythm in a part- or whole-word repetition, one can examine the proportion of the total time during the disfluency that the speaker spends talking and in silence. Thus, in a part-word repetition like |o-|*open*, one could measure the duration of the first [o], the duration of the pause following the first [o] (i.e., the editing phase), and perhaps the duration of the second [o] in what ends up as the fluent version of the word.

Throneburg and Yairi (1994) examined the temporal structure of children's part- and whole-word repetitions. They found that, in typically developing children, the "silent segment" (i.e., the editing phase) of a repetition was much longer than either the word or the portion of the word leading up to the moment of interruption. For a word repetition such as |*he-*|*he,* for example, the pause following the moment of interruption was about 65% longer than the duration of the first production of *he.* For a part-word repetition such as |*s-*|*some,* the pause was about 48% longer than the aborted attempt at *some* was. Throneburg and Yairi (1994) also found that, in a word repetition, the first word attempt (the one preceding the moment of interruption) was about 30% longer than the second, successful attempt at the word. For part-word repetitions, the first attempt was about 50% longer than the second, successful attempt. They also reported that repetition structure differed between typical children and children who stuttered. The average duration for the editing phase during typically developing children's repetitions was 2.5 to 3 times *longer* than it was for children who stutter. This contributed to the finding that the part- and whole-word repetitions produced by typically developing children were significantly longer than those produced by the children who stuttered. Interestingly, Throneburg and Yairi (1994) also demonstrated that the timing structure of single-unit, part- and whole-word repetitions predicted children's diagnostic classification ("stutterer" versus "nonstutterer") with at least 85% accuracy.

Effort in Typical Speakers

Perspectives on Effort

One can examine the construct of speaking effort from both physical and psychophysical perspectives. In a general sense, physical effort corresponds to the degree with which some parameter of speech production occurs—the force with which a muscle contracts, for example, or the amount of intraoral or subglottal air pressure during production of a speech sound. From these perspectives, effortful speech occurs when the value for a speech production parameter lies beyond its typical value for the task. Several sources discuss the methods that researchers and clinicians use to measure physical parameters of speech production (e.g., Behrman, 2007; Hixon, Weismer, & Hoit, 2008; Orlikoff & Baken, 1993). Examples of instruments that measure effort-related aspects of speech include strain gauges and electromyography. We discuss instruments such as these in later chapters that deal with research findings from studies of speakers who exhibit impaired fluency.

Psychophysical measurement of speaking effort consists of an observer's perceptions of the speaker's exertion while talking. In speech-language pathology research, perceptions of speaking effort usually are made using equal-interval rating scales, where one end of the scale corresponds with minimal effort and the other with maximal effort. Either the speaker or an observer can make the ratings. Both the speaker and the observer can rate speaking effort from either a physical perspective such as muscle tension or from a mental perspective such as the amount of attention being devoted to speech production. Although psychophysical assessments of speaking effort are not a routine component of contemporary fluency assessments (Al-Ghamedei & Logan, 2012), the American Speech-Language-Hearing Association (1995) does mention them in its guidelines for fluency assessment. Some researchers recently have shown renewed interest in conducting such measurements with speakers who stutter, as well. Thus, we focus our discussion on them in this section.

Psychophysical Assessments of Effort

Several studies have examined listeners' perceptions of the effort associated with producing various consonants within either VCV or CV contexts (e.g., Locke, 1972; Malecot, 1955; Parnell & Amerman, 1977; Young 1981). Young (1981) addressed some of the methodological shortcomings of previous research on the perceived effort of consonant production and reported that the following set of consonants was rated as being most effortful: [ʒ, ð, z, v, θ, g]. Young essentially discounted these findings, however, because of the poor reliability that raters showed when asked to re-rate their effort perceptions. He concluded that a listener's ability to evaluate the effort associated with the production of individual consonants is limited and that listeners likely base their perceptions of consonant effort on a range of physiological and psychological dimensions.

Other researchers have elicited effort ratings for longer samples of speech. For example, Ingham, Warner, Byrd, and Cotton (2006) examined 12 typical adults' self-ratings of speech-related physical effort during a 1-minute-long oral reading task. The participants recorded their self-ratings on a 9-point rating scale (1 = very effortless, 9 = very effortful) on three occasions during a single session. Their average effort rating was 1.59, indicating a perception of relatively effortless speech. The group's averages became more positive over time (rating 1 = 1.94, rating 3 = 1.30) and at all stages, the self-ratings from the typical speakers were much more favorable than self-ratings from a comparison group of adults who stutter.

In a follow-up study, Ingham et al. (2009) reported additional data on typical adults' self-ratings of speaking effort during eight 1-minute-long oral reading samples. On a 9-point scale (1 = very effortless), the average effort rating for the group was 2.98 (SD = 0.33), which was more favorable than the ratings from

a comparison group of adults who stuttered. Across trials, the average effort ratings varied from a low of 2.65 to a high of 3.68. In addition, the effort ratings reported in Ingham et al. (2009) were one scale point higher (indicative of more effortful speech) than the ratings reported in Ingham et al. (2006). The researchers hypothesized that the difference in ratings may have been due to the relatively fast articulation rate that participants in the 2009 study used. Findings such as these suggest that the construct of effort may be challenging to rate precisely, even with access to relatively long samples of speech. Nevertheless, effort ratings do seem to differentiate impaired speakers from unimpaired speakers reliably.

Naturalness in Typical Speakers

The construct of speech naturalness is routinely used in the fluency disorders literature. As with effort, naturalness data often are collected using equal-interval rating scales: a listener uses the scale to assign a numerical rating to a speech sample. The assigned rating reflects the listener's assessment of the relative amount of naturalness that the speaker exhibits within the sample. Rated samples in research studies range from single sentences (Logan, Roberts, Pretto, & Morey, 2002) to 1-minute stretches of running speech (Martin & Haroldson, 1992; Martin, Haroldson, & Triden, 1984).

Although researchers usually do not define naturalness for research participants, in a very general sense, it can be viewed as a measure of the extent to which a person's speech sounds like the speech of typical people. Put another way, it is a measure of the extent to which a speech sounds "normal." Of course, many factors can potentially affect a listener's perception of speech normalcy. Included among them are speech-based variables such as rate, disfluency frequency, disfluency duration, rhythm, and intonation. Markers of communicative competence such as message accuracy could conceivably enter into the construct as well, as could aspects of phonation such as fundamental frequency or intonation. In short, the basis for a listener's assessment of naturalness is unclear.

In Table 4–8, we present data from three studies of naturalness ratings for samples of speech from nondisordered speakers. In each study, listeners had to rate both fluent and disfluent samples of speech. As shown in Table 4–8, normally fluent speakers were not assigned perfect naturalness ratings. Rather, in all three studies, the mean naturalness ratings fell about 26% of the total scale length away from the best possible rating. Still, speakers with impaired fluency, even those who had received treatment, consistently earned less favorable naturalness ratings than the typical speakers did (Martin et al., 1984).

Talkativeness in Typical Speakers

The focus in this section is on the dimension of *talkativeness* as it pertains to verbal output, conversational participation, and communicative flexibility.

Verbal Fluency in Word-Generation Tasks

One index of talkativeness is *verbal fluency*. There is a large literature on word-level verbal fluency performance. Some of the studies in this area deal with *semantic fluency*, which is the ability to generate words within a specific semantic category such as animals (Rodríguez-Aranda & Martinussen, 2006). Many other studies, however, deal with *phonemic verbal fluency*, which frequently is assessed using the *Controlled Oral Word Association Test* (COWAT; Benton, 1967; Benton, Hamsher, & Sivan, 1994) or tasks similar to it. With the COWAT, an examinee attempts to name as many words as possible that begin with a certain letter. The examiner

Table 4–8. Mean Ratings (and Standard Deviations) of Speech Naturalness for Fluent Speech Samples From Adults With Typical Fluency

Study	Naturalness Rating		
	M	*SD*	±1 *SD*
Martin et al. (1984)	2.12	1.17	0.95–3.29
Martin & Haroldson (1992)[a]	2.30	1.21	1.09–3.51
Logan et al. (2002)[b]	2.15	1.14	1.01–3.29

Note. Ratings are based on a 9-point scale where 1 = highly natural speech and 9 = highly unnatural speech.

[a] Data are from the Audio condition.

[b] Data in this row were originally reported on a 7-point rating scale and converted to fit a 9-point scale.

presents the examinee with three letters in sequence—usually *F*, *A*, and *S*—and allows the examinee 1 minute per letter to generate the words. The examiner sums the total number of words produced across the three 1-minute trials to obtain a verbal fluency score.

Phonemic verbal fluency tasks like the COWAT are widely used in neuropsychological evaluations of cognitive functioning because they are sensitive to frontal lobe dysfunction and the detection of dementia (Rodríguez-Aranda & Martinussen, 2006). Through the mid-1990s, normative data for the COWAT were somewhat limited and distributed across numerous narrowly focused research reports. Since then, several research groups (e.g., Cerhan et al., 1998; Loonstra, Tarlow, & Sellers, 2001; Rodríguez-Aranda & Martinussen, 2006; Ruff, Light, Parker, & Levine, 1996) have bolstered the normative data for the task by conducting large-scale studies and by synthesizing previously published data through meta-analysis or the construction of "meta-norms."

Several factors affect adults' verbal fluency. One of these is education level. That is, on average, people with more education obtain higher verbal fluency scores than people with less education (Loonstra et al., 2001). Age affects the COWAT scores of healthy adults, as well. Porter, Collins, Muetzel, Lim, and Luciana (2011) demonstrated that young adults perform better on phonemic verbal fluency tasks than children do. The neuroimaging data that they collected in their study of children, teens, and young adults suggested that improvement in verbal fluency performance was associated with reduction in the thickness of cortical tissue within language-related regions of the left temporal and inferior frontal lobes. Porter et al. (2011) reported that reductions in cortical thickness begin during mid-childhood,

and they hypothesized that the changes reflect the development of efficient, adult-like neural organization patterns.

Results from one recent meta-analysis (Rodríguez-Aranda & Martinussen, 2006) suggest that phonemic verbal fluency increases modestly from early adulthood though roughly age 40. Between ages 40 and 60 years, however, performance gradually declines, and after age 60, the performance decline accelerates even more noticeably. Consequently, 70- to 79-year-olds perform worse than people who are 60 to 69 years old but better than people who are age 80 or older. Loonstra et al. (2001, p. 164) aggregated data from 32 studies of adults' FAS performance to generate "meta-norms" for verbal fluency performance at various points in the adulthood. According to their analysis, which pools data from more than 17,000 healthy adults, typical verbal fluency scores are as follows:

- Under age 40: M = 43.51 words, SD = 9.44 words,
- Age 40 to 59: M = 34.24 words, SD = 12.48 words,
- Age 60 to 79: M = 32.31 words, SD = 12.70 words, and
- Over age 80: M = 29.37 words, SD = 13.05 words.

Verbal Participation in Discourse

Another aspect of talkativeness involves verbal output during connected speech activities like conversation. Here, the focus is on the extent to which a speaker contributes to an interaction. The challenge is to determine how much a speaker typically says in any given situation. Much of the research in this area focuses on gender differences in verbal output. In the United States, the stereotypical view is that females talk more than males do. As we will see, though, this is not always the case.

Leaper and colleagues (Leaper & Ayres, 2007; Leaper & Smith, 2004) conducted two large meta-analyses to examine talkativeness patterns in children and adults. In both studies, the authors interpreted verbal output differences using Cohen's d statistic, an effect size measure that captures the magnitude of mean differences, in standard deviation units. With regard to adults' talkativeness, Leaper and Ayres (2007) unexpectedly found that, across the 62 studies that they analyzed, adult males talked more than adult females did. Although the difference was statistically significant, Leaper and Ayres noted that the magnitude of the difference was negligible ($d = |.14|$). Thus, they concluded that the overall difference in talkativeness that they detected between genders was unlikely to have practical sig-

nificance. With regard to children's talkativeness, Leaper and Smith (2004) found that, across the 61 studies in their analysis, girls talked more than boys did. Again, however, the researchers noted that the effect size associated with the statistically significant difference was negligible ($d = |.11|$). Thus, the statistical difference in talkativeness between girls and boys was unlikely to have practical significance.

In both studies, the researchers also examined the impact of numerous "moderator variables" (i.e., aspects of the research method) on talkativeness. Examples of moderator variables that affect adults' talkativeness are presented in Table 4–9. As shown, many factors affect adults' talkativeness. In some contexts, females talk more than males, but in other contexts, the opposite pattern exists. Conclusions about male and female verbosity also vary depending on how one defines talkativeness. For instance, in studies where talkativeness was defined by the number of

Table 4–9. Examples of Speaking Contexts in Leaper and Ayres' (2007) Meta-Analysis That Elicited Substantial Differences in Talkativeness Between Adult Males and Females

Males Talk More Than Females		Females Talk More Than Males	
Small Effect Size	**Moderate Effect Size**	**Small Effect Size**	**Moderate Effect Size**
Talking with mix of familiar and unfamiliar adults	Talking with a spouse or partner	Self-disclosure topics	Talking with male classmates
Talking with mix of male and female adults	Expressing disagreement	Talking with a dating partner	Talking with a child
Talking with others in the presence of a researcher	Discussing nonpersonal topics[a]	—	Engaging in a child-oriented activity

Note. The examples indicate contexts in which one gender talked significantly more than the other gender did (e.g., in studies of spousal interactions, males talked more than females). Effect sizes that ranged from $|.20|$ to $|.34|$ are considered small, while those that ranged from $|.35|$ to $|.56|$ are considered medium. Leaper and Ayres regarded effect sizes below $|.20|$ (not shown in this table) as negligible.

[a]The effect size for this context was –.79, which is moderate to large.

total conversational turns, females talked more than males did. In studies where talkativeness was defined by the mean length of utterance, however, males talked more than females did.

Methodological factors had less impact on children's talkativeness. Leaper and Smith (2004) reported that age was the only one of the many moderators they studied to have a substantial impact on talkativeness differences between boys and girls. More specifically, a meaningful gender effect existed only in studies involving 12- to 35-month-old children, where girls talked more than boys did. Comparisons of male-female talkativeness at other age levels yielded only negligible differences.

Patterns of Utterance Function

A third way of studying talkativeness is through examination of the communicative functions that speakers express through their conversational utterances. In Fillmore's (1979) view, a fluent speaker is one who uses speech for a variety of communicative purposes. In Chapter 1, we introduced Fey's (1986) speech-act classification system as a tool for evaluating the kinds of communicative functions a speaker expresses. The two fundamental communicative functions in Fey's system are *assertion* (e.g., unsolicited statements and comments) and *responsiveness* (e.g., answers to others' requests). Based on this, Fey proposed four types of communicative patterns:

1. Active communicators (i.e., people who consistently produce both assertive and responsive speech acts);
2. Passive communicators (i.e., people who consistently produce many responsive speech acts but few assertive speech acts);
3. Verbal noncommunicators (i.e., people who consistently produce many assertive speech acts but few responsive speech acts); and
4. Inactive communicators (i.e., people who consistently do not produce either assertive or responsive speech acts).

Normally, a speaker will show evidence of being able to produce both assertive and response acts (Type 1, above) consistently across a range of situations. However, some speakers with fluency impairment develop a "speak only if spoken to" style of communication (Type 2, above), which corresponds to the notion of participation restrictions. Styles 3 and 4 are less common in people who have impaired fluency, but they are associated with certain types of language-based impairments that can co-occur with fluency impairment. We discuss the latter issue in Chapter 8, under the discussion of cluttering.

Stability in Typical Speakers

Stability refers to consistency of performance. Clinicians can examine stability either within an individual or across a group of individuals. Researchers usually quantify performance stability with descriptive statistics such as the *range* or the *standard deviation*. When examining performance stability within a normally functioning person, it is expected that the speaker will perform in nearly the same way each time he or she performs a particular task. It also is expected that the person will perform with a similar level of competence across all of his or her daily activities (e.g., ordering food in a restaurant, talking on the telephone, conversing with friends). At a group level, it is expected that all people who are classified as having "normal fluency" will perform similarly to one another. That is, they should fall into a relatively narrow range of performance in terms of speech continuity, rate, rhythm, effort, and naturalness.

As was alluded to above, normal levels of talkativeness are more challenging to define, at least when it comes to measures of verbal output like the total number of words produced in a specific situation. Thus, for talkativeness, we may need to be satisfied with broader measures of verbal participation, such as the number of different situations a person speaks in or the extent to which a person feels satisfied with how much he or she says in a specific situation. In any event, the talkativeness levels among normally functioning speakers are more likely to be much more similar to one another than the talkativeness levels among impaired speakers are. Furthermore, normally functioning speakers usually attain even greater stability in performance when given the opportunity to practice or repeat a particular task. As we will see in later chapters, impaired speakers are less likely to benefit from practice and repetition than typical speakers are.

Summary

In this chapter, we have discussed several characteristics of "normal fluency." We have summarized data from studies on the types of disfluency that normally developing speakers produce and the frequency with which they produce them. We also have examined factors that affect speech rhythm, such as disfluency duration and repetition timing. Speakers who exhibit normal functioning in fluency usually will produce infrequent and relatively brief disfluencies, and disfluency frequency and duration will be similar across tasks. Speakers with disordered fluency will perform much differently, however. They typically will show more disfluencies and, sometimes, much longer disfluencies than typical speakers will, and their scores for these variables will be much more variable than those of typical speakers.

Among typical speakers, speech-related effort and naturalness will show patterns that are similar to those seen for disfluency frequency and duration. That is, scores will cluster tightly near the positive end of a rating scale, indicating a relative absence of effort and speech production that sounds very natural. Most speakers with disordered fluency will perform quite differently: Speech is apt to be rated as more effortful and less natural than the speech of typical speakers. Perceptions of effort and naturalness are associated with disfluency frequency, disfluency duration, and speech rate.

Researchers have identified a long list of factors that influence fluency performance in normal speakers. This means that a speaker will talk more fluently in some situations than in others. A key feature of normal fluency is that the speaker's performance variability is much more limited in comparison to that of disordered speakers. A normally fluent speaker talks in nearly the same way from one task to the next, and from one day to the next. Thus, normally fluent speakers exhibit stable fluency—a dependable speech pattern. Speakers with disordered fluency lack such dependability. Their speech may sound rather fluent in one situation but rather disfluent in another. This lack of fluency dependability is a source of frustration and distress for many people who have impaired fluency. In the remaining sections of the text, we address issues related to the characteristics and consequences of fluency disorders in greater depth, and we explore common methods that clinicians use to assess fluency performance and help speakers improve their fluency functioning.

SECTION

II

Etiologies and Characteristics of Fluency Disorders

5

Developmental Stuttering: Basic Fluency Characteristics

Developmental stuttering is the type of stuttering that emerges during childhood —for no obvious or outwardly observable reason—in the context of what otherwise appears to be normal development. In many textbooks and research articles, authors routinely refer to developmental stuttering simply as *stuttering*, which reflects the fact that this disorder is more common that any of the nondevelopmental forms of stuttering are. In this chapter, we review an assortment of findings that pertain to the nature and characteristics of developmental stuttering. Such information is necessary for planning and implementing essential clinical activities related to assessment, treatment, and client counseling.

Terminology

Most beginning clinicians are likely to be familiar with the term *stuttering* and the style of speech that typifies it. Another term that clinicians may encounter in the contemporary fluency disorders literature is *stammering*. The latter term is essentially a synonym for stuttering. Although the term *stammering* is not widely used in the United States, people use it with some regularity in other predominately English-speaking nations (e.g., New Zealand, England). However, even in those countries, the term *stuttering* is encountered frequently.

As a side note, it appears that contemporary usage of *stammering* is quite different from the usage of the term in the 1800s and early 1900s. Fletcher (1914) reported that, in 1830, the German author Schulthess described *stammering* (*Stammein*, in German) as being a distinct "speech defect" from stuttering (*Stottern*, in German). Makeun (1909) also made a distinction between the two terms, with *stuttering* referring to the notion of "difficult speech" (which perhaps implies excessive effort), while *stammering* referred to "incorrect" speech, which perhaps implies errors in speech sound production. Whatever the connotations for those terms may have been, the distinction between them seems to have been lost throughout the years, and today, one can consider the two terms as equivalent in meaning.

Also worth noting, the word *stutter* has several different connotations. For instance, in sports settings, it describes certain hesitant or choppy moves that an athlete makes (e.g., a "stutter step"). In speech settings, it can refer to certain isolated occurrences of disfluent speech—even in speakers who are regarded as having normal fluency. When people use the term in the latter way, it can leave the impression that everyone is a "person who stutters" at times. Terms like *stutterer* or *person who stutters*, however, are diagnostic labels that refer to cases wherein a person produces characteristic patterns of disfluency—at a frequency and in a manner that indicates the presence of a disorder (Sander, 1963). The main point for a speech-language pathologist to grasp is that although there occasionally may be superficial similarities between the disfluent behaviors of typical speakers and speakers who are diagnosed with developmental stuttering, one should not assume that the underlying nature of their disfluent speech patterns are equivalent.

Historical Perspective

Based on historical records, it appears that awareness of stuttering dates back to ancient times. Descriptions of the disorder are noted in clay tables from ancient Mesopotamia, 2,500-year-old writings of the Chinese poet Laotze, and Old Testament passages in the Bible (Van Riper, 1982). Systematic study of developmental stuttering did not begin in earnest, however, until the early decades of the 1900s. A search through English-language journals prior to the 1920s reveals a smattering of published research reports. Interestingly, some of the research questions from that era resemble those that modern-day researchers are tackling. For instance, Fletcher (1914) conducted a multistep experimental investigation of respiratory, laryngeal, and articulation functioning with adolescent and young adult speakers who stuttered. Issues related to speech motor control and coordination continue to be of interest to researchers today.

The pace of stuttering-related research increased steadily during the 1920s and the early 1930s (Mathews, 1986). In the late 1920s and early 1930s, Travis (1927, 1931, 1934) published a series of studies in which he examined physiological performance in speakers with developmental stuttering. Brown (1937, 1938, 1945) published several studies that examined the linguistic contexts within which stutter-like disfluencies were most apt to occur. At this same time and in the following years, Johnson and colleagues (e.g., Johnson & Associates, 1959; Johnson & Colley, 1945) published a wide range of studies on the characteristics of stuttering during childhood and adulthood. As speech-language pathology became increasingly established as a profession during the middle part of the 20th century, the volume of stuttering-related research increased dramatically. As we move into the 21st century, it is apparent that research on stuttering now occurs on a global scale and these research efforts have led to an increasingly accurate and detailed understanding of the causes, characteristics, and effects of the disorder.

Defining Developmental Stuttering

A definition is a concise statement about the meaning(s) associated with a word or term. Thus, an effective definition for the term *developmental stuttering* should provide a concise statement of the nature and characteristics of the disorder. Although definitional issues might seem inconsequential within the big scheme of providing effective clinical services for people who stutter, a definition is, in many ways, the basis for everything a clinician does in clinical practice. After all, one's definition of stuttering has the potential to affect downstream issues such as which clients are and are not considered to stutter, which symptoms are and are not considered to be characteristic of the disorder, and which clinical measures are best suited to capture changes in speech disability. One's definition of stuttering also might affect how the prevalence of stuttering is measured. For instance, it is plausible that under some definitions, a stutter-like disfluency pattern in a person with Down syndrome might be viewed as something other than stuttering. For these reasons, it is critical to create a clear, comprehensive, and valid definition of stuttering.

Defining developmental stuttering has proven to be challenging. Mostly, this is because of limitations in researchers' ability to determine what causes the disorder and, to a lesser degree, what the primary symptoms of the disorder are. Wingate (1964a), writing some 50 years ago, noted that an acceptable definition of developmental stuttering is one which adheres to basic scientific principles and is based strictly on observable features of the disorder. Scientific practice is rooted in *hypothesis testing* and the principles of *empiricism* (i.e., building knowledge through direct experience and observation) and *rationalism* (i.e., logical thought and deductive reasoning) (Maxwell & Satake, 2006). Wingate argued that conjecture about the etiology of developmental stuttering has no place in a definition of developmental stuttering. Rather, etiology should be mentioned only after it has been reliably determined through rigorous scientific investigation.

Early Attempts at Defining Stuttering

At the time Wingate presented his criteria for "a standard definition of stuttering," there were many competing definitions of developmental stuttering. Many of these definitions were lacking in rigor because they principally were based on the author(s) intuition and/or authoritative opinion. From a scientific perspective, such definitions were flawed and bound to result in misdirected conceptions about the disorder. For example, some early definitions included behavioral characteristics, which upon subsequent scientific study, were not essential features of the disorder. Other definitions made no mention whatsoever of the chief symptoms of the disorder and, instead, consisted mostly of an author's beliefs about the etiology of stuttering. Compounding the shortcomings of the latter approach was the fact that the evidence base for such beliefs was often poor.

Coriat's (1943) psychoanalytic explanation of stuttering illustrates the type of definition to which Wingate (1964a) objected. Writing from a psychoanalytic perspective, Coriat stated that "(stuttering) is a psychoneurosis caused by the persistence into later life of early pregenital oral nursing, oral sadistic, and anal sadistic components" (p. 27), and went on to link stuttering to "oral nursing" and "oral cannibalistic" dreams. Note that Coriat (1943) described developmental stuttering in relation to assumptions about what caused the disorder (i.e., psychoneurosis) and that the salient characteristics of stuttered speech were not mentioned. Note also the presence of constructs such as "oral nursing" and "oral sadistic" components. Many definitions from this era had similar shortcomings. In each case, it raises questions such as the following: Would a researcher be able to measure the constructs included in the definition?; and, if so, what do the constructs tell us about the speech disorder known as stuttering?

Contemporary Definitions

Most contemporary definitions for stuttering are organized around behaviors or qualities that are both observable and measureable, and they make no mention of causality except, perhaps, to acknowledge that the cause of stuttering is not fully understood. Given the pace at which scientific knowledge about developmental stuttering has progressed in recent years, however, we are optimistic that gaps in our understanding about the cause of stuttering will be filled in the not-too-distant future. Until then, however, we are left with interim definitions for developmental stuttering—ones that, as Wingate (1964a) said, are "phenotypic" in character and based on observable features of the disorder. Such definitions, while admittedly incomplete, still can be of use to researchers and clinicians.

In Table 5–1, we present stuttering-related symptoms from Wingate's so-called "standard definition" of developmental stuttering along with the primary stuttering-related symptoms included in five more recent definitions. As can be seen, the symptoms mentioned included in the definitions offered by the World Health Organization (WHO, 2010) and Logan (2011) are largely consistent with those in Wingate's (1964a) definition. Both definitions primarily focus on the disfluency types that commonly are observed with developmental stuttering, i.e., repetition of short elements of speech and fixed articulatory postures that result in prolonged or "blocked" sounds. Logan's (2011) definition focuses on the most common, observable manifestations of disfluency and adds descriptive information about the onset of the disorder and its developmental course. Van Riper's (1982) definition is less constrained than the others in terms of the types of disfluency that are said to characterize stuttered speech, whereas the WHO's (2010) definition is a bit broader than the others in terms of the disfluency types it includes and its inclusion of a criterion for disorder identification.

Not everyone is satisfied with symptom-based definitions such as these, however. For instance, some (Einarsdóttir & Ingham, 2005) have argued, correctly, that part-word repetitions and sound prolongations are not the only symptoms of developmental stuttering and, in some clients, may not even be the primary symptoms. Bloodstein and Bernstein Ratner (2008) made a similar point when they stated that the symptoms of stuttering are apparent not only in speech disruptions, but in many other speech parameters as well, including rate, pitch, loudness, and inflection, and that stuttering symptoms

Table 5–1. Examples of Symptoms Noted in Definitions for Developmental Stuttering

Author	Symptoms
Wingate (1964a, p. 488)	Disrupted speech fluency, involuntary repetitions or prolongations of sounds, syllables, and single-syllable words; disruptions are frequent or marked and not easily controlled; disruptions may be accompanied by other behaviors in speech system or other body structures, or by use of stereotyped speech and evidence of speech-related struggle or emotional arousal. (Wingate added that the "immediate source of stuttering is some incoordination expressed in the peripheral speech mechanism" but the ultimate cause is presently unknown.)
Van Riper (1982, p. 15)	"Stuttering occurs when the forward flow of speech is interrupted by a motorically disrupted speech sound, syllable, or word or by the speaker's reaction thereto."
Perkins, Kent, & Curlee (1991, p. 734)	" . . . a disruption of speech that is experienced by the speaker as loss of control."
Bloodstein and Bernstein Ratner (2008, p. 9)	" . . . whatever is perceived as stuttering by a reliable observer who has relatively good agreement with others."
World Health Organization (2010, p. 227)	Frequent repeating or prolonging of sounds, syllables, or words, as well as "frequent hesitations or pauses that disrupt the rhythmic flow of speech"; disruptions may be accompanied by associated movement of the face or other body structures. (The WHO added that these disfluent behaviors are often transient during early childhood and are considered a disorder when they lead to marked disturbance in speech fluency.)
Logan (2011, p. 2420)	Frequent and/or excessively long disruption in the forward flow of speech; common disfluency types include repetition of sounds, syllables, words (particularly monosyllabic words) and audible or inaudible fixed articulatory postures. (Logan added that these symptoms usually appear between age 2 to 5 years and they may persist across the lifespan.)

frequently extend beyond the bounds of speech such that they are manifested in things such as facial expression and body posture. Bloodstein and Bernstein Ratner also remark that the notion of stuttering "moments" is flawed. For some speakers, evidence of stuttering can be observed across entire utterances.

Remarks such as these suggest the need for developing a definition of stuttering that goes beyond how a client "sounds" to include other salient but often subtle markers of the disorder (Smith, 1992; Smith & Kelly, 1997). For instance, there are clients who can attain fluent-sounding speech by using word avoidance and word substitution. Although the speech of such individuals sounds fluent to the casual listener, most of these speakers continue to view themselves as having impaired fluency because of the frequent need to scan speech plans for words that might be difficult to produce fluently. A definition of stuttering that is based solely on overt disfluency misses cases like these.

There also is the matter of clients who have attained *controlled fluency*; that is, the ability to circumvent the overt disfluencies that characterize stuttering by actively monitoring and/or altering the timing and tension of speech movements (Guitar, 2006). Controlled fluency generally is viewed positively in the context of fluency treatment programs because the speaker sounds relatively smooth when talking; however, the client may again retain the self-concept of a "person who stutters" if the act of controlling fluency requires inordinate conscious effort. In these cases, speech may sound fluent to the listener, but it does not feel fluent to the speaker (Finn & Ingham, 1994). Thus, smooth speech is not always "normal speech" from the client's perspective. There clearly is a need to develop a definition of stuttering that better captures the multidimensional nature of the disorder.

The remaining definition of stuttering in Table 5–1 comes from Perkins, Kent, and Curlee (1991). The symptom profile mentioned in this definition is markedly different from most of the others in that the authors define stuttering from the speaker's perspective rather than the listener's perspective. Certainly, there is some appeal to the idea that the speaker knows better than the listener does if stuttering has occurred. After all, the speaker has access to internal feelings, sensations, and thoughts that the listener does not. As such, the speaker is positioned to comment on his or her internal speech experiences and the extent to which they feel like stuttering.

Speaker-based definitions of stuttering have not received widespread acceptance among experts who study stuttering, however (for a discussion of this issue, see Smith, 1992). The main reason for this is that the approach rests exclusively on the client's self-reports, and, to date, another researcher or clinician cannot corroborate such reports empirically. We can readily recall a host of first-hand experiences throughout the years, both in the role of clinician as well as client, where the speaker and listener's judgments about stuttered speech were mismatched. In some instances, the clinician clearly heard an utterance as stuttered, but the speaker experienced it as disfluent but not stuttered. In other instances, the clinician heard a fluent utterance, but the speaker experienced the utterance as stuttered. And, in still other instances, the clinician heard an utterance as stuttered, but the client had not detected any problem with fluency at all. Mismatches of this sort underscore the limitations associated with the use of a definition that is rooted solely in either the listener's observations or the speaker's subjective experience. Given these issues, it seems that a clinician certainly should ask a client about his or her speech experiences but should not rely on such reports as a sole source of clinical data. Perhaps in the future, if some of these stuttering measurement issues are resolved, we will see the development of definitions that reflect the multiple factors that are associated with the disorder itself as well as the speaker's associated experiences.

Characteristics of Stuttered Speech

Continuity Characteristics

One way to describing the characteristics of stuttered speech is to examine the kinds of continuity interruptions speakers who stutter produce.

Overall Disfluency Frequency

Developmental stuttering is characterized by frequent interruptions in speech continuity. In nearly all cases of developmental stuttering, the speaker's overall disfluency frequency (all disfluency types combined) will be greater than the frequency that is observed in the general population. Disfluency frequency can range from only slightly greater than normal (a slight deviation) to much, much greater than normal (a profound deviation), and, in general, the more disfluencies a speaker produces, the more his or her communicative functioning will be limited.

Frequency of Repetitions, Prolongations, and Blocks

When one closely examines the disfluency profiles of speakers who stutter, it becomes apparent that they usually produce only *certain types* of disfluency more frequently than normal. Most speakers who stutter produce two classes of disfluency excessively. The first type is disfluency that features repetition; that is, part-word repetition, whole-word repetition, and multiword or phrase repetition. The second type is disfluency that features fixed, held or physically tense articulatory postures. The latter type of disfluency leads to either *audible sound prolongations*, which occur when a sound source is present and exhaled air continues to move through the vocal tract, or so-called *inaudible prolongations*, which occur when the speaker constricts the vocal tract—usually at a place of articula-

tion—such that exhaled air is prevented ("blocked") from moving through the vocal tract. Some speakers who stutter may produce both repetitions and fixed articulatory postures excessively, while other speakers who stutter may produce only one of these forms of disfluency excessively. In most people who stutter, it is the excessive frequency of repeating and/or prolonging/blocking that makes the overall disfluency frequency greater than normal.[1] Bloodstein (1960) reported on the characteristics of stuttered speech in children aged 2 to 16 years. According to his analysis, about one-third of the preschoolers who stuttered featured "slow, easy repetitions" as the sole speech symptom of stuttered speech, but, by the age of 16 years, only 8% of the cases who stuttered did.

In many contemporary studies of stuttered speech, researchers define stuttering-related behavior narrowly as consisting of part-word repetitions and prolongations/blocks. In some studies, the researchers add monosyllable word repetitions to the mix. During the past 20 years or so, some researchers have used the term *stutter-like* disfluency to characterize these disfluency types. Although these disfluency types tend to be the most prominent ones in the speech of many speakers who stutter, they are not the only kinds of disfluency that, from a statistical standpoint, differentiate speakers who stutter from speakers who do not stutter. Evidence for the latter claim comes from studies such as the one by Ambrose and Yairi (1999), in which the researchers compared speakers who stutter to typical speakers in terms of

---

[1]The term "block" has been used in several ways in the speech-language pathology literature. Some use it generically; that is, as a label for any type of stuttering-related disfluency. In this text, we use it in the way Guitar (2006) did, which is as a label for disfluencies that result in a fixed and/or excessively tense articulatory posture as well as cessation of sound. The articulatory posture may be held for an excessive length of time and/or may be accompanied by excessive physical tension. Thus, *a block* includes the concept of *inaudible prolongation* along with disfluencies that feature tense articulatory postures either with or without notable prolongation.

the frequency with which they produced specific types of disfluency. In that study, the researchers examined the disfluency patterns of 90 children who stuttered and 54 children who did not stutter during parent-child conversational speech samples. The researchers found statistically significant differences between the two groups of children for all three categories of repetition they analyzed: part-word repetitions, single-syllable word repetition, and repetitions of multisyllable words or multiple words (i.e., phrase repetition). For each comparison, there was a less than 1 in 1,000 chance that the observed differences were due to sampling error. Thus, it appeared likely that the children's fluency status (stuttering versus nonstuttering) explained the differences in disfluency frequencies between the groups.

In addition to comparing the mean number of disfluencies that speakers who stutter and speakers with typical fluency produce, researchers also attempt to evaluate the *magnitude* of difference between groups. One can evaluate the magnitude of the difference between two group means using the *d* statistic (Cohen, 1988), which, in the arena of statistics, is one of several measures of *effect size*. The *d* statistic essentially adjusts the difference between two group means by taking into account the extent to which individual scores within each group vary about the group means. In a more practical sense, the *d* statistic provides information about the extent to which the difference between two means is likely to have practical significance. For example, in the context of stuttering, effect size measures can provide information about issues such as the extent to which a particular disfluency pattern would be noticeable to listeners. Thus, a researcher may discover statistical significance between two groups in terms of a fluency-related behavior, but

after examining the size of the statistical effect, the researcher may conclude that it has very little practical significance.

In Table 5–2, we present estimates of effect sizes that we computed using data that Ambrose and Yairi (1999) presented in their study. The effect sizes are the *d* statistics associated with each of the disfluency comparisons that were statistically significant in that study. For each of the *d* values, we also include a test-based interpretation based on information in Cohen (1988). As indicated in the table, the *d* values are of sufficient magnitude to suggest that each of the differences in disfluency frequency is likely to have clinical relevance.

Also in Table 5–2 are disfluency frequency ratios that we computed from the frequency data that Ambrose and Yairi (1999) reported. The ratios provide a sense for how much more often one group produces a certain type of disfluency compared to the other group. This ratio measure is rather crude in comparison to the *d* statistic because it does not account for the variation of individual scores within a group. Nonetheless, it offers another way of thinking about how different the two groups of children were. As shown in Table 5–2, at a group level, the children who stuttered produced twice as many multiword/phrase repetitions, 5 times as many single-syllable words repetitions, 9 times as many part-word repetitions, and 19 times as many disrhythmic phonations (e.g., prolongations/blocks) as the children who did not stutter. Interestingly, however, when the magnitude of the difference between the groups for disrhythmic phonation is expressed in terms of effect size, it is less than that for either part-word repetition or single-syllable word repetition. This is because of the relatively large variability that children exhibited in the frequency of disrhythmic phonation.

Table 5–2. Disfluency Frequency Ratios and Effect Sizes Associated With Comparisons Between Children Who Stutter and Children Who Do Not Stutter From Ambrose and Yairi (1999) for Disfluency Types That Differed Significantly in Frequency Between Groups

By Disfluency Type	Disfluency Frequency Ratio[a]	Effect Size	
		d	Interpretation
Part-word repetition	9:1	2.06	Much larger than typical
Single-syllable word repetition	5:1	1.93	Much larger than typical
Multisyllable word and phrase repetition	2:1	0.84	Larger than typical
Disrhythmic phonation	19:1	1.57	Much larger than typical
By Location of Speech Interruption			
Within a word boundary	11:1	—	—
At a word boundary	4:1	—	—

Note. The present author computed these effect sizes based on data reported from Ambrose and Yairi (1999).

[a]Ratios were computed by dividing the disfluency frequency for children who stuttered by the disfluency frequency for children who did not stutter. For example, children who stuttered produced 9 times as many part-word repetitions as children who did not stutter.

As described above, substantial differences between the groups were evident for all repetition types—even multisyllable word and phrase repetitions (*d* = .80). Other researchers (e.g., LaSalle & Conture, 1995) have reported this pattern as well. Although Ambrose and Yairi (1999) regarded multisyllable word and phrase repetitions as a form of "other (nonstuttered) disfluency," the data in Table 5–2 clearly show that, based on effect size, the children who stuttered performed very differently than the children who did not stutter on this type of disfluency. Thus, even though multisyllable word and phrase repetitions do not seem to be as strong of a marker for stuttered speech as, say, part-word repetitions or sound prolongation (disrhythmic phonation), it nonetheless appears to be relevant to the stuttering experience. More recently, Reilly et al. (2013) examined stuttering patterns in a large sample of preschool-aged children. They found that children

who produced whole-word repetitions—a disfluency type that is characterized as "normal" in many research studies—at the time of stuttering onset were *less likely* to recover from stuttering within 12 months of onset than those children who did not produce whole-word repetitions at onset. Thus, on the basis of this study and others discussed in this section, there seems to be clinical value in assessing *many* types of disfluency and, when doing so, to avoid assuming that certain types of disfluency (e.g., whole-word repetitions, phrase repetitions) are inherently "normal" and thus less relevant to stuttered speech.

Frequency of Interjections and Revisions

Results from a host of research studies indicate that, on average, speakers who stutter produce interjections and revisions at about the same frequency as typical speakers do. Thus, frequency data for these two disfluency types usually are not a reliable marker of stuttered speech.[2] As with most "rules-of-thumb" that pertain to communication disorders, however, there are clients who do not follow the general pattern. For instance, some speakers who stutter report that they routinely produce interjections such as *um*, *uh*, and *like* in reaction to the expectation of continuity interruptions that otherwise would lead to repeating or prolonging/blocking. At such times, the speaker essentially "slips in" an interjection just before the point within a planned utterance where the stuttering-related continuity interruption is expected to occur. In this context, the interjection seems to be an attempt to compensate for a disfluency that might be disruptive to communication and perceived as unusual by the listener. This process is illustrated in the example below:

Example 5–1:

Intended utterance: *We're holding a fundraiser on Saturday.*

Unfolding utterance: <u>*We're holding*</u>[(!)] *a f*[(#)]*undraiser on Saturday.*

Final spoken utterance: *We're holding a |um| fundraiser on Saturday.*

In the example above, the speaker first formulates an intended utterance. The "unfolding utterance" illustrates the error detection process midway through the utterance. In the example, the underlined text represents portions of the utterance that the speaker is in the process of saying, and the superscript (!) indicates the point during the utterance when the speaker detects the impending speech production problem. The second superscript (#) represents the point where the speaker expects continuity interruption to occur. So, as the speaker is saying *holding,* he anticipates a continuity interruption in the transition from the onset to the rime of the first syllable in *fundraiser.* As noted above, the boundary between syllable onset and rime is a common location for continuity interruption in stuttered speech (for detailed discussions of this phenomenon, see Chapter 3 in this text and Wingate, 1988). The speaker reacts to the anticipated interruption by stopping speech just before the word *fundraiser* and inserting the *um.* The editing time associated with this "filled pause" apparently enables the speaker to repair the covert error that triggered the interruption. In any case, the speaker proceeds through utterance without repeating, prolonging, or blocking and, with the use of interjection, the utterance sounded less atypical than it would have sounded if a repetition, prolongation, or block had occurred. In summary, while interjections are not a routine symptom of stuttered speech, some speakers who stutter may use them routinely in reaction to the expectation of being unable to advance an utterance toward its completion due to stuttering. In such cases, interjection is relevant to the stuttering experience.

Location of the Moment of Interruption

Another way to compare the disfluency patterns of children who stutter and

---

[2]This dissociation in the frequency of occurrence among speakers who stutter suggests that interjection and revision typically arise from speech production problems that differ from those associated with repeating and prolonging/blocking.

children who do not stutter is through examination of where the speaker interrupts speech continuity during disfluency (Conture, 2001). One option is to interrupt speech at a word boundary. When a speaker attempts to repair interruptions of this sort, it leads to the repetition of words and phrases (e.g., |*Jarvis-*|*Jarvis went* |*to the-*|*to the library*).[3] Another option is to interrupt speech within a word boundary. When a speaker attempts to repair interruptions of this sort, it leads to part-word repetition and sound prolongations/blocks (e.g., |*Ja-*| *Jarvis* |*wwww*|*went to the library*).

If we reanalyze the data from Ambrose and Yairi (1999) in this way (refer to the lower portion of Table 5–2), we see that, among the disfluency types that differentiated the two groups, the children who stuttered produced 11 times as many disfluencies that featured *within-word* interruption as the children with typical fluency did. In contrast, the children who stuttered produced 4 times as many disfluencies that featured interruption at a word boundary. Although both ratios are impressively large, it is apparent that speakers who stutter are especially prone to interrupting speech continuity in mid-word when they are disfluent (for further discussion of within- and between-word disfluency, see Conture, 2001). Of course, this is just another way of saying that speakers who stutter produce more part-word repetitions and sound prolongations/blocks than those with typical fluency do. Nonetheless, this type of description offers an additional perspective into how the patterns of stuttered and typically fluent speech differ. The underlying expla-

nation for this pattern of frequent within-word continuity interruption is unclear. Nonetheless, frequent within-word interruption in speech continuity is a reliable marker of stuttered speech.

Ratio of Repetitions and Prolongations to Interjections and Revisions

Based on the information in the preceding sections, it should be apparent that the majority of disfluency types observed in speakers who stutter feature some form of repeating, prolonging, or blocking in speech. Accordingly, for cases that fit this general pattern, one can summarize the disfluency frequency data of speakers who stutter by combining into one superordinate category all of the specific disfluency types that they produce more frequently than normal. Given research findings like those discussed earlier in this chapter, we have adopted the practice of placing the following disfluency types into this "super" category when evaluating cases of suspected stuttering: part-word repetitions, single- and multisyllable word repetitions, repetitions of multiple words and phrases, and sound prolongation/blocks. In recent years, we have adopted the descriptive, albeit inelegant, moniker "repetitions, prolongations, and blocks" (abbreviated as RPB) for this category. Conversely, we have assigned disfluency types that *do not* reliably differentiate speakers who stutter from speakers with typical fluency—namely interjections and revisions—into a separate superordinate category.[4] We have adopted the descriptive, and equally inelegant, moniker "interjections

---

[3]Continuity interruption at word boundaries also is associated with interjection and revision, but the latter disfluency types typically do not differentiate children who stutter from children who do not stutter.
[4]If a clinician happens to analyze pause frequency, it would fit into this category as well.

and revisions" (abbreviated as IR) for this category.

Also included in the RPB category are any unusually structured or behaviorally complex instances of disfluency that feature repeating, prolonging, or blocking. An example of the latter is the following part-word repetition with a filled editing phase: |*Oak- Oak- um* | *Oakland clinched a playoff spot.* One might argue that this disfluency could just as easily be assigned to the IR category; however, we would counter that the within-word interruption (a behavior that is unusual among typical speakers) makes it more appropriately placed among the disfluency types that typify stuttered speech. The multi-iteration repetition, which also is unusual among typical speakers, is a second reason for doing so.

In Figure 5–1, we contrast the fluency profile that a clinician would commonly observe in a speaker who stutters with one that a clinician would see in a speaker with typical fluency. As shown in the figure, speakers who stutter are likely to produce more total disfluencies than speakers with typical fluency and the majority of their disfluencies will fit into the RPB category. Typical speakers, in contrast, will show the opposite pattern: Fewer total disfluencies than speakers with typical fluency and the majority of their disfluencies will fit into the IR category.

Yairi (1997) reviewed a number of research studies in which the authors presented information about the frequency with which children produced specific types of disfluency. In study after study, the group results for children who stutter were the same: the combined frequency of

part-word repetitions, single-syllable word repetitions, and disrhythmic phonations (e.g., sound prolongation/blocks) was greater than the combined frequency of other types of disfluency such as interjections and revision.[5] In contrast, children with typical fluency showed the opposite pattern: The majority of their disfluencies fit into a superordinate category of "other disfluency" that included interjection, revision, multisyllable word repetition, and phrase repetition. Across the studies, the short-element repetitions and disrhythmic phonations comprised between 60 to 75% of all disfluencies the children produced. Although Yairi's (1997) classification approach was slightly different from the one we described in Figure 5–1 (the main difference is that he separated multisyllable word repetitions and repetitions of multiple words and phrases from the part-word and single-syllable word repetitions), the general pattern he uncovered was the same as we described in Figure 5–1.

Yairi's (1997) rationale for putting multisyllable word repetitions and repetitions of multiple words and phrases with the "other disfluencies" was that those disfluencies occurred infrequently and constituted a relatively small proportion of children's overall disfluency. We might add a second reason: Multisyllable word repetitions and repetitions of multisyllable words and phrases are not the kinds of disfluency that listeners typically regard as "stuttered" (Williams & Kent, 1958; Zebrowski & Conture, 1989). Still, as we suggested earlier in this chapter, one also can make a good case for including multisyllable word repetitions and repetitions of multisyllable words and phrases into

---

[5]Yairi (1997) used the term *short-element repetition* as a superordinate term for part-word and single-syllable word repetitions and *stutter-like disfluency* as a superordinate term for short-element repetition and disrhythmic phonation (e.g., prolongations and blocks).

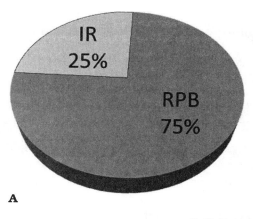

Speaker who Stutters: Disfluency data (by type)
- **Total disfluencies:** 16 per 100 syllables

- **RPBs:** 12 per 100 syllables (75% of total)
  - Part-word repetitions: 8 per 100 syllables
  - Whole-word repetitions: 2 per 100 syllables
  - Prolongations/blocks: 2 per 100 syllables

- **IRs:** 4 per 100 syllables (25% of total)
  - Interjections: 2 per 100 syllables
  - Revisions: 2 per 100 syllables

A

Typical Speaker: Disfluency data (by type)
- **Total disfluencies:** 6 per 100 syllables

- **RPBs:** 2 per 100 syllables (33% of total)
  - Part-word repetitions: 0 per 100 syllables
  - Whole-word repetitions: 2 per 100 syllables
  - Prolongations/blocks: 0 per 100 syllables

- **IRs:** 4 per 100 syllables (67% of total)
  - Interjections: 1 per 100 syllables
  - Revisions: 3 per 100 syllables

B

Figure 5–1. Pie charts illustrating the ratio of repetitions, prolongations, and blocks (RPBs) to interjections and revisions (IRs) in a hypothetical speaker who stutters and a speaker with typical fluency. The tables to the right of each pie chart contain data about the total number of disfluencies per 100 syllables, the number of RPBs and IRs per 100 syllables (and % of total disfluency), and, within each of those categories, the frequency with which each specific disfluency type is produced per 100 syllables. **A.** As indicated by the pie chart and accompanying table in this portion of the figure, most of the disfluencies produced by speakers who stutter fit into the RPB category. **B.** As indicated by the pie chart and accompanying table in this portion of the figure, most of the disfluencies produced by typical speakers fit into the IR category. Speakers with typical fluency usually produce less total disfluency than speakers who stutter, as indicated by the data in the two tables and the differences in the diameters of the two pie charts.

the same category as short-element repetitions and prolongations/blocks. This is because each of these repetition types differentiates between children who stutter and children with typical fluency in both a statistical and a practical (i.e., effect size) sense. Consequently, we place them in the RPB category in this chapter and elsewhere in this text.

Deviations in Disfluency Structure or Distribution

As we explained in Chapter 3, the disfluencies that typical speakers produce usually are quite consistent in form. For example, in a typical speaker, interjections usually contain only one editing term; word repetitions usually contain only one additional iteration of a word and no editing terms; overt speech errors usually require only one attempt to revise; and so forth. The standard or prototypical forms for disfluency essentially are those that appear in the various disfluency classification systems that we described in Chapter 3. When typical speakers produce disfluency, they usually do so using one of the forms described in these disfluency classification systems.

In our experiences with transcribing stuttered speech, however, speakers who stutter are more likely than typical speakers to exhibit disfluencies that deviate from the prototypical forms. In some of our past work (Logan, 2009; Logan & LaSalle, 1999), we have used the terms *behaviorally complex disfluency* and *clustering* to characterize such instances of disfluency; that is, disfluent segments of speech that contain elements of two or more of the standard behavioral descriptors for disfluency. We list examples of such disfluencies below:

Example 5–2: *|N- n- Neal| David bought my old guitar.* {part-word repetition within a word that subsequently is revised}

Example 5–3: *| They- um |They should finish the job by noon.* {use of an interjection within the editing phase of a word repetition}

Example 5–4: *. . . over at |nnnn- um nnnn- um |Newberry High School . . .* {prolonging a sound that is repeated + interjecting during the editing phase of a repetition}

Researchers also have used the term *clustering* to refer to instances in which a speaker produces disfluency on adjacent syllables or within adjacent words. This is illustrated in the following examples:

Example 5–5: *|N- n-|Nancy |and- |and |Ma-|Mary drove into town.*

Example 5–6: *|I-|I |um| think they will be back in time for lunch.*

In Example 5–5, three consecutive target words within the utterance feature forms of repetition. In Example 5–6, the adjacent syllables *I* and *think* either contain or are preceded by disfluency.

Disfluent segments like those in Example 5–2 through 5–6 occur regularly in the conversational speech of people who stutter, and at a frequency that is much greater than that for typical speakers (Hubbard & Yairi, 1988; LaSalle & Conture, 1995; Logan & LaSalle, 1999). In studies of conversational interactions between children who stutter and a parent (Hubbard & Yairi, 1988; LaSalle & Conture, 1995), the children who stuttered produced about 3 to 6 times as many irregularly structured or complex disfluencies as the children with typical fluency did, and some of the children with typical fluency did not produce *any* irregularly structured or behaviorally complex disfluencies at all. Logan and LaSalle (1999) found that 17% of the conversational utterances from children who stuttered contained at least one instance of irregularly structured or complex disfluency, compared to 3.5% of the utterances from children who did not stutter.

Not only do children who stutter produce more behaviorally complex disfluencies than children who do not stutter, but the disfluencies feature more behavioral descriptors, as well (Hubbard & Yairi, 1988; LaSalle & Conture, 1995). For example, Hubbard and Yairi (1988) reported that 40% of all behaviorally complex disfluencies from the children who stuttered featured three to four disfluency descriptors, whereas only 20% of behaviorally complex disfluencies from the typically developing children did so. There also seem to be categorical differences between the groups in the structure of their behaviorally complex disfluencies. For example, LaSalle and Conture (1995) reported that *none* of the 30 children with typical fluency in their study produced a cluster that consisted of classic stutter-like disfluency types (i.e., part-word repetitions, sound prolongations/blocks) on immediately adjacent syllables or words. In contrast, about one-third of all disfluency clusters from children who stutter assumed that form. Based on this categorical difference between the groups, LaSalle and Conture suggested that "stutter-stutter" clusters (e.g., |*Y-*|*you* |*b-*|*better hurry up.*) might be a robust diagnostic marker for developmental stuttering and that their presence in a speech sample might justify the diagnosis of stuttering in cases where other markers of the disorder are ambiguous. This possibility warrants further investigation.

Finally, Logan and LaSalle (1999) examined the linguistic contexts within which children who stutter produced behaviorally complex disfluency. They found that utterances containing behaviorally complex disfluency had more syllables and more syntactic phrases than utterances containing only behaviorally simple disfluency. In turn, utterances containing behaviorally simple disfluency had more syllables, clauses, and syntactic phrases than fluent utterances. Based on these findings, Logan and LaSalle concluded that the most complex forms of disfluency occur in the most complex utterances.

Relationship Between Disfluency Frequency and Stuttering Severity

We have established that speakers who stutter produce more total disfluency than typical speakers do and that the difference in total disfluency between the groups usually arises from excessive production of repetitions and prolongations/blocks. Several other issues related to disfluency frequency warrant consideration, however. One main issue concerns the relationships between disfluency frequency and stuttering severity. In other words, what kind of disfluency frequency scores would speakers with mild, moderate, and severe stuttering obtain, and how disfluent are the most severe cases of stuttering likely to be?

In research contexts, researchers often specify some minimum number of disfluencies that a participant must demonstrate in order to qualify for inclusion in the study's "stuttering group." Often, the criterion for inclusion is 3 "stutter-like" disfluencies per 100 words, with the term stutter-like defined as the combined frequency of part-word repetitions, sound prolongations/blocks, and, in many studies, single-syllable word repetition (e.g., Anderson, Pellowski, Conture, & Kelly, 2003; LaSalle & Conture, 1995). This does not mean that every speaker with typical fluency produces fewer than 3 RPBs per 100 words or that every person who stutters produces more. However, it does provide a sense for the point at which the two groups begin to separate; that is, where upper boundary of nonstuttered speech often ends and the lower boundary of stuttered speech often begins.

As indicated in Chapter 4, speakers with typical fluency seldom produce the kinds of disfluency that are most characteristic of stuttered speech; that is, part-word repetition, sound prolongation, and blocking. Thus, in absolute terms, once a speaker produces more than just a few of these disfluency types per 100 syllables of speech, he or she already has moved, in a statistical sense, beyond the bounds of what is normal. On the other hand, it would be highly unusual for a speaker who stutters to exhibit repeating, prolonging, or blocking in conjunction with *all*, or even half, of the syllables they speak. Rather, for most people who stutter, disfluency frequency falls within a somewhat restricted range, where roughly 2 to 3 RPB disfluencies per 100 words constitutes the low end of the range, and 30 to 40 disfluencies per 100 syllables constitutes the high end of the range.

One way to get a sense for what constitutes mild, moderate, and severe amounts of disfluency in stuttered speech is to look at norms from an assessment tool like the *Stuttering Severity Instrument* (SSI; Riley, 1994, 2009). In its third edition (SSI-3; Riley, 1994), stuttered speech was defined " . . . repetitions or prolongations of sounds or syllables (including silent prolongations) . . . " as well as repetition of one-syllable words that sound "abnormal" (which Riley defined as "shortened, prolonged, staccato, tense, etc."). In Riley's approach, single-syllable words that speakers do not repeat "abnormally" are not included in the scoring.[6] On the SSI, one determines stuttering severity, in part, by computing a speaker's percentage of stuttered syllables during conversation and, when applicable, during reading as well. After computing the stuttering frequency, the clinician converts it to a weighted "Task Score," which can range from 2 to 9 (i.e., eight possible weighted scores in all). The Task Score for stuttering frequency then is combined with similarly derived weighted scores for disfluency duration and concomitant behaviors to yield a total weighted score and an accompanying stuttering severity rating (e.g., mild, moderate, severe).

As with many other sources of normative data for stutter-like disfluency, the stuttering frequency scores on the SSI-3 (Riley, 1994) are skewed in a positive direction. This means that, given a distribution of the stuttering frequency scores, the right tail would be much longer than the left tail. A distribution of this sort comes about when many of the speakers in a population exhibit stuttering frequency scores that are concentrated just above zero (say, from 1 to 5 stuttering-related behaviors per 100 syllables) and the remaining speakers in the sample exhibit scores that are spread out over a much wider range (in this example, from 6 to 100). Thus, the higher the stuttering frequency score is, the fewer the number of speakers who would have that score.

The pattern described above is similar to what is seen on the SSI-3. Based on information in the conversational speaking portion of the SSI-3 (see the "Reader's Table" on the test's score form), about one-half of the speakers who comprised the norming sample exhibited 5 or fewer stutter-like disfluencies per 100 syllables. The remaining speakers in the norming sample were spread out over the remain-

---

[6]The manual for the fourth edition of the SSI (SSI-4; Riley, 1994) no longer includes this definition of stuttering. Instead, stuttering appears to be undefined. However, because the norm reference information for the two editions seems to be identical, it appears that the same definition was in force during both editions.

der of the range of possible stuttering frequency scores; that is, scores that extend upwards from 6 stutter-like disfluencies per 100 syllables. On the SSI-3, only a small percentage of the norming sample exhibited more than 22 stuttered disfluencies per 100 syllables.

The pattern of stuttering-related disfluency seen on the SSI-3 norms is consistent with data from other sources. For example, Yaruss, LaSalle, and Conture (1998) reported overall SSI scores on 81 children who stuttered. In that study, about 40% of the children presented with very mild to moderate stuttering, about 50% presented with moderate stuttering, and only about 10% presented with severe or very severe stuttering. Similarly, stuttering-related disfluency scores on the *Test of Childhood Stuttering* (Gillam, Logan, & Pearson, 2009) also skewed positively in a manner similar to that on the SSI-3. That is, many cases in the norming sample had disfluency scores that clustered toward the low end of the continuum of possible scores. The remaining, more severe cases were spread out over a much broader range of disfluency scores, and very few cases exhibited disfluency scores that fell at the very upper end of the continuum of possible scores. Simi-

larly, Ambrose and Yairi (1999) reported data on a weighted measure of stutter-like disfluency that they developed for use with preschool-aged children. The score was computed summing the number of part- and single-syllable word repetitions that the children produced per 100 syllables and then multiplying the sum by the mean number of repetition units that the child exhibited during those repetitions. Thus, the weighted measure captured elements of disfluency frequency and duration. As with the sources discussed above, the results showed that the distribution of the weighted score was positively skewed; that is, 38% of the 90 preschoolers who stuttered had weighted scores between 4 and 9.99; 47% had scores between 10 and 29.99; and only 15% had scores equal to or greater than 30.00. So, as with other metrics of stuttering-related behavior, cases were more apt to obtain scores that fell toward the low to middle region of the score continuum than they were to obtain scores that fell toward the high- or upper-end of the score continuum.

Another way to gain perspective on stuttering frequency is to read transcripts of speech that feature varying amounts of disfluency. An example of this is presented in Box 5–1.

Box 5–1: Examples of Minimal, Moderate, and Frequent Disfluency in a Printed Passage Used for Sampling Fluency During Oral Reading

Commonly, when disfluency frequency increases, other dimensions of speech fluency deviate from normal in a more severe or extreme manner as well. Below, in the paragraphs that feature 10 and 25 disfluencies per 100 words, note that disfluency duration is longer and disfluency structure is more behaviorally complex than that seen in the paragraph with 3 disfluencies per 100 words. Disfluent segments are in bold text.

100-word sample; 3 disfluencies with stuttering-related behavior

- A |s-|**sinkhole** is a depression in the surface soil that develops suddenly. Sinkholes occur in places that have limestone bedrock. |**LLLL**|**imestone** is a soft rock. When acidic water contacts it, the limestone dissolves. Over time, this creates pockets in the limestone—places where the limestone has dissolved completely. The underground pockets can affect the surface soil if they collapse. Sinkholes often form after heavy rain. |**The-**|**The** soil is soaked with rainwater and the pockets in the limestone collapse from the extra weight. When a pocket collapses, the soil above it collapses too and a depression in the surface soil forms.

100-word sample; 10 disfluencies with stuttering-related behavior

- A |s-|**sinkhole** is a |d----|**epression** in the surface soil that develops suddenly. |**SSSS**|**inkholes** occur in places that have limestone bedrock. |**LLLL**|**imestone** is a soft rock. When acidic water contacts it, the limestone dissolves. Over time, this creates pockets in the limestone— |p- p-|**places** where the limestone has dissolved completely. The |u- u-|**underground** pockets can affect the surface soil if they collapse. |**SSSS**|**inkholes** often form after heavy rain. |**The-**|**The** soil is soaked with |r- r-|**rainwater** and the pockets in the limestone collapse from the extra weight. When a pocket collapses, the soil above it |c-----|**ollapses** too and a depression in the surface soil forms.

100-word sample; 25 disfluencies with stuttering-related behavior

- A |s-|**sinkhole** is a |d----|**epression** in the |ssss|**surface** soil that develops |ssss|**uddenly**. |**SSSS**|**inkholes** occur in places that have |l- l- l-|**limestone** bedrock. |**LLLL**|**imestone** is a soft rock. When |a----|**cidic** water contacts it, the |l- l-|**limestone** dissolves. Over |t- t-|**time**, this creates pockets in the limestone— |p- p-|**places** where the limestone has dissolved completely. The |u- u-|**underground** |p- um p- um|**pockets** |c- c- can-|**can** affect |the- the-|**the** surface soil if they collapse. |**SSSS**|**inkholes** often form after |hhhh|**eavy** rain. |Th- The-|**The** soil is soaked with |r- rrrr- r-|**rainwater** and the |p- p-|**pockets** in the limestone collapse from the extra weight. When a |p- p-|**pocket** collapses, the soil above it |c-----|**ollapses** too |and-|**and** a |de- de-|**depression** in the |s-|**surface** soil forms.

Note: Vertical lines mark disfluency boundaries; a single dash after a typed character indicates a part-word repetition (e.g., |s-|sink); a sequence of repeated characters indicates audible prolongation of a sound (e.g., |ssss|ink); a sequence of repeated dashes after a character indicates inaudible prolongation of a sound (e.g., |c-----|ollapse).

As shown, increases in disfluency within a sample have a disruptive effect on the delivery of information, and the extra time spent during disfluency makes the overall duration of the passage noticeably longer. It also is possible that disfluency duration may increase along with disfluency frequency. One also may observe a greater occurrence of disfluent segments that feature behaviorally complex structure as disfluency frequency increases (Logan & LaSalle, 1999). Examples of the latter types of disfluency appear in the third transcript shown in Box 5–1.

Not surprisingly, changes in disfluency frequency have consequences that go beyond perceptions of severity. For instance, research has shown that listeners react less favorably to frequent stutter-like disfluency than they do to occasional stutter-like disfluency. Susca and Healey (2001) reported that speakers who produce a high frequency of stuttering (15%, in their study) were rated as less competent and less comfortable to listen to than speakers with mild to moderate amounts of stutter-like disfluency. In a related study, Panico and Healey (2009) found that stuttering frequencies of as low as 5% had a negative impact on listeners' ability to recall information from a story.

Rate and Rhythm Characteristics

Rate-based measures of speech can be viewed as an index of a speaker's communicative productivity. That is, rate measures provide a sense of how many linguistic units a speaker typically generates per unit of time. That said, faster rates are not necessarily better than slower rates, particularly if speaking rate becomes so fast that listeners are unable to process what the speaker has said.

A common notion among laypeople is that the fluency problems of people who stutter result from talking too fast. Consistent with this, many parents encourage their children who stutter to "slow down" during times of disfluent speech (Dickson, 1971; Lankford & Cooper, 1974). Some questions to consider, then, are whether speakers who stutter do indeed talk faster than speakers with typical fluency do, and whether talking fast is a necessary trigger for stuttered speech. As we noted in Chapter 4, speaking rate can be measured during stretches of perceptibly fluent speech (i.e., articulation rate) or during randomly selected utterances, which for most speakers will include a mix of both fluent and disfluent utterances (i.e., speech rate). As a rule, articulation rate is faster than speech rate. This is because speech rate measurements often include disfluent segments of speech, whereas articulation rate measurements do not.

Rhythmic properties of speech are associated with "localized" factors such as the duration of speech sound segments, syllables, pauses, and disfluencies, each of which affects speaking rate. Many of the studies that examine speaking rate and rhythm with speakers who stutter focus on children. Thus, in this section, we focus our discussion mainly on this segment of the population.

Articulation Rate

Results from a number of studies are consistent with the view that the articulation rates of children who stutter are similar to those of children who do not stutter. For example, Logan, Byrd, Mazzocchi, and Gillam (2011) examined articulation rate performance in two age groups of elementary-school children, using the Modeled Sentences, Structured Conversation, and Narration tasks from the *Test of Childhood Stuttering* (TOCS; Gillam et al., 2009). Across all three tasks, the articulation rate characteristics for the two fluency groups were similar and, thus, not statistically different. Reported articulation rates across all three tasks from the TOCS included the following:

- Younger subgroup
  - Children with typical fluency: *M* = 3.76 syll/s (*SD* = 0.42)
  - Children who stutter: *M* = 3.56 syll/s (*SD* = 0.38)
- Older subgroup
  - Children with typical fluency: *M* = 4.16 syll/s (*SD* = 0.49)
  - Children who stutter: *M* = 4.16 syll/s (*SD* = 0.64)

For both fluency groups, older children exhibited significantly faster articulation rates than younger children did, and among the older children, articulation rates were fastest during the Modeled Sentences task. The lack of a difference between the fluency groups in articulation rate, obviously, goes against the idea that children who stutter speak "too fast"—at least in any absolute sense. Another possibility is that speakers who stutter may articulate at rates that exceed their capacity for doing so. The latter hypothesis fits with a more generalized view that stuttered speech happens whenever task demands exceed one's "capacity" or "resources" for performing the task (the so-called Demands–Capacity model of stuttering; for more on this view, see Adams, 1990; Starkweather, Gottwald, & Halfond, 1990). Although the hypothesis is interesting, it is challenging to test from a scientific perspective because of the difficulties inherent in objectively defining a speaker's "resources" or the "capacity" that a speaker has for speaking rapidly. Others (e.g., Navon, 1984) have raised similar concerns with respect to the use of resources as a construct in models of human information processing.

Studies with preschool-aged children who stutter also have failed to support the idea that speakers who stutter articulate at an excessive rate. For instance, Meyers and Freeman (1985) reported significantly *slower* conversational articulation rates for a group of children who stutter (Group with stuttering: 3.51 syll/s [*SD* = 0.65]; Group with typical fluency: 4.04 syll/s [*SD* = 0.50]). Others (e.g., Kelly, 1994; Kelly & Conture, 1992) have found no significant differences in articulation rates between children who stutter and children who do not stutter, and the reported articulation rates in those studies are consistent with those in the Logan et al. (2011) study. Some researchers, however, have reported rather subtle differences between speakers who stutter and speakers with typical fluency in regard to aspects of speech timing within syllables and in the quickness with which a speaker initiates articulatory movements. We discuss this work in Chapter 6, in the section on speech motor control.

Speech Rate

Speech rate measurements are sensitive to both disfluency frequency and disfluency duration. In general, the more disfluent a speaker is, and the longer the disfluent segments last, the slower the speech rate is. Given this, it is clear that people who stutter usually will have slower speech rates than people who do not stutter, and the amount of rate difference between the groups will depend on the disfluency frequency and duration characteristics of the group under study.

Johnson (1961), in an analysis of oral reading data, reported that the speech rates of adults who stuttered were 30% to 50% slower than the speech rates of typical adults. Logan et al. (2011) reported that the mean speech rate of school-aged children who stuttered was 12% slower than the mean speech rate of typical children—a difference that was statistically significant and indicative of a large effect size (Group with stuttering: 2.52 syll/s; Group with typical fluency: 2.87 syll/s). The speech rate differences were apparent in both the younger and older subgroups within the study and across each of the three speaking tasks that the researchers examined.

Several researchers have studied the relationship between stuttering severity ratings and speech rate. In such studies, the correlation coefficients for the two variables suggest that a moderate-to-strong association exists between the variables (e.g., Minifie & Cooker, 1964; Prins & Lohr, 1972). Thus, although stuttering severity seems to reflect attributes of speech rate, the two constructs are by no means identical. Other researchers (Prosek, Walden, Montgomery, & Schwartz, 1979; Young, 1961) have reported that speech rate correlates more strongly with severity ratings than do measures of disfluency frequency. From this perspective, speech rate might be a more sensitive measure of a speaker's fluency performance than disfluency frequency, because it captures information about both disfluency frequency and disfluency duration.

Effects of Altering Speaking Rate

It is well known that the overt symptoms of stuttering are markedly reduced when speakers slow their articulation rate (Adams, Lewis, & Besozzi, 1973; Andrews et al., 1983; Bothe, Davidow, Bramlett, & Ingham, 2006). Speech-language pathologists commonly refer to this style of speech, which is akin to speaking in "slow motion," as *prolonged speech*. In many older studies, researchers induced prolonged speech by having speakers who stutter talk under delayed auditory feedback; however, in our experience, speakers can easily reduce articulation rate and attain "prolonged speech" without the use of delayed auditory feedback. Either way, the effects of prolonged speech are immediate and reliable; that is, in laboratory settings, stutter-like disfluency usually decreases dramatically on the speaker's first attempt at implementing the prolonged style of speech. Perhaps this is the reason that prolonged speech is a staple of many treatment programs for stuttering.

We will discuss prolonged speech as an intervention for stuttering in Section IV of the book. For now, however, it suffices to say that a clinician can expect the frequency of stuttering-related interruptions to decrease markedly when a speaker deliberately slows articulation rate. Explanations for why slowed articulation rate enhances speech fluency are largely speculative, but whatever it is, it clearly seems to facilitate the speaker's ability to execute speech movements continuously (Perkins Bell, Johnson, & Stochs, 1979).

Findings from some research studies have yielded results that are counterintuitive to common assumptions about the relationship between articulation rate and stuttering frequency. For example, Kalinowski, Armson, and Stuart (1995) reported that adults who stuttered demonstrated no significant difference in stuttering frequency between conditions that involved reading aloud at a typical rate and reading aloud while talking as fast as possible. In other words, rapid articulation did not reliably aggravate the symptoms of stuttering despite the fact that, on average, the adults' articulation rates were about 35% greater in the fast-reading condition compared to the typical-reading condition. Furthermore, some participants in the study actually showed substantial improvement in speech fluency during the fast-articulation-rate condition. The latter finding matches results from other researchers (e.g., Ingham, Martin, & Kuhl, 1974). It may be that general processes, such as increasing the amount of attention that one devotes toward speech parameters, is a common ingredient for many fluency-enhancing behaviors, including reduced articulation rate.

A variety of others researchers have examined the effects of "slow speech" on stuttering frequency. With this approach, researchers typically ask speakers to attempt talking at a rate that is a certain percentage slower than their customary rate. Andrews, Howie, Dozsa, and Guitar (1982) found that talking in this manner reduced stuttering frequency substantially and to roughly the same extent that prolonged speech did. In a study with typical adult speakers, Logan, Roberts, Pretto, and Morey (2002) found that when participants were asked to slow speech by 10%, they roughly doubled the frequency and the duration of their pauses, and their articulation rate slowed by about 20%. This led to an overall decrease in speech rate of about 33%.

Disfluency Duration

Comparative studies of disfluency duration are challenging to accomplish because speakers with typical fluency seldom produce the disfluencies that characterize stuttered speech and, in some research studies, some typical speakers do not produce any of the disfluencies types that are common to stuttered speech. Most of the disfluency duration data comes from descriptive studies of children. We summarize findings from eight different studies in Table 5–3. With the exception of the Johnson and Colley (1945) study, all of the studies primarily are based on preschool-aged children.

As shown in Table 5–3, researchers have reported disfluency data in different ways. Some researchers (e.g., Kelly & Conture, 1992; Logan & Conture, 1997; Yaruss, LaSalle, & Conture, 1998) collapsed the classic stutter-like disfluency types (part-word repetition, monosyllable word repetition, and prolongations) into a single category, while others (e.g., Throneburg & Yairi, 1994, 2001) reported durations for these types of disfluency separately. Across all of the child-based studies in Table 5–3, the overall mean duration for all disfluency types combined is consistently less than 1 second. As would be expected, disfluency duration increases somewhat as the number units within a repetition increases (Throneburg & Yairi, 1994, 2001). Somewhat surprisingly, however, the average disfluency duration for children who stutter does not seem to be greater than that for children with typical fluency (Zebrowski, 1991, 1994). In fact, in the Throneburg and Yairi (1994) study, children who stutter had shorter disfluency durations than children with typical fluency. In the latter study, the researchers attributed this finding to differences between the groups in the duration of the editing phase within the repetitions (i.e., it was significantly shorter among the children who stutter). Some researchers (Yaruss et al., 1998; Zebrowski 1991, 1994) reported the minimum and maxi-

Table 5–3. Characteristics of Disfluency Duration in Studies Of Children, Teens, and Adults Who Stuttered

Study	Age	Main Results	Other Findings
Kelly & Conture (1992)	Preschool	• PWR, MWR, PRO: *M* = 0.65 s (*SD* = 0.20)	No difference in duration between S and NS
Logan & Conture (1997)	Preschool	• PWR, MWR, PRO: *M* = 0.90 s (*SD* = 0.19)	Duration not correlated with syllable complexity
Throneburg & Yairi (1994)	Preschool	• PWR (1 unit): *M* = 0.63 s (*SD* = 0.13) • MWR (1 unit): *M* = 0.74 s (*SD* = 0.17) • MWR (2 units): *M* = 1.38 s (*SD* = 0.45)	NS have longer disfluencies than S
Throneburg & Yairi (2001)	Preschool	• PWR (1 unit): *M* = 0.58 s; 2-unit = 1.02 s • MWR (1 unit): *M* = ~0.80 s; 2-unit = ~1.30 s • PRO: *M* ~0.67 s	PS & RS have similar duration
Yaruss, LaSalle, & Conture (1998)	Preschool	• PWR, MWR, PRO: *M* = 0.82 s (*SD* = 0.53) • Max: 3.38 s	Duration not a predictor of treatment recommendations
Zebrowski (1991)	Preschool	• PWR: = *M* = 0.56 s; (*SD* = 0.37) • PRO: *M* = 0.44 s (*SD* = 0.27) • Min-Max: PWR = 0.16–1.88 s; PRO = 0.12–1.58 s	No difference in duration between S and NS
Zebrowski (1994)	Preschool	• PWR: *M* = 0.72 s (*SD* = 0.15) • Prolongation: *M* = 0.71 s (*SD* = 0.30) • Min-Max: PWR = 0.40–1.00 s; PRO = 0.44–1.06 s	Duration not correlated with age, time since onset, or disfluency frequency
Johnson & Colley (1945)	Teens & adults	10 longest stuttered disfluencies = 4.32 s 10 shortest stuttered disfluencies = 0.41 s	Stuttering duration and frequency show low to moderate correlation

Note: *PWR* = Part-word repetition; *MWR* = Monosyllable word repetition; *PRO* = prolongation and inaudible blocking; *Min-Max* = minimum and maximum mean durations among participants in the study. *S* = speakers who stutter; *NS* = speakers who do not stutter; *PS* = cases with persistent stuttering; *RS* = cases who recovered from stuttering.

mum mean scores for participants in their studies. As shown in Table 5–3, some individuals do have mean disfluency durations that exceed 1 second and, in some cases, the participants' mean duration greatly exceeds 1 second.

Johnson and Colley (1945) took a different approach to reporting disfluency duration. Rather than focusing on average duration, they reported the 10 longest and 10 shortest segments of stuttered speech in a group of adolescents and adults who stuttered. As shown in Table 5–3, the longest stuttering "moments" averaged more than 4 seconds, while the shortest were less than 0.5 seconds. Although 4 seconds may not seem particularly long in an absolute sense, consider that a speaker with typical fluency will produce at least four to five syllables per second. Thus, in the time it takes to produce a 4-second-long disfluency, the typical speaker can execute about 16 to 20 syllables of productive speech. In the context of normal speech production, 4 seconds clearly is a relatively long time. Johnson and Colley also examined whether the production of long disfluencies led to a spike in disfluency severity in the words that immediately followed. In this study, it did not appear to do so, because there was no difference in the cumulative duration of stuttering in the 30 seconds that followed long versus short disfluencies

Of course, data such as those reported in Johnson and Colley (1945) reflect only a slice of the population of people who stutter. In clinical practice, it is not uncommon to see cases in which the client's longest stuttered segments greatly exceed 4 seconds. Occasionally, we have seen cases in which disfluent segments have routinely lasted for 15 to 30 seconds or more. Disfluency of this sort is quite disruptive to communication and when a client produces it often, the clinician will likely wrestle with the question of whether it is better to let the client continue in disfluency or, instead, to gently interrupt and redirect him or her toward alternate speaking patterns that may shorten the interruptions. The answer to this question will vary with client and the stage of treatment, but eventually it will need to be addressed.

Reiterations Within Repetitions

As discussed previously, one can characterize part- and whole-word repetitions in terms of the number of repetition units they contain. Each repetition unit that occurs after the original moment of interruption constitutes an attempt on the part of the speaker to repair the disfluency. In Chapter 4, we indicated that speakers who do not stutter usually repair disfluencies on the first attempt after interrupting speech (e.g., *b- boy*). In contrast, speakers who stutter often require two or more attempts to advance the utterance beyond the original point of interruption (e.g., *b- b- b- boy*). Multi-iteration repetitions are likely to last longer than single-iteration repetitions. Thus, analysis of the number of iterations within a repetition provides information about the speaker's disfluency duration as well as his or her adeptness in repairing speech production problems.

Yairi (1997) reviewed several studies that contained data on repetition units. In six studies, the mean number of units per repetition for nonstuttering children ranged from 1.03 to 1.16. Because the means are slightly greater than 1.0, it tells us that nonstuttering children occasionally produce more than 1 unit per repetition, but it does not occur commonly. In contrast, in three studies that included children who stutter, the mean number of units per repetition ranged from 1.35 to 1.70. Mean values that exceed 1.50 tell us that many of a speaker's repetitions are likely to contain two or more repetition units.

Yairi and colleagues (e.g., Throneburg & Yairi, 1994, 2001) also have studied the temporal structure of repetitions using spectrographic analysis. In several studies, they measured the overall duration of the repetition, as well the durations of the editing phase, the duration of original utterance that leads into the moment of interruption, and the duration of unsuccessful repair attempts. These analyses revealed that the duration of the editing phase was significantly *shorter* in children who stutter than it was in nonstuttering children.

Effort, Awareness, and Compensation

Physical Tension

Excessive physical tension may accompany stuttering-related disfluency. This pattern occurs most often in conjunction with disfluency that features fixed articulatory postures (e.g., audible sound prolongation, silent blocks). When a speaker prolongs or blocks consonant sounds, the excessive physical tension is likely to be most apparent within the muscles that are involved with creating the vocal tract constriction associated with the particular sounds. Thus, when a speaker prolongs [t] inaudibly in a word like "team," he or she is likely to feel excessive tension in the tongue blade (because it acts as the primary organ of articulation for that sound). In contrast, inaudible prolongation of [p] (e.g., |p---|en) is likely to feature a feeling of excessive tension in the muscles surrounding the mouth. Inaudible prolongation of vowel sounds, in contrast, would likely feature excessive tension in the laryngeal musculature, as the speaker constricts the glottis to phonate. Of course, excessive tension is by no means limited to these regions and may be evidenced throughout the neck, shoulders, and/or

face. However, such patterns are not present in all speakers who stutter, nor are they apparent during all developmental stages of the disorder or during all utterances that a speaker says (Kelly, Smith, & Goffman, 1995).

It is important for clinicians to realize that the excessive physical tension does not arise from a problem, per se, in articulating the particular consonant or vowel sound that the speaker is prolonging or repeating. Consider, for example, the prolonged [s] in the word *sorry* (e.g., *ssssorry*), wherein the speaker *is* saying the [s] sound distinctly. In this instance, the [s] sound is not necessarily what the speaker experiences difficulty saying. Rather, the fluency difficulty observed for this particular word instead may reflect the speaker's situational inability to integrate the [s] sound with whatever sound or sounds that happen to follow. Excessive physical tension in the speech muscular may reflect the speaker's reaction to or attempt to cope with this break in speech continuity.

Kelly et al. (1995) studied orofacial muscle activity in children who stutter. Previous research by Smith and colleagues (e.g., Smith et al., 1993) indicated that a significant proportion of adults who stutter exhibit tremor-like oscillation in the speech musculature, particularly during stuttering-related disfluency. Kelly et al. sought to determine whether similar patterns appeared in children's speech. Overall, their results revealed evidence of tremor-like oscillation only among the oldest children in the study (ages 10 to 14 years). On this basis, they concluded that tremor-like oscillations are an emergent pattern in stuttered speech. They speculated that such a pattern might result from age-related increases in the duration of stuttering-related disfluency, the development of a chronically unstable speech motor control system as a result of accumulated experiences with stuttering, and/or the effects of autonomic nervous arousal associated with emotional reactions to the speech disruption.

Awareness of Impairment

The extent to which a speaker is aware of his or her stuttering has been an area of considerable interest in speech-language pathology. For much of the 1900s, one of the arguments against early intervention for stuttering was that the treatment activities would heighten a child's awareness of stuttering and, in doing so, exacerbate the symptoms of the disorder (see Bleumel, 1932, for example). Since then, the results from numerous treatment studies with preschoolers who stutter suggest that direct acknowledgement of a child's stuttering does not seem to worsen stuttering severity. In fact, when done properly, it seems to have a facilitative effect (Onslow, Packman, & Harrison, 2003).

In recent years, professional interest has turned to identifying how and when young children become aware of stuttering. Yairi and colleagues (Ambrose & Yairi, 1994, Ezrati-Vinacour, Platzky, & Yairi, 2001) examined the emergence of stuttering awareness in children between the ages of 3 to 7 years. A group of typically developing children and a group of children who stuttered listened to two puppets as they produced sentences. One of the puppets exhibited stuttered speech and the other exhibited typical fluency. The experimenters asked each of the children to point to the puppet "that talks the way you do." The results suggested that some 3-year-old children clearly were aware of their stuttering and that, by age 5, most of the children had a good sense for whether they spoke with a fluent or a stut-

tered speech pattern. Thus, self-awareness of one's speech fluency seems to emerge during the preschool years. Interestingly, self-awareness of stuttering was not associated with measures of children's stuttering severity (Ambrose & Yairi, 1994). However, by the age of 4 years, most of the children evaluated stuttered speech negatively, as demonstrated by their tendency to describe it as something that is "not good" (Ezrati-Vinacour et al., 2001). The latter findings are consistent with studies that have examined preschoolers' reactions to disorders and differences in speech-language functioning among their peers (Gertner, Rice, & Hadley, 1994).

More recently, Boey and colleagues (Boey et al., 2009) reported data on stuttering awareness from more than 1,100 2- to 7-year-old children who stuttered. The children's parents were asked to report whether their children exhibited indicators of stuttering awareness such as self-directed remarks about speech fluency ("I can't say it.") or nonverbal behaviors (e.g., sighing) that clearly coincided with fluency difficulties. On this basis, more than 60% of 2-year-old children demonstrated awareness of their stuttering and nearly 90% did so before their 7th birthday. The children's most common sign of awareness was to ask a parent for help with speaking, while the least common sign was to show sadness. Boys were no more likely than girls to show awareness of stuttering. Boey et al.'s findings are consistent with those of Culatta and Sloan (1977), who found that primary grade children could reliably recognize stuttered speech even though they might not have had a formal label for it.

Another way to assess stuttering awareness is to examine the extent to which speakers who stutter can anticipate instances of disfluency on specific words when asked to read a printed passage aloud. This phenomenon has been termed *expectancy*. Research on the expectation of stuttering has been conducted primarily with adults who stutter, and the general finding is that adults are quite accurate at anticipating where disfluency will occur. In some reports (Knott, Johnson, & Webster, 1937), adults correctly anticipated more than 90% of their stuttered words. Studies with children show that they can accurately anticipate stuttering-related disfluency also. For instance, Bakker, Brutten, Janssen, and van der Meulen (1991) used eye-tracking equipment and found that during a preliminary silent reading of a printed passage, children who stuttered fixated longer on the words that they subsequently stuttered on when reading the passage aloud.

For many speakers who stutter, the sense that speech may become disfluent seems to come a few syllables in advance of the syllable upon which stuttering is anticipated. People who do not stutter often have difficulty understanding how a speaker can know that stuttering might happen before it actually has occurred. The phenomenon of stuttering expectancy is not at all surprising, however, when viewed within the context of contemporary speech production models, wherein a speaker is said to plan utterances incrementally, with each increment consisting of about a phrase-length stretch of speech. The developing speech production plan is evaluated and updated through internal monitoring mechanisms and, through this process, the speaker can assess whether the utterance is developing in such a way that it is likely to result in fluent speech.

The experience of hiking down a mountain on a rain-slickened trail offers a rough analogy of the stuttering expectancy phenomenon. When descending a

trail, the hiker is continually looking at the upcoming terrain in order to plan the types of movements (in the case of hiking, a gait pattern) that will allow for safe, smooth, continuous locomotion. By analyzing critical characteristics of the upcoming segment of the trail (e.g., its steepness, slickness, and rockiness), the hiker readily identifies specific locations that—given the hiker's current hiking speed, stride length, and general physical fitness—are likely to induce a slip, stumble, or fall. The hiker also may take into account past experiences that have occurred on similar terrain and be acutely aware of experiences that resulted in painful falls. Thus, the hiker "knows" in advance which portions of the trail that he or she is likely to have difficulty walking through in a smooth, steady manner and is keenly aware of the consequences that a slip or fall can have. In speech production, an utterance is a bit like the hiking trail in that it constitutes the "terrain" through which the speaker must move. Each utterance offers unique challenges in terms of the movement sequences that are required in order to execute it successfully. Just as a hiker often can anticipate which parts of a mountain trail are most likely to induce a slip, stumble, or fall, the speaker who stutters often can anticipate which parts of an articulatory sequence are most likely to induce speech-based problems that equate with disfluency. The speaker also may be keenly aware of the negative consequences that come with disfluency, such as loss of a speaking turn or being laughed at by the conversational partner.

Extraneous Physical Movements

The symptoms of stuttering often go beyond disfluency to include various physical movements that are extraneous to speech production. Such behaviors are labeled by some as "secondary" or "associated" behaviors. Terms such as these serve to distinguish the behaviors from the ostensibly "primary" or "core" behavior of stuttering—the disfluency. Researchers have examined an assortment of other stuttering-related variables, as well. Among these are the number and variety of nonspeech movements that speakers who stutter produce while talking. Studies in this area have revealed that children who stutter produce more nonspeech movements while talking when compared to children who do not stutter, with the most notable differences occurring in conjunction with disfluent words (Conture & Kelly, 1991). Such movements can be relatively subtle and difficult for casual observers to detect. Included among them are head turns, eye blinks, and upper lip raising (Conture & Kelly, 1991).

Traditionally, authorities have viewed these nonspeech movements as an emergent feature of stuttering, meaning that they supposedly develop well after the onset of stuttering symptoms. Bloodstein (1960) provided some support for this view when he reported that associated behaviors occurred in conjunction with stuttered speech in about 33% of 3-year-olds, 57% of 6-year-olds, and 65% of 16-year-olds. This may be true for only the most obvious forms of stuttering-associated behavior, however, as subsequent research with young children who stutter has uncovered evidence of atypical and excessive nonspeech movements in preschoolers who stutter shortly after the time of onset for stuttered speech (Conture & Kelly, 1991; Yairi, Ambrose, Paden, & Throneburg, 1996). These findings suggest that some atypical nonspeech behaviors may not develop secondary to disfluency after all but are, instead, intrinsic to it.

With some clients, the nonspeech behaviors that coincide with stuttering-related disfluency are anything but subtle. Some speakers exhibit rhythmical movement of body parts that ordinarily are not involved in speech production (e.g., a finger, an arm, a foot). Typically, such movements occur during either the editing phase of stuttering-related disfluency or in advance of an anticipated stuttering-related interruption in speech production. In our experience, speakers typically use the rhythmic movement as a means of facilitating speech fluency. That is, rhythmical movements such as finger tapping, foot tapping, or head nodding function as a sort of timing template—akin to a metronomic beat—around which the speaker tries to sequence syllable production. In this sense, the rhythmic movements are a type of compensatory response to fluency impairment. With most speakers, however, these self-generated timing templates facilitate fluency inconsistently, and over time, the movements may become exaggerated or feature the sort of excessive muscle tension that characterizes stuttering-related disfluency. In some cases, they can become so exaggerated in appearance that they detract from communication to an equal or greater extent than speech disfluency does. Consequently, these extraneous movements generally are not adaptive, in the sense that they significantly facilitate communication.

Compensation and Concealment

Speakers who are sensitive to how others react to them may attempt to conceal their fluency impairment and its effects by either *avoiding* or *postponing* speech. Speakers also may devise their own strategies for improving speech continuity. To the extent that the latter behaviors facilitate fluency, they can be regarded as *compensatory* in nature. The list of behaviors that speakers who stutter have used toward these ends is lengthy. The discussion here is intended to highlight a few of the most common behaviors that speakers exhibit.

- *Use of (rhythmic) body movements to facilitate speech initiation or speech continuity.*

Many speakers who stutter report that they experience difficulty initiating articulatory movements. In other words, they know which muscles need to be moved; however, as is sometimes the case in a bad dream, movement initiation simply will not commence. The speaker may compensate for this difficulty by attempting to link speech initiation with the movement of some other nonspeech-related body part. Often, such movements are rhythmic (e.g., tapping a hand, finger, or foot; producing a series or sequence of head nods, eye blinks, or teeth clicks). Speakers also sometimes attempt to time speech initiation with time-based physiological sensations such as muscle tensing. For example, a speaker may plan to initiate a syllable when the muscles in the left forearm reach maximal contraction. In such instances, the bodily movements seem to function similarly to the actions of metronome in that they provide a temporal reference point for certain articulatory goals (e.g., the onset of phonation, the release of an articulatory constriction).

- *Use of altered phonation and/or articulatory patterns to facilitate fluency.*

A speaker might talk in a whisper, attempt to "sing" words, use exaggerated inflec-

tion, reduced intensity, or a nonhabitual pitch, or perhaps even feign a foreign accent or regional dialect in an effort to talk more fluently. The speaker may find that such behaviors sometimes do reduce the occurrence of stuttering-related disfluency. In the long term, however, these types of compensatory actions rarely are highly effective at improving fluency.

- *Use of word substitution or situational avoidance to conceal stuttered speech from others.*

A speaker may respond to the expectancy of stuttered speech on an upcoming word by substituting a synonym of that word. Although this strategy may prevent a stuttering-related disfluency from occurring, it sometimes can alter or obscure the speaker's intended message. For example, an intended utterance like, *"I'd like a croissant"* ends up being said as, "I'd like a soft, flaky kind of bread," after which the store clerk may end up saying, "Oh, do you mean a croissant?" Speakers who stutter also may attempt to conceal their disfluent speech by pretending to be disinterested in conversation or engaged in some other activity. In this way, the speaker reduces the likelihood that he or she will be asked to talk. Situational avoidance offers speakers short-term relief from whatever negative listener reaction may occur, but over the long term, it has numerous negative consequences (e.g., lack of social contact, inability to efficiently meet one's daily objectives).

- *Use of strategies that lead to stalling or postponement of speech.*

Some speakers who stutter find that they speak more fluently when they are able to initiate speech at a time of their choosing. Consequently, the speaker may deliberately attempt to stall or postpone the start of a speaking turn or an utterance. In one sense, the strategy is compensatory, but when it is accompanied with shame or embarrassment about stuttering, it more accurately is viewed as a form of avoidance or concealment—both of which generally are regarded as maladaptive behavior. Examples of such behaviors include the following: intentionally clearing one's throat to delay the start of an utterance, pretending as if one has forgotten what was about to be said, again, to delay the start of an utterance, and inserting superfluous words into a sentence in order to postpone the production of a word upon which stuttering is expected. Strategies such as these may offer the speaker temporary relief from the negative feelings that come from listener reactions, yet over the long term, they are unlikely to offer an effective way to compensate for fluency impairment. This is because stalling and postponement can negatively impact a speaker's conversational participation and lead to sentences that are less effectively formulated than they otherwise might be.

Not all speakers who stutter attempt to conceal stuttered speech from listeners. Bloodstein (1960) conducted a retrospective analysis of clinical records to document the emergence of stuttering-related avoidance behaviors from childhood through adolescence. He found that none of the children exhibited active avoidance of stuttering prior to age 3 and that only 17% did so by age 9. By age 16, however, avoidance of stuttering behaviors was apparent in 45% of the cases. Thus, the use of concealment strategies did appear to be an emergent aspect of stuttering and perhaps it was linked to associated developmental changes in social cognition that led to an increased awareness of how one is perceived by others.

Performance Variability

Many speakers who stutter exhibit variability in fluency performance. Some of the factors that have been linked to performance variability include the following: speaking task, communicative partner, physical setting, and developmental age.

Task and Setting Effects

It is well known that the overt symptoms of stuttering are substantially reduced or absent during tasks such singing, chorus reading, prolonged speech, slowed speech, and speaking in time to a metronome (Andrews et al., 1982). Of course, speakers who stutter rarely communicate in these ways during daily activities. Accordingly, the data obtained under these speaking conditions perhaps are more useful for understanding the nature of stuttering than they are for documenting the sorts of fluency fluctuations that people normally experience.

Several researchers have examined fluency variations using more ordinary speaking tasks. For example, Yaruss (1997) examined stuttering variability in 45 children who stuttered during story retelling, picture description, and three types of play-based conversation (with parent, with clinician, with clinician who purposefully introduced communicative pressures such as verbal interruption and use of a fast speaking rate). The children who produced the most stutter-like disfluency exhibited the most variability in disfluency across the speaking tasks. Analysis of group data showed that the children stuttered most often during the pressured conversation task and least often during the picture description task; however, the children demonstrated considerable individual differences in terms of which tasks were most and least disfluent. Thus, not all children experienced the most fluency difficulty when faced with communicative pressures.

In another study with preschoolers who stutter, Johnson, Karrass, Conture, and Walden (2009) examined the effects of speaking partner (parent, clinician), physical setting (home, clinic), and speaking task (narration, conversation). In this study, only speaking task had a significant effect on stuttering frequency: The preschoolers stuttered more during conversation than narration. In a study with school-aged children, however, Byrd, Logan, and Gillam (2012) reported the opposite pattern—more stuttering during narration than conversation. They attributed the result to the fact that school-aged children produce narratives that are substantially more complicated than preschoolers do. Thus, while the group data suggest that some types of speaking tasks are more challenging than others for speakers who stutter, clinicians should be mindful of the substantial variability that exists across individual research participants in these studies. Tasks that evoke relatively large amounts of disfluency for many children will not necessarily do so for all children.

Numerous factors have been examined with respect to variations in the frequency of stuttered speech in adult speakers. Included among these are the following: listener reactions to stuttering, the social status of the communication partner (e.g., speaking to an employer versus speaking to a child or a pet), or the gender of the communication partner (Bloodstein & Bernstein Ratner, 2008). Several researchers have examined the effect that audience size has on the fluency of speakers who stutter. Porter (1939) asked adults who stutter to read a passage aloud in various settings. She found that stuttering frequency increased progressively across the following conditions: reading alone, reading to the experimenter, reading to two strangers, and reading to four strangers. Audience sizes larger than four people did not lead to a reliable increase in stuttering frequency (16% of words stuttered with four people in the audience, 16.7% of words stuttered with eight people in the audience). The greatest proportionate increase in stuttering frequency occurred as the speaker went from reading alone (2.8% of words stuttered) to reading in front of one person (9.5% of words stuttered). Porter also asked the speakers to rate their expected stuttering frequency prior to each condition, and for the most part, the speakers' performance during the condition was consistent with their expectations; however, the estimated stuttering frequencies for several conditions were greater than they actually turned out to be.

For most speakers who stutter, stuttering frequency seems to be much less when they speak alone versus when they speak in front of a listener. Fluency while speaking alone is subject to variation, however, depending on what the person is speaking about. In clinical settings, we have heard some clients who stutter report that they stutter while they are orally rehearsing a speech they are about to deliver. No one else is present at the time of rehearsal but the act of saying words that eventually will be presented to a particular audience is apparently sufficient to trigger stuttering-related disfluency. Disfluency at such times may illustrate the effect that language formulation can have upon the stability of the speech motor system.

People who stutter may report speaking more fluently when interacting with children than they do when interacting with adults. Ramig, Krieger, and Adams (1982) examined variations in speech fluency among nine adults who stuttered and nine adults with typical fluency. Participants in each of the groups read aloud to one of the experimenters, another adult, a child, and the adult and the child. The adults who stuttered exhibited a significant reduction in stuttering frequency while reading to a child (about 9% of syllables stuttered when reading aloud to the adult or the adult and the child versus about 4.5% of the syllables when reading aloud to the child). Both speaker groups demonstrated predictable changes in fundamental frequency, fundamental frequency variability, speaking rate, and peak vocal sound pressure level in the two conditions that included a child. Thus, the presence of these vocal changes was not sufficient to explain the improvement in fluency that occurred when reading only to a child.

Utterance Characteristics

Many researchers have examined factors that affect fluctuations in fluency performance *within* a speaking task. In studies with both children and adults who stutter, the data suggest that the more linguistic units (e.g., syllables, clauses, morphemes, syntactic phrases, prosodic phrases) an utterance contains, the more likely it is that the utterance will contain stuttered speech (e.g., Klouda & Cooper, 1988; Logan, 2001, 2003a; Logan & Conture, 1997; Silverman & Williams, 1967a; Tsiamtsiouris & Cairns, 2013; Yaruss, 1999; Zackheim & Conture, 2003). The age at which a syntactic structure emerges seems to affect the fluency of children's sentences as well. The main effect is that the presence of a developmentally advanced language form within an utterance increases the likelihood that the utterance will contain stuttering-related disfluency (Bernstein Ratner & Sih, 1987; Logan & Conture, 1995).

Utterance complexity effects like these do not seem to be a case of a speaker simply having more opportunities to stutter within a long utterance than in a short utterance, because the stuttering-related disfluency within long utterances most often occurs at or near the start of an utterance rather than being randomly distributed throughout the utterance (Brown, 1945; Buhr & Zebrowski, 2009; Gaines, Runyan, & Meyers, 1991; Logan & Conture, 1995; Logan & LaSalle, 1999). In an analysis of children's stuttering patterns during conversation, Logan (2003a) found that utterances within multiple-utterance conversational turns were no more likely to contain stuttering than utterances within single-utterance conversational turns. This suggests that, within a conversation, speech fluency is affected more by utterance formulation and production demands than it is with issues that span utterance boundaries such as pronoun referencing and other elements of linguistic cohesion.

In children who stutter, there also is evidence that stuttering frequency may vary during the time course of a conversation. Sawyer and Yairi (2006) reported that preschoolers exhibited higher frequencies of stuttering-related disfluency in latter portions of a play-based conversation than they did in the early portions of conversation. In a follow-up study, Sawyer, Chon, and Ambrose (2008) found partial support for the idea that the increase in stuttering frequency resulted from the children's use of longer, more complex utterances as the conversation progressed. In a related study, Logan and Haj-Tas (2007) examined variations during the course of 1,800-syllable-long narratives produced by 10 adults who stutter. After the samples were elicited, the researchers parsed them into 300-syllable increments, which resulted in six 300-syllable subsamples of speech. Analysis of the subsamples revealed no significant differences in stuttering frequency across the subsamples. Participants were compared as to which 300-syllable subsample evoked the most and the least disfluency, and again, no consistent patterns were noted. The findings also indicated that a speaker's stuttering frequency score after 300 syllables of narration was not significantly different than his or her stuttering frequency score after 1,800 syllables. Thus, adults who stutter appear to show less variation within laboratory-based speech samples than children do.

Epidemiology

Epidemiology involves the study of how diseases or, in this case, *disorders* are manifested in a population. Some areas of concern in epidemiological research include the following: (a) how often a particular disorder occurs in a population, (b) patterns of persistence and recovery for a disorder, (c) factors that affect disorder frequency and outcome, and (d) whether a disorder affects some segments of the population more than others (Coggon, Rose, & Barker, 1997).[7]

Epidemiological data for developmental stuttering have been reported in a number of studies. Data such as these are helpful on many levels, such as determining whether developmental stuttering is more or less common than other speech disorders, examining whether the disorder is more common among some populations than others, examining whether the disorder has become more or less common over time in a population, and so forth. In the remainder of this section, we review some of the main findings about the epidemiology of developmental stuttering.

Age of Onset

It is widely agreed that the symptoms of developmental stuttering first appear during childhood. Indeed, developmental stuttering sometimes is referred to as *childhood stuttering*. A number of researchers have attempted to identify when in childhood the symptoms of stuttering are most likely to appear. This has proven to be a bit more difficult to do than one might think.

Cumulative Frequency Data

One can collect age-of-onset data via either retrospective or prospective methods. Typically, the onset data are part of a broader project in which the researcher also explores the prevalence, incidence, and/or recovery rates for stuttering. Onset data that come from prospective studies are considered more accurate than those that come from retrospective studies, because the prospective approach allows

---

[7]Many authors have used the term *recovery* when referring to the abatement of overt stuttering symptoms. To our way of thinking, the notion of recovery implies restoration of some previously held facility or level of performance that once was normal or, perhaps, resolution of the underlying impairment that caused the symptoms to appear in the first place. At present, there is no empirical support for either position. Accordingly, we prefer the term *remission,* which allows for the possibility that the symptoms—although absent at present—could return at some time in the future. Nonetheless, we use both terms in the discussion here and elsewhere in the text.

the documentation of the date of onset to occur relatively close in time to when the symptom onset actually occurred (Yairi & Ambrose, 1992b). There have been only a few prospective studies into the epidemiology of stuttering, however. Perhaps this is because such studies are both time- and resource-intensive and expensive to conduct.

Perhaps the best-known prospective study of stuttering epidemiology took place in England beginning in 1947, in a city named Newcastle-upon-Tyne. Researchers attempted to follow the speech development of 1,142 babies who were born in the city during May and June of that year, tracking them from birth through 16 years of age. A team of trained health care workers and speech clinicians met regularly with the children and their caregivers and reported their findings in a series of publications (e.g., Andrews, 1984; Andrews & Harris, 1964; Morley, 1957). During the course of the study, 43 children showed symptoms of developmental stuttering. The researchers collected data such as how old the children were when stuttering symptoms first appeared, whether the symptoms eventually resolved and, if they did resolve, how long the symptoms had been present before they finally resolved.

Selected results from this research are presented in Table 5–4, where they

Table 5–4. Cumulative Frequency Data for Age of Stuttering Onset

Study	Sample[b]	Design[c]	Age[a]										
			2	3	4	5	6	7	8	9	10	11	12
Andrews & Harris (1964)	Persist (n = 9)	P & R	14	42	58	**70**	77	82	88	92	95	96	100
	Remit (n = 34)		6	22	50	**70**	79	91	98	100	—	—	—
Dickson (1971)	Remit (n = 196)	R	16	50	**73**	86	92	96	98	99	100	—	—
	Persist (n = 168)	R	19	41	59	**74**	88	92	95	97	97	98	100
Seider et al. (1983)[d]	Persist (n = 269)	R	5	26	43	65	**72**	80	92	95	95	98	99

Note. The number in a cell represents the percentage of all stuttering cases in a particular study that had experienced stuttering onset by a particular age. For example, 14% of the persistent cases reported in Andrews & Harris (1964) began to stutter at age 2, and another 28% of cases began to do so by age 3, bringing the cumulative total to 42% of all cases. The percentages in this table are estimates that were derived from figures presented in the original manuscripts. Bolded numbers highlight the age at which at least 70% of the participants in the study had begun to stutter.

[a] Age is reported in years.

[b] Persist = participants whose stuttering persisted throughout the duration of the study; Remit = participants whose stuttering eventually remitted.

[c] P = prospective design; R = retrospective design.

[d] Data are for male participants in the study only.

are compared against data from other studies. In the table, the data represent cumulative percentages. This means that the number in each column of the table reflects the percentage of cases that began to stutter by a particular age. So, in the Andrews and Harris (1964) study, 58% of all cases of stuttering in that study evidenced symptoms of stuttered speech by age 4, and 77% of all cases did so by age 6. There were no cases in that study with a reported onset after age 12. Based on these data, Andrews (1984) concluded that virtually all of the risk for an individual to develop stuttering has passed by age 12 years. In other words, if a person has yet to exhibit symptoms of developmental stuttering by age 12, it is very unlikely that he or she will do so in subsequent years.

Researchers have used retrospective research strategies to determine the age of onset as well. With a retrospective approach, a researcher identifies a group of people who stutter and then asks each of them (or their caregivers) when stuttering symptoms first appeared. This method works best when all of the participants under study have passed the age when the risk for developing symptoms of stuttered speech has largely passed (~12 years). Several retrospective studies like this have been conducted. One such study was conducted by Andrews and Harris (1964), using a different set of participants than those who participated in their prospective study. Age-of-onset data from their retrospective study appear in Table 5–4. As shown in the table, the age-of-onset patterns for Andrews and colleagues' retrospective and prospective studies were generally consistent.

Dickson (1971) conducted a retrospective study of developmental stuttering in which questionnaire responses were examined for 3923 elementary- and junior

high school-aged students from Williamsport, New York, USA. Of these participants, 364 were reported to have shown symptoms of developmental stuttering. Age-of-onset data for these participants are presented in Table 5–4, as well. These data are mostly consistent with findings from the other studies. Of note, all of the students in Dickson's cohort who ever stuttered had begun to do so by the age of 10 years. Interestingly, there were no cases with a reported age-of-onset after age 10. The upper limit for stuttering onset in Dickson's study is somewhat younger than the age that Andrews and Harris (1964) reported but still is consistent with the idea that few cases of stuttering will feature an onset after childhood.

The third study listed in Table 5–4, Seider, Gladstien, and Kidd (1983), consisted of a retrospective examination of stuttering patterns in males and females who had either recovered from or persisted with stuttering. The data shown in the table are from the 269 males with persistent stuttering, and the general pattern of findings for their ages of onset is, again, similar to those in the other studies. Also consistent with the studies in Table 5–4 is a report from Wingate (1964b), who collected data from 50 persons who stutter, age 17 and older. Most of these participants (79% of males, 61% of females) reported stuttering onset as being before age 7, and all but one participant reported an onset between the ages of 2 and 13.

This is not to say that the onset for developmental stuttering *never* occurs after a child reaches 10 to 12 years. After all, not *every* person who has ever stuttered was included in these studies. However, based on these studies, it is safe to say that such a scenario is highly uncommon; so uncommon in fact that, based on data from the Newcastle-upon-Tyne study,

Andrews (1984) proposed that cases with an onset beyond age 12 be classified as "acquired stuttering." During the past two decades, we have evaluated several college-aged clients who reported that the onset for their stuttering symptoms occurred during early to mid-adolescence (e.g., age of 13 to 15 years). Each of these cases exhibited what we would regard as classic symptoms of developmental stuttering. Still, given how uncommon it is for stuttering onset to occur so late in development, it is prudent to carefully consider the possibility of an acquired form of stuttering. Thus, with such cases, it is important to inquire about at some length the client's neurological functioning and overall health and about any changes that have occurred with regard to stuttering symptoms over time. If there is any suspicion that the client presents with an acquired form of stuttering, then a medical referral is warranted.

One limitation with relying on client or caregiver reports for information about stuttering onset is that the informant may fail to recognize subtle symptoms of the disorder that existed prior to what they regard as the age of onset. It is quite possible that in cases of so-called "late-onset stuttering," the individuals exhibited symptoms of developmental stuttering much earlier in life, but the symptoms were not severe enough to attract the notice or concern of anyone but a speech-language pathologist.

Mean Age of Onset

Another way to think about onset is in terms of the average age when children begin to stutter. In Table 5–5, we present age-of-onset statistics from several studies. In all of the studies, the data come from retrospective reports. In some retrospective studies (Ambrose & Yairi, 1999;

Table 5–5. Mean Ages of Onset and Associated Standard Deviations for Developmental Stuttering in Several Studies of Children Who Stutter

| Author(s) | Sample | Reported Age-of-Onset (in Months) | | | | | |
| | | Male | | Female | | Male + Female | |
		M	SD	M	SD	M	SD
Ambrose & Yairi (1999)	N = 90 (59 boys, 31 girls); Age range: 23–59 mos.; M age: 37 mos. (SD = 9 mos.)	34	8	33	9	34	8
Yaruss et al. (1998)	85 males, 15 females; M age: 55 mos. (SD = 12.2 mos.).	36	11	30	10	35[a]	—
Yairi & Ambrose (1992b)	N = 87 (59 boys, 28 girls); Age range: males = 20–69 mos.; females = 21–43 mos.	34	9	29	6	33	8
Seider et al. (1983)	223 adult males and 82 adult females with persistent stuttering	62	—	57	—	—	—

Note: Dashes indicate data that were not reported in the original study.

[a]Mean was computed by present author based on reported data from original source.

Yairi & Ambrose, 1992b), the data were collected very near the age of reported onset, an approach which presumably yields more accurate information than, say, a study such as the one by Seider et al. (1983) wherein adults were asked about the age of onset for their stuttering. As shown in Table 5–5, the mean ages of onset in 3 of the 4 studies are roughly 2;6 for females and 3;0 for males.

Reilly et al. (2013) recently reported prospective data related to the cumulative incidence of stuttering, based on a sample of 1619 children from Melbourne, Australia. Although the authors did not report data for stuttering in terms of mean age of onset, their data on cumulative incidence indicated that a large majority of the 181 children who eventually developed stuttering, began to do so between the ages of 2;0 and 3;0. Because the Reilly et al. (2013) study only reports on children through age 48 months, new cases that might emerge later in life are not captured in the data. This is a limitation of the onset-age values in many other studies, particularly those in which the researchers' focus is on young children who stutter. For example, in the Yairi and Ambrose (1992b) study, the focus was on cases with stuttering onset *before* age 6. In the Reilly et al. (2013), it was on children between birth and age 48 months. In such studies, there obviously is no opportunity to incorporate cases with later ages of onset into the statistics. This may not be a major limitation, however, as both Yairi and Ambrose (1992b) and Reilly et al. (2013) remarked on the apparent diminution of new cases beyond roughly 40 to 48 months. This view is supported by data in Table 5–4, where roughly 10% to 20% of all cases of developmental began after age 6. Obviously, when these cases are factored into the age-of-onset calculations, the mean

would be somewhat higher than it would when the cases are excluded. Results from the Seider et al. (1983) study bear this out as well. The latter study was based on retrospective reports of adults who stutter (a method that allows for inclusion of late-onset cases), and the reported mean ages of onset for both males and females were closer to age 5. In the prospective study by Andrews and Harris (1964), stuttering onset for more than 70% of cases occurred by age 5. So, in all, it seems safe to say that symptom onset for stuttering most often occurs during early childhood, at or before age 5, and for many of those cases, onset occurs between the ages of 2;6 and 3;6.

Yairi and Ambrose (1992b) questioned 87 parents of children who had experienced onset of stuttering symptoms during the previous year. The parents characterized stuttering onset as "gradual" in 56% of the cases and as "sudden" in 44% of the cases. In 57% of the cases, stuttering onset did not occur in the context of unusual or excessive physical or emotional stress, whereas in 43% of the cases, it did. In most (70%) of the cases, the parents characterized their child's stuttering severity as mild at the time of onset. In the remainder of cases, it was moderate or severe. In 66% of the cases, there was a positive family history of stuttering; that is, there were others who stuttered in the family beside the child, and in the remainder of cases (34%), there was not. Overall, the most common profile (25% of all cases) was for a child to exhibit gradual onset of stuttering in the context of a positive family history and the absence of marked physical or emotional stress.

Before concluding this section, it is important to remember that age-of-onset data only tell us about when the symptoms associated with developmental stuttering are first overtly manifested in speech. Thus, the reported age-of-onset for a case does not necessarily correspond to the age at which the underlying cause of the disfluent speech first developed. For instance, a child may present with subtle neurodevelopmental abnormalities that eventually lead to stuttered speech but can be detected only through the use of sophisticated neuroimaging techniques. In this view, it is possible that many children who stutter have effectively "had" stuttering well before the overt symptoms of the disorder became apparent to listeners.

As we will see in the section on the speech production skills of people who stutter, some of the symptoms of developmental stuttering are detectable only through the use of sophisticated instrumentation. Thus, it also is important to remember that "fluent sounding speech" is not necessarily normal in terms of its underlying physiology or movement coordination.

Incidence and Prevalence

Incidence is an epidemiological statistic that captures the number of unique or newly diagnosed cases of a disorder within a population during a particular time frame. *Prevalence*, in contrast, is an epidemiological statistic that captures how many cases of a disorder exist within a population at a specific time. As such, it can include recently diagnosed cases as well as long-standing cases. Each statistic typically is expressed as a percentage. The relationship between incidence and prevalence is affected by several factors, including the following: (1) the developmental course of a disorder (i.e., age-of-onset patterns for the disorder; whether the

disorder usually is transient or chronic); (2) the cohort under study, (i.e., does the analysis focus on a narrow demographic segment of the population or on a broad segment?); and (3) the time frame that is being studied (i.e., does the analysis focus on the entire lifespan or on a shorter time span, such as the past year?).

In the stuttering literature, researchers most often have examined *lifetime incidence* (i.e., how many people have stuttered at some time during their life) and *point prevalence* (how many people stutter now). As we will see, many cases of developmental stuttering are transient, meaning that the speech-related symptoms of a person's disorder do not persist throughout the person's entire life but instead *remit* or *resolve*. In cases where the symptoms of developmental stuttering *persist*, the symptoms usually first appear during childhood and remain with the person for some significant length of time, perhaps even throughout the lifespan. Remission of stuttering symptoms is most likely to occur during childhood. This means that the lifetime incidence of developmental stuttering (i.e., how many individuals have stuttered at some point during life) will be greater than the prevalence of developmental stuttering (i.e., how many individuals stutter right now), because some individuals who formerly had the disorder have experienced remission of symptoms.

Lifetime and Cumulative Incidence

Data for the lifetime incidence of stuttering are most accurate when the participant pool includes individuals who are past the age at which new cases of stuttering are likely to arise. Because the onset of developmental stuttering seldom occurs after about age 10 to 12, incidence data that are based on reports from individuals who are older than this are most appropriate, at least when a retrospective design is being used. Other factors that can affect the reporting of incidence statistics include the following: how the researcher has defined developmental stuttering; how well the researcher has conveyed his or her definition of developmental stuttering to participants; the length of time that has elapsed between when a participant showed the symptoms of stuttering and when a participant is being asked to report on those symptoms; the size and representativeness of the participant sample; and the extent to which the researcher can corroborate a participant's report of stuttering. Differences in these factors across research studies probably account for much of the variance in reported lifetime incidence rates for developmental stuttering across research studies.

Overall, estimates of the lifetime incidence for developmental stuttering have ranged from about 3% to 6%. For example, Sheehan and Martyn (1970) reported 2.9% incidence; Cooper (1972) reported 3.7% incidence; and Porfert and Rosenfield (1978) reported 5.5% incidence. Andrews and Harris (1964) reported a lifetime incidence rate of 4.8% in their retrospective study of adults from Newcastle-upon-Tyne, England. Interestingly, the incidence rate from that study was very similar to the one reported in their prospective study, 4.9%. In turn, the incidence rate in Andrews and Harris's prospective study was similar to the reported lifetime incidence, 5.1%, in a prospective study by Månsson (2000). The latter study involved more than 1,000 children who were natives of the same Danish island and were followed from birth through about age 10.

Although lifetime incidence rates fall within the 3% to 6% range in most studies, others have reported somewhat different results. For example, Craig and colleagues (Craig, Hancock, Tran, Craig, & Peters, 2002) interviewed a randomized and stratified group of individuals from New South Wales, Australia, to obtain information about incidence, prevalence, and recovery rates for stuttering across the lifespan. In that study, the incidence rate for the entire sample was 2.2%, which is somewhat below the mean reported in most other studies. As expected, incidence rates varied depending on the age of the person who was being analyzed. In Craig et al. (2002), incidence rates for subsets of the overall sample varied as follows:

- 2.8% in 2- to 5-year-olds,
- 3.4% in 6- to 10-year-olds,
- 2.2% in 10- to 20-year-olds, and
- 2.1% in 21 to 50 years.

At the other end of the continuum, Dickson (1971), in a large sample of students from Williamsport, New York, USA, reported incidence rates of 10% for elementary-school-aged students and 8% for junior high school students. As noted, such differences may arise due to methodological differences such as the way in which stuttering was defined in a particular study or the challenges associated with collecting such data retrospectively.

More recently, Reilly et al. (2013) reported data on the incidence of stuttering in a sample of 1619 children. Reilly et al. tracked the children longitudinally from age 7 months through age 4. They reported that 181 children (11.2% of the total sample) developed stuttering prior to age 4. Unlike many other studies, a speech-language pathologist confirmed the diagnoses of stuttering through direct observation of the children and then subsequently monitored the children's fluency performance through monthly visits. The incidence estimate that Reilly et al. (2013), 11.2% is substantially higher than percentages reported in most of the other studies reviewed in this section. It is possible that the use of speech-language pathologists in identifying cases of stuttering explains some of this difference, as they presumably would be more attuned to the symptoms of stuttering and thus more likely to recognize children who have the disorder.

In contrast to the studies mentioned in the preceding paragraphs, some researchers have investigated stuttering incidence rates in specific subpopulations. As might be expected, this approach leads to quite different results than studies based on general population samples. For instance, Seider et al. (1983) examined patterns of stuttering in relatives of individuals who were diagnosed with developmental stuttering. They reported lifetime incidence rates of 13% among relatives of the male participants who stuttered and 18% among relatives of the female participants who stuttered, findings that support the notion that developmental stuttering tends to "run in families." Along these lines, MacFarlane, Hanson, Walton, and Mellon (1991) reported an incidence rate of 14% for developmental stuttering in a 1,200-member, five-generational family from the western United States. Finally, Kloth, Kraaimaat, Janssen, and Brutten (1999) examined the incidence of stuttering in a prospective study of children who had a parent who stuttered. Overall, 28% of the children developed symptoms of stuttering during the six-year course of the study. Results such as these are thought to reflect the role of genetic factors in shaping one's predisposition for developmental stuttering—an issue that we discuss later in this section.

Overall, these incidence data suggest that developmental stuttering is not a rare disorder, at least when examined during the course of the lifespan and when compared to some other developmental disorders. On the other hand, these data argue quite strongly against the view—often held by laypeople—that "everybody stutters." As described above, everybody does not stutter—if that were true, the incidence of developmental stuttering would be 100%. It *is* true that nearly everyone produces *stutter-like* disfluencies on isolated occasions, but that is very different from being diagnosed with the speech disorder called stuttering. To reiterate, current best estimates are that 2% to 6% of the general population will present with developmental stuttering at some time during the lifespan, with the risk for ever having stuttered increasing in segments of the population that are at a unique risk for the disorder.

Prevalence

As noted, prevalence involves the percentage of a population that currently exhibits a disease or disorder. As with incidence data, estimates of prevalence for developmental stuttering vary depending on the age and representativeness of the research participants and assorted other methodological factors such as how stuttering is defined, who is making the primary diagnosis of developmental stuttering, and whether reports of developmental stuttering are corroborated by researchers. Results from several studies that have examined the prevalence of developmental stuttering are presented in Table 5–6. Perhaps the most comprehensive of these

Table 5–6. Prevalence Estimates for Developmental Stuttering at Various Age Levels

Study	Sample	Preschool	School	Adult	All
		Age Level			
Proctor et al. (2008)	N = 2,223; Illinois, USA; preschoolers	2.52	—	—	—
McKinnon et al. (2007)	N = 10,425; Sydney, Australia; kindergarten to 6th grade	—	0.33	—	—
Van Borsel et al. (2006)	N = 21,027; Belgium	—	0.58	—	—
Craig et al. (2002)	N = 2,553; New So. Wales, Australia; all ages	1.40	0.90	0.37	0.72
Okalidou & Kampanaros (2001)	N = 1,113; Patras, Greece; kindergartners	—	1.71	—	—
Brady & Hall (1976)	N = 18,420; Illinois & Pennsylvania, USA; kindergarten to 12th grade	—	0.35	—	—
Gillespie & Cooper (1973)	N = 5054; Tuscaloosa, AL, USA; Grades 7 to 12.	—	2.12	—	—
Andrews & Harris (1964)	N = 7,358; Newcastle-upon-Tyne, England	—	—	—	1.20

Note. Dashes indicate that the authors did not examine the age interval.

studies is that by Craig et al. (2002), which involved telephone interviews with a large and stratified sample of individuals from one Australian state. The interviews included corroborative conversations with the people who were reported to have stuttered. The prevalence of developmental stuttering was highest among the cohort of preschool-aged children (1.40%) and then gradually decreased during the school-aged years (0.90%) and into adulthood (0.37%). Such a pattern is expected, given the observation that some people who stutter go on to exhibit remission of stuttering symptoms sometime after onset. The overall prevalence for devel-

opmental stuttering across all age levels in the Craig et al. (2002) study was 0.72 %. Thus, slightly less than 1% of the population exhibited active stuttering at the time the researchers conducted the study.

Findings from several other studies are roughly consistent with those from Craig et al. (2002). That is, the highest prevalence rates tend to be reported among preschool-aged cohorts (e.g., Okalidou & Kampanaros, 2001; Proctor, Yairi, Duff, & Zhang, 2008), and the reported prevalence rates among school-aged children tend to be somewhat lower (e.g., McKinnon, McLeod, & Reilly, 2007; Van Borsel, Moeyaert, Mostaert, Rosseel, Van Loo, &

Van Renterghem, 2006) than those for preschoolers. Not every study has yielded prevalence estimates that fit within this pattern, however. For instance, Gillespie and Cooper (1973) sampled more than 5,000 junior and senior high school students in Tuscaloosa, Alabama, USA, and found a 2% prevalence rate for developmental stuttering, which is roughly twice as high as that in other studies. It is difficult to assess the extent to which methodological factors contributed to this unusual finding, as neither the criteria for diagnosis of developmental stuttering nor the qualifications of the examiner(s) who made the diagnoses were detailed in the published report of the study. It is possible (though in our estimation, unlikely) that the prevalence of developmental stuttering was particularly high in that community.

As with the incidence of developmental stuttering, the prevalence of the disorder varies from the general population mean when certain subgroups of people are examined. For example, Montgomery and Fitch (1988) surveyed 77 residential/specialized schools for children with hearing impairment and obtained data on the fluency performance of more than 9,900 students. Based on survey responses, only 12 of the students (0.12% of the total) exhibited symptoms of stuttering. Each of the 12 students had at least severe hearing loss. Half (6 of 12) stuttered during manual communication; five during both oral and manual communication modes, and one during only oral communication. In contrast, Cooper (1986) summarized findings from 14 studies of stuttering prevalence among individuals with mental retardation/developmental disabilities. Nearly all of the studies that he reviewed reported prevalence rates substantially higher than those for the general population. That is,

in 8 of the 14 studies, the prevalence estimate fell in the range of 2% to 8%, and in three other studies, it fell between 10% and 20%. Similarly, Van Borsel and Tetnowski (2007) summarized research on stuttering characteristics associated with various genetic syndromes. In the studies they reviewed, the prevalence of stuttering among people with Down syndrome ranged from 15% to 48%, although in some studies (e.g., Otto & Yairi, 1975), the authors argued that the speech patterns were not entirely consistent with those seen in developmental stuttering. Proctor et al. (2008) examined the prevalence of developmental stuttering among more than 3,000 preschool-aged American children of European and African descent. Data were collected using teacher and parent reports and clinician screenings. Results indicated the prevalence of stuttering for both groups was similar (2.6% for African-American children; 2.44% for European-American children). Thus race was not a significant predictor of stuttering, but for all of the children, the child's sex was (males were more likely to stutter than females). Finally, in a study of school-aged children from Belgium, Van Borsel et al. (2006) reported a prevalence rate of 2.28% for a sample of children who were enrolled in a special education setting but a prevalence rate of 0.58% for children who were enrolled in regular education.

Sex Differences

It is well accepted that males are more likely to exhibit symptoms of developmental stuttering than females are. The ratio of males to females who stutter is not fixed, however. Instead, it varies somewhat depending on the age of the cohort under investigation. For example, Yairi and Ambrose (1992a, 1992b, 1999) reported information on the age of onset and stuttering remission patterns in a large group of preschoolers. They found that girls began to stutter at an earlier age than boys did and that girls demonstrated remission of stuttering symptoms more often than boys did. Given this, one would expect the ratio of males to females who stutter to be smaller among a cohort of, say, 33-month-old children than that of a cohort of 60-month-old children. Indeed, this is precisely what Yairi and Ambrose (1992b) found. The male-to-female ratio was relatively small among children who were younger than 27 months old (1.2 males to 1 female), and it was substantially greater when the age interval was expanded to consider children between the ages of 2;0 and 5;9 (2.1 males to 1

female). Craig et al. (2002) found a similar pattern when they examined the sex ratio for stuttering in preschool- and school-aged children (Figure 5–2), along with a steady increase in the ratio through early adulthood. Somewhat unexpectedly, however, they also reported a decline in the magnitude of the sex ratio with older segments of the population (e.g., 1.4 males per female after age 50).

In recent decades, explanations for why males appear to be at greater risk for stuttering than females has centered on genetic factors. In contrast, strong forms of environmental explanations (e.g., factors such as societal and cultural expectations for males versus females) have fallen into disfavor (Kidd, Kidd, & Records, 1978; Yairi & Ambrose, 2005). Support for genetic-

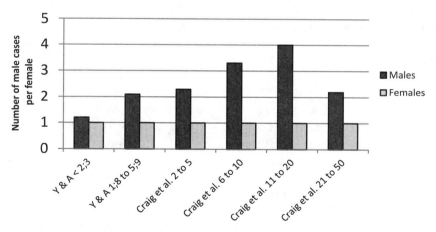

Figure 5–2. A bar graph that is based on data from two studies in which researchers reported male-to-female ratios for cases of stuttering they identified during data collection. Yairi and Ambrose (1992b) reported such data for a sizable group of preschoolers who stuttered. When they examined only the youngest children in their study (see "Y & A < 2;3"), the ratio was 1.2 males to every 1 female who stuttered. When they included older children in the analysis, the ratio of males to females increased to 2.1:1 (see "Y & A 1;8 to 5;9"). Craig et al. (2002) reported sex ratio data for age subgroups across the lifespan and found a gradual increase in the male to female ratio through age 20, after which the male-to-female sex ratio decreased to values similar to what was observed in preschool-aged cohorts (51+ group not shown).

based explanations of the sex ratio data come from examination of stuttering patterns within families. For example, Kidd et al. (1978) examined epidemiological patterns of stuttering among the immediate relatives of the *probands* (i.e., the participants under direct examination) in their study. Their findings included the following:

- Male relatives of probands who stuttered were nearly three times as likely to stutter as female relatives were (Ratio = 2.93 males:1 female);
- Male probands who stuttered had more than twice as many sons who stuttered as they did daughters who stuttered (Ratio = 2.3 sons who stuttered:1 daughter who stuttered); and
- Female probands who stuttered were more than twice as likely to have a daughter who stuttered than a son who stuttered (Ratio = 2.44 daughters who stuttered:1 son who stuttered)

Kidd et al. (1978) interpreted their findings as evidence that stuttering is a sex-modified trait. MacFarlane et al. (1991) reported similar findings, although smaller in magnitude (sex ratio (1.8 males: 1 female) in a study of developmental stuttering patterns within a 1,200-member, multigeneration family living in the western United States.

Developmental Course of Stuttering Symptoms

Both researchers and clinicians have studied how the symptoms of developmental stuttering change over time. Such information is useful when counseling clients and their family members and when making decisions about when to assess and treat clients.

Developmental Paths for Stuttering

At a very basic level, one can think of developmental stuttering as a disorder that can follow one of two paths. The first path, which we will term *persistent developmental stuttering*, features the onset of stuttering symptoms during childhood. The speaker then continues to manifest the symptoms for a significant length of time in an unabated manner that suggests chronic impairment. The classic profile of persistent stuttering is one in which a person begins to stutter during childhood and continues to do so throughout the remainder of his or her lifespan.

The second path, which we will term *transient developmental stuttering*, features onset of stuttering symptoms during childhood, and then subsequent remission of the symptoms sometime later. In such cases, the changes in symptom expression are such that the speaker comes to regard him- or herself as a normally fluent speaker, and other people do so as well. Thus, in this developmental path, the symptoms of stuttering are temporarily present in the speaker's speech.

The dichotomy between the *persistent* and *transient* paths for developmental stuttering suggests a degree of order and simplicity in the clinical outcomes that, unfortunately, is not present in real life. In reality, there are many ways that developmental stuttering can unfold, and this can make it difficult for clinicians to be confident about which path the client is travelling and where the client will ultimately land. One main problem is that the remission of stuttering occurs on various timescales, a situation which makes it difficult to define terms such as *persistent, chronic,* and *transient* precisely. In Figure 5–3, we offer a sense of the possible paths that developmental stuttering assumes, and we briefly elaborate on their characteristics below:

- In some cases, remission occurs relatively soon after onset—a scenario that we might term *early remission*. In such cases, symptom expression is measurable in terms of weeks, or months, and extending, perhaps, to two years from onset. Early remission occurred relatively often among the cases of childhood stuttering that Ambrose and Yairi (1999) and Andrews (1984) discussed.

- In other cases, symptom remission occurs several years after onset, but prior to adolescence—a scenario we might term intermediate remission. Researchers have noted

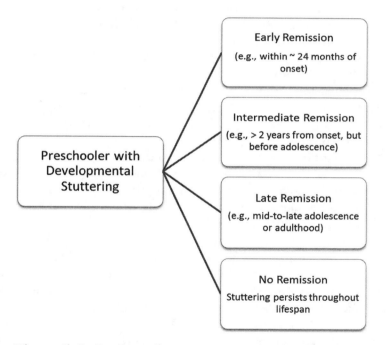

Figure 5–3. Diagram illustrating possible paths for developmental stuttering. Among children who begin to stutter during the preschool years, if symptom remission (recovery) occurs, it often will happen relatively soon after onset. The clearest cases of persistent stuttering are those in which symptoms continue throughout the lifespan. Cases in which stuttering symptoms remit many years after onset perhaps are most appropriately regarded as a variant of persistent stuttering, given the potential for a long-standing history of stuttering-related disability and the potential for that history to impact the speaker even after recovery occurs.

this pattern routinely, as well, although based on Andrews (1984), it seems to be less common than the early remission scenario described above.

- Lastly, there are cases, which according to research data are not very common, wherein remission from stuttering occurs many years after onset, such as during late adolescence or adulthood. To our way of thinking, it is questionable whether one should consider such cases as transient in any conventional sense of the word. Thus, given the current level of understanding for this phenomenon, a purely descriptive label for this type of developmental path—late remission—seems more appropriate.

A second challenge in specifying developmental paths for stuttering involves the definition of *remission* or, as it often is termed in the fluency disorders literature, *recovery*. Although the term can refer to notions such as improvement or a lessening in symptom severity, in most applications to developmental stuttering during early childhood, it refers to a complete absence of symptoms and an apparent resolution of the disorder. When using the word *remission* in the latter sense, the essential question concerns the length of time stuttering symptoms must be absent before one can be confident that speech fluency has truly normalized and stuttering symptoms will not return at some time in the future. Of course, the best way to answer this question would involve documenting fluency performance in cases of remitted stuttering across the lifespan. Given the impracticalities associated with that approach, researchers instead typi-

cally specify some minimal length of time that symptoms are absent. For example, in the Ambrose and Yairi (1999) study, symptoms of stuttering had to have been absent for at least one year for a case to be classified as remitted. Obviously, the longer the symptoms of stuttering have been absent, the more confident one can be in the use of the label *remission*.

Remission of Stuttering During Childhood

It is has long been known that a significant portion of the children who begin to stutter during childhood eventually stop doing so (e.g., Andrews & Harris, 1964; Martin & Lindamood, 1986; Sheehan & Martyn, 1970). In the literature, researchers have referred to this process as *recovery* or *remission*. Many have used the term *spontaneous recovery*, as well, when referring to cases in which symptom remission occurs in the absence of formal intervention. In addition, various colloquial expressions appear in the literature and among laypeople to describe this process of stuttering abatement. These include terms such as *outgrowing stuttering* and *overcoming stuttering*.

One focus of research efforts in this area has been to determine the percentage of children who in fact do stop stuttering. Such data are important, in large part, because of their implications for clinical intervention practices (Andrews, 1984; Martin & Lindamood, 1986). For instance, if a large percentage of children do indeed recover from stuttering, this creates questions about whether clinicians should treat developmental stuttering during childhood and, if they do, which children should they treat and when should they provide the treatment (Andrews, 1984; Martin & Lindamood, 1986). High recovery rates also create challenges for interpreting treatment outcomes research (Curlee & Yairi, 1997; Saltuklaroglu & Kalinowski, 2005). That is, if a child's stuttering resolves following a course of treatment, how is one to know whether the improvement resulted from the treatment as opposed to developmental processes unrelated to treatment?

Researchers have examined remission rates for developmental stuttering using both retrospective and prospective approaches. Survey data from large-scale retrospective studies of college students during the 1960s and 1970s (e.g., Sheehan & Martyn, 1966, 1970) suggest that stuttering symptoms remit in up to 80% of cases. Results from these studies also suggest that individuals who had stuttered severely at some time in the past have lower remission rates (about 50%) than those with milder stuttering do. In Dickson's (1971) retrospective survey of nearly 4,000 parents, approximately 70% of all children who had stuttered experienced spontaneous recovery by 9th grade. In addition, most cases of stuttering were relatively brief—lasting two years or less. Recovery was most likely to occur early in life, usually before age 7. Wingate (1964b), in contrast, reported data in which participants indicated that recovery occurred on a more protracted scale. In that study, however, about half of the participants reported that they still stuttered occasionally, making it difficult to compare the findings with those of some other studies. Some authors (e.g., Martin & Lindamood, 1986; Young, 1975), citing the limitations associated with retrospective research and the possibility that caregivers' comments about their speech to children who stutter may have therapeutic benefits, questioned whether the remission process for stuttering is as "spontaneous" as it some-

times is made out to be and, accordingly, whether spontaneous remission rates are as high as the past data had suggested. Findings from several prospective studies (discussed below) suggests that remission/recovery from childhood stuttering is quite common. The extent to which it is spontaneous, however, remains to be determined.

One such prospective study (i.e., Andrews & Harris, 1964) tracked the speech performance of a large cohort of infants (1,142 at the time the study began) from birth through age 15. During the 15-year course of the study, 43 showed symptoms of stuttering at one time or another. The broad findings on remission rates generally were similar to those from the retrospective studies cited above. That is, 34 of the 43 children (79%) evidenced remission of stuttering symptoms prior to the conclusion of the study (i.e., before the children reached age 16). For many of these cases, stuttering proved to be a short-lived phenomenon. That is, for 24 of the 34 cases (about 71% of the total), remission occurred within one year of onset. Less commonly (6 of 34 cases; 18% of the total), remission occurred two or more years after onset, including one case (3% of the total) in which remission occurred 11 years after onset. There were 9 cases (21% of the total) who continued to stutter at the conclusion of the study. Andrews (1984), in a review of his earlier study, noted that some of these long-standing cases eventually may have remitted as well in the years after the conclusion of the study. If so, this would put the remission rate somewhat higher than 79%.

Yairi and colleagues (e.g., Yairi & Ambrose, 1999) conducted a series of studies during a long-running project at the University of Illinois that focused primarily on recovery patterns in cases of early childhood stuttering. They used a longitudinal design to follow the fluency performance of youngsters who had begun to stutter prior to age 6. The researchers evaluated the children at 6-month intervals, with the initial evaluation occurring within 6 months of stuttering onset (and often much less than 6 months). Yairi's team published (and continues to publish) numerous papers summarizing various facets of the research. We will summarize some of that work very briefly here. In addition, Yairi and Ambrose (2005) published a detailed summary of the primary project outcomes in a textbook. Readers who are interested in reading more about the project should consult that source in addition to the various individual research publications they authored.

Yairi et al. (1996) examined changes in the children's disfluency patterns during the first few years after stuttering onset. By 7 to 12 months post-onset, the children who eventually recovered from stuttering showed a clear divergence in terms of the number of stutter-like disfluencies they produced when compared to the children with persistent stuttering. Thus, it appeared that a trend toward recovery was evident within one year of onset. On this basis, children who do not show signs of such a trend during this period might be considered "at risk" for persistent stuttering. Also of note, Yairi et al. (1996) found that, at the time of the initial evaluation for the study, the children who eventually recovered from stuttering had a higher frequency of stutter-like disfluency than the children who eventually exhibited persistent stuttering did. On this basis, they concluded that disfluency frequency at or near the time

of onset is not a sensitive predictor of whether stuttering symptoms will remit. This was consistent with findings from Yairi, Ambrose, and Niermann (1993), who reported that some cases with very severe stuttering at the time of the initial evaluation went on to recover.

Other markers of persistent stuttering reported by Yairi et al. (1996) included the percentage of a child's relatives who exhibited persistent stuttering. In that study, children with persistent stuttering had a greater percentage of relatives who exhibited persistent stuttering than the children who recovered from stuttering did, with the difference being about 5.5% to 1%. In contrast, children who recovered from stuttering had more relatives who had recovered (about 4.5%) than the persistent children did (about 1.5%).[8] Finally, both the persistent and recovered cases exhibited more movements of the head and facial muscles while talking than children in a control group did. In both stuttering groups, the movements were apparent near the time of stuttering symptom onset; thus, they did not appear to be an emergent feature of the disorder. Both the recovered and persistent cases produced the movements with similar frequency; thus, these extraneous movements did not appear to be a good predictor of recovery.

Ambrose and Yairi (1999) reported recovery data for 84 children who they had observed for at least four years. Overall, 74% of children demonstrated remission of stuttering symptoms during the course of the study. Each of the children had met the researchers' recovery criteria for at least 12 months, and most (92%) had met the criteria for 18 months or longer. Criteria for recovery consisted of

---

[8]The latter finding is consistent with results from Kloth et al. (1999), who reported that recovery from stuttering took place in only 62% of children who had a parent who also stuttered.

experimenter and parent judgments of stutter-free speech, ratings of less than 1 on multipoint stuttering severity rating scales, and fewer than 3 stutter-like disfluencies per 100 syllables of conversational speech, all for a period of at least 12 months (Throneburg & Yairi, 2001). In a related study, Finn, Ingham, Ambrose, and Yairi (1997) examined the perceptual assessments of speech normalcy using samples of speech produced by children who had recovered from stuttering as well as children who had never stuttered. Three types of judges (sophisticated, unsophisticated, experienced) rated the participants in terms of speech naturalness. Across all three judging groups, the children who recovered from stuttering received comparable ratings to the children who had never stuttered. Thus, the speech of children who recovered from stuttering was indistinguishable from the speech of children who never had stuttered.

Yairi and Ambrose (1999) also found that girls were significantly more likely to recover than boys were (85% of girls versus 69% of boys; ratio of 1.22 girls to 1 boy). Both boys and girls demonstrated varying amounts of time between onset and remission; however, with most cases, recovery took place within 24 to 30 months of onset, and in many cases, it was much sooner than that. Interestingly, the children who exhibited persistent stuttering showed a trend toward decreased stuttering during the course of the study, as well; however, the magnitude of their decrease was not nearly as marked as that of the children who recovered. The latter finding and a similar one by Throneburg and Yairi (2001), with a smaller group of children, go against the traditional view that stuttering gradually worsens as the time from symptom onset increases. Rather, the data suggested that children

who showed no reduction or only minimal reduction in stuttering severity during the first year or two after onset were less likely to exhibit remission than children who showed substantial reductions in stuttering severity during that time.

Reilly et al. (2013) also examined patterns of recovery in a longitudinal study of children from birth to age 4. In their study, only 6.3% of the children who had begun to stutter exhibited recovery within 12 months of onset. In addition, recovery was more likely to occur within this time frame among boys than it was among girls, and the initial parent ratings of stuttering were lower (more favorable) for cases that did recover than for cases that did not. Interestingly, none of the 54 girls included in the analysis showed recovery from stuttering within 12 months of onset. The findings from Reilly et al. are different in some respects (e.g., recovery rates for boys versus girls) from those reported by Yairi and colleagues (e.g., Throneburg & Yairi, 2001; Yairi & Ambrose, 1999). The reasons for these differences are not entirely clear but may in part reflect differences in the time scales of research methods used by the two research groups.

Yairi and colleagues conducted several other studies in which they examined the role of language-related factors in predicting recovery from stuttering. One such study (Watkins, Yairi, & Ambrose, 1999) examined the extent to which a child's expressive language performance predicted recovery. Watkins et al. analyzed 84 children's conversational speech in terms of structural complexity and lexical diversity. They found that both the children who recovered and the children who did not recover exhibited average to above-average skills in expressive language. However, a subgroup of children who began to stutter between the ages of 2 to 3 years exhibited expressive language skills that significantly exceeded age-level expectations. Overall, the results suggested expressive language performance was not a strong predictor of which children recovered from stuttering; however, it did offer insight into factors that might precipitate stuttering onset. In this view, precocious language development during the early years of life may be something of a double-edge sword: advantageous for rich and varied communication but a potential liability for communication fluency. Reilly et al. (2013) reported a similar finding in their prospective study of 1,619 children from birth to 4 years. At the end of the study period, children who had begun to stutter exhibited significantly better scores on standardized tests of language development and nonverbal cognition than children who did not stutter. In the study, however, the children's language development at age 2 was not a strong predictor of which children began to stutter prior to age 4, and language performance at age 4 was not a good predictor of recovery from stuttering.

Paden, Yairi, and Ambrose (1999) examined the role of phonological development in recovery from stuttering in a study of the same 84 children included in the Watkins et al. (1999) study. Analysis of data from the children's initial evaluations showed that the children who eventually recovered from stuttering exhibited phonological skills that were superior to those of the children who persisted. In general, however, the types of errors that all of the children who stuttered made were similar to those of typically developing children. Thus, children who stutter seemed to be following the same developmental course as typical children, but some children who stutter (i.e., those who eventually exhibited persistent stuttering) were developing

at a slower-than-typical pace. These concerns about phonological development were short-lived, however. In a follow-up study of the children, Paden, Yairi, and Ambrose (2002) found that, by one year after stuttering onset, the children who eventually exhibited persistent stuttering effectively "caught up" with the children who eventually recovered from stuttering in terms of phonological development. Thus, phonological development distinguished the two subgroups of children who stuttered near the time of symptom onset but failed to do so in later stages of the disorder.

Other researchers have examined aspects of consonant-vowel coarticulation as potential predictors of recovery from stuttering during childhood. Results from some of these studies suggest that motor-based measures of speech production have the potential to distinguish between children who will and will not recover from stuttering. We outline two examples of research studies that have incorporated this method below:

- Brosch, Häge, and Johansenn, (2002): In this study, children produced a variety of target utterances. The researchers then analyzed aspects of speech such as voice onset time, vowel duration, fundamental frequency, jitter, and articulation rate. When the mean scores of the two groups were compared, none of these measures reliably differentiated the children whose stuttering persisted from the children who recovered from stuttering; however, the children who eventually exhibited persistent stuttering showed greater *variability* for many of these measures, and especially for voice onset time, than the children who eventually recovered from stuttering did.

- Subramanian, Yairi, and Amir (2003): In this study, the authors measured the duration and frequency changes associated with second formant (F2) transitions during children's perceptibly fluent productions of specific CV syllables. Kent and Read (1992) explain that a formant is a pattern of vocal tract resonance, and that F2, during vowel production, provides information about anterior-posterior tongue movement (e.g., front vowels are associated with relatively high F2 frequency values; back vowels are associated with relatively low F2 frequency values). In Subramanian et al.'s (2003) study, the children who persisted with stuttering showed smaller frequency shifts than the children who stuttered did. The authors interpreted the finding to mean that the persistent group used relatively restricted or constrained movements when shifting from one vocal tract configuration to another during syllable production. Transition duration, in contrast, did not differ between the two groups of children. Thus, analysis of F2 patterns in young children might provide clues about whether the stuttering will follow a persistent or transient course.

Late Recovery From Stuttering

The term *late recovery* can be used to refer to cases in which stuttering symptoms either resolve or improve substan-tially sometime after childhood (i.e., during adolescent or adulthood). There are data from several studies, most of them retrospective in nature, that shed light on this phenomenon.

Wingate (1964b) studied 50 individuals who reported having stuttered earlier in life and then experiencing remission of the stuttering symptoms. Participants ranged in age from 17 to 54 years (mean age = 34 years). Half of the participants described themselves as "normally fluent," while the other half reported that they usually spoke with normal fluency; however, in some stressful situations, they still exhibited minimal stuttering, which they reported being able to usually control. Across all cases in Wingate's (1964b) study, onset most often occurred before age 7, and significant stuttering symptoms were present for an average of 12 years. Among males, the age at time of recovery ranged from 9 to 26 years and 60% of the males experienced recovery during adolescence. Among females, the age at time of recovery was more variable and only 28% of females experienced recovery between the ages of 14 to 20 years. Individuals attributed their recovery to factors such as attitude change, speaking practice, symptomatic speech therapy, and environmental change. It is difficult to compare results from Wingate's (1964b) study with results from the studies by Yairi and colleagues, however. This is because Wingate included many participants whose stuttering still was apparent in some situations. Accordingly, it perhaps is safer to think of Wingate's data, at least in part, as providing information about the ages at which stuttering no longer presents a significant disability for speakers who stutter.

Other studies of recovery from stuttering have featured participants that are similar in fluency functioning to those in

Wingate's (1964b) study (e.g., Anderson & Felsenfeld, 2003; Finn, 1997; Shearer & Williams, 1965; Sheehan & Martyn, 1966). Finn, Howard, and Kubala (2005) reported on 15 cases of unassisted recovery from stuttering. Overall, 7 of the 15 cases reported that they no longer stuttered at all. The remaining 8 participants reported that they still stuttered on occasion; however, stuttering no longer presented a significant handicap for them. In a previous study, Finn (1997) compared speech samples from these recovered speakers with speech samples from speakers who never had stuttered. Raters assigned lower naturalness ratings to the recovered group, and naturalness ratings correlated moderately with speech rate and part-word repetition frequency. In 11 of the cases, unassisted recovery occurred at or after age 15. In five of those cases, recovery happened between age 20 and 26, and in one case, at age 42. It is impossible to say how representative of the overall population these ages of recovery are. Nonetheless, data such as these underscore the fact that, although complete recovery from stuttering seems to be less likely as one ages beyond childhood, instances of complete remission apparently do occur. Moreover, instances of near-complete remission occur as well and, in the latter cases, a person may be quite satisfied with his or her level of functioning despite having speech that sounds somewhat different than someone who never has stuttered.

Each of the studies cited in this section contains participants' impressions of factors that led to their recovery from stuttering. Common themes that participants mentioned included the following: *changes in confidence and motivation, making a conscious decision to change, making overt or explicit changes in speech* (e.g., talking slower, thinking before

speaking) *either within or apart from speech therapy*, and *remaining focused or vigilant about speech fluency over time*.

Speech Characteristics Near the Time of Onset

The onset of stuttering can assume a range of behavioral presentations. Van Riper (1982, pp. 94–108) proposed a four-part classification system for capturing the unique symptom profiles that children who stutter present in the earliest stages of the disorder and, with persistent cases, in years that follow. Van Riper developed these "tracks," as he called them, by studying 300 case files. All but 69 of those cases (23% of the total) fit into one of the four tracks. Van Riper associated numerous characteristics with each of the tracks. Some characteristics pertained to stuttering onset and others to the developmental course of the disorders. Some of the main characteristics associated with each of the tracks are listed below to provide a sense for how the cases differed at onset.

- *Track 1*—Gradual onset between ages 2;6 and 4;0 following an earlier period of fluent speech, with cyclic symptom presentation consisting mostly of relatively effortless part-word repetitions on utterance-initial function words and little associated awareness, frustration, or fear.
- *Track 2*—Onset is relatively late (i.e., at the time of sentence development), is gradual in nature, and follows a period in which speech never was very fluent. Speech is characterized by relatively effortless repetitions of syllables and words, revisions, and "gaps" that are scattered

throughout content words within sentences. A comorbid delay in speech sound production is present, as is rapid articulation. There is little associated awareness, frustration, or fear.

- *Track 3*—Sudden onset at any time after "consecutive speech" develops, often following trauma. Speech is characterized by slow rate, effortful inaudible prolongations and blocks, particularly in sentence initial contexts. The child shows keen awareness, frustration, and fear toward the fluency difficulties.
- *Track 4*—A sudden onset that occurs after the age of 4 years following an earlier period of fluent speech. Speech is characterized by excessive repetition of words and phrases and production of long, behaviorally complex disfluency. Speech symptoms change little over time. The child is highly aware of the disfluent speech but with no frustration or fear.

One limitation of highly delineated classification approaches like this is that a client can present many, but not all, of the characteristics associated with a particular track. In such cases, it can be challenging to know how the client should be classified. Although Van Riper's (1982) tracks are not used routinely in stuttering assessment and diagnosis today, they nonetheless offer a useful reminder of the range of clinical profiles that a clinician will see when providing services to children who stutter.

Research from Yairi and colleagues' University of Illinois Stuttering Research Program (for a summary, see Yairi & Ambrose, 2005) has included several analyses of fluency characteristics of preschool children at or near the time of onset. Among the findings to emerge from this work are the following:

- Gradual symptom onset (56% of cases) was more common than sudden onset (44% of cases), and the proportion of boys and girls with sudden onset was similar (Yairi & Ambrose, 1992b);
- In most cases (70%), stuttering severity was mild near the time of onset, and in the remaining cases, it was either moderate or severe (Yairi & Ambrose, 1992a, 1992b);
- Across 87 preschoolers, the most common profile for onset of stuttering (25% of all cases) was gradual onset in the context of a positive family history of stuttering and no obvious or overt stress in the child's life (Yairi & Ambrose, 1992b); and
- Near the onset of stuttering symptoms, a substantial number of children presented with relatively high stuttering frequency scores; however, a child's stuttering frequency score from the weeks immediately following symptom onset was not a sensitive predictor of whether the child's stuttering remitted (Yairi et al., 1993).

Developmental Course of Stuttering Symptoms

Experts in stuttering have long had an interest in documenting the developmental course of the disorder in terms of stages or phases. Some of the earliest efforts in this regard came from Bleumel (1932), who made the distinction between "primary" and "secondary" forms of stuttering.

Bleumel used *primary stuttering* in reference to the disfluent speech that is observed at the outset of the disordered speech, prior to when a child becomes aware of the speech pattern and views it negatively. Bluemel used *secondary stuttering* in reference to the speech patterns that appear once a child is aware of his or her stuttering and actively attempts to cope with it through the use of various compensatory behaviors and/or conceal it from others through the use of various speech avoidance and concealment strategies.

There seems to be a general agreement that, in cases of chronic or persistent stuttering, the severity of the disorder and/or its consequences gradually worsens as the length of time from symptom onset increases. In other words, the longer one stutters, the more severe the stuttering and/or its consequences become. Clinical authorities have presented this position in several ways. One well-known approach is the one that Bloodstein outlined (see Bloodstein & Bernstein Rater, 2008). He proposed four phases of stuttering, which he organized around the type, manner, and frequency of disfluency produced, the speaker's reactions to disfluency, and the contexts in which stuttered speech occurred most often. Bloodstein described the symptoms at stuttering onset in a manner consistent with Van Riper's (1982) Track 1 and claimed that as the stuttering symptoms persist, a speaker's concern level increases, and with it, the use of strategies for actively concealing, avoiding, and coping with stuttering-related disfluency. In Bloodstein's conceptualization of stuttering development, the symptoms of stuttering are said to unfold as follows:

- *Phase One*—(mainly ages 2 to 6) stuttered speech can be episodic and is largely situational in nature.

It is characterized by utterance-initial repetition of content words and relatively little concern about speech disfluency.

- *Phase Two*—(mainly elementary school-aged children) stuttered speech becomes chronic and may increase in severity when the speaker is excited or speaks rapidly. The speaker has a self-concept of being a "stutterer," yet he or she remains relatively unconcerned about the disfluent speech. Stuttering-related disfluency continues to occur mostly on content words, but the stuttered words are less restricted to the utterance-initial context.
- *Phase Three*—(mainly ages 8 to adulthood) stuttering symptoms continue to vary in frequency and severity across situations; however, the speaker begins to view some words as harder to say than others. The child may avoid or delay such words through word substitution and/or circumlocution but still does not exhibit substantial situational avoidance or speech-related fear and embarrassment.
- *Phase Four*—(mainly adolescents and adults) the speaker is acutely aware of his or her stuttered speech as evidenced by "vivid, fearful anticipation of stuttering . . . feared words, sounds, and situations" . . . and frequent use of word and situation avoidance. Stuttering symptoms continue to vary in frequency and severity across situations, and the speaker becomes increasingly aware of the social penalties that come with stuttering and how others react to stuttered speech, which results in the speaker going to extreme

lengths "to maintain a pretense as a normal speaker."

Although stage-based conceptualizations of stuttering such as the ones described above offer a general sense for how the expression of stuttering evolves over time, the approach has somewhat limited clinical application because there always will be clients who fit some, but not all, of the characteristics that are attributed to any particular stage. As Bloodstein noted (Bloodstein & Bernstein Ratner, 2008), these phases are best regarded as "typical" patterns, rather than as "universal" patterns.

Conture (1990) offered a more circumscribed account of symptom progression in his *alpha-delta hypothesis*, which was designed to capture changes in stuttered speech during the years immediately following symptom onset in early childhood. He proposed that the earliest symptoms of stuttered speech (*alpha behavior*) consist of brief inefficiencies in speech production. These inefficiencies are manifested as brief "laryngeal catches," which mostly are imperceptible to the listener. Support for Conture's hypothesis came, in part, from previous investigations of laryngeal movements during stuttered speech (e.g., Conture, Schwartz, & Brewer, 1985). Under the alpha-delta hypothesis, speakers are said to compensate for the laryngeal glitches by producing oscillatory behavior such as part-word repetitions (*beta behavior*), which over time lead to rigid, fixed articulatory postures associated with sound prolongation (*gamma behavior*), and finally to various coping or reactive responses to the preceding forms of disfluency (*delta behavior*). There is some support for the idea that sound prolongations are an emergent aspect of stuttering. For example, Pellowski and Conture (2002) reported that the proportion

of "disrhythmic phonations" (a category that includes sound prolongation) a child produces is positively correlated with the amount of time that has elapsed since the onset of stuttering symptoms. Others (e.g., Yairi et al., 1996), however, point out that a sizable proportion of children who stutter exhibit sound prolongation near the time of symptom onset for stuttering.

More broadly, research does not fully support the notion that stuttering severity increases as a function of how long a speaker has stuttered. For example, Andrews and Harvey (1981) conducted repeated measurements of adults who stutter as they waited for treatment during a period of several months. During the first three months on the wait list, stuttering showed modest but significant *improvement*, and after that period, it remained stable. Thus, with those adults, the passage of time did not necessarily correspond to a worsening of speech disfluency. Yairi and colleagues (Yairi et al., 1996) reported a similar pattern among preschool-aged children who they followed over time but did not enroll in active treatment. Similarly, in our experience with developing norms for the *Test of Childhood Stuttering* (Gillam et al., 2009), we found that there was no significant correlation between a child's chronological age and his or her stuttering severity. There is relatively little research on the stuttering-related experiences of older adults. In one study (Manning, Dailey, & Wallace, 1984), older adults who stuttered showed similar communication-related performance and attitudes as younger adults who stuttered, but they perceived stuttering as less handicapping. Together, these findings suggest that although gradual worsening in stuttering severity certainly may happen with some individuals, it is by no means a universal feature of the disorder.

Summary

Stuttering has been documented in writings that date back to ancient times. In the past half-century, the pace of research on the disorder has accelerated greatly, and this has led to a much more complete understanding of the nature and characteristics of the disorder. Most definitions of stuttering are symptom-based and center on the tendency for affected speakers to produce part-word repetitions and sound prolongations/blocks much more frequently than the typical speaker does. Although stuttering definitions tend to emphasize these disfluency types, in a statistical sense, it has been shown that speakers who stutter produce *all* types of repetition more often than typical speakers do and that the disfluency types that are indicative of stuttering do not always assume the structural form of classic disfluency types. Repetitions, prolongations, and blocks are common symptoms of stuttered speech; however, there are cases in which a speaker is able to cope with his or her fluency impairment adroitly, such that impending repetitions, prolongations, and blocks are effectively hidden from listeners through the use of strategies such as word avoidance or circumlocution, or through production of more common types of disfluency such as interjection and pausing. Thus, current definitions for stuttering describe the behavior of most people who stutter but certainly not all of them. Accordingly, it seems clear that disfluency-based definitions offer a constrained perspective on the disorder because they generally only focus on what a listener *hears* during speech. As discussed in the next chapter, there are many other markers of stuttering, some of which can be detected only through the use of sophisticated instrumentation.

Stuttering frequency is commonly used as an index of stuttering severity; however, research findings have shown repeatedly that stuttering frequency is only partly predictive of a speaker's stuttering severity score. Other factors that contribute to stuttering severity include the duration of stuttering-related disfluency, speech rate, the amount of effort that a speaker exerts when talking, and the naturalness of his or her speech. Stuttering severity is variable both within and across speakers. Some speakers may find that they are able to speak with relatively high levels of fluency during some situations, but in other situations, their speech fluency performance may be much less proficient. In contrast, other speakers who stutter may exhibit a relatively constant amount of stuttered speech across most tasks and situations. Speaking tasks that evoke a lot of disfluency for one speaker may evoke relatively little disfluency for another speaker. For most speakers who stutter, speech fluency is greatly improved or perhaps even normalized during singing, choral speaking, and speaking in a slowed or rhythmic manner. When compared to solo speech, it appears that these facilitative tasks are associated with changes in the temporal/prosodic aspects of speech and, by inference, their corresponding patterns of neural activation. The differences in fluency performance between solo speech and speech during fluency-facilitating contexts may provide insight into the nature of stuttering.

Children seem to develop an awareness of stuttering gradually, and most children who stutter exhibit awareness of their own stuttering by the time they enter elementary school. At that time, children who stutter also are likely to have developed the sense that stuttered speech is undesirable. As children who stutter become aware of their fluency difficulty, they are apt to react to it through the use of various coping strategies. These coping strategies are commonly oriented toward reducing the frequency or severity of speech disfluency and, with it, the extent of speech disability. In most cases, these self-devised coping strategies are only partially effective and, in some cases, they can detract from verbal communication more than the speech disfluency.

Stuttering is considered a developmental disorder, as the overt symptoms of the disorder emerge during childhood in the context of neuromaturation. For most children, stuttered speech first is noted during the preschool years; however, cases with onset during later childhood have been documented as well. Stuttering is a fairly common problem in that approximately 3% to 5% of the population reports having stuttered at some point during the lifespan. Males are more than three times as likely to stutter as females, although the male-to-female ratio for stuttering varies somewhat depending on the age of the cohort that is being studied. In cases where onset occurs during the preschool years, "recovery" from the disorder seems to be common—current estimates are that approximately 75% of preschoolers who exhibit stuttered speech eventually will experience remission of the atypical fluency patterns that characterize the disorder. If recovery from stuttering symptoms does occur, it often seems to do so within roughly 18 to 24 months after onset. Still, there are reports of recovery taking place in children who are several years removed from symptom onset. Researchers have searched extensively for reliable predictors of which children will recover from stuttering. Thus far, such efforts have yielded limited results.

Stuttering sometimes is conceptualized as developing in stages or phases. In such conceptualizations, the speaker's degree of communication disability is said to worsen with age, such that fluency difficulties become a fixed or stable part of speech, and the speaker becomes increasingly sensitivity to how others' reaction to stuttered speech. As speakers become aware of their fluency impairment and others' reactions to it, they are more likely to implement coping strategies either to facilitate fluency or conceal fluency impairment from others. In some cases, such as when a speaker attempts to conceal fluency impairment by electing not to participate in verbal communication, the coping responses may hinder the speaker's communication functioning more than the disfluent speech does. Thus, a key treatment goal for many speakers who exhibit persistent stuttering will be to help them cope with or compensate for fluency impairment as effectively as possible. The latter topic is discussed in Section IV of this text.

6

Developmental Stuttering: Correlates, Causes, and Consequences

In the previous chapter, the focus was on what one might call the "surface features" of stuttering; that is, the way in which stuttered speech sounds and is manifested in various speaking contexts and at different points in the lifespan. In this chapter, the focus shifts toward three main topics: (1) past and current theories on the causes of stuttering; (2) factors that are correlated with stuttering; and (3) the social, emotional, and communicative consequences of stuttering. It is essential for clinicians to develop a thorough understanding of such information, as it is fundamental to both evidence-based practice and the ability to establish a strong therapeutic alliance with clients. Simply put, it is difficult for a clinician to construct an effective treatment plan and provide effective counsel for a person who stutters if the clinician's "map" of the disorder is incomplete, outdated, or inaccurate. With this in mind, the goal in the present chapter is to dig below the surface of stuttered speech and explore the finer details of what researchers have discovered about stuttering and people who stutter.

Historical Perspective

Scientific research on the characteristics and etiology of stuttering began in earnest during the 1930s. Since then, the pace of research has accelerated markedly. At times, it seems as if researchers have examined stuttering from every possible angle. Bloodstein and Bernstein Ratner (2008) summarized much of the early research on stuttering, including findings from studies in which researchers examined the following variables for their potential role in the disorder:

- Breathing patterns,
- Hand-eye coordination,
- Manual strength and steadiness,

- Cardiovascular functioning (e.g., blood pressure, basal metabolic rate),
- General biochemistry characteristics (e.g., blood oxygen levels, pH levels in saliva),
- Reflexive responses to environmental stimuli,
- Peripheral and central auditory system functioning,
- Visual perception, and
- Oral and peripheral sensory functions (e.g., vibrotactile detection, weight estimation, spatial discrimination).

At some time in the past, each of the variables listed above was hypothesized to have potential relevance to stuttering. Through research, some of these variables have been found to have relatively little role in stuttering and, consequently, have dropped off the scientific agenda. The current landscape of scientific research into stuttering has been fueled in large measure by technological advances that allow for increasingly reliable and precise study of genes, neuroanatomy, neurophysiology, and movement coordination. Another factor that has been important in shaping the research agenda for stuttering pertains to conceptualizations about the nature of the disorder itself. In the 1960s, learning-based theories of stuttering were influential, as were models that explained the disorder from a psychosocial perspective. Competing neurophysiological explanations for stuttering became more common and gained increasing acceptance toward the late 1960s as the shortcomings of learning- and emotion-based theories became more apparent. Along with this came a growing call for researchers to integrate stuttering-related research into mainstream research dealing with nor-

mal speech production processes, rather than continuing to study it from the perspective of arcane and poorly supported alternatives (see, for example, MacKay & McDonald, 1984; Smith & Weber, 1988; Starkweather, 1987).

In the remainder of the chapter, the primary focus is on how people who stutter compare with normally fluent speakers on a host of variables that are relevant to speech production. The intent is not to review *all* of the comparisons that have been made between these groups but instead to offer a thorough description of most of the main ways in which the two groups differ.

Correlates of Stuttering: An Overview

In the context of speech-language pathology, the term *correlate* refers to a factor that is associated with a disorder. Thus, when one talks about the "correlates of stuttering," he or she is referring to behaviors, traits, or patterns that relate in some way to the disorder. The nature of this relationship varies with the factors under consideration. Some factors are associated with the etiology of stuttering. Other factors are associated with the way in which the disorder manifests itself. Still, other factors are associated with the effects of stuttering on a person's quality of life; particularly, his or her ability to communicate. Thus, in a general sense, the correlates of stuttering are those factors that influence a speaker's experience of stuttering. As will be seen, the extent to which any one factor contributes to a speaker's stuttering experience varies across individuals, and factors that have a large impact on one person's stuttering experience may have little impact on another person's stuttering experience. The more a clinician understands about the dynamic nature of stuttering, the better positioned he or she will be to develop effective treatment plans for people who stutter.

So, what are the main correlates of stuttering? There probably are many ways this question could be answered; however, in this chapter, the discussion is organized around seven themes:

1. Genetic correlates—the role of genetic factors in the etiology and expression of stuttering;
2. Anatomical correlates—aspects of body structure that seem to affect the expression of stuttering, with a particular emphasis on neuroanatomical correlates;
3. Physiological correlates—aspects of body function that seem to affect the expression of stuttering, with a particular emphasis on neurophysiological correlates;
4. Linguistic and cognitive correlates—the role of linguistic and cognitive factors in stuttered speech;
5. Motor correlates—the role of the motor system in stuttered speech and motor system functioning in speakers who stutter;
6. Psychological, social, and emotional correlates—the roles of attitudes, beliefs, thoughts, and feelings in stuttering;
7. Environmental correlates—the effects of other people's actions and beliefs on the speaker's experience of stuttering.

In the present chapter, selected research findings from each of these areas are reviewed to illustrate the ways in which they relate to the causes, characteristics, and consequences of stuttering.

Genetic Correlates

One topic that has attracted considerable interest among researchers is the possibility that stuttering is a heritable disorder. Research methods in the field of genetics have advanced considerably in recent decades, and with these advances have come an increasingly clear picture of the manner and extent to which genes are involved in developmental stuttering.

Approaches to Researching Genetic Factors

In Table 6–1, the primary approaches that researchers have used to study genetic influences in fluency disorders are outlined, along with the basic research methods and frameworks for data interpretation that accompany them. In each of these approaches, researchers construct information that provides insight into the genotype (i.e., the sum total of specific variants of genes) associated with stuttered speech.

Twin Studies

Interest in the epidemiology of stuttering among twins is longstanding. Berry (1937) noted a relatively high occurrence of stuttering among families with twin children. A common analysis in twin research is to compare monozygotic (identical) and dizygotic (nonidentical) twin pairs on their concordance for a trait. The notion of *pairwise concordance* refers to instances in which both members of the twin pair exhibit the same trait (e.g., stuttering). In contrast, the term *discordance* refers to

Table 6–1. Research Approaches Used to Study the Role of Genetic Factors in Stuttering

Approach	Method	Data Interpretation
Twin studies	Comparing monozygotic and dizygotic twin pairs for the presence of stuttering	If concordance for stuttering is greater in monozygotic pairs than dizygotic pairs, it suggests that genetic factors influence the trait more than environmental factors do.
Adoption studies	Comparing a child against his or her biological and adoptive parents for the presence of stuttering	If the child and the biological parents are more similar than the child and the adoptive parents, it suggests that genetic factors influence the trait more than environmental factors do.
Pedigree analysis (Familial incidence, Familial aggregation)	Examining patterns of stuttering across members of a family (e.g., proband, siblings, parents, grandparents, aunts, uncles)	The number of shared genes across a given pair predicts the extent to which a trait should co-occur across pair members.
Linkage studies (Molecular genetics)	Identification of chromosomal regions and, perhaps, specific genes, that are associated with stuttering	Genes in identified chromosomal regions are sequenced and compared in affected and unaffected speakers to identified genetic variants that are unique to stuttering.
Epigenetics	Examining patterns of gene expression over time.	Focus shifts from study of DNA sequence to factors that affect gene expression, such as environmental interactions

Note. Based on Drayna, 2011; Kraft & Yairi, 2012; Yairi, Ambrose, & Cox, 1996.

instances in which one member of the twin pair exhibits the trait, but the other does not.

Between the 1940s and the 1960s, several research studies explored pairwise concordance patterns for stuttering. The general finding from these studies was that monozygotic twin pairs were more likely to be concordant for stuttering than dizygotic twin pairs were (Graf, 1955; Nelson, Hunter, & Walter, 1945). That is, in roughly 80% of the cases where one member of a monozygotic twin set stuttered, the other

member did too. For dizygotic twins, the concordance rate fell into the 7% to 10% range. Such findings were taken as support for the idea that genetic factors play a role in developmental stuttering.

In subsequent years, researchers implemented increasingly refined research methods when studying concordance for stuttering and, consequently, they were able to control several extraneous variables that limited the results of early research. In recent decades, researchers also have reported data in terms of *probandwise concordance*[1], a statistic that captures the probability of a twin stuttering given that his or her co-twin stutters (van Beijsterveldt, Felsenfeld, & Boomsma, 2010). Several authorities have argued that probandwise concordance is preferable to pairwise concordance as a measure of hereditability, because it is less likely to be distorted by data collection methods and it fits better with the types of questions that researchers ask about stuttering (Dworzynski, Remington, Rijsdijk, Howell, & Plomin, 2007).

In Table 6–2, concordance findings from several twin studies are presented. As can be seen, both the pairwise and probandwise rates are consistently higher for monozygotic twins than for dizygotic twins. Thus, in a large percentage of cases in which stuttering is present in a monozygotic twin pair, both twins within the pair are affected. With studies that have utilized adult samples, the probandwise concordance rate is roughly .50 to .80 for monozygotic twins (meaning, that if one member of a twin pair stutters, there is as much as an 80% chance that the co-twin will stutter too). Conversely, the risk for a co-twin to develop stuttering drops considerably when the twins are diyzgotic. Thus, when one twin stutters, the likelihood that the other also will stutter is predictable on the basis of how similar the twins are genetically.

As shown in the table, Dworzynski et al. (2007) reported comparatively

Table 6–2. Selected Findings From Studies of Concordance for Stuttering in Twin Pairs

Study	Pairwise Concordance		Probandwise Concordance	
	Monozygotic	Dizygotic	Monozygotic	Dizygotic
Howie (1981)	.64 (males)	.29 (males)	.78 (males)	.45 (males)
	.60 (females)	0.0 (females)	.75 (females)	0.0 (females)
Felsenfeld et al. (2000)	.45	.15	.62	.26
Dworzynski et al. (2007)	.15 (age 3)	.04 (age 3)	.26 (age 3)	.09 (age 3)
	.17 (age 7)	.02 (age 7)	.29 (age 7)	.03 (age 7)
van Beijsterveldt et al. (2010)	—	—	.53 (males)	.36 (males)
			.61 (females)	.34 (females)

Note. Numbers under the pairwise heading represent the proportion of twin pairs in which both members stutter; numbers under the probandwise heading represent the proportion of individual cases that can be expected to stutter when a co-twin stutters. Data from Howie (1981), Felsenfeld et al. (2000), and Dworzynski et al. (2007) are based on direct interviews of research participants. Data from van Beijsterveldt et al. (2010) are based on parents' responses to a questionnaire. The questionnaire only required parents to report on the children's disfluency behaviors. Parents were not asked directly whether their children stuttered. Hence, van Beijsterveldt et al. (2010) labeled the children as "probable stuttering."

---

[1]In genetics research, the term *proband* refers to the person who is being studied directly. For example, if a researcher asks a woman who stutters whether she has any siblings who have ever stuttered, the woman who stutters is regarded as the proband.

low probandwise concordance rates in a study that involved preschool-aged probands. Even so, the concordance rate for monozygotic preschool-aged twins in that study was much greater than it was for dizygotic preschool-aged twins and the pattern is seen as evidence that genetic factors influence the expression of stuttering very early in life (Dworzynski et al., 2007). Despite all of the evidence for a relatively high degree of concordance for stuttering among monozygotic twins, one must remember that in each of these studies, there have been monozygotic twin pairs who are discordant for stuttering. This suggests that environmental factors interact with genetic factors to influence the expression of stuttering (Dworzynski et al., 2007; Howie, 1981).

In some twin studies, researchers have used statistical modeling to determine the extent to which genetic and environmental factors contribute to the expression of stuttering. Using this approach, Felsenfeld et al. (2000) concluded that additive genetic factors accounted for about 70/% of the variance in a person's liability to develop stuttering, with the remaining 30% attributable to environmental factors. Others (e.g., Andrews, Morris-Yates, Howie, & Martin, 1991; Dworzynski et al., 2007) have reached very similar conclusions based on their findings. Overall, data from twin studies suggest that developmental stuttering is a moderately to strongly heritable disorder (Dworzynski et al., 2007; van Beijsterveldt et al., 2010).

Familial and Pedigree Studies

It has long been known that stuttering seems to run in families. This has led to studies of the familial patterns of stuttering. One basic analysis involves the com-putation of the percentage of cases that have other relatives who stutter. Yairi and Ambrose (2005) noted that much of the early research on familial incidence is flawed because researchers did not control for the family size. They indicated that this is problematic because a large family has a higher probability of having an affected member than a small family does.

Yairi and Ambrose (2005) reported that, in their longitudinal research with preschoolers who stutter, 69% of the preschoolers who stuttered had a positive family history of stuttering (i.e., at least one other affected family member). The children who recovered from stuttering were less likely to have a positive family history than the children who exhibited persistent stuttering (63% of the recovered cases had a positive history versus 88% of the persistent cases).

A second line of research entails examination of family aggregation patterns. This approach leads to information about which relatives of a proband are most at risk for exhibiting stuttering. Yairi and Ambrose (2005) reported on familial patterns of stuttering in children with persistent stuttering. They found that the observed frequency of stuttering was significantly greater than the expected frequency for each of the four possible basic patterns of aggregation. That is, stuttering was observed in:

- 24% of the immediate male relatives of a male proband who stuttered (which is 16 times greater than the expected percentage),
- 33% of the immediate male relatives of a female proband who stuttered (which is 22 times greater than the expected percentage),
- 7% of the immediate female relatives of a male proband who

stuttered (which is 14 times greater than the expected percentage), and

- 12% of the immediate female relatives of a female proband who stuttered (which is 24 times greater than the expected percentage).

These findings are generally consistent with findings from other studies. That is, other researchers (e.g., Andrews & Harris, 1964; Kidd, 1984; MacFarlane, Hanson, Walton, & Mellon, 1991) also have reported that the risk for stuttering is greatest among male relatives of female probands and that it is lowest among female relatives of male probands.

Kloth and colleagues (Kloth, Janssen, Kraaimaat, & Brutten, 1995,, 1998; Kloth, Kraaimaat, & Brutten, 1995; Kloth, Kraaimaat, Janssen, & Brutten, 1999) conducted a unique prospective examination of familial patterns of stuttering. Participants in their studies were 93 preschool-aged children whose parents had a history of stuttering. Because of their positive family history for the disorder, the children were presumed to be at greater risk for developing stuttering than the typical child. The researchers tracked the children's development between the ages of 2 to 8 years. None of the children stuttered at the start of the project; however, during the first two years after enrollment, 26 of the children (28% of the total) began to stutter (Kloth et al., 1998). This percentage is much greater than what one would expect from a sample of the general population.

Kloth and colleagues (Kloth et al., 1995, 1998, 1999) examined various aspects of the children's performance prior to the time of symptom onset, with the hope of finding markers that precipitated the onset of stuttering symptoms. Among the many variables they examined, the only ones that differentiated the groups significantly were articulation rate and articulation rate variability. That is, the group that began to stutter had a faster articulation rate prior to symptom onset and more variable articulation rate over time than the group that did not begin to stutter.

Chromosomes and Genes

Recent advances in technology have made it increasingly feasible to search for specific genetic markers of stuttering. The basic approach is to identify chromosomes, regions on chromosomes, and, ultimately, specific genes that seem to be associated with the disorder. If researchers can establish a *linkage* between stuttered speech and specific genes, the function of those genes then can be investigated to delineate the biological mechanisms that underlie the disorder. Several studies have been conducted in recent years toward this goal.

One research strategy in these early-stage studies was to focus the genomic analyses on subgroups of people that are closely related to one another and have a relatively high incidence of stuttering. If genetic markers exist, they most likely are to be detected within samples of this sort. Examples of such subgroups include members of an extended Hutterite family from South Dakota (Wittke-Thompson et al., 2007) and members of "highly-inbred" Pakistani families (Riaz et al., 2005). Other researchers have based their analyses on what seem to be more genetically diverse samples. Although the initial results from such research seem promising, most would agree that there still is much work to be done before any definitive statements can be made about which genes are mostly strongly linked to the etiology of stuttering.

As noted above, an initial goal in this line of research is to isolate chromosomes that are most strongly associated with the disorder. To date, research findings have yielded divergent findings in this regard. Chromosomes (C) that have been flagged as having the strongest association to developmental stuttering include the following:

- C 9 (Suresh et al., 2006),
- C 12 (Kang et al., 2010; Riaz et al., 2005),
- C 13 (Wittke-Thompson et al., 2007),
- C 15 (Suresh et al., 2006), and
- C 18 (Shugart et al., 2004).

It is not possible at present to explain precisely why the studies yield such different results. It may be that the findings from any one study are unique to that specific sample and thus are not representative of the entire population. For the most part, the samples from the studies that are discussed in this section come from nonoverlapping populations that were widely separated in geographical and environmental terms. To the extent that each of the implicated chromosomes is relevant to stuttering, it may be that there are several genetic pathways to stuttered speech.

In each of these studies, researchers also identified several "secondary" chromosomes of interest; that is, chromosomes with regions that were less strongly associated with stuttering but still potentially relevant to the disorder. The flagged chromosomes have varied across studies as well, with the exception that in three studies (Riaz et al., 2005; Shugart et al., 2004; Wittke-Thompson et al., 2007), chromosome 1 was identified as containing a region of potential relevance to stuttering.

In recent years, attempts have been made to isolate specific genes that are linked with stuttering. Based on findings from Riaz et al. (2005), Kang et al. (2010) searched for genetic mutations within chromosome 12 that possibly were related to stuttering. They identified three candidate genes, each of which featured mutational variations that were, in large measure, unique to speakers who stuttered. The genes are labeled with letter sequences: GNPTAB, GNPTG, and NAGPA. All three genes were identified through previous research to have an association with metabolic functions, specifically those associated with lysosomal functioning within cells.[2] Kang et al. noted that certain mutations in GNPTAB and GNPTG are associated with a metabolic disease called mucolipidosis. The disease is characterized by various skeletal, cardiac, and ocular disorders, as well as deficits in speech production. The mutations observed in Kang et al.'s sample were different in nature from those that are associated with mucolipidosis. Kang et al. speculated that this might explain why the speakers who stuttered did not exhibit any of the nonspeech disorders that characterized mucolipidosis.

Kang et al. (2010) noted that mutations in NAGPA previously had not been associated with human disorders; however, previous research with mice had revealed that both NAGPA and GNPTAB are strongly associated with functioning and/or development in the hippocampus and cerebellum. These brain regions are associated with emotions and motor control, and Kang et al. noted that emotional

---

[2]The lysosome is an organelle within a cell body. It contains enzymes that degrade and digest waste products and other unnecessary materials associated with the cell's functioning (Cooper, 2000).

states often have a significant effect on speech fluency in speakers who stutter. Mutation of the NAGPA gene was noted only among speakers of North American-British descent, while mutation of the GNPTAB and GNPTG genes were noted only in speakers of South Asian and European descent. Kang et al. cautioned that, although these particular mutations did seem to be linked with stuttering, they were present in only about 10% of the stuttering cases in their study. This suggests that other types of genetic mutations may be relevant to stuttering as well. Yairi and Ambrose (2005) pointed out that an individual's liability for developing stuttering can be conceptualized as the summation of both genetic and environmental factors, and that, from this perspective, it is plausible that an individual can present with a number of stuttering-related factors yet still not exhibit observable symptoms of the disorder.

Anatomical Correlates

It is intuitively appealing to suppose that stuttered speech is associated with anatomical differences in the speech production system. In recent years, improvements in methods of neuroimaging have enabled researchers to explore this possibility in ever-increasing depth. Results from such studies support the broad hypothesis that certain neuroanatomical anomalies are associated with stuttered speech.

Gray Matter Volume and Hemispheric Asymmetry

In some studies, researchers have measured the volume of key left hemisphere cortical regions that are involved in speech production and compared it to measures from homologous areas within the right hemisphere. Foundas et al. (2003) examined the volume of right and left frontal and temporo-parietal lobe regions in adults who stuttered and adults with typical fluency. They found significant differences between the groups in the relative sizes of these brain regions. That is, speakers with typical fluency showed larger cortical volume in the right frontal lobe versus the left frontal lobe, whereas speakers who stutter either showed no difference in the sizes of these regions or a reversed pattern (i.e., larger cortical volume in the left frontal lobe relative to the right frontal lobe). A similar pattern existed for comparisons of the temporo-parietal lobule. That is, speakers with typical fluency showed larger cortical volume in the left temporo-parietal lobule than in the homologous right hemisphere lobule. In contrast, the speakers who stuttered either failed to show this cortical asymmetry or they exhibited reversed cortical asymmetry (i.e., larger right temporo-parietal cortex than left).

In a separate analysis, Foundas, Bollich, Corey, Hurley, and Heilman (2001) detected several additional differences between speakers who stuttered and speakers with typical fluency. Specifically, the speakers who stuttered showed:

- More gray matter volume in both the right and left planum temporale in comparison to typical speakers;
- A less prominent right versus left hemispheric asymmetry in the planum temporale volume in comparison to speakers with typical fluency; and
- More than three times as many anomalies in gyral structure (including some gyral anomalies that fluent speakers never exhibited).

Although these neuroanatomical characteristics differed significantly at a group level, the researchers (Foundas et al., 2001, 2003) cautioned that not all speakers who stuttered exhibited atypical neuroanatomy and that some of the speakers with typical fluency exhibited neuroanatomical anomalies as well. Among the speakers who stuttered, the magnitude of the anomaly did not predict their stuttering severity; however, it did predict the speakers' performance in a language-processing task.

In a subsequent study, Foundas and colleagues (Foundas et al., 2004) found that stuttering speakers who had the atypical rightward asymmetry pattern in the planum temporal demonstrated greater fluency enhancement when talking under delayed auditory feedback (DAF) in comparison to those stuttering speakers who exhibited the typical leftward asymmetry pattern. On this basis, Foundas et al. (2004) suggested that the neuroanatomical anomaly in the planum temporale negatively affected components of the speech production process that are critical for fluent speech.

Although the preceding findings are intriguing, other researchers have failed to replicate them exactly in subsequent studies. For example, in a study with adults who stuttered, Cykowski et al. (2008) found no evidence of either anomalous rightward asymmetry in the temporoparietal region or atypical sulcal or gyral patterning in the left perisylvian region. However, in their study, the adults who stuttered did show evidence of atypical sulcal and gyral patterns in the right perisylvian region. In a study with children, Chang and colleagues (Chang, Erickson, Ambrose, Hasegawa-Johnson, & Ludlow, 2008) found no evidence of an anomalous rightward asymmetry in the planum temporale in either children with persistent

stuttering or children who recovered from stuttering. However, they did find that both subgroups of children who stutter had reduced gray matter volume in cortical regions associated with speech production (i.e., left inferior frontal lobe, left and right temporal lobe). On this basis, Chang et al. (2008) hypothesized that the neuroanatomical differences reported in some recent studies with adults who stutter may represent a consequence of having stuttered for many years, rather than a cause of the disorder.

White Matter Integrity

In recent years, several research teams (e.g., Chang et al., 2008; Kell et al., 2009; Sommer, Koch, Paulus, Weiller, & Büchel, 2002) have used *diffusion tensor imaging* (DTI) to collect information about axonal integrity in the speech production system. Axon fibers project from nerve cell bodies and allow nerve cells to communicate with one another. A myelin sheath covers each axon fiber. The myelin functions in a manner that is similar to insulation around an electrical wire; that is, it increases the speed or efficiency with which electrical signals propagate along the axon. The DTI technology allows researchers to make inferences about an axon's diameter and structural integrity, including its myelination characteristics.

In each of the DTI studies conducted with speakers who stutter to date, researchers have detected evidence of compromised white matter integrity. Although the specific findings have varied somewhat across studies with regard to where the differences between speakers who stutter and typical speakers exist, one finding that has emerged consistently from this research is evidence of abnormal white matter integrity in the left, ventral perisylvian area.[3] Other findings to emerge from this line of research include the following:

- Sommer et al. (2002) reported significant differences between adults who stuttered and adults with typical fluency in axonal integrity within the rolandic operculum of the left hemisphere. Differences were particularly apparent in the portion of the sensorimotor cortex involved in representation of oropharynx.
- Watkins, Smith, Davis, and Howell (2008) reported evidence of reduced white matter integrity in the ventral premotor cortex. The researchers noted that white matter tracks in this area project to the temporo-parietal lobule and allow for integration of articulatory planning and sensory feedback. Watkins et al. reported evidence of atypical myelination in other regions of the brain, as well.
- Chang et al. (2008) reported evidence of reduced white matter integrity among children with persistent stuttering but not among children who recovered from stuttering or children with typical fluency. The anomalies existed in the left anterior perisylvian cortex, particularly in areas associated with motor functions for the face and larynx.
- Cykowski, Fox, Ingham, Ingham, & Robin (2010) reported evidence of reduced white matter integrity in a group of adults who stuttered.

As with the studies above, the differences were consistent with a pattern of dysmyelination. Areas of difference included the ventral perisylvian region and the body of the corpus callosum. The most robust finding implicated abnormal white matter development in the ventral subdivision of superior longitudinal fasciculus, deep to Brodmann area 44. Consistent with Sommer et al. (2002) and Chang et al. (2008), the authors noted that this fiber tract allows for two-way communication between the speech production area of the premotor cortex and the somatosensory area in the inferior parietal lobule. Both of these areas play an integral role in speech articulation.

- In a comparison of adults who stuttered and adults with typical fluency, Choo et al. (2011) detected differences between the groups in the structure of the corpus callosum, a large fiber tract with connections between the left and right hemispheres. The analysis focused on regions of the corpus callosum that are involved in informational exchange between the hemispheres. These regions of the corpus callosum were significantly larger in the adults who stuttered than they were in the adults with typical fluency. Choo et al. suggested that the differences were related to differences in how language-related processes are distributed in adults who stutter versus adults with typical fluency.

---

[3]The sylvian fissure (lateral sulcus) forms a boundary between the frontal and temporal lobes. In a lateral view of the brain, it appears as a prominent fissure that courses along the anterior-posterior dimension of the cortex.

In sum, the white matter abnormalities observed in the preceding studies are consistent with the notion of a dysfunctional connection between speech motor planning and sensorimotor feedback centers in the brain (Cykowski et al., 2010; Sommer et al., 2002). One would expect that impairment in this portion of the speech production system would lead to difficulty in fluently producing novel, infrequent, or motorically complex words (Chang et al., 2008; Cykowski et al., 2010)—and this is precisely what happens with many speakers who stutter.

Cykowski et al. (2010) noted that the superior longitudinal fasciculus does not normally begin to myelinate until 4 to 6 postnatal months. Thus, they suggested that the anomaly in this axonal tract is consistent with the idea of a disruption in the developmental course of myelination (i.e., disrupted *myelogenesis*). They proposed that the dysmyelination leads to degradation in connectivity between the premotor and auditory association regions of the cortex. Cykowski et al. (2010) also noted that the dysmyelination pattern observed in speakers who stutter may be consistent with the recent discovery that some people who stutter exhibit genetic variations that are associated with metabolic dysfunction that affects nerve cell development. Others (e.g., Fisher, 2010) have challenged this view. Whether genetic factors are involved in some, most, or all cases of dysmyelination remains to be determined. Other factors may contribute to myelination development in early life, as well. For example, Mahurin-Smith and Ambrose (2013) reported that the mothers of preschoolers with persistent stuttering breastfed their children for a shorter duration than did the mothers of preschoolers who recovered from stuttering. They noted that the fatty acid profile of human milk affects gene expression and contributes to neural development and hypothesized that the differences in breastfeeding patterns between the groups may have contributed to the eventual developmental course of the speech production system and, along with it, the expression of stuttering.

Physiological Correlates

Early Studies of Brain Activation and Language Dominance

Studies into the role of the central nervous system in stuttered speech began in earnest during the early 1930s. Up through the early 1980s, many of the brain-based research questions pertaining to stuttering addressed rather broad issues. One question that received extensive attention from researchers from the 1960s though the early 1980s was whether speakers who stutter were less apt to show left hemisphere dominance for language processing than speakers with typical fluency. Moore (1984) summarized findings from a variety of research methods that were used to address this question. One of the more unusual approaches to the study of language dominance in speakers who stutter involved the use of *sodium amytal* as a means of anesthetizing either the right or left cortical hemisphere in order to determine whether a patient is right or left hemisphere dominant for language. Wada (1949) originally described the procedure; hence, it came to be called the Wada test. The sodium amytal is injected into either the right or left carotid artery, whereupon it leads to a loss of ipsilateral hemispheric function for about 2 to 3 minutes. Jones

(1966) reported Wada test results for four speakers who stutter and were about to undergo brain surgery for medical problems unrelated to stuttering and reported that these individuals seemed to exhibit bilateral control for speech-language functions, rather than the typical pattern of left-hemisphere dominance. Moore (1984) reviewed several other studies in which the Wada test was used to assess language lateralization in speakers who stutter, and in each of the latter cases, the findings from Jones were not corroborated.

A second approach to examining hemispheric activation with speakers who stutter involved the use of the *dichotic listening* paradigm (Kimura, 1961). During dichotic listening tests, competing auditory stimuli are presented simultaneously to the right and left ear at an equal intensity. Research participants must tell the experimenter what they have heard. After many trials, an ear preference emerges. That is, the participants report what they have heard in one ear more often than what they have heard in the other ear. Most people show a preference for stimuli that are presented to the right ear. This is because information presented to the right ear is routed to the left hemisphere, which in most people is the dominant hemisphere for language processing. In contrast, stimuli that are presented to the left ear take a more circuitous route in most people, traveling first to the right hemisphere and then to the left hemisphere for processing. Therefore, information presented to the left ear takes longer to process than information that is presented to the right ear. If speakers who stutter do indeed show a bias toward processing linguistic information in the right hemisphere, then they would be expected to exhibit the right ear advantage during dichotic listening less often than speakers with

typical fluency. Results from several studies are consistent with this prediction (Curry & Gregory, 1969; Sommers, Brady, & Moore, 1975); that is, individuals who stutter seem to show the anomalous *left-ear* preference during dichotic listening, particularly when meaningful stimuli are presented.

A third approach involved the study of language processing through the visual system. In several studies, researchers made use of an instrument called a *tachistoscope* to examine hemispheric dominance for language. The tachistoscope is a device that is capable of presenting visual information to either the right or left visual field. Information presented to the right visual field is routed to the left hemisphere, whereas information presented to the left visual field is routed to the right hemisphere. Thus, similar to the dichotic listening paradigm, when linguistic information is presented to the right visual field, it is processed faster than when it is presented to the left visual field. As with the dichotic listening studies, the data suggest that speakers who stutter show a left visual field (right hemisphere) bias for language processing during tasks that utilize the tachistoscope (e.g., Hand & Haynes, 1983; Moore, 1976).

Findings From Electroencephalography (EEG)

A fourth approach used in early studies of the neural events associated with stuttering made use of the electroencephalogram (EEG), an instrument that measures electrical activity at the surface of the brain. Several researchers have examined changes in alpha wave activity during speech and nonspeech activities. The alpha wave has a characteristic frequency—8 Hz to 13 Hz—and it is prominent when the brain is in a relaxed state (Moore, 1984). When a region of the brain is actively involved in the processing of a particular task, the alpha wave is absent ("suppressed"). Thus, the study of alpha wave suppression during language-related tasks can yield information about which regions of the brain are actively involved in particular tasks. Moore summarized several studies that he and his colleagues conducted with this method. In each of the studies, they found anomalous right hemisphere alpha wave patterns during language-processing tasks among adults who stutter. The alpha wave suppression was most notable on the right posterior temporal-parietal lobe, an area that is the homologue of the auditory association cortex in the left hemisphere. This pattern differed from that of the fluent speakers in the control group.

Researchers have continued to use EEG throughout the ensuing decades to study various facets of speech-language performance in speakers who stutter. For example, Weber-Fox and colleagues (Cuadrado & Weber-Fox, 2003; Weber-Fox & Hampton, 2008; Weber-Fox, Wray & Arnold, 2013) have conducted a series of studies in which they examined event-related brain potentials (ERPs) in both adults and children who stutter. ERPs are peaks of electrical activity that can occur in either a negative (N) or positive (P) direction during the time course of an activity such as sentence processing. Weber-Fox and colleagues examined two characteristic peaks in electrical activity (N400, P600) that are associated with the processing of semantic and syntactic information, particularly information that is anomalous (e.g., subject-verb disagreement). In each of the studies, they found that speakers who stutter exhibited an atypical response profile compared to fluent controls. For example, adults who stuttered exhibited peaks in event-related potentials during simple sentences that fluent speakers exhibited only during complex sentences (Weber-Fox & Hampton, 2008). Children who stutter were slower to respond to semantic anomalies than children with typical fluency, and when presented with syntactic anomalies, they showed differences in brain electrical activity throughout the course of sentence processing. In the later stages of processing syntactically anomalous sentences, the children who stuttered showed ERP responses that were right hemisphere lateralized—the opposite pattern that the children with typical fluency showed. Interestingly, in all of these studies, the children and adults who stuttered scored *within the normal range* on traditional tests of language competence. Findings from studies such as these illustrate that the differences and deficits that people who stutter exhibit sometimes are subtle and detectable only with the use of sophisticated measurement tools.

Neuroimaging Findings

Advances in neuroimaging technology during the past two decades have led to a number of imaging studies of the central nervous system in speakers who stutter. As noted in the previous section, neuroimaging has been used in recent years to analyze *structural* aspects of the speech-language system. The focus in this section is on the application of neuroimaging approaches to describe *functional* aspects of the speech-language system; specifically, the patterns of neural activation that occur in fluent and stuttering speakers during various types of speech tasks. In some recent studies, researchers have adopted a two-pronged strategy of linking structural anomalies to functional impairments. Together, the structural and functional neuroimaging studies create a portrait of how a "stuttering brain" compares with a "fluent brain," and in doing so, provide a mechanism for linking behavioral data about the surface features of stuttered speech to its neurological substrates.

Findings from seven studies that have utilized neuroimaging to study neurophysiological functioning are summarized in Table 6–3. A common goal in these studies has been to isolate regions of the nervous system that distinguish speakers who stutter from speakers with typical fluency. After such areas are identified, one then can examine the functions of those areas for the purpose of specifying the types of impairment that underlie stuttered speech.

Brown, Ingham, Ingham, Laird, and Fox (2005) conducted a meta-analysis of eight previously published neuroimaging studies. In these eight studies, a host of neuroanatomical regions were associated with stuttered speech. Brown et al. sought to determine the common areas of anomalous activation across the studies. As can be seen in the table, the areas of overactivity common to all eight studies are all integral to motor functioning, and the common region of underactivity, the left primary auditory cortex, plays a role in sensorimotor guidance during speech production. Brown et al. described the left primary auditory cortex as being "essentially undetectable" (i.e., deactivated) during speech production in each of the eight studies. The latter pattern is, of course, markedly different from what is seen in speakers with typical fluency. Interestingly, the dramatic stuttering reductions that are observed during fluency enhancing conditions such as choral speaking are accompanied by increased activation in the left auditory association cortex among speakers who stutter (Stager, Jeffries, & Braun, 2003).

Brown et al. (2005) also reported several right hemisphere areas that were much more active among speakers who stutter than they were among speakers with typical fluency. Some of these areas are homologues to the classic left hemisphere premotor regions. Other researchers (e.g., Blomgren, Nagarajan, Lee, Li, & Alvord, 2003; Watkins et al., 2008) also have reported underactivity among speakers who stutter in left hemisphere regions involved in premotor functions and auditory representation of spoken syllables and words. Brown et al. also reported overactivation of the right anterior cingulate cortex, a region that is involved in error monitoring, attention, decision-making, and emotional responses.

Other researchers have reported patterns of excessive right hemisphere activation in speakers who stutter, as well (e.g., Blomgren et al., 2003; Chang, Kenney, Loucks, & Ludlow, 2009; Chang, Horwitz, Ostuni, Reynolds, & Ludlow, 2011). In these cases, the overactive areas are homologous to left hemisphere regions that are associated with premotor and auditory association functions. In current models of speech production (e.g., Guenther, 2006; Max, Guenther, Gracco, Ghosh, & Wallace, 2004), these areas assume crucial roles in the creation of the internal motor models and the sensory models for movement goals that, respectively, are necessary for the attainment of fluent speech. This pattern of rightward overactivity is viewed by most as compensatory in nature. This view is supported by data such as that described in the previous section, in which structural anomalies in left hemisphere regions of the speech motor system are found in speakers who stutter much more often than in speakers with typical fluency.

Table 6–3. Examples of Studies That Used Neuroimaging to Examine Neurophysiology in Speakers Who Stutter

Study	Method	Findings for Stuttering Group
Blomgren, Nagarajan, Lee, Li, & Alvord (2003)	Examined neural substrates of lexical activation by presenting participants with descriptions of target words in the context of fMRI imaging.	Controls primarily used left hemisphere speech-language areas; stuttering group showed bilateral activation and right hemisphere activation of Broca's area homologue, the precentral gyrus, and the auditory association area.
Jeffries, Fritz, & Braun (2003)	Compared neural activation during fluency-evoking conditions, typical solo speech, and a resting state using $H_2{}^{15}O$ PET imaging.	Areas linked to fluency-enhancing speech conditions included the auditory association cortex for laryngeal and oral articulators, particularly in the left hemisphere.
Brown, Ingham, Ingham, Laird, & Fox (2005)	Conducted a meta-analysis of eight studies that featured coordinate-based analysis of all or most of the brain and overt speaking tasks.	• Areas of overactivity: primary motor cortex, supplementary motor area, cingulate motor area, and cerebellar vermis. • Rightward laterality: frontal operculum and Rolandic operculum and anterior insula. • Auditory cortex activations were "essentially undetectable."
Watkins, Smith, Davis, & Howell (2008)	Compared stuttering and fluent speakers during speech using fMRI.	• Areas of bilateral overactivity in stuttering: anterior insula, cerebellum, and midbrain. • Areas of bilateral underactivity in stuttering: ventral premotor area, Rolandic operculum and sensorimotor cortex, and L Heschl's gyrus. • Overactivity in midbrain nuclei; underactivity of motor and premotor cortex associated with speech articulation.
Chang, Kenney, Loucks, & Ludlow (2009)	Compared stuttering and fluency speakers during speech perception, planning, and production using fMRI.	• Underactivity in L superior temporal gyrus and L premotor areas. • Overactivity (during speech) in right superior temporal gyrus, bilateral Heschl's gyrus, insula, putamen, and precentral motor cortex. • Females showed greater differences than males. • Abnormal activation present during speech perception, planning, and production.

Table 6–3. *continued*

Study	Method	Findings for Stuttering Group
Chang, Horwitz, Ostuni, Reynolds, & Ludlow (2011)	Compared functional and structural connections in corticocortical and thalamocortical loops during speech and nonspeech tasks using fMRI and DTI.	• Deficits in functional connectivity between left BA 44 and BA 6 (left premotor region); connectivity in homologous right hemisphere region was increased. • No functional connectivity differences between BA 44 and auditory cortex.
Ingham, Grafton, Bothe, & Ingham (2012)	Compared stuttering and fluent speakers during oral reading and monologue using PET.	• At rest, L and R basal ganglia and posterior insula were more activated than controls. • During speech, less activation in L globus pallidus and L and R posterior insula. • Stuttering frequency was associated with activation in the thalamus, supplementary motor area, caudate, and globus pallidus (cortico-striatal-thalamic loop); speech rate, in contrast, was negatively correlated with these regions.

Note. BA = Brodmann's area; *L* = left; *R* = right.

In some reports (e.g., Chang et al., 2009; Ingham, Grafton, Bothe, & Ingham, 2012; Watkins et al., 2008), anomalous patterns of neural activity have been detected in subcortical structures among speakers who stutter. Regions such as the basal ganglia and the thalamus are associated with motor regulation and sensory integration, respectively—aspects of performance that are integral to stuttered speech. In contrast to the other studies in Table 6–3, Chang et al., 2011 studied the axonal connectivity between key processing regions in the speech production system and found evidence of reduced connectivity between Broca's area and the supplementary motor area, areas that are involved in syllable preparation during speech production. Unlike some other studies, however, there did not appear to be a deficiency in the connectivity between the inferior frontal cortex and the auditory cortex. To the extent that the connectivity problems between brain regions reflect disruptions in the neurodevelopmental processes that lead to axon development, it may be that there are individual variations in the number, type, and extent of neural connections that are anomalous across individuals who stutter.

Linguistic and Cognitive Correlates

Researchers have studied the linguistic and cognitive correlates of stuttering extensively. With regard to linguistic correlates, much of the research addresses issues related to the developmental competence of speakers who stutter and the effects that linguistic context has on their speech fluency. With regard to cognitive variables, research has focused mainly on the effects that increases in cognitive load have on the production of stuttering-related disfluency.

Language Form and Stuttering-Related Disfluency

The effect of language form (i.e., syntax, phonology, morphology) on disfluency frequency and location has been examined in many studies.

Location of Stuttering-Related Disfluency

A main purpose in many studies has been to identify which words are most likely to feature stuttering-related disfluency. In the earliest studies of stuttering, researchers hoped that the description of the *loci* for stuttering would lead to insights about the nature of the disorder. The general finding from this line of research is that stuttering-related disfluency is not a random event. Rather, it occurs in some linguistic contexts more often than it does in others (Brown, 1945; Logan & Conture, 1995; Taylor, 1966). In Table 6–4, five factors that researchers have examined in relation to the loci of stuttering-related disfluency are presented.

Most researchers (e.g., Bloodstein & Grossman, 1981; Logan & LaSalle, 1999) have interpreted the tendency for stuttering-related disfluency to occur at or near the onset of an utterance as an effect of utterance-planning demands. A common view is that articulating the beginning stages of an utterance while simultaneously planning or holding in memory upcoming portions of an utterance promotes instability in the speech production system, which is manifest as disfluency (Jayaram, 1984; Logan, 2001; Tsiamtsiouris & Cairns, 2013; Wall, Starkweather, & Cairns, 1981). Thus, the simultaneous act of sentence planning and sentence production seems to aggravate the effects of whatever primary speech production impairment speakers who stutter may present. As we will see later in the chapter, the biomechanics of syllables that occur in utterance initial contexts differs from that of utterance final syllables. Thus, motoric factors may explain this phenomenon as well.

From a speech planning standpoint, the word length and word position factors are similar in that both pertain to the amount of material the speaker attempts to produce. The general pattern is this: The more a speaker has to say within an utterance, the more he or she is likely to produce stuttering-related disfluency at the onset of that utterance. In speakers who stutter, the *amount* of motor planning to be coordinated seems to have more of an impact on speech fluency than the *content* of motor plan does (i.e., the specific speech sounds that the speaker is planning to say). For example, Wingate (1967) asked adults who stutter to read two types of word lists. One list contained pairs of one-syllable words (e.g., *fan—sea*) and the other contained two-syllable words that were composed of the syllables in the one-syllable word pair condition (e.g., *fan—sea → fancy*). Overall, 22% of the two-syllable words featured symptoms of stuttering versus only 9% of the one-syllable words.

Several researchers (e.g., Soderberg, 1966, 1967) have noted that low frequency words evoke stuttered speech more often

Table 6–4. Some Factors That Affect the Occurrence of Stuttering-Related Disfluency Within Spoken Utterances

Factor	General Finding(s)	Supporting Studies
Word location	Stuttering-related disfluency occurs more often in conjunction with words that are located near the beginning of clauses or sentences than it does in conjunction with words located elsewhere within an utterance.	• Jayaram (1984) • Logan & LaSalle (1999) • Buhr & Zebrowski (2009)
Word stress	Stuttering-related disfluency is more apt to occur within words that carry the primary stress in a phonological phrase.	• Klouda & Cooper (1988) • Wingate (1988) • Prins, Hubbard, & Krause (1991)
Word length[a]	Stuttering-related disfluency is more likely to occur at the onset of polysyllabic words than it is at the onset of monosyllabic words, even when controlling for phonetic content of the words.	• Soderberg (1967) • Wingate (1967)
Word frequency	Stuttering-related disfluency is more apt to occur in conjunction with low-frequency words than it is with high-frequency words.	• Soderberg (1967)
Word class	A relatively high proportion of preschoolers' stuttering-related disfluency occurs in conjunction with function words. With older children and adults, the opposite pattern in noted (a high proportion of stuttering-related disfluency in conjunction with content words).	• Bloodstein & Grossman (1981) • Howell, Au-Yeung, & Sackin (1999)

[a]In contemporary research, word length usually is defined as the number of syllables per word.

than high frequency words do. Cykowski et al. (2010) suggested that when speakers produce low frequency words, they rely on corrective auditory feedback more than they do when saying high frequency words. Presumably, this is because the motor movements associated with low frequency words are less practiced than the motor movements for high frequency words. As such, novel or infrequent words might require a greater degree of moment-to-moment sensory guidance and the risk of disfluency increases if this guidance system is impaired.

Other researchers have examined the effects of word frequency and ordinal sequence[4] on vowel duration during connected discourse. Low frequency words feature longer vowel duration than high frequency words do (Wright, 1979) and, independent of that, the first mention of a specific word within connected dis-

---

[4]This term pertains to any word that a speaker uses more than once during a task. Researchers especially have been interested in comparing the articulatory properties of the first mention of a word with a spoken passage to subsequent mentions of the word. In this way, newly introduced information is contrasted with previously introduced information.

course features a longer vowel duration than subsequent mentions of that word do (Fowler & Housum, 1987). To complicate matters further, Munson and Solomon (2004) found that the density of a word's phonological neighborhood[5] affects vowel duration as well, such that high-neighborhood-density words feature a more expansive vowel space than low-neighborhood-density words do. Thus, it may be more than a lack of practice that make certain words prone to stuttering-related disfluency. That is, the need to create a prosodic contrast between one word and another may place unique stress on the speech motor control system.

Speakers seem to modify the prosodic pattern of a word if it is (a) rare, (b) mentioned for the first time, or (c) phonologically similar to other words. The speaker stresses these words to make them "stand out' from surrounding words or from other words with which it might be confused. Several authors have noted the association between linguistic stress and stuttered speech (Klouda & Cooper, 1988; Prins, Hubbard, & Krause, 1991; Wingate, 1984b). It seems plausible that the prosodic adjustments a speaker makes when saying such words would necessitate greater reliance on sensorimotor guidance from the speech motor control system. In this view, speakers who cannot readily or fully incorporate such feedback into a speech motor plan due to impairment in the speech production system are at risk to produce the word disfluently.

The grammatical class of a word is another language-based factor that researchers have examined extensively in relation to stuttered speech. The traditional view has been that, with adults and older children, stuttering-related disfluency occurs more often during the production of "content" words (i.e., nouns, verbs, adjectives, adverbs) than it does during production of "function words." For example, Brown (1937) examined disfluency location during an oral-reading task with adults who stutter. The median percentages of adverbs, nouns, and adjectives stuttered were each greater than 7%, while the median percentages for stuttered pronouns, prepositions, conjunctions, and articles were all less than 2.5%. Verbs, in contrast, fell between these two groups, with a median stuttering frequency of 3.75%. Preschool-aged children, in contrast, appear to exhibit a relatively high proportion of stuttering disfluency in conjunction with function words (Bloodstein & Gantwerk, 1967; Bloodstein & Grossman, 1981). However, some authors (e.g., Bloodstein & Grossman, 1981) have argued that the function word effect is confounded with sentence planning effects (i.e., many of the stuttered function words that children produce are in sentence-initial contexts). Thus, the stutter-like disfluency that occurs in conjunction with function words actually may be a reflection of sentence planning demands more so than word-based effects.

Au-Yeung, Howell, and Pilgrim (1998) reexamined the content word versus function word distinction using Selkirk's (1984) concept of phonological words. In Selkirk's view, the distinction between "content" and "function" words is not meaningful in most phonetic contexts, because the unstressed function words attach to host content words to form prosodic units called phonological words. Au-Yeung et al. (1998) found that preschool-aged chil-

---

[5]Munson and Solomon (2004, p. 1049) defined this as "the number of words that differ from a target word by a single phoneme."

dren only exhibited relatively high levels of "function word disfluency" if the function word led off a phonological word. For instance, the word *after* would have a significantly higher probability of attracting stuttering-related disfluency in the first sentence from Example 6–1 (below), where it initiates a phonological word, than it would in the second sentence from Example 6–2, where it terminates a phonological word. (The asterisks below indicate phonological word boundaries.)

Example 6–1: **We looked**after the movie ended.

Example 6–2: **We looked after**my little brother.

Some researchers have worked diligently to determine which linguistic factors are "strongest" in terms of triggering disfluency. The results of these efforts have yielded mixed answers (cf. Hubbard & Prins, 1994; Soderberg, 1967; Taylor, 1966). Ultimately, it perhaps is most productive to adopt a view similar to the one that Brown (1945) used. That is, the probability that a speaker will produce stuttering-related disfluency at any particular point within an utterance is the product of multiple factors (e.g., a word's frequency, stress characteristics, syllable length, and position within a sentence or phrase), and words that feature relatively many of the triggers for stuttered speech are more likely to feature stuttering-related disfluency than words that have relatively few of the triggers.

Linguistic Complexity and Stuttering-Related Disfluency

The effect of linguistic complexity on stuttering-related disfluency is another area that researchers have studied extensively. Research has focused mainly on the notions of syntactic and phonologic complexity. Some of the approaches researchers have used to examine this issue are explored below.

In some studies, researchers have defined *syntactic complexity* from a developmental perspective. With this approach, early-emerging syntactic forms are seen as less complex than late-developing syntactic forms. (See Chapter 4 for examples of variations in the syntactic complexity of sentence types.) In other studies, researchers have defined syntactic complexity in strictly quantitative terms by counting the number of syntactic elements within an utterance. Examples of the latter approach include analysis of either the number of clauses or the number of syntactic phrases (i.e., clause constituents) within an utterance. An utterance that contains relatively many syntactic elements is seen as more complex than an utterance that contains relatively few syntactic elements.

Researchers commonly use sentence imitation, conversation, and narration tasks when analyzing effects of syntactic complexity on fluency. Sentence-modeling tasks have been implemented frequently as well. With sentence modeling, a participant attempts to produce a novel sentence that is similar in syntactic form but different in content from a sentence that an examiner has just spoken (e.g., Examiner: *The boy gave the girl a pencil*. Child: *The girl gave the boy a crayon*. Picture stimuli usually are used to model and elicit the sentences.

In Table 6–5, findings are presented from several representative studies of the effect of syntactic complexity on the fluency of people who stutter. As shown in the table, the syntactic complexity effect is quite reliable in studies with children,

Table 6–5. Findings From Selected Studies of Syntactic and Phonologic Effects on Stuttering-Related Disfluency

Study	Groups	Complexity Focus	Complexity Measure(s)	Findings
Bernstein Ratner & Sih (1987)	CWS; CWTF	S; P	Sentences ranked for developmental difficulty and number of syllables	Late-developing sentence forms elicited more stuttering-related disfluency than early-developing sentence forms did; syntactic complexity correlated more strongly with disfluency than syllable-length complexity did.
Gaines, Runyan, & Meyers (1991)	CWS	S	Language complexity score[a] and number of words per utterance	Stuttered utterances had more words and higher language complexity scores than fluent utterances did.
Logan & Conture (1995)	CWS	S; P	Language complexity score[a] and number of syllables per utterance	Stuttered utterances had more syllables and higher language complexity scores than fluent utterances did.
Logan & Conture (1997)	CWS; CWTF	S; P	Syllable structure, syllable complexity, and number of syntactic phrases per utterance	When controlling for the number of syllables per utterance, stuttered utterances contained more syntactic phrases than fluent utterances did.
Silverman & Bernstein Ratner (1997)	TWS; TWTF	S	Syntactic complexity in sentences	Complex sentences elicited more interjections and revisions, but not more stuttering-related disfluency, than simple sentences did.
Throneburg, Yairi, & Paden (1994)	CWS; CWTF	P	Phonological complexity of selected words	The proportion of phonologically complex words that featured stuttering was not significantly greater than the expected proportion.
Tsiamtsiouris & Cairns (2013)	AWS; AWTF	S	Syntactic complexity in sentences	High complexity sentences elicited more disfluency than low complexity sentences did.

Table 6–5. *continued*

Study	Groups	Complexity Focus	Complexity Measure(s)	Findings
Yaruss (1999)	CWS	S; P	Syllables, words, morphemes, syntactic phrases, and clauses per sentences	Stuttered utterances had more syllables, words, and grammatical units than fluent words did. The number of syllables per sentences was the strongest predictor of stuttered speech.
Zackheim & Conture (2003)	CWS; CWTF	S, P	Number of syllables and morphemes per utterances	Utterances above a child's MLU elicited more disfluency than utterances below a child's MLU did. Long, complex sentences elicited the most disfluency.

Note. CWS = children who stutter, *CWTF* = children with typical fluency. For the other abbreviations in the Groups column, *T* = teens and *A* = adults; *S* = syntax and *P* = phonology; *MLU* = mean length of utterance.

[a]Language complexity scores were based on Lee's (1974) *Developmental Sentence Scoring* procedure.

regardless of how one defines complexity. In studies with adolescents and adults who stutter, the effect seems less reliable. Silverman and Bernstein Ratner (1997), for example, found no difference in the frequency with which teens who stuttered produced stuttering-related disfluency while imitating sentences that featured syntactic forms of varying difficulty but a similar number of syllables. Syntactic complexity did affect the frequency with which both fluency groups produced interjections and revisions, however.

Logan (2001)—not shown in Table 6–5—presented teens and adults who stutter with four categories of sentences. The sentences varied in the number of syntactic constituents within the subject-noun phrase. The participants read the sentences silently and then repeated them aloud a short time later when given a sig-nal to speak. The frequency of stuttering-related disfluency was similar across the four sentence types; thus, the syntactic form of the subject noun phrase did not affect the participants' speech fluency. Logan also reported that the frequency of stuttering-related disfluency was less during the sentence production task than it was during length-match sentences from a conversational task. The latter finding suggested that, with older speakers, syntactic form might affect fluency only when the speaker is required to self-formulate sentences. Findings from Tsiamtsiouris and Cairns (2013) challenged this notion, however. In the latter study, syntactic complexity effects on stuttering-related disfluency were obtained during an elicitation procedure similar to that of Logan but with sentences that were a bit longer and more syntactically challenging.

Researchers also have examined phonologic complexity as a possible correlate of stuttering. Throneburg, Yairi, and Paden (1994) defined phonological complexity in terms of syllable shape, phonemic content, and word length:

- Words that featured syllables with clusters (e.g., CCVC) were considered more complex than words that featured syllables with singleton consonants (e.g., CVC);
- Words with late-emerging phonemes were considered more complex than words with early-emerging phonemes; and
- Words with multiple syllables were considered more complex than words with single syllables.

Some words, of course, contained more than one of these characteristics. Throneburg et al. found no significant effect for phonological complexity—at least when defined in the way they did —on the frequency with which children produced stuttering-related disfluency on words during conversation. Howell and Au-Yeung (1995) defined phonological complexity in the same way and conducted a similar analysis with children who stuttered while also controlling for other word-level factors such as grammatical class that influence stuttering-related disfluency. They too found no evidence that the phonological complexity of a specific word affected the likelihood of stuttering-related disfluency on a particular word. Accordingly, measures of phonological complexity that are based on the presence or absence of clusters and/or the developmental difficulty of consonants within words do not seem to be particu-

larly sensitive at flagging the words upon which a speaker will stutter. Conversely, the number of syllables within an utterance does seem to be a reasonably strong predictor of which utterances will contain stuttering-related disfluency.

In more recent studies, researchers have defined phonological complexity in different ways. Anderson and Byrd (2008) reported that children who stutter were more likely to produce whole-word repetition when saying words that contained low frequency speech sound segments or low frequency sequences of speech sounds. These phonotactic word properties were not associated with other types of stuttering-related disfluency, however. Anderson (2007) found that children tended to stutter on low frequency words (a finding that many other researchers have reported) and on words that have a low "neighborhood density frequency." (Neighborhood density refers to the frequency of those words that are phonologically similar to a target word, e.g., dog → hog, bog, log.)

Language Functioning in Speakers Who Stutter

Researchers have shown a long-standing interest in studying the language functioning of speakers who stutter (e.g., Berry, 1938; Silverman & Williams, 1967; Westby, 1979). For the most part, results from these studies suggest that, as a group, children who stutter perform less adequately than children with typical fluency do. For example, based on parent-report data, Johnson and Associates (1959, p. 36) reported that children who stutter tended to be "slower in speech development and less adequate in current vocabulary."

Performance on Tests of Language Performance

One way to examine children's language-related functioning is through administration of formal, norm-referenced tests. Researchers have used this approach extensively in studies with children who stutter and have detected evidence of substandard performance among children who stutter in many different facets of language. For example,

- Westby (1974) reported that kindergarten and first-grade children who stuttered scored significantly lower than age-matched children with typical fluency on formal tests of vocabulary comprehension, expressive sentence complexity, and semantic skills.
- Ryan (1992) administered a battery of formal language tests to preschoolers who stuttered and found the group's mean score on 7 of 8 measures to be below that of age-matched children with typical fluency.
- In a review of diagnostic data from nearly 100 preschoolers who stuttered, Yaruss, LaSalle, and Conture (1998) reported that significant percentages of the children scored below normal limits in the following areas: receptive language performance (15% of the children), expressive language performance (29% of the children), and speech sound development (37% of the children).
- Several researchers have reported anomalous performance among speakers who stutter on tasks that involve nonword repetition. In several studies, children who stuttered made more errors than typical children during nonword repetition (Anderson & Wagovich, 2010; Anderson, Wagovich, & Hall, 2006; Hakim & Bernstein Ratner, 2004). Adults who stuttered displayed similar accuracy to nonstuttering adults during nonword repetition; however, kinematic data revealed atypical variability in articulatory coordination when saying nonwords, and stuttering speakers' movements became more variable as the length and complexity of the nonword targets increased (Smith, Sadagopan, Walsh, & Weber-Fox, 2010).

Ntourou, Conture, and Lipsey (2011) conducted a meta-analysis of language-related findings from 22 studies in which language performance data were reported for young children who stuttered. They computed effect sizes for mean performance differences (children who stuttered versus children who do not stutter) across the 22 studies. The results of their analysis are summarized below:

- The receptive vocabulary scores for children who stuttered were 0.52 standard deviation units below those of children with typical fluency. Thus, Ntourou et al. (2011) explained, 70% of the children who stuttered had a lower receptive vocabulary score than the average child with typical fluency.
- The expressive vocabulary scores for children who stuttered were 0.41 standard deviation units below those of children with

typical fluency. Thus, 66% of the children who stuttered had a lower expressive vocabulary score than the average child with typical fluency.

- The overall language performance scores (receptive + expressive language) for children who stuttered were 0.48 standard deviation units below those of children with typical fluency. Thus, 68% of the children who stuttered had a lower overall language performance score than the average child with typical fluency.

In summary, results from studies of language-related functioning on norm-referenced instruments suggest that children who stutter tend to perform more poorly than children with typical fluency. Of course, group data are built from averaging the scores of many children. This means that some children who stutter are likely to score better on these measures of language functioning than the average child who does not stutter. Based on Ntourou et al.'s (2011) analysis, the percentage of stuttering children who do so is relatively small (i.e., roughly 30% to 35%).

At first glance, this performance profile appears to be inconsistent with findings from studies of children's language performance around the time of onset for stuttering symptoms (e.g., Watkins & Yairi, 1997), wherein children who stutter seem to perform similarly to, if not better than, children with typical fluency. However, Watkins and Yairi (1997) noted that preschoolers who ultimately exhibited persistent stuttering displayed more variable language performance than the children who ultimately recovered from stuttering. They also noted that poor language performance was more closely associated with persistent cases of stuttering than with recovered cases. Thus, it may be that many of the children studied in Ntourou et al.'s (2011) analysis were on track for persistent stuttering. This interpretation seems plausible because, in nearly all of the 22 studies included in Ntourou et al.'s analysis, the average age of the children who stuttered was 48 months or older. If one assumes a typical age of onset for the children, this means that many of them had stuttered long enough to meet criteria for "persistent stuttering" or at least to be "at risk" for doing so. Nippold (2012a) suggested that impairment in speech motor functioning might account for some of the deficiencies that children who stutter seem to exhibit in expressive language. Although this is a possibility, problems in speech motor functioning cannot easily account for the receptive language deficiencies found among stuttering children in several studies. Additional research is needed to clarify the nature of the relationship between children's language functioning and speech motor functioning.

Narrative Production

Narrative production is a form of oral discourse in which the speaker constructs an extended account of an event or a series of interrelated events (Liles, 1993). Narrative discourse emerges during the preschool years, and children gradually develop the ability to produce increasingly elaborate stories. By the start of elementary school, children can construct stories that contain both background setting information and one or more episode. With age, the episodes within children's stories gradually increase in complexity such that they eventually feature structural elements such as an initiating event, the character's physical, emotional, and cognitive responses to the initiating event, the character's attempts to resolve a problem or challenge, and the effects of the character's action (Stein & Glenn, 1979). In addition, narrative discourse requires a speaker to reference information clearly across sentences using devices such as pronouns and prosodic markers.

Not surprisingly, children often find narrative construction to be relatively demanding. For instance, children who present with delays in aspects of sentence form also are likely to exhibit delays with aspects of story grammar (Paul & Smith, 1993). Furthermore, both children who stutter and children with specific language impairment produce more disfluency than typical children do during narrative production (Byrd, Logan, & Gillam, 2012; Guo, Tomblin, & Samelson, 2008). Several authors (e.g., Byrd et al., 2012; Trautman, Healey, & Norris, 2001) also have reported that children who stutter produced more stuttering-related disfluency during narrative tasks than they do during other forms of discourse. In addition, certain types of narratives (e.g., story-retelling narratives) evoke more disfluency from children who stutter than other types of narratives (e.g., story-generation narrative; Trautman, Healey, Brown, Brown, & Jermano, 1999). In the latter case, language complexity differences between the two narrative tasks appear to drive the children's disfluency pattern.

Given the tendency for children who stutter to perform more poorly than typical children on various norm-referenced tests of language performance, one would expect children who stutter to exhibit deficits in narrative production as well. Several researchers (e.g., Nippold, Schwarz, & Jescheniak, 1991; Trautman et al., 1999; Weiss & Zebrowski, 1994) have examined this issue and, to date, they have uncovered relatively few differences between the groups. For example, Weiss and Zebrowski (1994) reported that children with typical fluency produced longer, more elaborate narratives than children who stuttered did but only when interacting with listeners who were unfamiliar with content of the narrative. Both Nippold et al. (1991) and Trautman et al. (1999) reported that children who stuttered produced narratives that were similar to those of children with typical fluency in terms of structural complexity and use of cohesive devices. One limitation of these studies of narrative production is that most have featured relatively small sample sizes and accompanying limitations in statistical power. Because of this and the evidence of language performance deficits in other types of studies with children who stutter, narrative production is an area that may warrant additional examination in the future.

Coexisting Communication Disorders

Throughout the years, a number of clinical researchers have noted that children who stutter often seem to exhibit coexisting difficulty with speech sound production (Bloodstein & Bernstein Ratner, 2008). In studies based on analysis of the researchers' clinical caseloads, the estimated percentage of cases with co-occurring fluency and speech sound production difficulties has ranged between 20 to 40% (e.g., Louko, Edwards, & Conture, 1990; Yaruss, LaSalle, & Conture, 1998). Another approach is to survey school-based speech-language pathologists on the characteristics of their caseloads (Table 6–6). This approach is likely to offer a more representative sample of the population of people who stutter. Although surveys of school clinicians do not necessarily provide information about

Table 6–6. Occurrence of Concomitant Disorders Among Children Who Stutter

Study	Both Speech Sound Disorder and Language Disorder	Speech Sound Disorder Only	Language Disorder Only	Any Type of Accompanying Disorder
	Percent of Cases			
Blood & Seider (1981)	4	16	10	68[a]
Arndt & Healey (2001)	14	14	15	67[b]
Blood, Ridenour, et al. (2003)[c]	—	—	—	63[a]

[a]Includes all types of communication disorders plus noncommunication-based disorders.

[b]Includes confirmed disorders of speech sound production and language functioning, plus other suspected or confirmed communication- and noncommunication-based disorders.

[c]Data were collected for specific types of speech sound production and specific areas of language disorder. Because individual cases could present with more than one of these problems, it is not possible to complete the first columns in this table.

the prevalence of coexisting disorders among all children who stutter (Nippold, 2012a), they do yield a good sense for the types of cases school-based clinicians are likely to encounter in that work setting.

The main finding from these survey studies is that many of the children who receive treatment for stuttering in school settings also meet their school district's criteria for other disorders. As shown in Table 6–6, data from Blood and Seider (1981) and Arndt and Healey (2001) indicate that roughly 15% of the children who stutter present with co-occurring disorders that affect speech sound production and about the same percentage present with co-occurring disorders that affect language functioning. Blood, Ridenour, Jr., Qualls, and Hammer (2003) reported that articulation disorders were more likely to co-occur with stuttering (33% of all cases) than were voice disorders (2% of all cases) or cluttering (1% of all cases). About 13% of the children who stutter met school

district criteria for language impairment that affected semantics and/or syntax, and 10% met criteria for language impairment that affected syntax.

If one expands the focus to include any type of accompanying disorder, the percentage of affected cases jumps to more than 60% (see Table 6–6). This is, of course, much higher than what one sees in the general population and is consistent with data from some smaller scale studies as well (e.g., Brazell & Logan, 2001; St. Louis, Murray, & Ashworth, 1991). The presence of concomitant communication disorders among children who stutter has led some authors (e.g. Seery, Watkins, Mangelsdorf, & Shigeto, 2007; Yairi, 2007) to discuss the possibility of subtypes of stuttering. Yairi (2007) reviewed a number of research studies spanning several decades and developed a framework of potential factors that might facilitate the identification of stuttering subtypes. The potential bases for subtype identification that Yairi (2007) identified included the following:

- Co-occurring disorders (e.g., presence or absence of a co-occurring disorder, type of co-occurring disorder);
- Speech characteristics (e.g., disfluency types produced, frequency of disfluency, changes in disfluency in response to speech motor rehearsal;
- Biological characteristics (e.g., gender, brain morphology, genetics);
- Response to drugs (e.g., presence or absence of a fluency response, type of fluency response [positive, negative, neutral]); and
- Developmental course (e.g., age of onset, changes in symptom expression over time, eventual outcome).

Another issue that bears examination is whether the presence of a concomitant communication disorder results in patterns of speech production that are substantially different from those that are observed when a disorder exists in isolation. The issue has not received extensive attention in the research literature to date, and most of the available evidence concerns cases in which phonological disorder co-occurs with stuttering. Louko et al. (1990) reported that children who stuttered were more likely to exhibit phonological disorder than children in a control group with typical fluency (40% versus 7%, respectively). In addition, the children who stuttered exhibited a greater variety of phonological processes. Some of the phonological processes that the children who stuttered produced (i.e., glottal

replacement, backing, lateralization) were not produced at all by the children in the control group, and other processes, such as cluster reduction, occurred in about 33% of children in the stuttering group but less than 5% of the children in the control group.

Wolk, Edwards, and Conture (1993) compared speech sound production and fluency characteristics of children who stuttered, children with disordered phonology, and children who exhibited both disorders. They found that the presence of disordered phonology did not markedly alter the frequency or duration of stuttering-related disfluency, stuttering severity, or speaking rate. The only difference between the two groups was that the children who exhibited both stuttering and disordered phonology had a significantly greater proportion of sound prolongations in their disfluency profiles (37% of all disfluencies) than children who only stuttered (19% of all disfluencies). Similarly, the presence of stuttering did not markedly alter the symptoms of phonological disorder. That is, children with both stuttering and disordered phonology were similar to children with only disordered phonology in terms of phonetic inventory, percent of consonants correct, percent of process occurrence, and most frequent types of processes produced (i.e., vowelization, gliding, cluster reduction, and velar fronting). Logan, Louko, Edwards, & Conture (1995) compared the phonological skills of mild and severe cases of childhood stuttering using many of the same measures that Wolk et al. (1993) used. Logan et al. (1995) reported no difference in the number or types of phonological errors produced across the two levels of stuttering severity. On this basis, the presence of coexisting fluency and phonological disorders does not seem to result in performance patterns that are markedly different from those that occur when either disorder exists in isolation.

Language Processing

Several studies have examined the language performance of speakers who stutter during tasks that involve word or sentence production. Most of these studies have focused on functioning in the area of phonological processing. In one study, children who stuttered performed similarly to typical children with respect to their response initiation times on a naming task that included words from "low density" and "high density" phonological neighborhoods (Arnold, Conture, & Ohde, 2005). However, there is evidence of immaturity in phonological encoding, as children who stuttered did not realize the benefit that children with typical fluency did when presented with *incremental primes* of phonological words (Byrd, Conture, & Ohde, 2007). In the latter study, 3- and 5-year-old children who stuttered increased naming speed only when presented with a phonological model of an entire target word (i.e., a *holistic prime*). In contrast, 5-year-old children in the control group showed a developmental change in the type of phonological prime that facilitated their response initiation times. At age 3, they benefited from holistic primes; however, at age 5, their naming speed increased when they received *incremental* primes; that is, a model of the initial consonant and a small portion of the transition to the following vowel of the target word.

Wijnen and Boers (1994) reported a similar result in a priming study with children who stuttered. In that study, the priming benefit was present when the CV portion of a target word was primed, but it was not present when only the initial consonant was primed—a pattern that differed from that of the control group. However, in a follow-up study (Burger & Wijnen, 1999), they did not replicate the result. The children who stuttered did, however, exhibit slower response initiation times than the control group.

Cognitive Functioning and Stuttering-Related Disfluency

Results from several studies suggest that people who stutter experience an increase in stuttering frequency when asked to perform a concurrent cognitive task while speaking. Bosshardt (2002) found that adults who stuttered were significantly more disfluent when asked to repeat a series of three words at the same time that they performed either a reading or a memorization task than they were when repeating the words without performing a concurrent task. Interestingly, exacerbation of fluency was observed only when the concurrent task featured words that were phonologically similar to the words that participants were repeating. Adults with typical fluency showed no difference in fluency between the concurrent- and single-task conditions of the study. Bosshardt hypothesized that, in speakers who stutter, the functioning of the phonologic and/or articulatory systems is prone to disruption when attentional resources are diverted toward other goals.

In a similar study, Bosshardt (1999) examined the effect of a concurrent mental addition task on speech fluency during a word repetition task. He found that the speakers who stutter demonstrated a temporary improvement in speech fluency immediately after receiving a cue that the mental addition task was about to be presented, but speakers' fluency then worsened when they performed the simultaneous tasks. Nonstuttering controls showed no change in fluency during the experimental task. In this study, the increase in disfluency was limited to a subgroup of participants. Findings again demonstrated that stuttering behavior is affected by the extent to which the speaker's attentional resources are devoted to speaking.

Jones, Fox, and Jacewicz (2012) also found evidence of an interaction between phonological- and cognitive-processing demands in a study with adults who stuttered. In this study, the participants made rhyme judgments and recalled letter strings of varying lengths. Although the adults who stuttered performed as accurately as the nonstuttering controls in the rhyme judgments at all levels of cognitive load, their response times were on average about 250 ms slower than those for the control group, and response lags were most prominent in conditions that involved the most cognitive load.

Caruso and colleagues (Caruso, Chodzko-Zajko, Bidinger, & Sommers, 1994) examined the effects of cognitive load on the performance of adults who stuttered using the Stroop Color Word Test. In their study, participants produced speech samples during a series of tasks in which they either read printed words (i.e., "red," "yellow," "blue," and "green") or stated the ink color in which the color words were printed. In one condition, the ink color was congruous with the color word (e.g., the word "red" was printed in red ink), in another it was neutral (all words were printed in white font against a

black background), and in another condition, the ink color was incongruous with the color word (e.g., the word "red" was printed in blue ink). Tasks were performed under speeded and self-paced conditions. Caruso et al. measured the participants' cardiovascular responses, speech motor timing and coordination, and fluency across the conditions. Results showed that the presence of cognitive stress (e.g., naming incongruous ink colors under time pressure) had significant effects on heart rate, word and vowel duration, speech rate, and response latency for the speakers who stuttered. Similar evidence of speed-accuracy trade-offs have been demonstrated in studies where speakers who stuttered perform a concurrent task while producing complex manually sequenced movements (Webster, 1990).

In another study, Weber-Fox, Spencer, Spruill, III, and Smith (2004) found that adults who stuttered had slower response initiation times than fluent controls during the most complex conditions of a rhyme judgment task in which the experimenters manipulated phonologic and orthographic congruency (e.g., *thrown-own*; *cake-own*; *gown-own*; *cone-own*). In that study, the adults who stuttered also showed an anomalous cognitive-processing strategy, which was characterized by greater right hemisphere activation than what was observed in the control group.

Motor Correlates

Issues related to speech motor control have been examined extensively in speakers who stutter. Some representative studies from this literature are summarized in this section.

Manual Coordination

It is intuitive to think that speakers who stutter might present with motor control difficulties in the speech production mechanism. It is less intuitive to think that speakers who stutter might present with a generalized impairment in motor performance; that is, impaired functioning during speech and nonspeech tasks. Several researchers have examined this issue and have uncovered some interesting differences between speakers who stutter and typical speakers. Webster (1986) demonstrated that speakers who stuttered were less accurate and slower at initiating manual responses than speakers with typical fluency while performing a speeded sequential finger-tapping task. In a subsequent study (Webster, 1989), it was demonstrated that the response initiation lags in speakers who stuttered were present only under speeded conditions. When the experimenter gave the people who stuttered control over response preparation time, the between-group differences in response initiation times dropped dramatically. Even with control over response preparation time, however, the participants who stuttered continued to demonstrate more errors than the controls. Findings such as these have been reported in other studies (e.g., Starkweather, Franklin, & Smigo, 1984) and extended in other studies wherein adults who stutter have been found to exhibit greater variability in the timing of complex sequential finger tasks (Smits-Bandstra, De Nil, & Rochon, 2006). Tasks that involve bimanual coordination (i.e., coordination between two hands) seem especially likely to elicit evidence of manual-timing deficits in people who stutter relative to fluent speakers (Hulstijn, Summers, van Lieshout, & Peters, 1992; Zelaznik, Smith, Franz, & Ho, 1997).

It is conceivable that lags in response initiation could somehow reflect more general compensatory strategies that people who stutter develop as a consequence of speaking disfluently for many years. This does not seem to be the case, however, as deficits in manual movements are present in young children who stutter as well. For example, Olander, Smith, and Zelaznik (2010) examined timing patterns during clapping in 4- to 6-year-old children who stuttered and children with typical fluency. The researchers introduced the children to a target clapping rhythm by having them clap in time to a metronome. They then asked the children to continue clapping at that beat when the metronome was turned off. They found that the two groups were similar in terms of clapping speed and "accuracy" (i.e., the number of usable clapping trials); however, significant differences existed between the groups in a measure called *interclap interval,* which captured the extent to which the children could maintain a *consistent* rate of clapping. The children who stuttered exhibited significantly more variability in the interclap interval than the children with typical fluency did. Overall, 10 of 17 children who stuttered exhibited this limitation in the ability to time repeated, rhythmic, bimanual movements.

Reaction Time and Speech Initiation

There is a large research literature in which people who stutter are compared to fluent controls in the ability to initiate spoken target responses as quickly as possible. Researchers have referred to this performance measure variably as speech reaction time (SRT), vocal initiation time (VIT), and laryngeal reaction time (LRT), depending on the type of target response and the researchers' main focus in a study. Examples of response targets used in this research include lip-closing gestures, isolated vowels, single syllables and words, short phrases, and simple and complex sentences. Several representative studies from this part of the research literature are summarized in Table 6–7. Overall, the general finding from this research is that people who stutter are slower than people who do not stutter in their ability to initiate speech-based targets (e.g., Cross & Olson, 1987; Dembowski & Watson, 1991; Logan, 2003b; Starkweather et al., 1984). In many of these studies, the average initiation times of speakers who stutter lag those of speakers with typical fluency by roughly 150 ms, and response complexity tends to exacerbate the extent of the difference in initiation time between the groups (Tsiamtsiouris & Cairns, 2013; Watson, Pool, Devous, Sr., Freeman, & Finitzo, 1992).

Lags in speech initiation also have been documented for nonspeech targets like throat clearing (Starkweather et al., 1984), during tasks that examine vocal termination time (Adams & Hayden, 1976; Cullinan & Springer, 1980), and in tasks that permit participants to rehearse the response target many times prior to performing the test trial (Adams & Hayden, 1976). Initiation lags also have been demonstrated in both adults and children who stutter (Anderson & Conture, 2004; Bishop, Williams, & Cooper, 1991; Cross & Luper, 1979; Cullinan & Springer, 1980; McKnight & Cullinan, 1987). Thus, it appears that the initiation time lag is not simply the result of a speaker's anticipated difficulty in speaking fluently or compensations for stuttered speech that develop across many years. Rather, it seems to be rooted in the neurophysiological integrity of the speech production system. Indeed, in a study of adults who stuttered, Watson et al. (1992) found that slow laryngeal reaction times were observed mainly in a subgroup of participants who exhibited reduced cerebral blood flow to left hemisphere areas associated with speech-language processing. Others (e.g., McKnight & Cullinan, 1987) have reported that slow initiation times were present mainly in a subgroup of children who presented articulation and/or language disorders concomitantly with stuttering.

Speech Motor Control

Another approach to studying the role of motoric factors in stuttering is to compare speakers who stutter and speakers with typical fluency in terms of their ability to coordinate and control speech movements. Conture and colleagues (Caruso, Conture, & Colton, 1988; Conture, Colton, & Gleason, 1988) examined this issue by studying children's temporal coordination of muscles in the respiratory, laryngeal, and articulatory systems during fluent repetitions of simple target sentences. They found no significant difference in the sequence of muscle activation between children who stuttered and children with typical fluency during fluent target responses. In utterances that contained stuttered speech, the coordination of the respiratory, laryngeal, and articulatory muscle systems again was similar in terms of the sequence in which muscle systems activated in comparison to fluent utterances from children with typical fluency. During stuttered trials, however, the

Table 6–7. Results From Selected Studies of Response Initiation Times With Speakers Who Stutter

Study	Participants			Results
	Sample Size	**Age**	**Target Response**	
Cross & Luper (1979)	9	C, A	"uh"	S slower than NS at age 5, 9, and in adulthood; response initiation time decreases with age for both groups.
Cullinan & Springer (1980)	20	C	"ah"	S had slower response initiation times than NS; the effect resulted from a subgroup of children who stuttered and had co-occurring articulation and/or language disorders.
Hand & Hayes (1983)	10	A	"ah," key press	S had slower response initiation than NS for both targets; S manual response times were slower than their vocal response times.
Bakker & Brutten (1989)	24	A	"pa," "uh"	S had slower voice initiation time than NS across all stimulus presentation conditions.
Watson, Pool, Devous, Sr., Freeman, & Finitzo (1992)	16[a]	A	"ah," "Oscar," sentence starting with "Oscar"	S slower than NS in response initiation; effect strongest for participants with reduced cortical blood flow to middle and superior temporal gyri in left hemisphere; stuttering severity did not affect response initiation.
Maske-Cash & Curlee (1995)	18	C	1 and 4 syllable targets; words, nonwords	S slower than NS in response initiation across all response types; effect attributable to a subgroup of children who stuttered and had co-occurring articulation and/or language disorders.
Logan (2003b)	11	T, A	Sentences	S slower than NS group for 3 of 4 sentence types; response initiation time not correlated with stuttering severity.
Tsiamtsiouris & Cairns (2013)	21	A	Sentences	S slower than NS across sentence types; increased syntactic complexity was associated with increased response initiation time for both groups.

Note. S = speakers who stutter, NS = speakers who do not stutter; C = children, T = teenagers, A = adults. Numbers in the sample size column indicate the number of participants per group within a study.

[a]There were 16 adults who stuttered in this study. Control group characteristics varied across analyses. Minimum sample size for control groups was 30.

children who stutter initiated the onsets of key words within the target sentences significantly earlier than children with typical fluency did during fluent trials. Thus, the children's timing structure for the stuttered trials was subtly different from that of typical, fluent speech, even though the gross pattern of coordination was normal.

Other researchers have uncovered differences between speakers who stuttered and typical speakers in the relative sequence of upper lip, lower lip, and jaw muscle activation during lip closure for [p] within the context of target words like *sapapple* (e.g., Caruso, Abbs, & Gracco, 1988; Gracco & Abbs, 1985). Speakers with typical fluency show a predictable activation sequence when speaking at habitual rates: upper lip → lower lip → jaw. There is evidence that speakers who stutter are less likely than fluent speakers are to produce the lip-closing gesture in this sequence (Caruso et al., 1988). Whether this coordination difference is the direct consequence of fluency impairment or, perhaps, a *compensation* for impairment remains to be determined (Namasivayam & van Lieshout, 2008). A variety of other relatively subtle differences have been discovered in speakers who stutter when compared with fluent controls. These include the following:

- Differences in the timing structure of consonant-vowel transitions during perceptibly fluent speech (Howell, Sackin, & Rustin, 1995; Zebrowski, Conture, & Cudahy, 1985);
- A greater magnitude of error in tasks that involve tracking the movement of a stimulus using lip movement (Howell et al., 1995);

- Differences in the relative speeds with which the tongue and lower lip move in relation to the jaw during speech (McClean & Runyan, 2000). (The tongue and lip moved with excessive velocity while the jaw moved with insufficient velocity. Velocity disparities were greatest in speakers who stuttered severely); and
- Evidence of tremor in lip muscles during disfluent speech (McClean, Goldsmith, & Cerf, 1984).

Smith and colleagues (Denny & Smith, 1992; Smith, 1989; Smith, Denny, Shaffer, Kelly, & Hirano, 1996; Walsh & Smith, 2013) examined patterns of lip, jaw, and neck muscle activation using electromyography (EMG) in samples of fluent and stuttered speech. They found evidence of characteristic *tremor-like oscillations* during muscle activation in speakers who stutter that none of the typical speakers exhibited. The frequency characteristics of the tremor-like oscillations all fell within a characteristic range (5 to 15 Hz), which suggested that they resulted from a common neural source (Smith, 1989). Not all stuttered disfluencies exhibited the atypical EMG activation, however, and some segments of fluent-sounding speech showed evidence of the tremor-like oscillation that was present during stuttered speech. Furthermore, the tremor-like oscillations were present in differing extents across speakers. Thus, there was no single common physiological pattern that characterized all stuttered disfluencies, and there was evidence of abnormality during speech that sounded fluent. The source of the tremor across speech-related muscles was unclear, but Smith (1989) speculated that it might relate to speech-related anxiety or autonomic nervous system arousal. Results from other studies showed no differences in the EMG activity of preschool- and early-elementary-school-aged children who stutter (Kelly, Smith, & Goffman, 1995; Walsh & Smith, 2013); however, tremor-like oscillations have been detected in the speech of 10- to 14-year-old children who stutter, which suggests that tremor is an emergent feature of stuttered speech (Kelly et al., 1995).

In another line of studies, Smith and colleagues have compared the *stability* (i.e., coordinative variability) of motor movements in speakers who stutter with those of fluent controls (see, for an example, Kleinow & Smith, 2000). The research paradigm they have used examines the timing and spatial characteristics of lip and jaw movements during repeated productions of a target utterance that features multiple bilabial consonants (e.g., *Buy Bobby a puppy*). In these studies, variability in the spatial and temporal aspects of articulatory movement is condensed into a single numerical value (the *spatiotemporal index* or STI) through the use of a mathematical equation. In some of the studies, the target utterance has been embedded in longer and/or linguistically complex contexts. In other studies, the researchers have used nonword response targets (e.g., mabshibe, mabfieshabe).

The general finding from this research is that the articulatory movements of speakers who stutter show significantly *greater spatiotemporal variability* than those of fluent speakers (e.g., Kleinow & Smith, 2000; Smith, Goffman, Sasisekaran, & Weber-Fox, 2012; Smith, Sadagopan, Walsh, & Weber-Fox, 2010). The utterance productions of typical speakers are relatively stable; that is, in trial after trial, the articulatory movements of the typical speakers are nearly the same in terms of

their spatial properties and temporal patterning (as measured by markers such as the time and manner in which lip closing occurs on target bilabial consonants within the target utterance). With the speakers who stutter, however, the articulatory movements are "messy," meaning that the spatiotemporal organization for the first trial in a series of repeated productions of *Buy Bobby a puppy* can be rather different from that in the second trial, which in turn can be rather different from that in the third trial and so on. Although these repeated productions all *sound* fluent, they all are significantly different from those of fluent speakers in terms of their coordination, and therefore, they are characteristic of stuttering. From this perspective, one might argue that *most*, and perhaps *all*, of the utterances that a speaker who stutters produces—including those that "sound fluent"—are atypical and indicative of the impairment that results in stuttering. The discrepancy between the sound of an utterance and its underlying coordination characteristics can create difficulties in the clinical assessment of stuttering. That is, an utterance can sound fluent to a clinician, but it can feel stuttered to a client. Thus, one must be mindful that listener-based acoustic measures of speech disfluency offer only a crude sense of motor system functioning in speakers who stutter (Smith & Kelly, 1997).

Motor Learning

Another facet of research in stuttering has focused on the motor-learning abilities in people who stutter. In this research, speakers who stutter and speakers with typical fluency repeat target utterances numerous times in succession. This generally results in improved fluency such that disfluency frequency decreases and speech rate increases. In older studies of stuttering, the immediate improvement in fluency was labeled "the adaptation effect" and early explanations for the adaptation tended to center on presumed changes in a speaker's beliefs or anxiety about stuttering-related disfluency (see, for example, Williams, Silverman, & Kools, 1968). Since then, however, several researchers (e.g., Frank & Bloodstein, 1971; Max, Caruso, & Vandevenne, 1997) have demonstrated that the effect is better explained in terms of motor learning; that is, the speaker learns how to produce the articulatory movements with increased proficiency after having practiced them many times.

The notion of motor learning goes beyond immediate changes in performance to include durable or long-lasting improvements in performance. Thus, in studies of speech motor learning, participants typically will practice a target utterance dozens, if not hundreds, of times in succession, and then leave the research laboratory and return hours or days later to perform the task again. If a speaker is able to resume the task during these follow-up sessions at a level that is substantially better than his or her baseline performance at the first session, then motor learning is said to have taken place. Several researchers have examined whether speakers who stutter exhibit evidence of motor learning on speech-related tasks and, if so, whether the amount of learning they attain is comparable to that of fluent speakers. Several representative studies from this part of the research literature are summarized in Table 6–8. As shown, in each of the studies presented in the table, speakers who stuttered exhibited evidence of motor learning. In all but two of the studies, the improvements were demonstrated during a retention task that occurred some time

after the initial practice phase. Nonetheless, speakers who stuttered consistently failed to attain a comparable degree of improvement in the speed and/or coordination of motor movements as speakers with typical fluency did (Bauerly & De Nil, 2011; Smits-Bandstra, De Nil, & Rochon, 2006; Smits-Bandstra, De Nil, & Saint-Cyr, 2006) and, even after practice, continue to exhibit anomalous movement patterns (Namasivayam & van Lieshout, 2008). So, although motor learning takes place, speech motor control does not fully normalize—a finding that would be expected if one assumes that stuttered speech is, in part or in whole, a manifestation of impairment in the speech motor system.

Psychological and Social/Emotional Correlates

Having discussed the many communication-related differences and deficits that people who stutter present, the next issue to consider relates to the stuttering-related feelings, attitudes, beliefs, and thoughts. Stuttering can have a marked impact on a person's ability to communicate. The extent of a person's communication disability is not always an accurate indicator of the broader effects of the disorder such as a person's psychological and social-emotional functioning. For example, a person who appears, outwardly, to exhibit relatively mild stuttering, can feel a range of intense negative emotions (e.g., embarrassment, shame) about being a person with impaired fluency and about stuttering openly in front of other people. This can lead the person to limit participation in social settings and possibly lead to changes in speech motor behavior that result in more severe stuttering than the

Table 6–8. Findings From Selected Studies of Motor Learning in Speakers Who Stutter

Study	Method	Results
Frank & Bloodstein (1971)	Speakers read a paragraph 6 times in succession. In one condition, all 6 trials were read solo; in the other, the first 5 trials were read chorally, and the 6th trial was read solo.	Stuttering frequency gradually declined across the trials in the solo condition. Stuttering frequency was near zero during the 5 choral trials. Speakers attained similar improvement on the 6th trial of both conditions.
Max & Caruso (1998)	Study 1 replicated Frank & Bloodstein (1971); Study 2 involved production of multisyllable target words embedded in a paragraph.	After reading the passage consecutively, stuttering frequency decreased, as did word duration, vowel duration, consonant-vowel transition duration, and movement duration for lip closure on select consonants.
Max & Baldwin (2010)	Participants read a paragraph 5 times in succession during three different sessions. Half of the paragraph sentences were consistent across trials (repeated sentences), and half varied (novel sentences).	Repeated sentences showed more fluency improvement than novel sentences after the first 5 readings, and again, after 5 more readings two hours later. After 24 hours, the repeated sentences showed evidence of retaining the motor improvements from the previous day, but novel sentences did not.
Namasivayam & van Lieshout (2008)	Participants repeated nonsense words at fast and slow rates during three sessions (session 1 and 2 on one day, session 3 one week later).	After practice, speakers who stuttered were similar to controls on several motor measures but had significantly larger amplitude for upper lip movements and a trend toward greater variability in lip movement and less tightly coupled coordinative patterns.
Bauerly & De Nil (2011)	Participants produced 100 repetitions of a monosyllable nonsense word sequence (*baz dob jeb zot gak vud daf bup jeg tup*). They then returned the following day to produce 50 additional repetitions.	Speakers who stutter had longer durations than controls for the target syllable sequence after both sessions. The effect was confined to a subgroup of participants. The stuttering group showed retention of practice effects one day later (i.e., motor learning).
Smits-Bandstra & De Nil (2006)	Participants produced 30 repetitions of a monosyllable nonsense word sequence (*ta ba pa ta ga pa ga ta pa ba*). Pre- and post-task measures of motor performance were obtained.	Speakers who stutter showed less improvement than controls and, unlike controls, no change in response initiation time.
Smits-Bandstra, De Nil, & Saint-Cyr (2006)	Studied finger-tap sequence learning. Participants typed a number sequence (e.g., *4 2 1 3 1 2 4 1 3 4*) on a response pad featuring horizontally placed buttons.	Speakers who stutter showed slower reaction times and less improvement in movement sequencing after practice and did not maintain gains in reaction time during a retention task as well as the control group did.

person otherwise might exhibit. As Johnson and Associates (1959) noted many years ago, stuttering is a dynamic disorder, and a speaker's experience of the disorder is shaped by four main factors:

- The speech behaviors that characterize the disorder called stuttering;
- The way in which the speaker reacts to his or her stuttered speech;
- The way in which listeners react to the speaker's stuttered speech; and
- The way in which the speaker reacts to the listeners' reaction to his or her stuttered speech.

The interactions among these factors can exacerbate the basic fluency difficulties that a speaker experiences from stuttering (Conture et al., 2006). For example, a speaker may have personal expectations for performance that are unrealistic ("I can *never* let other people hear me stutter"). This expectation might lead to heightened anxiety and/or muscular tension during situations where it is challenging to manage impending stuttering-related disfluency and, in doing so, increase the frequency and/or duration of any stuttering-related disfluency that occurs. A speaker's beliefs and feelings about stuttering do not develop in a vacuum, of course. Listeners react to stuttering in any number of ways, some of which may convey negative evaluations such as disapproval or rejection of the individual. Thus, a speaker's seemingly high internal standards for performance may originate in the standards that another person has for the speaker. Over time, the speaker may come to internalize another person's reactions or expectations and begin to develop unhelpful thoughts, negative

emotions, and unrealistic expectations regarding how he or she should speak. In doing so, the speaker creates a perspective toward speaking that hinders fluency functioning.

Life Experiences of People Who Stutter

Several researchers have used qualitative research methods to learn about how people who stutter experience their speech disorder and the types of challenges they face during daily activities. Such research studies typically are based on a standard interview. After eliciting responses from participants, the researchers implement systematic analyses that are designed to identify response themes that are common across the participants. Corcoran and Stewart (1998) conducted a qualitative study of eight adults who stutter that centered on the participants' common emotional themes. Four interrelated themes emerged among the participants: *shame, helplessness, fear,* and *avoidance,* which together added up to an overall portrait of *suffering.* Corcoran and Stewart discussed the relationship between feelings of shame and the stigma that is attached to stuttering through an assortment of negative cultural connotations of stuttered speech and people who stutter. They noted that the experience of suffering, in medical spheres, often is accompanied by an individual's feelings of *lacking control* over and *understanding* of the situation (in this case, stuttering) and a sense of *feeling overwhelmed* at the prospect of *dire* or *unrelenting* negative outcomes. Data such as these provide a glimpse into the types of treatment outcomes that might be helpful to a speaker who stutters (e.g., learning more about the nature of stuttering, developing *helpful* strategies for responding to impending stuttering-related disfluency, learning about the positive outcomes that other speakers who stutter have attained).

Plexico, Manning, and DiLollo (2005) used qualitative methods to identify the processes that are involved in learning to manage stuttering successfully. They conducted in-depth interviews with seven adults who stuttered. Each of the adults had developed the ability to manage stuttering well enough that the disorder no longer resulted in significant communication disability. In Plexico et al.'s study, the participants discussed their speech and general experiences from childhood through adulthood. The common themes that the participants mentioned with regard to those periods in life when they did not manage stuttering successfully included the following: *experiencing negative emotions; experiencing negative reactions from listeners; leading a restrictive lifestyle, avoiding social and communicative situations; gradual awareness of communication disability;* and *receiving inadequate speech therapy.*

Based on comments from the participants, Plexico et al. (2005) also identified the "essential structure" of stuttering at three periods in the participants' lives: the period when stuttering was not successfully managed, the transition period toward successful management, and the (current) period when stuttering was successfully managed. The essential structure consisted of a concise narrative that captured the seven participants' common core experience. The essential structure that Plexico et al. reported for unsuccessfully managed stuttering included the following elements: (1) experiencing significant "struggle" and "suffering" due to

the challenges associated with stuttering; (2) enduring negative reactions toward stuttering from people within and beyond the immediate family; (3) attempting to conceal stuttering from others either by avoiding participation in social situations or by implementing coping strategies in order to minimize or prevent stuttering-related symptoms; and (4) experiencing a range of unpleasant and disabling emotions (e.g., helplessness, anxiety, poor self-esteem).

Daniels, Gabel, and Hughes (2012) completed a qualitative study in which 21 mainly middle-aged adults who stutter recounted their stuttering-related experiences during the school years. Experiences that the participants reported included the following:

- The use of physical (finger tapping), linguistic (word avoidance), and social-interactional (situational avoidance) coping strategies (86% of participants);
- Physiological consequences such as physical illness (e.g., vomiting from anticipation of public speaking), muscle tension, and anxiety (67% of participants);
- Psychological consequences such as feelings of hopelessness (33% of participants);
- Academic consequences such as limited verbal participation in learning activities and limited attention to lectures because of stuttering-related anxiety (90% of participants);
- Speech therapy that focused mostly on speaking techniques and rarely on speech-related feelings and emotions (76% of participants); and
- Persistent fear of speaking following completion of school and

development of a stuttering self-identity (81%) of participants.

Clearly, in cases of chronic stuttering, the memories of communication-related difficulties from childhood remain vivid into adulthood, and they seem to color a person's life experiences well after the school years end. Research with older adults who stutter indicates that speakers may continue to experience negative feelings concerning social interaction, concern about negative reactions from listeners, and less satisfaction than non-stuttering speakers about their general health (Bricker-Katz, Lincoln, & McCabe, 2009). These experiences seem to extend to people in a variety of cultural settings. For example, South African adults who stuttered reported similar histories of negative listener reactions and similar stuttering-related limitations for their academic performance and for occupational performance (Klompas & Ross, 2004). As an aside, student speech-language pathology clinicians who are required to complete pseudo-stuttering activities as part of their clinical training report many of the same reactions as speakers who stutter (McKeehan, 1994; Rami, Kalinowski, Stuart, & Rastatter, 2003).

Anxiety and Related Disorders

According to the American Psychological Association (APA, 2014), anxiety is "an emotion characterized by feelings of tension, worried thoughts, and physical changes like increased blood pressure . . . sweating, trembling, dizziness, or a rapid heart beat." The APA states that people with anxiety disorders also may present recurring intrusive thoughts and concerns and situational avoidance that is based in worry about how a situation will unfold. Included under the umbrella of anxiety disorders are conditions such as social phobia, generalized anxiety disorder, panic disorder, and obsessive-compulsive disorder (Iverach et al., 2010). Anxiety has been included as a variable in many studies of stuttering, where its role as a potential cause and/or consequence of stuttering has been examined.

State and Trait Anxiety

Some scientists make the distinction between *state anxiety* and *trait anxiety* (Spielberger, Gorsuch, Lushene, & Vagg, 1983). The notion of state anxiety refers to how a person experiences anxiety within specific situations or settings. Trait anxiety, in contrast, is a more general term, referring to a person's background level of anxiety across all activities; the level of anxiety that one experiences chronically or, perhaps, that is intrinsic to one's personality. Research of this sort has consistently detected differences between speakers who stutter and speakers with typical fluency. For instance, Ezrati-Vinacour and Levin (2004) reported that adults who stuttered had higher trait anxiety scores than fluent controls and that severe cases of stuttering had higher state anxiety scores than mild cases of stuttering.

Craig (1990) examined differences in state and trait anxiety for a large sample of adults who stuttered and nonstuttering controls (102 participants per group at the onset of the study; the average age was 32 years). Craig noted that much of the research that predated his study had reported no significant differences in anxiety levels between speakers who stuttered and speakers with typical fluency. However, he also noted that many of these studies featured small sample sizes and thus lacked the statistical power necessary to detect potentially meaningful differences between the groups. Craig obtained anxiety ratings for the speakers who stuttered in the context of recorded telephone conversations before and immediately after participation in a stuttering therapy program.

In the pretreatment assessment of Craig's (1990) study, both the state and trait anxiety scores for the speakers who stuttered were significantly greater (more severe) than those for the fluent controls. For the speakers who stuttered, pretreatment state anxiety was significantly correlated with stuttering frequency as well. Following the treatment, which resulted in a near complete elimination of stuttering-related disfluency during the phone calls, the trait anxiety scores were comparable to those of the control group and were not correlated to stuttering severity in either the pre or posttreatment condition. Thus, after the speakers developed skills for managing speech fluency more effectively, their anxiety scores improved markedly. On this basis, Craig suggested that anxiety is more likely a *consequence* of stuttering than it is a cause of stuttering. Craig interpreted the high pretreatment trait anxiety scores for the speakers who stuttered as a consequence of having had a speech handicap for many years. Similarly, he interpreted the elevated state anxiety as a consequence of the speakers' repeated exposure to negative reactions from conversational partners in this context and their expectation of receiving such reactions again in the future.

In some studies, researchers have failed to detect differences in either state or trait anxiety between speakers who stutter and speakers with typical fluency, but they have found evidence of anxiety-related differences between the groups using other measures. For instance, Blood and colleagues (Blood, Blood, Bennett, Simpson, & Susman, 1994) reported that speakers who stuttered showed higher levels of salivary cortisol (a hormone that is involved in glucose metabolism and the body's response to stress) than nonstuttering controls during self-rated "high stress" sessions in the experiment. Both groups reported comparable increases in state anxiety scores during the "high stress" condition relative to a baseline condition, but the groups did not differ in the amount of anxiety they reported.

Social Anxiety

Other research has supported the notion that the elevated anxiety found in many speakers who stutter is primarily socially based. Messenger, Onslow, Packman, and Menzies (2004) administered a comprehensive anxiety rating scale to both adults who stuttered and matched fluent controls. They found that the stuttering group exhibited elevated scores only on portions of the scale that pertained to social evaluation and participation in new or unfamiliar social situations. Scale items dealing with other anxiety-provoking contexts (i.e., exposure to physical danger, participation in certain daily routines) failed to differentiate the groups. In a similar study, Mahr and Torosian (1999) found that speakers who stuttered had higher (less favorable) ratings on a scale of social anxiety than a fluent control group did, but when the speakers who stuttered were compared to a group of people with social phobia, they scored lower (more favorably) with regard to social distress, avoidance, and fear of negative evaluation. The most common fears reported by speakers who stuttered dealt with speech-related issues. Findings from other research with adults who stuttered showed that they identified more daily activities as being stressful than speakers with typical fluency did, and they exhibited higher levels of stuttering on self-reported "high stress" days than on low stress days (Blood, Wertz, Blood, Bennett, & Simpson, 1997).

Elevated anxiety ratings also have been reported in some studies with adolescents who stutter (Blood, Blood, Maloney, Meyer, & Qualls, 2007; Mulcahy, Hennessey, Beilby, & Byrnes, 2008). Although self-reported ratings of self-esteem for adolescents who stutter do not necessarily differ from those for typically fluent adolescents, the self-esteem scores are significantly correlated with self-ratings of anxiety, such that highly anxious teens who stutter tend to have poor self-esteem (Blood et al., 2007).

Relatively little is known about how common social anxiety disorder is among people who stutter. In one recent study, Blumgart, Tran, and Craig (2010a) administered a battery of tests to 200 adults who stuttered and 200 fluent controls. As in other studies, they found evidence of elevated trait anxiety and social anxiety among the speakers who stuttered. In addition, 40% of the adults who stuttered met criteria for social phobia, and these individuals were judged to be at risk for a generalized phobia. Examples of fears that differentiated the groups included the following: "public speaking," "saying stupid things in a group," "asking questions in a group," "business meetings," and "social gatherings or parties." Iverach et al. (2009) used a statistical modeling approach to estimate the extent to which adults who seek therapy for stuttering are at risk for various anxiety-related disorders. Based on their analysis, they concluded that people who stutter have a 6 to 7 times greater chance than fluent controls of meeting a 12-month diagnosis for some type of anxiety disorder. The risk for social phobia was particularly high (16 to 34 times greater than the fluent controls), and there also was significantly higher risk for developing generalized anxiety disorder (4 times greater risk than the fluent controls) and panic disorder (6 times greater risk than the fluent controls). Iverach et al. (2010a) found that people who stutter were 2 times as likely as fluent controls to meet criteria for mood disorders (e.g., major depression) but no more likely than fluent controls to exhibit substance abuse. The latter findings differ from those in some other studies, wherein speakers who stutter were found to exhibit a similar degree of depression as fluent controls (Bray, Kehle, Lawless, & Theodore, 2003; Miller & Watson, 1992). Sample sizes in the latter studies were smaller than those in the Iverach et al. (2010a) study, however.

Personality Characteristics

Bloodstein and Bernstein Ratner (2008) summarized numerous studies from the mid- to late-1900s in which the research focus was on the personality, personal adjustment, and mental well-being of speakers who stutter. Based on this review, they concluded that the average person who stutters does not show evidence of severe maladjustment or neuroticism, nor do they show evidence of a specific "character structure" or personality profile. With respect to personal adjustment, they concluded that people who stutter show marked variability—some people are very well adjusted both to their communication impairment and to general life activities, while others clearly are not. They concluded that, on average, people who stutter "are not quite as well adjusted as are typical normal speakers." This conclusion was based on findings from many studies in which people who stuttered showed a tendency toward lower self-esteem and reduced willingness to take risks in comparison to typically fluent speakers. Still, Bloodstein and Bernstein Ratner concluded that the differences between people who stutter and typical speakers were a matter of degree, not kind. Thus, people who stutter may score lower than typical speakers on measures of personality and emotional health, but usually not so much lower as to create a categorical difference and the labeling of a disorder.

The personality characteristics of speakers who stutter continue to receive researchers' attention. Iverach et al. (2010b) examined five personality domains in speakers who stutter compared to speakers with typical fluency and found that the stuttering group was well within the normal range for all five domains (neuroticism, extraversion, openness, agreeableness, and conscientiousness); however, they had less favorable ratings than controls for three of these domains (neuroticism, agreeableness, conscientiousness). Manning and Beck (2013) also examined personality factors in a sample of 50 adults who were undergoing treatment for stuttering. They found that only 10% of the participants met criteria for personality disorder and that personality disorder was no more common among people who stutter than it is in the general population. Other recent research suggests that stuttering speakers who exhibit strong social support networks, healthy social relationships, and a high degree of "self-efficacy" (i.e., the belief that one can exert influence over circumstances in their life), are much less likely to experience adverse psychosocial effects than stuttering speakers who lack these markers of resilience (Craig, Blumgart, & Tran, 2011).

Temperament Characteristics

Temperament has been defined as "biologically based individual differences in behavioral characteristics or reactions that are present in infancy and are relatively stable across contexts and over time" (Anderson, Pellowski, Conture, & Kelly, 2003). The construct typically is conceived of as a collection of hereditable traits or dimensions pertaining to reactivity, sociability, self-regulation, agreeableness, positive or negative emotionality, and adaptability (Eggers, De Nil, & Van den Bergh, 2009; Rothbart & Bates, 1998; Seery et al., 2007). Recent estimates are that roughly 20% to 60% of the individual variation in temperament can be attributed to genetic factors, with the remainder attributable to environmental factors (Eggers et al., 2009). In recent decades, researchers have examined the temperament of children who stutter in an attempt to clarify its role in the development and expression of stuttering. In some studies, researchers have measured children's temperament using parent responses on formal rating scales of temperament (e.g., Anderson et al., 2003; Eggers et al., 2009; Karrass et al., 2006; Kefalianos, Onslow, Ukoumunne, Block, & Reilly, 2014). In other studies, researchers have examined children's verbal and nonverbal behaviors during experimental situations that are designed to elicit positive and/or negative emotions (Arnold, Conture, Key, & Walden, 2011; Johnson, Walden, Conture, & Karrass, 2010). In the Arnold et al. (2011) study, behavioral measures were supplemented by electrophysiological measures of brain activity.

The general pattern of findings from this research seems to be that although children who stutter and children with typical fluency show similarities in temperament profiles, in all studies, at least some differences have been detected between the groups (Seery et al., 2007). The nature of temperament differences between groups varies across studies, however, and the relationship between the group differences and stuttered speech sometimes is unclear. For example, some researchers (Kefalianos et al., 2014) have found that children who stutter are *less reactive* to environmental stimuli than children with typical fluency; others have found that they are *more reactive* (Karrass et al., 2006; Schwenk, Conture, & Walden, 2007); and still others have the two groups react similarly (Arnold et al., 2011). In several studies, children who stutter have been found to be more likely to manifest reduced attention and/or task persistence in comparison with nonstuttering children (Anderson et al., 2003; Karrass et al., 2006; Kefalianos et al., 2014). Schwenk et al. (2007) examined children's reactivity and distractibility by studying the way in which the participants reacted to movements of a remotely controlled video camera that the experimenters used to collect data during the experimental task. They found that when the camera moved, the children who stuttered were nearly three times as likely as the nonstuttering children to reorient attention toward it and, consequently, away from the toy or person to which they had been attending. The children who stuttered also showed a trend toward orienting more quickly toward the camera movement than the nonstuttering children did.

Differences between children who stutter and children with typical fluency in emotional regulation also have been reported. For example, children who stuttered produced more nonverbal expressions of negative emotion than children with typical fluency when presented with an undesirable gift in an experimental setting and, at such times, their speech became more disfluent (Johnson et al., 2010). Children who stutter are also less apt than children with typical fluency to implement overt emotional regulation strategies such as *distraction* (i.e., shifting attention toward another event or activity), *self-stimulation* (i.e., seeking comfort from another person), or *cognitive restructuring* (i.e., requesting more information about a situation) during communication contexts that are associated with discomforting emotions (Arnold et al., 2011).

Kefalianos et al. (2014) examined aspects of temperament in preschool-aged children for the presence of traits that are associated with anxiety. Among other variables, they examined whether children who stuttered were more reluctant to approach novel stimuli and novel social situations than children with typical fluency and whether they showed a greater tendency toward being viewed by their parents as being difficult to deal with in terms of child rearing. Neither variable differentiated the two groups of children, a finding that was consistent with other research (Anderson et al., 2003; Eggers et al., 2009). Based on these findings, Kefalianos et al. concluded that anxiety is not likely to be a causal factor at stuttering onset. Rather, it seems to be an emergent feature of stuttering and develops after preschool as a consequence of accumulated negative experiences with speaking. Given the nature of the findings in the temperament literature, Seery et al. (2007) proposed that there is not a single, common "stuttering temperament" but rather that temperamental differences are present to varying degrees in subgroups of children who stutter.

Autonomic Nervous System Functioning

One way of studying the physiological correlates of stuttering is to examine the functioning in the autonomic nervous system (ANS), a branch of the nervous system that regulates body activities that are largely "involuntary" in nature (e.g., heart rate, vasoconstriction, digestion, sweat secretion). Several researchers have examined ANS functioning in fluent speakers and speakers who stutter through examination of variables such as heart rate and pulse volume. One of the main findings is that high levels of autonomic arousal characterize speech production for *all* speakers—typical speakers and speakers who stutter, alike (Weber & Smith, 1990). The relationship between autonomic arousal and stuttered speech is complex, however. For example, Weber and Smith (1990) reported that high levels of autonomic nervous system activation were present prior to, during, and just after overtly stuttered speech; however, levels of autonomic arousal were not strongly predictive of stuttering severity or disfluency frequency. Further, speakers who stutter did not show more autonomic arousal than speakers with typical fluency.

Environmental Correlates

Listener Behavior

As noted in the previous section, many people who stutter report having received negative responses from listeners. Often, such responses result from the listener's failure to recognize stuttered speech as it is occurring. Thus, a speaker's brief delay in response initiation when asked, "What is your name?" is met with seemingly innocuous remarks such as "Oh, that's a tough question, huh?" or "Yeah, I've had a long day too." At other times, the listener may respond with a facial expression that conveys impatience or incredulity. Listener responses such as these may not seem particularly harmful on the surface; however, when a speaker is on the receiving end of such responses multiple times per week, for month after month, and is expending a considerable amount of effort to say even simple sentences, it can lead the speaker to become apprehensive or anxious about how the next speaking partner might respond and to feel frustrated or angry about the act of communication. Children who stutter may face listener reactions that are more intense than those that adults who stutter receive. Examples of the latter include teasing and bullying, topics that are discussed in the next section.

Bullying

The issue of bullying has received growing attention—both in school and in work settings—in recent years. The Workplace Bullying Institute (2014) defines bullying as "repeated, health-harming mistreatment of one or more persons (the targets) by one or more perpetrators." It is abusive conduct, often in the form of verbal abuse that is threatening, humiliating, or intimidating. The American Psychological Association (2014) adds that bullying "is a form of aggressive behavior in which someone intentionally and repeatedly causes another person injury or discomfort" and that it can take the form of "physical contact, words, or more subtle actions."

In most cases, the victim cannot defend him- or herself easily and has done nothing obviously wrong or threatening to the bully. When bullied, the victim may withdraw from social interaction and experience low self-esteem, as well as physical symptoms such as difficulty sleeping, loss of appetite, and anxiety. Research into the bullying experiences of people who stutter is limited, but data suggest that it is a significant problem for this population. In one retrospective study, about 89% of participants with a history of stuttering reported having been bullied during their school years (Hugh-Jones & Smith, 1999). In a study of adolescents, 44% of those who stuttered reported that they had been bullied, while only 14% of the control group did (Blood et al., 2011). Interestingly, in the Blood et al. study, 4% of the adolescents in the stuttering group met criteria for *being a bully*, as did 11% of the adolescents in the control group.

Davis, Howell, and Cooke (2002) interviewed school-aged children individually regarding their views about classmates. They showed the children a class roster and asked them to nominate the three children they liked most and least. Then they asked the children to pick three classmates who best fit each of the following eight adjectives: shy, assertive, cooperative, bully, bully victim, disruptive, leader, and uncertain. The results showed that peers rejected children who stutter more often than they did nonstuttering peers and that children who stutter were less likely to be viewed as popular or as leaders and more likely to be characterized as victims of bullying and as seeking help. Similar findings have been reported in studies that examine classmate nomination patterns for preschool-aged children with other types of speech-language disorders (Gertner, Rice, & Hadley, 1994). Langevin (2009) found that about 17% of 10-year-old children expressed somewhat

negative to very negative attitudes toward two stuttering children who they viewed on video. However, the participants who reported knowing someone who stuttered had more favorable attitudes toward the children on the video recordings than the participants who reported not knowing someone who stuttered. This suggests that educational programs that are geared toward building school-aged children's knowledge of stuttering may be an important component in programs that are designed to prevent bullying in schools.

Listener Attitudes

The issue of listener attitudes toward stuttering and people who stutter has been studied extensively (Bloodstein & Bernstein Ratner, 2008; Logan & O'Connor, 2012). One common approach is to present adult research participants (i.e., adults with typical fluency) pairs of contrasting adjectives such as *outgoing* and *withdrawn* and then ask them to use the adjectives to rate a hypothetical person who stutters and a hypothetical person who does not stutter. In many of these studies, the hypothetical speaker who stutters ends up being assigned less favorable or less desirable characteristics than the hypothetical fluent speaker. In other studies, subgroups within the population (e.g., teachers, nurses, prospective employers) are presented with descriptor-based rating scales and again are asked to rate hypothetical speakers. Once again, hypothetical people who stutter tend to be rated less favorably than hypothetical fluent speakers.

On this basis, it might appear that the raters in such studies have negative or stereotyped attitudes toward people who stutter. This conclusion is not necessarily warranted, however, because in many of the "rate the hypothetical person who stutters" studies, the rater has only one reference point (e.g., one hypothetical person who stutters). Thus, it is possible that the ratings they make are based upon an amalgamation of all people who stutter or perhaps one particularly severe case of stuttering that they have seen. However, Logan and Willis (2011) found that when participants are given multiple samples of speech containing varying degrees of stuttering-related disfluency, raters do demonstrate the ability to alter their perceptions of people who stutter. Logan and Willis concluded that adult listeners do not seem to adopt the view that "one stutterer is the same as the next." Rather, they seem capable of empathizing with types of communicative difficulties that speakers with varying degrees of stuttering severity might encounter.

Studies of employers suggest that they tend to view people who stutter as being less capable or less likely to be promoted than people who do not stutter (Bloodstein & Bernstein Ratner, 2008). Interestingly, studies with people who stutter tend to show similar findings, in that they sometimes report that their stuttering limits their performance in work settings (Logan & O'Connor, 2012). When speakers with typical fluency are asked to provide career advice to a person who stutters, they are much more likely to recommend occupations with low speaking demands than occupations with high speaking demands, whereas their occupational advice for speakers with typical fluency is primarily based on the raters' perceptions of the academic or training requirements associated with an occupation (Logan & O'Connor, 2012).

People who stutter are sometimes faced with the dilemma of whether to overtly acknowledge their stuttering in front of other people. Results from some studies suggest that listeners react to a speaker who stutters more favorably when the speaker acknowledges his or her fluency impairment in comparison to when the impairment is not acknowledged (Collins & Blood, 1990; Schloss, Espin, Smith, & Suffolk, 1987). A listener's attitudes toward stuttering are likely shaped by the amount of knowledge that he or she has about the disorder. Not surprisingly, research indicates that many of the people with whom speakers who stutter interact—including medical personnel, teachers, and speech-language pathologists—have only limited knowledge about the disorder (Bloodstein & Bernstein Rather, 2008). This lack of basic knowledge about stuttering among the general public may help to explain why stuttering is often depicted in a negative light in contemporary films and in a sometimes distorted and simplistic manner in fictional literature (Logan, Mullins, & Jones, 2008).

Other Environmental Factors

It is tempting to think that parents of children who stutter are, through their speech behaviors or expectations for the child, somehow the cause or trigger of their child's speech disfluency. This does not seem to be the case, however, as parents of children who stutter have been found to perform similarly to parents of typically fluent children on variables such as disfluency identification (Zebrowski & Conture, 1989); the type of verbal input that they provide to their developing child (Miles & Bernstein Ratner, 2001; Nippold & Rudzinski, 1995); and their judgments about their child's communicative functioning (Bernstein Ratner & Silverman, 2000). In addition, parents of children who stutter seem to use speech rates and turn-taking patterns that are similar to those observed in parents of typically fluent children (Kelly & Conture, 1992), and they express similar pragmatic functions during conversation (Weiss & Zebrowski, 1991). Meyers and Freeman (1985) found that mothers of both children who stutter and children with typical fluency talked more rapidly when interacting with a child who stuttered severely than they did when interacting with children who stuttered less severely or with children who did not stutter. Thus, there may be some aspects of stuttered speech that alter or disrupt the typical temporal course of conversation. Beyond this, however, studies of prenatal, developmental, and medical factors have failed to uncover any consistently compelling differences between the home lives of stuttering and nonstuttering children (Cox, Seider, & Kidd, 1984).

Etiological Considerations

Early Theories

Many of the early theories of stuttering featured a single "key factor" that the author(s) presented as an explanation for either the conditions surrounding stuttering onset or the occurrence of stuttering-related disfluency (Conture, 2001). The number of hypothesized explanations put forth for stuttering during the 20th century is, in retrospect, rather remarkable. That is, it seems as if there were nearly as many theories of stuttering as there were authorities on stuttering. Obviously, with a situation like that, some of the theories are bound to be incorrect or, at least, incomplete.

Bloodstein (1958) introduced a three-part classification system to describe the existing theories of that era (and, in later writings, he continued to use the framework to classify many of the theories that emerged after this time). According to

Bloodstein, most of the pre-1958 theories of stuttering fit into one of three categories: (1) stuttered speech as a symptom of *repressed needs*; (2) stuttered speech as a symptom of "breakdown" (i.e., impairment) in the speech production system; and (3) stuttered speech as a symptom of *anticipatory struggle*. These categories for stuttering theories are briefly explained below.

Stuttering as an Expression of Repressed Needs

As Bloodstein (1958) described, in the repressed needs view, stuttering-related interruptions in speech were thought to occur because the speaker unconsciously wished them to occur. Theories of this sort typically invoked explanations for stuttering that involved conflict in parent-child interactions, particularly during the early stages of development. In this view, stuttered speech was presumed to be a symptom of this conflict. Disfluent speech was said to represent an outward manifestation of aggression, anger, unresolved issues, and unspeakable feelings (cf. Coriat, 1943; Travis, 1971). Theories of this sort eventually fell out of favor, as they lacked robust empirical support (in fact, it is doubtful if some theories in this category could even be scientifically tested) and could not offer compelling explanations for many of the characteristics of stuttering. Today, they are not viewed as credible explanations for stuttered speech.

Stuttering as a Breakdown in Speech Production

In this view, stuttering-related interruption was thought to result from "temporary failures" in the speech production system. In many such models, the failures were presented as "moments" of disfunction (e.g., intermittent spasms or "rough spots") in the speech stream. Sometimes included in this view was the notion that individuals were predisposed to fluency difficulty (e.g., West, 1958). In the early to mid 1900s, authorities proposed a range of sources for fluency breakdown. Examples of these include the following:

- Discoordination of cerebral input to speech-related musculature (Travis, 1931),
- Brief, subtle convulsions that disrupt speech production (West, 1958),
- A psychophysiologic compulsion to adduct the vocal folds (Kenyon, 1943), and
- Discoordination among the respiratory, laryngeal, and articulatory muscle systems (Van Riper, 1982).

The notion of "breakdown" in speech production continues to appear in contemporary theories of stuttering; however, there is growing recognition (e.g., Smits-Bandstra & De Nil, 2007; Smith & Kelly, 1997) that the consequences of breakdown are not confined to discreet moments, but rather are apparent throughout the course of an utterance, and that there may be more than one aspect of speech production that is impaired.

Stuttering as a Learned, Anticipatory Struggle

In the anticipatory struggle view, stuttering-related interruptions in speech were said to arise from the speaker's fear of or concern with speaking disfluently. Examples of theories that Bloodstein (1958) placed into this category included the following:

- The *diagnosogenic theory* (Johnson et al., 1942) in which laypeople (e.g., parents) supposedly mislabel a child's ordinary disfluency as "stuttering" and the behaviors that typify stuttering are then the product of this (mis-)diagnosis and the child's reactions to the (mis-) diagnosis;
- The *approach-avoidance conflict* theory (Sheehan, 1958), in which stutter-like interruptions were modeled as the manifestation of competing urges to speak and to remain silent; and
- Bloodstein's (1958) *anticipatory struggle hypothesis* described stuttering essentially as a belief-based phenomenon. Bloodstein proposed that a child's early speaking experiences in language acquisition lead to the conviction that "speech is difficult" to do. Bloodstein claimed that this firm belief about the difficulty of speaking leads to a sense of feeling overwhelmed by the act of speaking, which, in turn, leads to excessive muscle tension and "fragmentation" of sequential motor movements. In this way, the classic stutter-like disfluencies (prolonging and repeating) were thought to be manifestations of excessive tension and fragmentation of motor movement—all due to the belief that speaking is difficult.

The construct of anticipatory struggle is rooted in the more fundamental notion that speakers learn beliefs and behaviors that either make them prone to stutter or that lead directly to stuttered speech. During the 1960s, other learning-based explanations for stuttering were hypothesized.

These accounts came under the headings of classical and/or operant conditioning. With operant conditioning, came the idea that the behaviors a person exhibits are shaped by the events or consequences that accompany those behaviors. In this framework, consequences (*contingencies*) that increase the frequency of a behavior are termed *reinforcers*, while consequences that decrease the frequency of a behavior are termed *punishers.*

The next issue to consider is whether operant conditioning explains the onset of stuttered speech. When followed to its logical conclusion, the theory would predict that parents and other caregivers must respond to speech disfluency, particularly part- and whole-word repetitions and sound prolongations, in ways that increase (*reinforce*) their occurrence. There is little evidence, however, that parents of children who stutter interact with young children who stutter in ways that are markedly different from the ways that parents of nonstuttering children interact with children, including children who stutter (Bernstein Ratner & Silverman, 2000; Kelly & Conture, 1992; Meyers & Freeman, 1985; Miles & Bernstein Ratner, 2001; Weiss & Zebrowski, 1991). For instance, Zebrowski and Conture (1989) compared the perceptual judgments that mothers of young children who stuttered and mothers of young typically developing children made about samples of fluent and stuttered speech. Both groups of mothers most often regarded instances of part- and whole-word repetition to be stuttered, while they regarded instances of sound prolongation as nonstuttered. The results also showed that disfluency duration affected parents' judgments of stuttering similarly: Longer disfluencies were more apt to be judged as stuttered by both groups. The findings of this study

present difficulties for an operant-based explanation of stuttering onset. For example, why would some mothers selectively reinforce instances of part-word repetition and others would not, even when they both considered part-word repetition to be symptomatic of stuttering? Further, why do some children who stutter develop excessive sound prolongation if their mothers are less inclined to regard that disfluency type as sign of stuttering? For reasons such as this, operant conditioning frameworks generally are considered to be better suited to explaining how stuttering-related disfluency changes over time than they are to explaining how stuttering-related disfluency develops in the first place.

Brutten and Shoemaker (1967) proposed a more elaborate learning-based model for stuttered speech (the so-called "two-factor" theory). They proposed that negative emotion is associated with disintegration of cognitive and motor processing. In their model, they proposed that children who stutter learn to associate speaking with "negative emotion" through classical conditioning such that, over time, the act of speaking is paired with the disintegration of the cognitive and motor processes that are necessary for fluent speech production. Once the link between disfluency and negative emotion is established, the speech disfluency is subject to the effects of operant conditioning in the manner described above. The theory attracted considerable attention at the time it was proposed, and was notable for linking physiological events associated with emotion to cognitive and motor processes associated with speech production. This is an area that continues to be researched today. In retrospect, one weakness of theory is that the proposed mechanism for the onset of stuttering is inconsistent with more recent findings on children's awareness of stuttered speech. That is, it has been shown that many young children have little awareness of their disfluent speech prior to age four (Ezrati-Vinacour, Platzky, & Yairi, 2001), a situation which seems inconsistent with the idea that children pair disfluency with "negative emotion" during the earliest stages of speech development. Further, studies of motor and autonomic nervous system activation of speakers who stutter also are inconsistent with this theory. For example, speakers who stutter, and particularly young children who stutter, do not consistently show heightened muscle activation or heightened autonomic nervous system arousal in conjunction with stuttered speech (Denny & Smith, 1992; Kelly et al., 1995; Smith, 1989; Weber & Smith, 1990). The model's mechanisms for explaining changes in stuttering behavior after onset continue to be plausible. This theory and others that have come before and after underscore the complexities associated with explaining speech disorders like stuttering.

Stuttering as a Psycholinguistic Impairment

In the late 1980s through the 1990s, several authors proposed explanatory models for stuttering that were rooted in psycholinguistic aspects of speech planning. Four such models are described in this section.

Prosody and Syllable Structure

Wingate (1988) described a model to account for the disfluency types that are most characteristic of stuttered speech (i.e., part-word repetition, sound prolon-

gation). He noted that many of the disfluencies in stuttered speech feature a break between the onset and rime of a syllable—a location he termed the "fault line." On this basis, as well as others, he proposed that people who stutter present impairment in the ability to retrieve syllable rimes. Wingate claimed that the deficit is particularly evident in linguistic contexts in which the rime conveys linguistic stress. With such syllables, the speaker assigns prosodic parameters to the rime in order to attain the desired changes in duration and vocal emphasis. In the model, the hypothesized deficit in rime retrieval results in abandoned syllable onsets. In other words, having retrieved the syllable onset, the speaker is left waiting for the sound segments that comprise the remainder of the syllable (i.e., the rime). The speaker presumably repeats or prolongs the syllable-initial sound until the remainder of the syllable is available for production. In this way, stuttering was modeled as a problem in making phonetic transitions.

Neuropsycholinguistic Theory

Perkins, Kent, and Curlee (1991) published a description of a neuropsycholinguistic theory. In this model, speech disfluency reflects dyssynchrony between the segmental processor, which generates the phonetic content (i.e., speech sounds) of an utterance, and the Paralinguistic-Prosodic (PP) system, which generates a timing "frame" for a spoken utterance and specifies paralinguistic parameters such as articulation rate and syllable durations. When time pressure coincides with dyssynchrony between the two systems, the speaker experiences the disfluency as "stuttering." In the model, dyssynchrony can originate with either part of the system (i.e., segments are activated, but the

PP frame is not "ready;" the PP frame is "ready," but the segments are not fully activated to allow insertion into the PP frame). Perkins et al. presented a number of other hypotheses associated with these basic claims.

Covert Repair of Phonological Errors

The Covert Repair Hypothesis (Postma & Kolk, 1993) is similar to the other psycholinguistic models of stuttering, in that the authors posit that impairment in phonological encoding is a primary source of stutter-like disfluency. Postma and Kolk presented phonological encoding within the context of Levelt's (1989) speech production model, wherein lexical selection occurs within a neural network. When a speaker attempts to access the lexical entry (i.e., lemma) associated with a specific semantic concept, the lexical entries associated with semantically similar and phonologically similar entries activate as well. This, in turn, leads to activation of the phonemes associated with those lexical items. For example, in a situation where a speaker intends to produce the semantic concept <mouse>, the semantic concepts <rat> and <gerbil> might activate as well during the selection process. In the model, activation of the latter semantic nodes spreads activation toward the lexical entries associated with <rat> and <gerbil>, as well as their associated phonemes. Selection of the target semantic concept <mouse> also leads to activation of phonologically similar words (e.g., "moose") and their associated phonemes. Consequently, the speaker must select the target phonemes associated with <mouse> from a field of other inapplicable phonemes.

The specific claim of the covert repair hypothesis is that people who stutter take longer than normal to select the phonemes that are unique to a lexical item. The slowness makes speakers who stutter prone to selecting inappropriate, off-target phonemes. In this model, the part-word repetitions and sound prolongations in stuttered speech are symptomatic of the speaker's attempts to "repair" the effects of the underlying lag in phoneme selection through either "restart" (repetition) or "postponement" (i.e., prolongation) strategies.

Multifactorial Models

The notion of multifactorial models of stuttering became increasingly attractive during the 1980s and 1990s as the limitations of key-factor theories became more and more apparent. Several authors (e.g., Smith & Kelly, 1997; Starkweather, Gottwald, & Halfond, 1990; Van Riper, 1982) offered accounts of stuttering that included multiple variables that interacted with one another.

Demands Versus Capacities

Starkweather et al. (1990) proposed a "demands-capacity" model for stuttering, in which stuttered speech was seen as the result of a mismatch between task demands and the skills and abilities that a speaker brings to the task. In this view, a speaker's abilities or performance in arenas such as motor control, language, and cognition must be sufficiently developed in order to attain fluent speech across the wide range of speaking activities that are encountered in everyday life. Stuttering-related disfluency was seen as an instance of mismatch between a speaker's "capacity" or "available resources" for speech production and the speech production demands of a particular task.

The demands-capacity model received considerable attention when it first was presented, and it provides a useful general framework for thinking about fluency performance, and in particular the relationship between one's neurophysiological functioning and the surrounding environment. Starkweather et al. (1990) identified four dimensions with potential relevance to fluency: *motoric*, *linguistic*, *emotional*, and *cognitive*. This framework leads to predictions about the communicative scenarios that might trigger stuttered speech (e.g., a child with a limited-capacity for speech motor control would be more likely to stutter when his or her parent speaks rapidly). As such, it provides a potentially helpful structure for organizing treatment activities.

References to the demands-capacity model continue to appear in contemporary literature on stuttering. Broad-based conceptualizations of "resource limitations" have been challenged, however, because of the practical difficulties associated with *quantifying* capacity and the amount of resources that a person has available at any particular moment during the production of a task (Navon, 1984). When a research participant or client performs poorly on a task, the explanation inevitably is that the task demands must have exceeded the person's capacity to perform the task. Beyond this explanation, the demands-capacity framework offers limited detail about *how* or *why* a person's capacity for the task has failed or exactly how limited capacity leads to breakdowns in speech production that result in disfluent speech. Also, research into parental interaction patterns with children who stutter has not supported the idea that parents of children who stutter routinely place inordinate communicative demands on their children (Nippold & Rudzinski, 1995). Thus, it appears that, with children who stutter, speech fluency routinely "breaks down" within the context of fairly typical communicative settings.

Dynamic, Multifactorial Model

Smith and Kelly (1997) proposed a "dynamic, multifactorial model" of stuttering, which was similar in some respects to the demands-capacity model described above. One main premise of the model is the notion that multiple factors contribute to the phenomenon of stuttering. In other words, there is not one key factor for every case or, necessarily, one constant, predominant factor within an individual during the course of a lifespan. Rather, Smith and Kelly (1997) envisioned stuttering as being dynamic in nature. Across individuals, different factors contributed in differing degrees to the disorder, and, within individuals, different factors contributed in differing degrees to the disorder at different phases of the lifespan. Another main premise is that the factors associated with stuttering interact with one another in a *nonlinear* manner. This means that the factors do not "add on" to one another in a neat, summative manner. Rather, a slight change in status of one factor can potentially lead to very large changes in the other factors with which it interacts.

Factors that Smith and Kelly (1997) identified for inclusion their model are as follows:

- Genetics—e.g., the biological context in which speech production develops and occurs;
- Emotions—e.g., the effects of emotional arousal on cognition, language, and motor performance;

- Cognition—e.g., the role of memory, information retrieval, attention, and other related cognitive functions on other aspects of functioning;
- Language—e.g., the speaker's ability to represent intentions via syntactic and lexical representations;
- Speech Motor System—e.g., the speaker's ability to articulate sequences of syllables in a stable, tightly coordinated manner; and
- Environment—e.g., the context within which the speaker lives and its impact on other factors within the model.

Smith and Kelly (1999) noted that each of these factors can be measured in multiple ways (e.g., acoustic, kinematic, electromyographic, perceptual, linguistic, psychological, and so forth). As such, Smith and Kelly's perspective on stuttering speech implied the need to look beyond the traditional method of studying "stuttered moments" within speech signals if one is to understand stuttering completely.

The Execution and Planning (EXPLAN) Model

Howell (2004, 2011) proposed the execution and planning model (EXPLAN) of stuttering. The model consists of two main components or processes. The PLAN component is involved with the generation of symbolic language representations. The EX component, in contrast, converts the language plan into an executable motor plan. Each of components is time dependent; that is, the language and motor plans take a certain amount of time to develop, and the time necessary to develop any specific plan varies with the complexity of its form and content. With regard to stuttering, Howell argued that neither component of the model is sufficient to create stuttered speech. Support for this view comes from the observation that nonstuttering individuals show some of the same motor and language deficits that speakers who stutter show, yet they do not stutter. Thus, in the EXPLAN model, stuttered speech comes about through the way in which the two components interact.

In the EXPLAN model, difficulty in language planning is defined in part at the word level by factors such as a word's stress designation (stress words are viewed as complex), phonological structure, frequency, and neighborhood density (defined as the number of similar entries that a target word has in the lexicon). Content words tend to include more of these complexity elements than function words do, and the assumption is that the more complex a word is, the longer it will take to plan. In the EXPLAN model, the motor plans that correspond to words are similarly affected; that is, complex words will result in motor plans that take longer to plan than the motor plans for simple words. Another facet of the EXPLAN model is the *disruptive rhythm hypothesis* (DRH). Disfluency (especially the types of disfluency that tend to typify stuttered speech) is viewed as instances of dyssynchrony between the language and motor components of the speech production system. Thus, if a speaker attempts to generate the motor output for a word prior to completing the planning for the word, it results in "fragmentary" types of disfluency such as part-word repetition, sound prolongation, and "broken words" (i.e., disfluencies that are characterized by a moment of interruption in mid-vowel and an initiation of the repair phase from the point of interruption). Such disfluencies essentially constitute a form of "stalling" until synchrony between the two components of the system is reestablished. Linguistically complex utterances may exacerbate the effects of any motor system deficit that a speaker exhibits. In this way, both the language system and the motor system are seen as integral to stutter-like disfluency.

With its basis in desynchronized planning, the EXPLAN model is similar in some ways to the psycholinguistic theories of stuttering that were outlined above. In contrast to those theories, which primarily are based on concepts associated with phonological planning, the EXPLAN model incorporates elements of broad-based language planning and speech motor control. As is explained elsewhere in this chapter, there is mounting evidence in support of the idea that speakers who stutter demonstrated deficits—albeit sometimes subtle ones—in various processes associated with both language planning and motor execution.

Motor-Based Models of Stuttering

A number of motor-based accounts for stuttering have been proposed during recent decades, and this perspective has received growing emphasis during the past decade in light of emerging findings about the motor system functioning of speakers who stutter. Some of the most recent "motor models" are multifactorial in the sense that the motor system is seen as interacting with other neural systems such as those involved in the processing of language, cognition, and emotion.

The idea that stuttering might be fundamentally a motor-control problem is by

no means a new one. In the early 1930s, Orton and Travis (e.g., Travis, 1931) proposed that stuttering results from asynchronous neural input to bilaterally innervated speech musculature. They proposed that the breakdown in synchronous neural input resulted from a lack of cerebral dominance that is necessary to keep neural input to the muscles properly timed. The hypothesized consequence of this lack of integrated timing was that a speech muscle on the right side of the body would receive neural input at a slightly different time than the paired muscle on the left side of the body—a situation that supposedly would lead to disfluency. Since then, a variety of motor-based explanations for stuttering have been proposed.

Stuttering and Movement Variability

Zimmermann (1980) suggested that stuttered speech is triggered by excessive variability in speech-related articulatory movements. His model for stuttering was based on previous research, some of which he conducted, that showed abnormalities in speech motor timing of perceptibly fluent speech produced by adults who stuttered (e.g., Zimmermann, 1980). In the model, he proposed that excessive variability in the velocity or spatial-temporal positioning of speech articulators could result from various sources including heightened emotional arousal. In his model, if movement variability exceeds critical thresholds, it triggers afferent nerve impulses that change the "tuning" of the brainstem reflexes that are involved in motor movement. The retuning would throw the articulatory system "off balance" by altering the typical "reflexological" interactions among the respiratory, laryngeal, and supra-laryngeal structures." This retuning was said to create instability in the motor system, which then would result in fluency breakdown, which would be manifested as either oscillatory movements (i.e., repetitions) or static posturing (i.e., sound prolongations).

Packman and colleagues (Packman, Onslow, Richard, & Van Doorn, 1996) also proposed a model for stuttering that incorporated concepts related to movement variability—the aptly titled "Vmodel." In their view, a speaker's need to realize syllable stress within multisyllable utterances is an immediate source of variability in speech motor movements. In other words, stressed syllables are longer, louder, and higher pitched than unstressed syllables, and the attainment of such syllables requires the speaker to alter temporal and spatial parameters of ongoing speech articulation movements in relation to surrounding syllables. In the Vmodel, the production of syllable stress is seen as a precipitator of speech disfluency; that is, it acts as a stressor that challenges the capabilities of an immature or impaired speech production system.

Packman et al. (1996) suggested that reduced movement variability is an underlying contributor to the fluency facilitation that occurs when speakers who stutter adopt a slow, prolonged style of speech or when they use syllable-timed speech, the pattern of speech that one exhibits when speaking in time to a metronome. They cited studies of syllable variability during both of these contexts that show a reduction in the variability of articulatory movements. Packman et al. state that the use of prosodic contrasts is an emergent feature in the development of speech during the preschool years. In other words, children must learn to create contrasts between syllables, and Packman et al. proposed that the attainment of this ability is an important developmental milestone in terms of fluency development. In the context of the Vmodel, children's repetitions are seen as a sign that speech production has been "destabilized" by the need to create a syllable that differs in its temporal properties in relation to surrounding syllables. In the Vmodel, Packman et al. stated that the repetitions that occur during disfluency provide a means of "reducing variability and stabilizing the system so that the child can move forward in speech."

Stuttering and Sensorimotor Processing

Another motor-based perspective on stuttering is centered on the ability to incorporate sensorimotor information into the motor plans that form the basis of speech-related movements. In this view, stuttering is a problem of updating movement plans with moment-to-moment information about the execution of an ongoing utterance. Such updating is needed to fine tune the minimally specified motor plans (i.e., gestural scores) to the dynamic conditions that are present during the course of an ongoing utterance. Several models of stuttering are based on hypothesized deficits in these aspects of motor planning. Neilson and Neilson (1987) viewed stuttering as a failure or weakness to utilize *adaptive feedback control*. In their model, adaptive control refers to events that establish a relationship between motor commands and the "sensorimotor motor consequences" that motor commands create, as well as the verification or modification of motor commands based on sensorimotor information.

Sensorimotor factors continue to play a prominent role in contemporary models of stuttering. For example, Max et al., 2004 presented a theoretical model for stuttering that was closely aligned with principles and concepts from the DIVA model (Guenther, 2006; Ghosh, Tourville, & Guenther, 2008). In Max et al.'s model, it is proposed that stuttered speech can result in one of two ways:

1. The speaker's internal motor models or sensory models for movement goals are either unstable (i.e. they do not remain activated for a sufficient length of time) or insufficient (i.e., they do not activate completely); or
2. The speaker relies too heavily on afferent (somatosensory) feedback, which creates instability in the speech production system due to the amount of time that it takes to incorporate the afferent feedback into the ongoing articulatory movements.

Max et al. (2004) noted that their model accounts for specific instances of stuttering-related disfluency but not necessarily for how certain people come to have the disorder. The authors offered several possible mechanisms that could lead to stuttering. For instance, they noted that abnormal levels of dopamine in the basal ganglia system could lead to problems in both motor planning and programming, along with difficulties in motor learning and sensorimotor integration. They also cited a number of studies in which speakers who stutter have been found to exhibit atypical patterns of cortical activation in brain regions that are involved with speech production, particularly those associated with motor planning and sensorimotor aspects of spoken sounds, syllables, and words.

Multifactorial Model Revisited: The Communication-Emotional (C-E) Model

Conture and colleagues (Conture et al., 2006; Richels & Conture, 2010) proposed a multifactorial model for stuttering that attempts to capture which persons are likely to stutter and, once the person is stuttering, which factors contribute to overt instances of stuttering-related disfluency. The model is organized around two main components: *distal contributors* and *proximal contributors.*

In the C-E model, the distal contributors are factors that play a role in determining which people will stutter. This part of the model consists of two factors:

- *Genetics*—a person inherits a propensity for inefficient speech-language functioning; and
- *Environment*—social, communicative, and emotional variables that can influence the expression of one's genetic predisposition for speech-language performance.

The proximal contributors to stuttering are those factors that have an immediate impact on the expression of stuttering. These include the speaker's functioning in the planning and production of speech, a speaker's life experiences, and a speaker's emotional functioning, particularly with regard to emotional reactivity and regulation.

- *Speech-language planning*—In the C-E model, speech-language planning is conceptualized as being incremental in nature. That is, utterances develop through a series of separate representations that allow for conversion of a preverbal intention into a syntactic, then morphophonologic, and then phonetic representation. This process is hypothesized to be inherently inefficient in speakers who stutter due to genetic influences on the development of the speech production system.

- *Experience*—In the C-E model, experience consists of a speaker's accumulated life experiences and with it, a history of genetic-environment interactions. Speakers who communicate in an environment that features frequent fluency stressors such as conversational interruption or requests to speak faster may develop stuttering-related behaviors that a child who was not reared in such an environment would not exhibit. In the C-E model, accumulated exposure to fluency stressors may exacerbate whatever speech-language planning problems the speaker presents.

- *Emotional contributors*—The C-E model also incorporates the notions of *emotional reactivity*, which refers to the frequency or intensity of emotional arousal, and *emotional regulation*, which refers to the act of controlling the expression of feelings and emotions and their underlying physiological substrates. In the C-E model, emotional reactivity and emotional regulation are hypothesized to influence stuttering-related disfluency.

- *Instances of stuttering*—The fourth proximal factor in the C-E model

is the occurrence of stuttering. It is hypothesized that the speaker's experiences with stuttering-related disfluency act in a "bottom-up" manner to influence a speaker's emotional functioning, interactions with other people, and speech-language planning.

Consequences: Disability and Quality of Life

In light of the many findings regarding the life experiences of people who stutter, it is not surprising to learn that, on a group level, adults who stutter report having a lower quality of life than speakers who do not stutter (Craig, Blumgart, & Tran, 2009; Yaruss & Quesal, 2006). Interestingly, Craig et al. (2009) found that stuttering affects life domains that go beyond verbal communication to include arenas such as *physical vitality, social functioning, emotional functioning,* and *mental health status*. They also found that the quality of life differences exhibited by people who stutter were similar in magnitude to those seen in people with chronic disorders such as spinal cord injury, heart disease, and diabetes. They also reported that individuals with severe stuttering were more likely to report limitations in quality of life than speakers with mild or moderate stuttering were (Craig et al., 2009).

Stuttering can have economic consequences as well (Blumgart, Tran, & Craig, 2010b). The disorder influences the occupational choices that people who stutter make (Hayhow, Cray, & Enderby, 2002), as well as the types of occupations that others deem to be suitable for people who stutter (Gabel, Blood, Tellis, & Althouse, 2004; Logan & O'Connor, 2012). Blumgart et al.

estimated the cost of stuttering-related services in Australia for adults to be about $5,500, and they found that individuals with high social anxiety tended to spend less on treatment than people with low social anxiety, possibly because of their discomfort with confronting stuttering-related issues. Clearly, the consequences of stuttering can be quite serious.

The quality of life differences in people who stutter are related, in part, to the presence of a communication disability. Although there seems to be a relationship between the severity of one's stuttering and the person's assessment of their quality of life (Craig et al., 2009), there are cases when the severity of the impairment is not clearly predictive of social and emotional consequences. Disability in people who stutter often goes beyond the surface-level interruptions in speech to include limitations and restrictions in participation. Both a person's activity limitations and participation restrictions are influenced by contextual factors, particularly the person's attitudes, beliefs, and feelings about having a communication disability and the way in which other people react or respond to the person because of the disability.

Summary

The main focus in this chapter was on the correlates of stuttering. As demonstrated in this chapter, researchers have examined stuttering from many perspectives. As scientific inquiry of stuttering progresses, researchers begin to develop an increasingly clear and detailed picture of what stuttering is. Stuttering seems to be a disorder that is rooted in genetic factors. Some people have a greater predisposition to develop the disorder than others, as evidenced by the high familial incidence of stuttering in comparison to the general population. In current models, environmental factors are thought to play a role in determining whether one's genetic predisposition to stutter will be expressed and, if so, how it will be expressed. A main focus of current research is to identify chromosomes and, eventually, genes that are associated with stuttering. Work of this nature is underway, and it has led to some initial insights into chromosomes and genes that might be relevant to the disorder.

After stuttering-related genes are reliably identified, the next step is to determine their relationship to speech-language development and speech production. It is possible that genetic factors are linked to certain neurodevelopmental differences in the speech production system that are key to stuttering. Preliminary evidence suggests that stuttered speech is associated with breakdowns in the development of white matter tracts—particularly those that connect brain regions that are involved in phonetic planning and the sensorimotor guidance of ongoing spoken utterances. An impairment of this sort might explain why speakers who stutter show patterns of anomalous (and, presumably, compensatory) neural activation in right hemisphere regions and why they have particular difficulty saying low frequency words and multisyllable words fluently. A deficit of this sort also might explain why many people who stutter experience more disfluency when engaged in dual-task activities, wherein they presumably must divert attention away from speech execution toward some other task. It also might explain some of the motoric deficits that people who stutter exhibit, particularly those that relate to the speed of response initiation, stability in speech motor movements, and the ability to learn new motor patterns. Clearly, further research is needed to examine these possibilities.

People who stutter also seem prone to deficits or disability in aspects of communication beyond speech fluency, as evidenced by findings related to syntactic, phonologic, and semantic processing. Surprisingly, language-related differences have been noted in people who stutter for both receptive and expressive language activities. In studies of school-based speech-language pathology caseloads, children who stutter are routinely found to present concomitant language and/or articulation difficulties. The association, if any, between these seemingly "peripheral" communication problems and the etiology and expression of stuttering is unclear at present.

Beyond its impact on speech fluency, chronic stuttering can affect the attitudes, feelings, and beliefs that a speaker has toward communication and, more broadly, his or her overall identity. Several studies have reported evidence of elevated anxiety among people who stutter, particularly with regard to speech-related tasks and social interactions. The general consensus is that "negative" emotions like these

are an emergent aspect of the disorder. Fortunately, speech-related anxiety seems amenable to change through effective speech therapy. Still, stuttering can have significant negative consequences on an individual's quality of life, and it can interfere with social interactions with friends, teachers, and employers. Indeed, research evidence suggests that the deleterious effects of stuttering can persist across the lifespan and influence the most basic activities of daily life, including when, how often, and how much one communicates, as well as the type of occupation that one chooses to pursue.

Based on this review, it should be apparent that stuttering is much more than simply a case of a person being "nervous" or "tense" while communicating. There is a physical basis for stuttering, and as the physical nature of the disorder becomes better understood, it should lead to the development of increasingly effective treatments. In the meantime, it is important to remember that many people who stutter possess resources to learn strategies for coping with and compensating for fluency impairment in ways that substantially reduce stuttering-related disability. The latter topic is explored in the following chapters.

7

Nondevelopmental Forms of Stuttering

The fluency patterns discussed in this chapter differ from those seen in the developmental form of stuttering that is familiar to most people. One main area of difference between the two types of stuttering concerns the conditions that are present at the time the symptoms of fluency impairment first become apparent in speech. That is, with nondevelopmental stuttering, the onset of symptom expression often can be confidently linked to some specific, precipitating event such as traumatic brain injury that adversely affects central nervous system functioning. This is unlike developmental stuttering, wherein the initial signs of fluency impairment occur during childhood, in the absence of any obvious injury or illness.

Another point of difference between developmental and nondevelopmental forms of stuttering concerns the individual's history as a fluent speaker. The individual who presents with a nondevelopmental form of stuttering typically has a well-established history as a "normally

fluent speaker" up until the time when the onset of stuttered speech occurs. In contrast, the individual who presents with developmental stuttering usually will have yet to establish a substantial history of speaking fluently at the time when onset of stuttered speech occurs. This is because he or she still is in the midst of developing the neural system that allows for fluent speech.

The purpose of this chapter is to review the basic features of nondevelopmental forms of stuttering. The chapter includes overviews of the following topics: (a) the suspected etiologies for nondevelopmental stuttering, (b) subtypes of nondevelopmental stuttering, (c) the speech characteristics that are associated with nondevelopmental forms of stuttering, particularly those forms that occur secondary to neurological trauma or disease, (d) the impact of concomitant disorders on speech fluency, and (e) similarities and differences that exist between developmental and nondevelopmental forms of stuttering. Issues concerning the assessment and treatment of nondevelopmental stuttering are addressed in later chapters in the text.

Developmental Versus Nondevelopmental Stuttering

Having outlined a few of the basic differences between developmental and nondevelopmental forms of stuttering in the introduction above, the distinctions between these types of stuttering are explored in greater detail within the present section.

Basic Features of Developmental Stuttering

Most cases of stuttering are developmental in nature. This means that the initial signs of fluency impairment emerge during childhood, at a time when the speech production system still is maturing. As discussed in previous chapters, developmental stuttering is characterized by excessive production of disfluency, particularly disfluency types that lead to part-word repetition, audible sound prolongation, and "blocks" in which the speaker assumes the articulatory posture for a speech sound but seemingly is unable to move through that sound and into the next speech sound. Other types of repetitions (e.g., word repetitions, multiword/phrase repetitions) often occur excessively as well; however, in most cases, the latter types of disfluency tend to occur less often than the part-word repetitions, prolongations, and blocks.

Historically, the factors that cause developmental stuttering have been poorly understood. To the caregivers of a child with developmental stuttering, the child's fluency difficulties seem to "come out of nowhere." That is, usually there are not any obvious injuries, illnesses, or diseases that a caregiver or clinician can name confidently as the precipitator of speech disfluency, nor is there typically any clear evidence of environmental factors that have harmed the child's fluency. Researchers' understanding of the factors that cause developmental stuttering has advanced markedly in recent decades, however. During this time, consensus has grown for a model that depicts stuttering as a heritable disorder and the disfluencies that characterize the disorder as symptoms of an impaired, weak, or immature speech production system. As outlined in Chapter 6, a host of relatively recent studies of genetic, neurophysiological, psycholinguistic, and motor variables support this view (e.g., Anderson & Conture, 2004; Brown, Ingham, Ingham, Laird, & Fox, 2005; Chang, Erickson, Ambrose, Hasegawa-Johnson, & Ludlow, 2008; Max & Baldwin, 2010; Smith, Goffman, Sasisekaran, & Weber-Fox, 2012). Speakers with developmental stuttering tend to exhibit an assortment of structural and functional differences that affect cortical and subcortical regions of the central nervous system that are involved in speech-language production. As noted in Chapter 6, in several studies, researchers have discovered evidence of anomalies in white matter tracts that connect regions of the nervous system that are integral to speech-language formulation and production. The presence of these anomalies suggests that the speech fluency problems observed in developmental stuttering are a predictable consequence of using an underdeveloped or abnormally developed neural system when speaking.

Basic Features of Nondevelopmental Stuttering

As noted in the introduction, with nondevelopmental forms of stuttering, the onset of fluency impairment can be reliably linked to the occurrence of a precipitating event that adversely affects the functioning of the speech production system. Thus, to the casual observer, the client's fluency difficulties do not seem to "appear out of nowhere" as they do with developmental stuttering. Instead, they can be linked in time to events such as stroke or traumatic brain injury that are known to alter the functioning of the speech production system.

The State of Research on Nondevelopmental Stuttering

Before discussing nondevelopmental forms of stuttering further, it is important to briefly discuss the state of the research literature in this area. Although medical and social science databases contain many published reports that deal with nondevelopmental stuttering, much of what is published consists of case reports. Although case-based reports have value in any research literature, the limitations associated with the research approach (e.g., small sample size, lack of experimental controls) are well known, and it generally is agreed that case reports should not be the primary source of evidence for any disorder. The reliance on case studies in this literature is, in part, a reflection of the fact that nondevelopmental stuttering is not very common in the general population and, in part, a reflection of the heterogeneity that exists among speakers with nondevelopmental forms of stuttering (Jokel, De Nil, & Sharpe, 2007; Theys, van Wieringen, Sunaert, Thijs, & De Nil, 2011). Variables that contribute to participant heterogeneity in this population include age, general health status, the presence and nature of co-occurring disorders and diseases, past medical history, and use of medications.

There are, however, several group-level descriptive studies of individuals with nondevelopmental stuttering (e.g., Aram, Meyers, & Ekelman, 1990; Ludlow, Rosenberg, Salazar, Grafman, & Smutok, 1987) and a handful of survey studies (e.g., Market, Montague, Jr., Buffalo, & Drummond, 1990; Theys, van Wieringen, & De Nil, 2008) that yield population-level perspectives on this type of fluency disorder. Encouragingly, in recent years, at least one research team (i.e., Theys et al., 2011) has utilized a prospective group design to collect much-needed information on the frequency with which stuttering develops following stroke. Another positive feature of the research literature on nondevelopmental stuttering is the relatively high degree of consistency in the fluency measures that are reported. That is, many researchers provide information about stuttering frequency, common and uncommon disfluency types, the location of stuttering-related disfluency within sentences, the extent to which content words and function words are stuttered, the extent to which stuttering frequency or severity varies across speaking tasks, speaking partners, and physical settings, the extent to which secondary (e.g., adaptive, reactive, compensatory) behaviors are present, and the extent to which the speaker shows acknowledgement of and/or emotional reactions to the stuttered speech. In some studies, researchers also report on the effect that repeated practice has on performance (i.e., adaptation). As data accumulate for these variables, they should provide researchers and clinicians with a better sense of which variables are most important to measure when documenting fluency performance in speakers with acquired forms of stuttering.

Terminology and Subtypes

Authors have used a wide range of terms to describe stuttered speech that results from processes other than those associated with ordinary development (De Nil, Jokel, & Rochon, 2007). In a general sense, nondevelopmental stuttering is an *acquired* impairment. Indeed, many authors use the term *acquired stuttering* as a general descriptor for individuals who have established a mature speech production system and a long-standing history of speaking fluently but then begin to stutter after a life event that adversely affects neural functioning (e.g., traumatic brain injury, neurodegenerative disease, use of drugs that affect the actions or availability of neurotransmitters). Although we will use the terms *acquired stuttering* and *nondevelopmental stuttering* interchangeably in the remainder of the chapter, we prefer the latter term because it offers a direct contrast with the term for the other main category of stuttering, i.e., developmental stuttering.

Another widely used term in this literature is *neurogenic stuttering*. This diagnostic label customarily is applied in cases where there is clear evidence of acquired brain injury near the time of stuttering onset. Although stuttering that arises under such conditions is certainly neurogenic in nature, research data suggest that the speech fluency problems associated with developmental stuttering are neurogenic as well. Thus, while there is general recognition among contemporary clinicians that the term *neurogenic stuttering* applies to cases *of fluency impairment that result from acquired neurological disfunction*, the term *neurogenic stuttering* is, itself, a somewhat imprecise label when it comes to differentiating between developmental and nondevelopmental forms of stuttering. Rosenbek (1984) made a similar point when he suggested that speech fluency professionals should declare a moratorium on the use of the term neurogenic stuttering because it is, at once, too specific and too vague. That is, the term implies that researchers and clinicians know the intricate neural mechanisms that lead to stutter-like disfluency, and, at the same time, it is too vague because disfluency that is associated with language-based disorders such as aphasia is neurogenic as well. We can go even further to say that all disfluency—even that produced by normally functioning speakers—is neurogenic. Although researchers and clinicians undoubtedly will continue to use the term *neurogenic stuttering* for the foreseeable future, it is important that newcomers to clinical practice fully grasp the limitations associated with the current usage of the term.

De Nil et al. (2007) noted that (acquired) neurogenic stuttering typically is contrasted with *psychogenic stuttering* in the fluency disorders literature, with the latter term usually referring to cases of adult-onset stuttering that occur in the absence of measurable neurological disfunction. De Nil et al. cautioned, however, that the occurrence of acquired stuttering in the absence of obvious neurological impairment does not necessarily mean that there is no neurological impairment. They supported this caution with a reference to a case study by Lebrun, Retif, and Kaiser (1983) wherein adult onset stuttering was the *first symptom* of what eventually was diagnosed as motor neuron disease.

Another potential pitfall that comes with making a distinction between psychogenic and neurogenic stuttering is that it can leave the impression that psychological states and psychiatric disorders are somehow "not neurological" or that they lack a physical basis. As anyone who is involved in the field of neuropsychology will say, this is inaccurate. Thus, there seems to be a need for reframing the terminology that is used to describe nondevelopmental forms so that "neurogenic" is not directly contrasted with "psychogenic." One simple approach would be to use terms that emphasize the fact that the stuttering is *acquired* (i.e., nondevelopmental) and then to indicate the conditions under which it is acquired. In the case of psychogenic stuttering, this approach would lead to a term such as *acquired stuttering following mental illness.* That latter term then could be contrasted with terms such as *acquired stuttering following traumatic brain injury, acquired stuttering following stroke,* or *acquired stuttering following neurodegenerative disease.* This approach allows for the possibility that neurological functioning is relevant to a client's disfluent speech in each of the scenarios.

Disfluency Characteristics

In most published accounts of nondevelopmental stuttering, the authors examine the extent to which the speaker's disfluency patterns are similar to those seen in cases of developmental stuttering. In some early reports (e.g., Canter, 1971), it was stated that the speech characteristics of speakers with nondevelopmental

forms of stuttering are markedly different from those observed in developmental stuttering. In many subsequent reports, however, researchers have noted many similarities between the two types of stuttering (De Nil et al., 2007; Helm, Butler, & Canter, 1980; Lebrun, Leleux, Rousseau, & Devreux, 1983; Rosenbek, Messert, Collins, & Wertz, 1978). In terms of the *types of disfluency* that are produced, it seems that the two forms of stuttering are similar. That is, as with developmental stuttering, speakers with nondevelopmental forms of stuttering typically exhibit excessive production of part-word repetitions, sound prolongations, and "blocks" in speech continuity.

Jokel et al. (2007) conducted a detailed analysis of the frequency with which "less typical" (i.e., stutter-like) and "more typical" (i.e., nonstutter-like) disfluencies occurred in the speech of six adults with acquired stuttering following traumatic brain injury and six adults with acquired stuttering following stroke. They found a mix of both categories of disfluency for both speaker subtypes. With the stroke group, the proportion of more typical disfluencies was somewhat greater than that for less typical disfluencies; however, with the traumatic brain injury group, the opposite pattern was observed: a greater proportion of less typical disfluency. The relative proportion of both categories of disfluency varied across group, depending on the nature of the speaking task. Also, the participants with traumatic brain injury had a greater frequency of total disfluency during conversation than participants with stroke did. In several case studies (Burch, Kiernan, & Demaerschalk, 2013; Tani & Sakai, 2010), however, some speakers appear to produce only stutter-like disfluency. Thus, as with other aspects of fluency, symptom presentation may vary across cases. Clinicians also should be mindful of the possibility of other types of fluency problems among patients with neurologic disease. For example, patients with various types of non-Alzheimer's dementia may exhibit deficits on language-based tests of semantic and phonemic fluency (see, for a review, Reilly, Rodriguez, Lamy, & Neils-Strunjas, 2010).

Listener Perceptions

Relatively little is known about the extent to which listeners can differentiate the speech fluency patterns associated with developmental and nondevelopmental forms of stuttering. In one study (Van Borsel & Taillieu, 2001), researchers asked experienced speech-language pathologists to evaluate samples of speech that had been produced by adults with developmental stuttering and adults with nondevelopmental stuttering. The clinicians were not easily able to differentiate the two types of speakers. The clinicians demonstrated 100% accuracy at categorizing the speech samples from only one of four speakers with nondevelopmental stuttering and only two of four speakers with developmental stuttering. Although the clinicians' judgments for most of the other speakers tended toward the correct diagnostic classification, the clinicians did not make clear, categorical distinctions between two types of speech samples. Thus, it appears that the disfluency patterns associated with developmental and nondevelopmental stuttering sometimes do sound quite similar. Still, as explained later in this chapter, there are many documented cases in which the disfluency patterns of speakers with nondevelopmental forms of stuttering are significantly different from those of speakers with devel-

opmental stuttering in terms of structure or severity.

The differences between the two speaker groups perhaps are more likely to be apparent when a listener hears the person speak on multiple occasions. For example, the fluency performance of brain-injured speakers may be more variable than that of speakers with developmental stuttering (Aram et al., 1990; Helm-Estabrooks, 1986; Meyers, Hall, & Aram, 1990), and in some cases, the frequency of speech disfluency is much greater than what is typical in speakers with developmental stuttering (Van Borsel, Van Lierde, Van Cauwenberge, Guldemont, & Van Orshoven, 1998). Speakers with nondevelopmental forms of stuttering also are less likely to benefit from repeated speaking practice and access to choral speech models than speakers with developmental stuttering are (Balasubramanian, Max, Van Borsel, Rayca, & Richardson, 2003; Market et al., 1990; Tani & Sakai, 2011; Theys, et al., 2008; Turget, Utku, & Balci, 2002). The listeners' ability to differentiate developmental and nondevelopmental forms of stuttering under such conditions warrants investigation.

Epidemiological Data

Epidemiological data for nondevelopmental stuttering are limited. Data on its occurrence in males versus females, at various points of the lifespan, and in conjunction with specific neuropathologies are discussed here.

Male-to-Female Ratio

Consistent with data for developmental stuttering, there is general agreement that nondevelopmental stuttering is more likely to occur in males than in females. Developmental stuttering affects males roughly three times as often as it affects females (Bloodstein & Bernstein Ratner, 2008). Overall, the male-to-female ratio for nondevelopmental stuttering appears to be similar to that for developmental stuttering. Clinicians' responses to surveys about patients with nondevelopmental stuttering have yielded male-to-female ratios that range from 2.23:1 to 3.76:1 (Market et al., 1990; Theys van Wierignen, & De Nil, 2008). Market et al. (1990) suggested that males may be more susceptible than females to experiencing nondevelopmental stuttering because they are more likely to engage in behavior that can cause brain injury.

Theys et al. (2008) reported male-to-female ratios according to the nature of the participants' neuropathology. Males were far more likely than females to acquire stuttering in conjunction with both traumatic brain injury (ratio = 10:1) and neurodegenerative disease (ratio = 8:1). The male-to-female ratio for nondevelopmental stuttering following stroke was smaller but still skewed toward males (ratio = 1.9:1). Females were more likely than males to acquire stuttering in conjunction with other sources of neurological disfunction such as epilepsy, encephalitis, and use of medication (ratio = 2:1). The sample sizes for all but the stroke subgroup ranged from 9 to 11 participants; thus, these data on male-to-female ratios should be considered preliminary.

Age Characteristics

On average, nondevelopmental stuttering appears to occur in middle-aged and older adults much more often than it does in children, teens, and young adults. Market et al. (1990) reported a mean age of 43.7 years (median = 43 years; range = 36 to 93 years) for their sample of 58 adults. In contrast, Theys et al. (2008) reported a mean age of 69 years (range = 16 to 86 years) for their sample of 81 adults with acquired neurogenic stuttering. That said, there are several published reports of young children who have acquired stuttering following neurological injury (e.g., Aram et al., 1990; Meyers et al., 1990). The distributional patterns of nondevelopmental stuttering across the lifespan are undoubtedly influenced by the fact that older adults have a greater risk than young adults to experience the kinds of neurological events (e.g., stroke, neurodegenerative disease) that precipitate nondevelopmental stuttering.

Theys et al. (2008) reported the mean ages for various participant subgroups within their report on survey data from 58 adults with acquired neurogenic stuttering. The mean age of people with stroke-related acquired stuttering was 69 years, and for acquired stuttering following neurodegenerative disease, the mean age was 72 years. In contrast, the mean age for people with stuttering following traumatic brain injury was 46 years. The age characteristics of the traumatic brain injury group are most likely a reflection of the fact that younger people typically are more active than older people and thus more likely to be in situations where traumatic brain injury (and, with it, acquired stuttering) can result.

Incidence and Prevalence

To date, relatively little known is about the extent to which individuals with brain injury or neurodegenerative diseases are at risk for acquiring stuttering. In one recent report (i.e., Theys et al., 2011), researchers tracked 319 adult stroke patients to see how many of them subsequently began to stutter. Of the total, 5.3% met criteria for a diagnosis of (acquired) neurogenic stuttering during the course of the study and 2.3% of the total exhibited symptoms of stuttering for at least six months. Thus, it appears that approximately 40% of the cases exhibited persistent forms of acquired stuttering. Individuals who developed aphasia following stroke were at a greater risk for acquiring stuttering than individuals who did not develop aphasia. In contrast, neither dysarthria nor cognitive impairment following stroke was associated with an increased risk for acquiring stuttering. Theys et al. (2011) cited data indicating that 17% to 35% of people who experience stroke will develop aphasia. Thus, overall, it seems that the acquisition of stuttered speech following stroke is not a common outcome. Based on results from their large-scale survey of clinicians' experiences with acquired stuttering, Theys et al. (2008) estimated that about 27% of the clinicians they had contacted about the study had provided clinical services to at least one patient with acquired stuttering during the five years preceding the study.

Although the presence of aphasia may increase the risk for acquiring stuttering, it is not uncommon for acquired stuttering to occur in the absence of other communication or cognitive disorders (Ardila & Lopez, 1986; Bhatnager & Andy, 1989; Lebrun et al., 1983; Ludlow et al., 1987). Ludlow et al. (1987) found that the severity of brain-injured patients' aphasia was not useful in predicting the stuttering severity. In addition, Meyers et al. (1990) found that speech disfluencies did not parallel the course of word-finding difficulties in a 7-year-old boy with a history of stroke, and they concluded that the two disorders were independent. Theys et al. (2008) did, however, report a significant positive correlation between the number of concomitant disorders a person had and the frequency with which he or she stuttered. Thus, the additive effects of concomitant disorders may be an important factor to consider in clinical settings. Finally, several of the participants in studies of acquired stuttering have had a history of childhood stuttering followed by recovery and, with it, several decades of ostensibly normal speech fluency, and then onset of stuttering in adulthood following neurological trauma. In such cases, it is unclear whether the stuttering that appears during adulthood represents a resurgence of the person's childhood stuttering or, instead, whether it is an independent occurrence. In many cases, the speech behaviors of the adult stuttering are unlike those that the person exhibited during childhood, which would suggest that the fluency problems are unrelated (Theys et al., 2008). Further research is needed to determine whether this is the case.

Neuropathology and Disfluency

Onset of Stuttered Speech

Several researchers have reported data on when the onset of acquired stuttering occurred in relation to the time of neurological insult. Market et al. (1990) reported survey results on 57 people with acquired stuttering. In 81% of the cases, stuttering onset began within one month of the neurological event, and in 93% of the cases, stuttering onset began within three months. Theys et al. (2008) reported similar data in their survey study. In the latter study, 69% of participants began to stutter within one week of experiencing a stroke, and in 73% of those cases, the onset was sudden. In some cases, onset of stuttering has reportedly occurred within the context of recovery from a coma (e.g., Abe, Yokoyama, & Yorifuji, 1993; Van Borsel et al., 1998) or stroke (Ardila & Lopez, 1986; Grant, Biousse, Cook, & Newman, 1999; Meyers et al., 1990).

Neuropathologies Associated With Nondevelopmental Stuttering

Nondevelopmental stuttering has been observed in conjunction with an assortment of neurologic conditions, including the following:

- *Left hemisphere lesions* following stroke or head trauma (Grant et al.,1999; Osawa, Maeshima, & Yoshimora, 2006; Rosenbek et al., 1978; Turget et al., 2002; Van Borsel et al., 1998);
- *Right hemisphere lesions* following stroke or head trauma (e.g., Ardila & Lopez, 1986; Balasubramanian et al., 2003; Burch et al., 2013; Lebrun & Leleux, 1985; Rosenbek et al., 1978);
- *Diffuse cortical damage* following stroke or head trauma (e.g., Aram et al., 1990; Ludlow et al., 1987; Rosenbek et al., 1978);
- *Lesions that impact white matter tracts* at cortical and subcortical levels (e.g., Burch et al., 2013; Ludlow et al., 1987);
- *Basal ganglia, thalamus, and brain-stem lesions* (Abe et al., 1993; Balasubramanian et al., 2003; Bhatnager & Andy, 1989; Tani & Sakai, 2011);

- *Cerebellar lesions* (Ludlow et al., 1987; Theys, van Wieringen, Tuyls, & De Nil, 2009); and
- *Neurodegenerative disease* (Lebrun et al., 1983; Louis, Winfield, Fahn, & Ford, 2001; Silbergleit, Feit, & Silbergleit, 2009).

As shown in the list above, stuttered speech, at least in its nondevelopmental form, has been linked to neurological damage in the left and right hemispheres, assorted white matter tracts, the cerebellum, basal ganglia, thalamus, and various brainstem regions. Case-based reports such as those cited above offer insight into the breadth of suspected etiologies that are associated with acquired forms of stuttering. However, given the possibility that only the most severe or unusual cases are submitted for publication, the case reports do not necessarily provide a sense for the extent to which any particular neurological condition is likely to be associated with the acquisition of stuttering, nor do they provide a sense for what sorts of fluency problems most speakers with acquired stuttering will present.

Survey studies offer a potential solution to this problem. With a survey study, researchers potentially can compile information about many cases of nondevelopmental stuttering and subsequently obtain a more accurate sense of the characteristics of the clinical population. In this chapter, results are reviewed from two relatively large-scale survey studies dealing with neurologically based forms of acquired stuttering. Market et al. (1990) contacted more than 100 speech-language pathologists in the United States, which resulted in data for 81 cases of acquired (nondevelopmental) stuttering. More recently, Theys et al. (2008) contacted more than 200 clinical sites in northern Belgium, which resulted in data for 58 adults who had acquired stuttering in the context of neurological injury or disease. In both of the surveys, the researchers inquired about the medical histories, speech-language characteristics, social and emotional characteristics, and treatment experiences of the individuals who stutter. A comparison of findings from the two studies with regard to the suspected etiologies for the acquired stuttering is presented in Figure 7–1. As shown, in both studies, acquired forms of stuttered speech were most commonly associated with either stroke or traumatic brain injury. Although the proportion of stuttering cases associated with the two conditions differed between the two studies, it is clear that, together, these conditions were much more likely to be associated with acquired stuttering than other neurological events were.

The relatively wide range of neuropathologies associated with acquired stuttering shows that the disorder cannot be readily localized to any one region of the central nervous system. For instance, in studies that have documented left hemisphere lesions in conjunction with acquired stuttering, lesion sites have included the temporal lobe, the parietal lobe, the inferior frontal lobe, and the supplementary motor area (Grant et al., 1999; Osawa et al., 2006; Rosenbek et al., 1978; Turget et al., 2002; Van Borsel et al., 1998). Grant et al. (1999) reported on a case of acquired stuttering in conjunction with a left occipital lobe infarction and concomitant right homonymous hemianopia. In this case, the role of the infarction in stuttered speech is unclear, as the occipital lobe typically is not implicated in speech fluency impairments.

In their survey study of neurogenic stuttering, Theys et al. (2008) found that, among 29 adults who began to stutter

following stroke, 17 had left hemisphere lesions, five had right hemisphere lesions, and five had bilateral cortical lesions (data were not available for the remaining two individuals). Among 11 adults who began to stutter following traumatic brain injury, four (36% of the total) had bilateral cortical lesions, and two had no detectable lesions. The findings from research on normal speakers and speakers with nondevelopmental forms of stuttering suggest that many neural areas are critical to the attainment of fluent speech. Speech production, even during seemingly simple tasks like CV syllable production, entails an extensive network of neural activation (Ghosh, Tourville, & Guenther, 2008). To the extent that this is true, speech fluency then can be conceived of as an index of the overall functioning of this neural network.

As noted, the brain injuries that follow stoke and head trauma often are diffuse, and this complicates researchers' attempts to identify specific nervous system regions that are critical to the occurrence of stuttered speech. The study of relatively focal lesions therefore is a potentially fruitful approach for gaining insight into the neural basis for stuttered speech. Ludlow et al. (1987) conducted a study in which they examined 10 adults who had received relatively discrete penetrating missile wounds during the Vietnam War. Each of the participants exhibited acquired stuttering and concomitant rate disturbance, which was characterized as consisting of "intermittent and unpredictable bursts of rapid and unintelligible speech." The participants' speech continuity was characterized by excessive production of repetitions and prolongations and "long silences without struggle." Statistical analysis of neuroimaging data showed that the participants who stuttered differed from a fluent control group and a nonstuttering head-injury

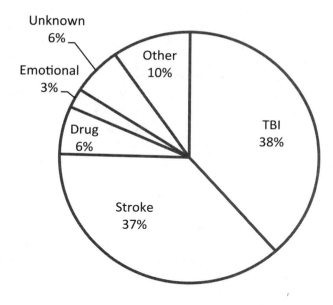

Market et al. (1990); *N* = 81

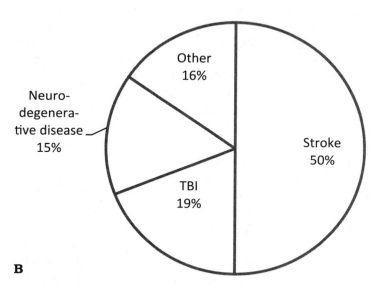

Theys et al. (2008); *N* = 58

Figure 7–1. A comparison of frequency-of-occurrence data from two survey studies that examined suspected etiologies associated with the onset of acquired (nondevelopmental) stuttering in adults. Findings from Market et al. (1990) (**A**) and Theys et al. (2008) (**B**) suggest that most cases of acquired stuttering occur in the context of stroke or traumatic brain injury. A range of other neurological events are associated with the remaining cases.

group on the extent of lesion involvement in the internal and external capsules, low frontal lobe white matter tracts, and the caudate and lentiform nuclei. Most of the participants with acquired stuttering had unilateral lesions that affected one or more of these areas. In five cases, the lesions were right lateralized, in four cases, they were left lateralized, and in one case, they were bilateral. Interestingly, the group with acquired stuttering and the group with head injury but no stuttering showed no differences in the frequency of presented lesions in Broca's area, the supplementary motor area, or the primary motor area—each of which has been linked to developmental stuttering in other research. Based on their findings, Ludlow et al. (1987) suggested that the motor system plays an important role in a speaker's ability to attain and maintain normal levels of speech fluency.

Several authors have documented nondevelopmental forms of stuttering that result from the use of certain drugs (Rentschler, Driver, & Callaway, 1984). This has led to the use of terms such as *pharmacogenic stuttering* and *drug-induced stuttering*. McClean and McLean, Jr. (1985) reported on a case of adult-onset stuttering in association with a drug-based treatment for seizures that occurred following a head injury. The patient's seizures developed about three months post injury, at which point the drug phenytoin was introduced to manage the seizures. At the initial speech evaluation, which took place several months after the introduction of phenytoin, the patient exhibited frequent disfluencies (about 20 to 30 per 100 syllables), most of which consisted of part-word repetitions. At this time, the patient showed symptoms of phenytoin toxicity, and consequently, he gradually was shifted to an alternate anti-seizure medication, carbamazepine. McClean and McLean, Jr. monitored the patient's speech fluency across roughly a one-month period during which the change in medications occurred. During this time, the patient's fluency improved markedly, as shown by a decrease in stuttering frequency from about 25% syllables stuttered while taking phenytoin to about 12% syllables stuttered while taking carbamazepine. Use of carbamazepine was associated with an increase in the proportion of sound prolongation in the patient's overall disfluency profile, however. Similarly, Makela, Sullivan, and Taylor (1994) reported a case of stuttering onset in an adult upon introduction of sertraline to treat work-related anxiety. The patient's stutter-like speech featured excessive silent blocks in speech, each of which lasted from 1 to 3 seconds. The patient's disfluent speech pattern resolved completely within two days after use of sertraline was discontinued. Case reports like this suggest a link between emotions, neurotransmitters, and speech fluency. Several researchers have explored the potential association between stuttered speech and the neurotransmitter dopamine. The latter topic is discussed further in Chapter 14, under the heading of drug-based treatments for stuttering.

Neuropathology and Disfluency Profiles

It is reasonable to consider whether the behavioral symptoms of acquired stuttering might differ according to the nature of the underlying neuropathology. Many of the published reports on acquired stuttering have examined this issue, and results from several such studies are summarized in Table 7–1. Findings from these and other studies are compared in the subsections below.

Table 7–1. Neurological, Speech Fluency, and Concomitant Disorder Characteristics of Adults With Nondevelopmental Stuttering

Study	Participant(s)	Neuropathology	Stuttered Disfluency		Concomitant Problems
			Frequency/Distribution	Types	
Rosenbek et al. (1978)	7 adult males	5 w/ LH stroke, 1 w/ RH stroke, 1 w/ diffuse stroke.	8% to 70% of words stuttered; mostly word initial, but 6/7 stutter on noninitial syllables.	Part-word repetition most common for 6/7 cases; 6/7 cases exhibit prolongations.	1 w/ none, 3 w/ aphasia, 1 w/ aphasia + apraxia, 1 w/ language disorder & dysarthria, 1 w/ suspected language & intellectual impairment.
Ardila & Lopez (1986)	Adult male	Right temporal lobe infarct following stroke.	Stuttering increased as a function of task demands (e.g., 37% of words during counting, 52% of words in conversation).	Sound and syllable repetition most common, word repetition noted but less frequent; repetition in all word positions.	Normal language functioning. Severe loss of verbal automatisms (songs, poems); dress apraxia, déjà vu phenomena, depersonalization, episodic amnesia.
Abe et al. (1993)	Adult male	Infarcts in the paramedian thalami and mid-brain; 3 months post coma.	58% of syllables stuttered in spontaneous speech, 28% in naming, 9% in reading, 5% in sentence repetition.	Syllable repetition (no word or phrase repetition).	Mild disorientation, memory impairment (recent memory, visual memory).
Van Borsel et al. (1998)	Adult male	Stroke affecting LH SMA, subarachnoid bleeding above corpus callosum, in coma for ~3 days.	100% syllables stuttered in all tasks except reading, where 70% to 82% of syllables were stuttered. Disfluency impairs speech intelligibility.	Mainly sound or part-word repetitions, occasional prolongations. No other disfluency types.	Mild comprehension deficits for abstract content and in reading; mild word finding difficulty. Stuttering onset occurred about 2 months post stroke.
Balasubra-manian et al. (2003)	Adult male	Pons, orbital surface of RH frontal lobe.	~5% syllables stuttered in solo and unison reading; ~6% to 8% under AAF.	Part-word repetitions, prolongations (ratio not reported).	History of childhood stuttering with subsequent recovery for several decades.

Note: RH = right hemisphere, *LH* = left hemisphere, *SMA* = supplementary motor area, *AAF* = altered auditory feedback, *w/* = with.

275

Disfluency Frequency and Type

As shown in Table 7–1, stuttering frequency varies widely across study participants. In some studies, adults with acquired stuttering exhibited stuttering frequency scores that are consistent with mild severity in cases of developmental stuttering. Sometimes, the fluency deviations are even subtler. For example, in a recent study of children with localization-related epilepsy (Steinberg, Bernstein Ratner, Gaillard, & Berl, 2013), the children with epilepsy displayed a higher overall frequency of disfluency and a higher proportion of sound prolongations than the typically fluent children did. The mean frequencies of total disfluency for both groups were not exceptionally high (epilepsy group: 6.0 per 100 words; control group: 4.6 per 100 words) but still of statistical significance. The difference between the groups in the frequency of stutter-like disfluency approached statistical significance as well.

In other studies, the participants exhibited frequency scores that correspond with profound impairment. The patient in the study by Van Borsel et al. (1998) reportedly produced stutter-like repetitions on 100% of the syllables during all speaking tasks except reading. This means that each syllable the speaker initiated, even those in the word-medial and word-final positions of multisyllable words featured repetition (e.g., the word *tricycle* would have been produced as follows: |tr- tr-|tri |cy- cy-|cy |c- c-|cle). The participant in the study by Abe et al. (1993) also showed very high stuttering frequency scores during both conversational discourse (>50% syllables stuttered) and picture naming (>25% syllables stuttered). Theys et al. (2008) also reported considerable intersubject variability across the 58 participants in their study.

For participants with a history of stroke and traumatic brain injury, stuttering frequency ranged from 3% to 50% of syllables, and for participants with a history of neurodegenerative disease, the stuttering frequency extended beyond 50% of syllables.

Repetitions of sounds, syllables, and parts of words seem to be the predominate type of disfluency noted in many of the studies of acquired stuttering. This is true of the studies outlined in Table 7–1 and also of a host of other studies as well (e.g., Grant et al., 1999; Meyers et al., 1990; Lebrun et al., 1983; Osawa et al., 2006; Silbergleit et al., 2009). Because repetitions are observed in cases with widely varying areas of neurological impairment, they do not appear to arise from a particular lesion type or location. Speakers with acquired stuttering seem to produce sound prolongations less often than part-word repetitions (Aram et al., 1990; Ardila & Lopez, 1986; McClean & McLean, Jr., 1985; Meyers et al., 1990; Theys et al., 2008). In some reports (Cipolotti, Bisiacchi, Denes, & Gallo, 1988; Marshall & Neuburger, 1987), prolongations were not observed at all. Aram et al. (1990) compared the fluency characteristics of 20 children with unilateral left hemisphere lesions and 13 children with unilateral right hemisphere lesions and found that both groups of children produced more total disfluency and more sound prolongations than normally fluent controls. Children with left hemisphere lesions exhibited more effortful speech production, as well. Further research into the types of disfluency that accompany specific patterns of brain injury or dysfunction is needed before any firm conclusions can be drawn with regard to the effect, if any, of lesion site on disfluency profiles. It is interesting to consider whether the structural form of a disfluency correlates with certain types of neuropathology.

In cases of nondevelopmental stuttering, the production of stutter-like disfluency appears to be independent of the so-called "normal" types of disfluency such as interjection and revision. Meyers et al. (1990) reported on a 7-year-old boy who began to stutter following a cerebrovascular accident that affected a diffuse region of the left hemisphere along with portions of the putamen, caudate nucleus, globus pallidus, and internal capsule. Meyers et al. had access to recorded samples of the boy's speech prior to the brain injury and thus could compute pre- and post-morbid frequencies for various disfluency types. They found that the frequency of the boy's stutter-like disfluencies increased dramatically following the stroke; however, the frequency of interjections and revisions remained almost constant. This pattern is consistent with data from several other studies reviewed in this chapter in which data for interjections and revisions are reported. In several studies, those disfluency types constitute a minority of all disfluencies that the speakers produced and, in some cases, interjections and revisions were not produced at all. Of course, not all cases follow this main pattern. For example, Marshall and Neuburger (1987) reported on a person with acquired stuttering following traumatic brain injury. The participant presented frequent whole-word and phrase repetitions, as well as prominent interjections and repetitions of sounds and syllables. As noted earlier, Jokel et al. (2007) reported frequent production of nonstutter-like disfluency such as revision and interjection in adults who acquired stuttering subsequent to stroke or traumatic brain injury.

Disfluency Location

Helm-Estabrooks (1986) reviewed several studies that were published between the 1960s and early 1980s and concluded that speakers with acquired stuttering "always" produced stutter-like disfluency in conjunction with word-initial phonemes, and "often" produced stutter-like disfluency in conjunction with word-medial phonemes. This pattern of disfluency is consistent with the results from the studies that are summarized in Table 7–1, as well as with findings from survey studies that include data from scores of speakers with nondevelopmental forms of stuttering (i.e., Market et al., 1990; Theys et al., 2008). Some authors have suggested that acquired and developmental forms of stuttering can be differentiated on the basis of whether noninitial syllables are stuttered. To our knowledge, this claim has not been subject to rigorous experimental testing. On the surface, it seems questionable that the presence of stuttering in conjunction with word-medial syllables is a unique feature of acquired stuttering. The main problem is that many speakers with developmental stuttering do indeed produce stuttering-related disfluency when saying word-medial syllables. Thus, a more pertinent question might be to examine whether the proportionate frequency of word-medial stuttering differs between the groups. Experimental research is needed in which speakers with each type of stuttering are compared on common stimuli. The stimuli should be matched for variables that are known to trigger stuttered speech (e.g., word- and sentence-level stress patterns, word frequency, the number of syllables per word, the syntactic structure of sentences).

Canter (1971) suggested that speakers with acquired forms of stuttering are prone to word-final stuttering, a behavior that rarely is observed in developmental stuttering. This claim has not been strongly supported by findings from subsequent research, however. For example,

Rosenbek et al. (1978) studied seven brain-injured patients with acquired stuttering and found that none of them exhibited repetitions of word-final syllables or sounds. Helm-Estabrooks (1986) summarized disfluency patterns reported in several studies from the 1960s through the 1980s. Interestingly, word-final phonemes were not mentioned in her summaries of "typical" acquired stuttering patterns following stroke, head trauma, and disease of the extrapyramidal system. Presumably, this omission reflected the fact that word-final phoneme repetition seldom, if ever, was mentioned in the studies she reviewed.

In several subsequent studies (Aram et al., 1990; Ludlow et al., 1987), researchers reported detailed disfluency data for groups of speakers with nondevelopmental stuttering but made no mention of word-final disfluencies. As with word-medial stuttering, experimental comparisons between speakers with developmental and acquired forms of stuttering are necessary to attain a satisfactory level of confidence in settling this matter. In such research, it will be important to define the notion of "final disfluency," as it can pertain to several distinct patterns of disfluency, including the following: interruption between the onset and rime of a word-final syllable (e.g., *pave|m-|ment*) and failure to terminate sounds within a word-final syllable after the syllable has been successfully spoken once (e.g., *pavement-|t- t- t-|*). The latter type of disfluency is very unusual in cases of developmental stuttering, although it has been noted occasionally in conjunction with individuals who are diagnosed with autism spectrum disorder.

Theys et al. (2008) reported that 5 of 58 (9% of the total) participants with acquired neurogenic stuttering produced stuttering-related disfluency in conjunction with final sounds. Final sound disfluency was noted in 2 of 29 (7% of the total) participants with a history of stroke, 1 of 9 (11% of the total) participants with degenerative neurological disease, and 2 of 11 (18% of the total) participants with traumatic brain injury. Three other studies included in the present review mentioned instances of word-final repetition. Two of these cases had histories of stuttering onset following right temporal lobe stroke (Ardila & Lopez, 1986; Helm-Estabrooks, Yeo, Geschwind, Freedman, & Weinstein, 1986). Of course, the participants in these studies exhibited repetition in the word-initial and word-medial positions as well. Van Borsel et al. (1998) reported a single instance of final sound repetition in a case of very severe stuttering subsequent to left supplementary motor area damage. That participant produced sound repetition in conjunction with 100% of the syllables spoken during all tasks except reading. Despite this extraordinarily high occurrence of stutter-like disfluency, virtually all of the participant's disfluencies involved difficulty in moving from the onset to the rime of a syllable.

Another variable that has been studied often is the grammatical class of stuttered words. Researchers accomplish this by comparing the proportion of function words (e.g., prepositions, articles) and content words (e.g., nouns, verbs) that feature stutter-like disfluency. Study results consistently indicate that speakers with nondevelopmental forms of stuttering exhibit stutter-like disfluency on both word classes (Market et al., 1990; Theys et al., 2008), and stuttered speech occurs in conjunction with a variety of speech sounds (Theys et al., 2008). Overall, however, most stuttered speech can be expected to occur in conjunction with content words (Jokel et al., 2007).

Task Effects

Speakers with developmental stuttering often exhibit variation in disfluency frequency across speaking tasks. The main pattern is that tasks with relatively high language formulation demands (e.g., conversation, narration) usually feature more disfluency than tasks such as oral reading, sentence repetition, counting, and alphabet recitation, wherein the content is fixed or predetermined. Several researchers have examined variations in disfluency frequency across tasks with speakers who have acquired stuttering following neurological injury. In Helm-Estabrooks' (1986) review of studies, she found that speakers who began to stutter following stroke, head trauma, and extra-pyramidal disease "always" exhibited disfluencies in conversational speech and "usually" exhibited stuttering during tasks such as sentence repetition and rote or automatic speech. Ludlow et al. (1987) studied 10 individuals with chronic acquired stuttering and found that stuttering frequency was greatest during conversational speech. In a case study of stuttering following a right hemisphere stroke, Ardila and Lopez (1986) reported that disfluency increased as a function of the formulation requirements associated with the task. For example, the participant in that study stuttered on 32% of the words during recitation, 37% of the words during counting, 42% of the words during reading, 44% of the words during sentence repetition, 46% of the words during picture description, and 52% of the words during conversation.

Rate Characteristics

Relatively few studies have reported rate data for speakers with acquired forms of stuttering, and when rate information is provided, it often consists of only subjective verbal descriptions how the speech sounded. Meyers et al. (1990) offered a more objective description of speech rate in their case study of a child with acquired stuttering following a left hemisphere stroke. A comparison of the child's pre- and post-morbid speech rates showed that his articulation rate had increased from 3.17 syllables per second to 4.37 syllables. Interestingly, the time period when the child stuttered most was marked by increases in his use of syntactically complex utterances and a gradually increasing speech rate. Ardila and Lopez (1986) reported similar findings for a patient with acquired stuttering following right hemisphere stroke. As the man recovered from the stroke, he began to produce longer and more complex sentences, and he began to speak at a progressively faster rate. His speech became increasingly disfluent at this time. Ardila and Lopez introduced a metronome to help the participant use a slower speech rate, but this approach was unsuccessful. As is the case with typical speakers and speakers with developmental stuttering, speech rate does not have a fixed affect on fluency. For instance, Aram et al. (1990) reported that children with unilateral left hemisphere lesions used a slower speech rate than both children with right hemisphere lesions and normally fluent children in a control group, yet both of the groups with brain injury were comparably disfluent.

Adaptation, Facilitative Contexts, and Response to Treatment

Normally fluent speakers and developmental stutterers have been observed to adapt (i.e., produce increasingly fewer disfluencies) when asked to say the same material repeatedly (Bloodstein & Bernstein Ratner, 2008). In addition, certain conditions (e.g., choral reading, rhythmic speech, singing, whispering, delayed auditory feedback) usually result in complete or near complete elimination of stuttering-related disfluency in cases of developmental stuttering (Andrews et al., 1983). Some experts have stated that speakers with acquired forms of stuttering are less likely than speakers with developmental stuttering to show fluency improvement in these contexts. The available data provide some support for this claim.

Market et al. (1990) found that 35 of 76 participants (46.1% of the total) in their survey did not show significant fluency improvement under the adaptation paradigm. Theys et al. (2008) reported a higher percentage of participants who did not show fluency improvement under adaptation (55% of total). It also is important to note that in these studies, some participants are unable to attempt adaptation tasks due to concomitant impairments. Adaptation generally is viewed as a measure of motor learning by contemporary speech scientists, and a lack of favorable response to the task has been noted in conjunction with a range of neuropathologies including stroke and brainstem infarction (Ardila & Lopez, 1986; Balasubramanian et al., 2003; Bhatnager and Andy, 1989; Jokel et al., 2007; Theys et al., 2008). Some participants do show favorable responses during adaptation tasks, however.

McClean and McLean, Jr. reported dramatic reduction of disfluencies in one person with acquired stuttering (from approximately 30% of words stuttered to 5% of words stuttered) during choral reading and delayed auditory feedback conditions. Facilitative effects have been reported in some individuals with acquired stuttering during singing and serial speech, as well (Rousey, Arjunan, & Rousey, 1986). Conversely, Ardila and Lopez (1986) reported severe stuttering across all contexts for a patient with a history of right hemisphere stroke in the following tasks: singing, choral reading, and metronome-paced speech. Similarly, Balasubramanian et al. (2003) reported a lack of fluency adaptation during choral reading, delayed auditory feedback, and frequency-altered feedback in an adult with lesions of the right hemisphere and the pons.

Secondary Behaviors, Emotional Reactions, and Outcomes

Secondary Behaviors

In developmental stuttering, moments of stuttering sometimes are accompanied by a variety of "secondary" or associated behaviors such as eye blinking, facial and limb movements, abrupt pitch changes, physical tension in the speech musculature, and disrupted speech-breathing patterns (Bloodstein & Bernstein Ratner, 2008). The presence of such behaviors typically is interpreted as evidence the speaker is aware of his or her fluency difficulties and, perhaps, is attempting to compensate for them.

Researchers have examined the extent to which these secondary or associated characteristics are present in the speech of speakers with nondevelopmental forms of stuttering. There has been speculation that speakers with nondevelopmental forms of stuttering are less likely to exhibit secondary behaviors than speakers with developmental stuttering. Some case reports support this idea. For example, Bhatnager and Andy (1989) reported the absence of associated behaviors in a patient with brainstem dysfunction, and Ludlow et al. (1987) described several of their participants' stuttering-related disfluencies as "effortless." However, group data suggest that secondary behavior is relatively commonplace among people with acquired stuttering. Market et al.'s (1990) survey results indicated that 31.6% of individuals with acquired stuttering displayed secondary behaviors with some regularity. Theys et al. (2008) reported that 55% of participants with acquired stuttering exhibited secondary behaviors. In a study of 12 adults with acquired stuttering, Jokel et al. (2007) concluded that the participants did not always seem aware that they produced secondary behavior, but the majority of them exhibited behaviors that were readily observable to clinicians.

When associated behaviors do occur, they seem to resemble the behaviors that occur in developmental stuttering (Ludlow et al., 1987). Examples of such behaviors include foot tapping as a strategy for timing speech initiation and the use of stereotypical interjections and phrases to start speech. Marshall and Neuburger (1987) reported muscle fixations, irregular breathing, and loss of eye contact that accompanied the disfluencies of an adult with acquired stuttering. Ardila and Lopez (1986) indicated that part-word repetitions in an adult with acquired stuttering sometimes were accompanied by visible muscle tension that resulted in blockage of speech.

Emotional Reactions

Another focus in research involves participants' emotional reactions to acquired

stuttering. In Market et al.'s (1990) survey, 67.1% of the participants with acquired stuttering were characterized as "annoyed but not anxious" with regard to their speech. Other patients have been described as "discontent but not anxious" (Ardila & Lopez, 1986) and as "stuttering easily" with "little overt anxiety" but yet expressing "concern" about speech (McClean & McLean, Jr., 1985). Ludlow et al. (1987) characterized 10 adults with chronic-acquired stuttering as "annoyed" and "surprised" by their disfluent speech, as making little effort to change speech because, as one patient expressed, "it's a problem that we can't control." Ludlow et al. used a behavior rating scale to compare acquired stuttering of patients' affective expression with that of nonstuttering brain-injured patients and normal controls and found no difference between the groups.

In other studies, participants are described as having stronger reactions to their stuttered speech. Patients have been reported as being "quite anxious" (Rosenbek et al., 1978) and as displaying "a great deal of fear and avoidance of speaking situations" (Rousey et al., 1986). In a few of the cases reviewed in this chapter, the onset of stuttered speech occurred in conjunction with stressful life events that occurred in the weeks and months after the neurological event. For example, Nowack and Stone (1987) reported a case of acquired stuttering wherein the symptoms markedly worsened during a period of great family stress and then markedly decreased following resolution of the family stress. Jokel et al. (2007) administered a communication attitudes scale to adults with acquired stuttering and found that the responses were similar to those seen in speakers with developmental stuttering. Whether a person reacts to acquired stuttering or not may depend on the type of neurological event. Theys et al. (2008) report that about 80% of individuals with a history of traumatic brain injury showed emotional reactions to their stuttered speech, versus about 60% of individuals with a history of stroke, and 33% of individuals with neurodegenerative disease. In light of such findings, clinicians should be mindful of the fact that, in some cases, a person's feelings and emotions about acquired stuttering can contribute as much to his or her communication disability as the stutter-like interruptions in speech do (De Nil et al., 2007).

Summary

Based on this review of the literature, it appears that the disfluency patterns associated with nondevelopmental stuttering are similar in several respects to those associated with developmental stuttering. Some of the characteristics that the two disorders share include the following: part-word repetitions, prolongations, and blocks tend to be the predominate type of disfluency produced; these disfluencies are most commonly associated with word-initial syllables but are sometimes produced in conjunction with word-medial syllables; and the disfluencies are not constrained by phoneme class, but they generally are most frequent during tasks that require relatively high language formulation demands (e.g., conversation, narration). For both developmental and nondevelopmental types of stuttering, the stutter-like disfluencies may be accompanied by excessive physical tension and/or the use of "secondary" behaviors such as rhythmic movement of nonspeech body

parts or head jerking. From a perceptual standpoint, the speech of some speakers with acquired stuttering sounds very similar to that of speakers with developmental stuttering. Many speakers with acquired stuttering seem aware of their fluency impairment and, those who are aware, may express concern, frustration, or other similar emotions in response.

There certainly are differences between developmental and nondevelopmental forms of stuttering, however. For example, as a group, speakers with nondevelopmental forms of stuttering appear to be less likely than speakers with developmental stuttering to exhibit fluency improvement during adaptation tasks, and they seem to be less likely to exhibit fluency facilitation during conditions such as choral reading, singing, use of delayed auditory feedback, and the production of rote or serial speech. Some cases of nondevelopmental stuttering are characterized by severely disfluent speech. This fluency pattern is not surprising, given the propensity for individuals to have other communication disorders and/or medical conditions that may exacerbate the effects of fluency impairment. The presence of concomitant problems seems to increase the risk that a speaker will acquire stuttering.

Acquired forms of stuttered speech have been documented in conjunction with a wide range of conditions that impact neurological functioning. Preliminary evidence suggests that some characteristics of acquired stuttering may vary with the type of neuropathology that is present. For example, speakers who acquire stuttering in conjunction with degenerative neurological diseases may be less likely to show emotional reactions to speech disfluency than speakers who acquire stuttering in conjunction with stroke. Nondevelopmental stuttering has been associated with a wide variety of lesion locations. This finding underscores the extent to which the processes that are integral to speech fluency are distributed throughout the nervous system.

8

Cluttering

The word "clutter" evokes images of messiness and disorganization. In its common usage, it most often refers to the organizational state of physical places such as a desktop, an office, or a garage. The term *cluttering* has a similar connotation in the field of speech-language pathology. A precise definition of cluttering is presented later in this chapter, but in general terms, it refers to a communication disorder that leads to messy and disorganized speech. Cluttered speech may be excessively fast and interrupted more often than normal, and listeners may have difficulty deciphering the speaker's intention because speech sometimes is unintelligible and ideas are presented in a disorganized or tangential manner. Scientific understanding of cluttering has progressed slowly during the past 50 years; however, speech-language pathologists' interest in the disorder seems to be on the upswing during the past decade, as evidenced by newly forged international collaborations among speech-language pathologists and recently published books and conference proceedings that focus on cluttering.

Historical Perspective

Weiss (1964) offered an overview of how cluttered speech has been conceptualized throughout the centuries. He noted that reports of clutter-like speech date back to ancient Greece and Demosthenes, a statesman who was said to have spoken indistinctly, misarticulated certain words, and displayed difficulty with topic maintenance. Weiss also discussed several texts from the Middle Ages in which speech disorders that seem consistent with contemporary notions of cluttering were discussed. According to Weiss, scholarly writing about clutter-like speech patterns increased in frequency and gradually became more refined during the 18th and 19th centuries. He noted, for instance, the writings of Bazin, who in 1717 documented a class of speakers in whom speech rate was rapid and several thoughts seemed to be "fighting for expression" at once. Weiss also mentioned the writings of Colombat, who in 1830 distinguished between speech disorders that featured excessive rate (which is consistent with contemporary notions of cluttering) and speech disorders that featured excessive hesitation (which is consistent with contemporary notions of stuttering).

Despite these and other writings from the late 1800s and early 1900s, clutter-like speech did not attract much scholarly attention until Weiss published his text, *Cluttering,* in 1964. The book was part of a series called the *Foundations of Speech Pathology*, which was edited by the eminent speech-language pathologist and expert on stuttering, Charles Van Riper. In the following decades, however, cluttering received relatively limited attention in fluency disorders research. The status of cluttering during this era perhaps is best exemplified by the title of Daly's (1993) review article on the disorder, in which he labeled cluttering the "orphan of speech-language pathology." More recently, Scaler Scott, Grossman, and Tetnowski (2010) reported results from a survey that they distributed to faculty of academic programs in speech-language pathology within the United States, Canada, and Europe. They found that although more than 90% of the programs included cluttering within their academic curriculum, the instructional time allotted to studying the disorder averaged only 100 minutes (mode = 60 minutes). It is no wonder that authorities on cluttering (e.g., Myers, 2010) have continued to argue for extending the research base of the disorder and for conducting activities that increase professional awareness and interest.

Efforts to expand professional awareness of cluttering and re-energize the research agenda for the disorder seem to have had some success. This is exemplified by activities such as the following:

- Publication of a special issue on cluttering in the *Journal of Fluency Disorders* in 1996;
- Establishment of the International Cluttering Association (ICA) in 2007 at the First International Cluttering Conference;
- Delivery of the first International Online Cluttering Conference in 2010 and the Second International Congress on Cluttering in 2014; and
- Publication of Ward and Scaler Scott's (2011) textbook, *Cluttering: A Handbook of Research, Intervention, and Education*—the only cluttering-specific textbook to be published in the United States since Myers and St. Louis' (1992) edited text on cluttering and only the second cluttering-specific book to be published since Weiss's classic text on cluttering in 1964.

Public Views on Cluttering

Results from studies of people in the United States, Bulgaria, Turkey, and Russia suggest that the general public seems to be aware of cluttering—at least when researchers provide them with a definition of the disorder—and that many people have interacted with people who clutter (St. Louis et al., 2010b). To date, however, there is relatively little research on public attitudes toward people who clutter. To address this gap, St. Louis and colleagues (St. Louis et al., 2010a) administered the Public Opinion Survey of Human Attributes (POSHA-E) to laypersons in the United States, Bulgaria, Turkey, and Russia. The POSHA-E is a comprehensive rating scale with items designed to measure the attitudes and beliefs that people have about speech disorders such as cluttering. Results from St. Louis et al.'s (2010a) research indicated that laypeople tend to have relatively neutral attitudes toward cluttering, a finding that perhaps reflects the limited experience that most people have with the disorder. Some of the items on the POSHA-E required responders to rate cluttering and other conditions in terms of how much they would want to have a specific condition themselves. On these items, participants in the St. Louis et al. (2010a) study rated cluttering less favorably than scenarios such as *using a wheelchair*, *having a mental illness*, and *being overweight*.

Factors Affecting Professionals' Views Toward Cluttering

It has been approximately three decades since St. Louis and Rustin (1986) surveyed speech-language pathologists in the United States and the United Kingdom with regard to their awareness of cluttering. The results from that study uncovered reluctance on the part of clinicians in both countries to treat people who clutter—an attitude that seemed to be driven, at least in part, by the clinicians' limited knowledge of the disorder. Although recent attempts to improve professional awareness and knowledge of cluttering may have improved this situation somewhat, on the whole, it is quite possible that professionals' views toward cluttering are not markedly different today than they were in 1986.

It is interesting to consider why cluttering has not attracted more attention than it has from researchers and clinicians. There are at least three factors that

seem to account for this situation. First and foremost, authorities have encountered considerable difficulty in constructing a suitable definition for cluttering (St. Louis, 1992; St. Louis & Schulte, 2011). The initial attempts to define cluttering (e.g., Weiss, 1964) included numerous symptoms, many of which applied to other disorders as well. This created questions about whether cluttering was a distinct disorder or, instead, merely a subset of some other disorder. The lack of a suitable definition for cluttering undoubtedly has undermined researchers' and clinicians' attempts to study the disorder systematically. After all, how can one study a phenomenon when he or she is unable to state precisely what the phenomenon is? Consequently, contemporary professionals have made it a high priority to develop a valid and agreed-upon definition for cluttering. In fact, the *International Cluttering Association* is leading such an effort presently (St. Louis, 2010).

Epidemiological factors also seem to have influenced the amount of research and clinical attention that cluttering has received. Although epidemiological data for cluttering are scarce, authorities generally agree that it is a low-incidence disorder and that it is less common than stuttering is. Because cluttering seems to affect a relatively small percentage of the population, it is challenging for individual research laboratories to conduct the kinds of group-level research studies that are useful for advancing scientific understanding of the disorder (Craig, 2010). With the establishment of the International Cluttering Association, however, speech-language pathologists, speech scientists, and related professionals now have a formal venue for forging collaborative research efforts. Such collaborations could lead to pooling of research participants across laboratories and, with that, a dependable way to conduct group-level research studies. As noted, group-level studies are necessary to make population-based inferences about the nature and treatment of cluttering. There also is agreement among authorities that cluttering can co-occur with stuttering. In other words, an individual can exhibit both disorders simultaneously. Given the relative prominence of stuttering as a communication disorder, it is possible that clinicians and researchers might be prone to regarding "stutter-clutter" cases as a variation of stuttering and, in doing so, push a speaker's cluttering-related behaviors into the background (Craig, 2010).

A third factor that seems to affect the standing of cluttering is the quality of the research base on the disorder. Notwithstanding the challenges associated with researching low-incidence disorders, the quality of cluttering-related research literature generally is regarded as weak (Craig, 2010; Curlee, 1996). Up until the mid-1990s, much of the data on the etiology and characteristics of cluttering was derived from anecdotal case reports. Although such information has a place in any research literature, it is regarded as a very weak form of evidence and certainly unworthy of being the primary source of knowledge for any disorder. Anecdotal case reports have a host of shortcomings, including the following: lack of control over observer bias and other extraneous variables; the inability to test hypotheses and make statements about cause-effect relationships; and the inability to generalize information to a broad population (in this case, people who clutter). Craig (2010) reported that, as of 2007, the research literature on cluttering continued to be based largely on clinical observations and

authoritative accounts and the occasional case-controlled study. On this basis, he argued that there was an urgent need for more robust forms of research, such as (a) well-controlled cohort studies (i.e., longitudinal designs and cross-sectional studies in which participants are well matched across groups on critical variables), (b) randomized controlled clinical trials (RCTs), and, ultimately, (c) systematic reviews of RCTs. Until such studies are conducted, scientific understanding of cluttering is unlikely to advance beyond its current level (Craig, 2010; Curlee, 1996).

Defining Cluttering

As noted in the preceding section, it is critical for professionals to reach consensus on the essential features and properties of a disorder if the research base for the disorder is to advance in a meaningful way. A definition provides a succinct summary of the essential features and properties of a disorder. To date, experts in speech-language pathology have found it challenging to define cluttering.

Approaches to Defining Cluttering

At the First International Conference on Cluttering in 2007, the meeting delegates made it a high priority to arrive at a valid definition for cluttering (St. Louis, 2010). Attainment of this goal is not as easy as it might seem. If cluttering is defined too narrowly, legitimate cases of the disorder will be missed. Alternately, if cluttering is defined too broadly, the disorder will be overidentified and variables that are superfluous to the disorder will be conflated with variables that are essential to the disorder. If a definition of cluttering is very broad, it is possible for two clinicians to say that they each are treating a person who clutters, yet the symptom presentation for the two cases is completely different (Myers & St. Louis, 1996).

St. Louis and Schulte (2011) described several approaches that speech-language professionals have used to define cluttering. *Expert definitions* are those that are written by a person who is an authority on cluttering. Such definitions are prone to incorporating the biases of the individual who composes the definitions. In contrast, c*onsensus definitions* are those that are written by a panel or committee of experts. Although such definitions are likely to reflect a broader perspective than expert definitions, they too may be limited by the need for committee members to compromise on key elements of the definition's content.

St. Louis and Schulte (2011) also noted that definitions for cluttering differ in their orientation or area of emphasis. They stated that some definitions are *symptom oriented*. Definitions of this sort may incorporate the essential characteristics of the disorder, but they also may include symptoms that are present in only a subset of people who clutter. As such, definitions of this sort are prone to including extraneous information. St. Louis and Schulte cited Weiss's (1964) definition for cluttering (presented in Table 8–1) as an example of a symptom-based definition. Other definitions are *continuum oriented*. With the continuum-oriented approach, cluttering is defined in terms of both the number of relevant symptoms a speaker has and the strength or degree to which those symptoms are present. Thus, cluttering is conceptualized as existing along a continuum or spectrum wherein one

speaker can present a stronger or more clear-cut case of cluttering than another speaker does. Ward (2006) proposed that cluttering should be defined in this manner. Lastly, other definitions aim to identify the *lowest common denominator* (LCD) for cluttering. St. Louis and colleagues (St. Louis, Myers, Bakker, & Raphael, 2007; St. Louis & Schulte, 2011) have argued that cluttering should be defined in terms of its most essential characteristics (i.e., the lowest common denominator). The LCD approach yields a narrower definition of cluttering than the previously described approaches do. If a particular LCD definition includes the critical or essential characteristics of a disorder, its use reduces the likelihood of incorrectly identifying cases of cluttering. According to St. Louis et al. (2007), the challenge with defining cluttering in this way lies in determining what the essential characteristics of the disorder are.

Some Definitions of Cluttering

In Table 8–1, we present several definitions for cluttering. As shown in Table 8–1, the earliest formal definition for cluttering is the one by Weiss (1964). Weiss's definition portrays cluttering as a multifaceted impairment, with some facets related to communication (i.e., impaired oral and written language, speech rate, speech articulation), other facets related to cognition (i.e., impaired attention, planning, problem awareness), and still other facets related to motor functioning and movement sequencing (i.e., impaired rhythm generation, musical performance). Based on Weiss's (1964) definition, it is unclear which—if any—of these symptoms he regarded as most essential to the diagnosis of cluttering. In the diagnostics chapter

Table 8–1. Examples of Definitions for Cluttering

Author	Definition
Weiss (1964)	Cluttering is a speech disorder characterized by the clutterer's unawareness of the disorder, by a short attention span, by disturbances in perception, articulation, and formulation of speech, and often by excessive speed of delivery. It is a disorder of the thought processes preparatory to speech and based on a hereditary disposition. Cluttering is the verbal manifestation of a Central Language Imbalance, which affects all channels of communication (e.g., reading, writing, rhythm, and musicality) and behavior in general.
Daly (1992)	Cluttering is a disorder of both speech and language processing that frequently results in rapid, dysrhythmic, sporadic, unorganized, and often unintelligible speech. Accelerated speech (or tachylalia) is not always present but impairments in formulating language almost always are.
St. Louis, Raphael, Myers, & Bakker (2003)	Cluttering is a syndrome characterized by a speech delivery rate that is either abnormally fast, irregular, or both. In cluttered speech, the person's speech is affected by one or both of the following: (a) failure to maintain normally expected sound, syllable, phrase, and pausing patterns; and (b) evidence of greater than expected incidents of disfluency, the majority of which are unlike those typical of people who stutter.
St. Louis, Myers, Bakker, & Raphael (2007)	Cluttering is a fluency disorder characterized by a rate that is perceived to be abnormally rapid, irregular, or both for the speaker (although measured syllable rates may not exceed normal limits). These rate abnormalities further are manifest in one or more of the following symptoms: (a) an excessive number of disfluencies, the majority of which are not typical of people who stutter; (b) the frequent placement of pauses and use of prosodic patterns that do not conform to syntactic and semantic constraints; and (c) inappropriate (usually excessive) degrees of coarticulation among sounds, especially in multisyllable words.
St. Louis & Schulte (2011)	Cluttering is a fluency disorder wherein segments of conversation in the speaker's native language typically are perceived as too fast overall, too irregular, or both. The segments of rapid and/or irregular speech rate must further be accompanied by one or more of the following: (a) excessive "normal" disfluencies; (b) excessive collapsing or deletion of syllables, and/or (c) abnormal pauses, syllable stress, or speech rhythm.

of his textbook, however, Weiss (1964, p. 63) suggested that lack of problem awareness, excessive speaking rate, and excessive or atypical speech disfluency were core symptoms.

As with many of the early definitions for stuttering, Weiss's (1964) definition for cluttering included a claim about etiology. He asserted that cluttering is a manifestation of "central language imbalance." Unfortunately, the construct of central language impairment was not well specified then and it has not been subject to extensive scientific scrutiny since then. Thus, Weiss's (1964) notion of central language imbalance as an etiology for cluttering should be regarded as an untested hypothesis.

Daly (1992) published a definition of cluttering that was narrower than Weiss's (1964) definition. Daly described cluttering as a speech and language disorder that affects speech rate, speech rhythm, speech intelligibility, and linguistic organization. Interestingly, the notion of fluency impairment was not mentioned explicitly in Daly's (1992) definition, although it is likely captured indirectly under the concept of impaired rhythm. Daly (1992) characterized cluttering primarily as a language disorder, a position that seemed to be based on his observation that neither impaired speech rate nor reduced intelligibility was present in all cases.

St. Louis, Raphael, Myers, and Bakker (2003) developed a definition for stuttering that was more speech-based than previous definitions. As shown in Table 8–1, St. Louis et al. (2003) defined cluttering primarily in relation to rate, rhythm, and disfluency. In contrast to Daly (1992) and Weiss (1964), St. Louis et al. (2003) did not mention the notion of language disturbance in their definition of cluttering. Subsequently, St. Louis and colleagues (i.e., St. Louis et al., 2007; St. Louis & Schulte, 2011) refined the St. Louis et al. (2003) definition by designating rate impairment as the primary characteristic of cluttered speech and attributing whatever disfluency and rhythm abnormalities a speaker might have as secondary to the rate impairment. St. Louis and colleagues (St. Louis et al., 2007; St. Louis & Schulte, 2011) also added the concept of *impaired coarticulation* to the definition of cluttering. In their view, impaired coarticulation underlies the common perception that cluttered speech sounds excessively fast and unintelligible. As with the St. Louis et al. (2003) definition, neither of the latter definitions explicitly mentioned language-related deficits. Overall, contemporary definitions for cluttering are quite different from the initial definition for cluttering that Weiss (1964) put forth.

St. Louis and Schulte (2011) summarized the details of a doctoral dissertation that Schulte conducted in 2009. Schulte studied various characteristics of 15 persons who previously had been diagnosed with cluttering by other speech-language pathologists. Among other things, Schulte examined how the behavioral profiles of the speakers who cluttered matched the characteristics contained in St. Louis et al.'s (2007) definition of cluttering. Schulte's analysis revealed that each of the individuals who cluttered (15 of 15) exhibited a rapid speaking rate (defined in the study as anything greater than 250 syll/min); however, only 5 of the 15 (33%) people exhibited irregular speaking rate (i.e., bursts of accelerated speech within an utterance). The combined frequency of interjections and revisions, both of which Schulte termed "normal disfluencies," was excessive in 6 of the 15 (40%) participants. Evidence of overly coarticulated speech was apparent in 6 of the 15 (40%) participants, as well.

Interestingly, none of the 15 participants in Schulte's (2009) study showed evidence of atypical pause use or atypical prosodic patterns in speech, characteristics that also are included in St. Louis et al.'s (2007) definition. Also of note, 2 of the 15 (13%) participants who had been diagnosed with cluttering by a speech-language pathologist exhibited only one of the symptoms from the St. Louis et al. (2007) definition (in both cases, the symptom was abnormally fast speaking rate). Given the findings from Schulte's (2009) study, it appears that some speech-language pathologists assign the label "cluttering" to a rather heterogeneous group of individuals.

An excessively fast speaking rate was the most common symptom. After that, however, the behavioral profile of identified individuals diverged, such that other definitional characteristics of cluttering were present only in subsets of speakers.

Although St. Louis et al.'s (2007) LCD definition since has been used as the basis for a number of studies and discussions about cluttering, not everyone agrees that it is the best way to define cluttering. For instance, van Zaalen-op't Hof and DeJonckere (2010) argued that cluttering fundamentally is a language-based problem and that the many symptoms commonly associated with the disorder arise from that basic etiology. The latter view is broadly consistent with the definition that Weiss proposed in 1964.

The difficulties that experts have faced in defining cluttering are not unique. For example, in recent decades, experts have struggled to define developmental forms of speech apraxia. As with cluttering, numerous behavioral characteristics have been associated with the diagnostic label "developmental apraxia," a situation that creates the potential for invalid or imprecise identification of the disorder. To complicate matters further, experts have debated what to call apraxic-like speech that affects young children. Candidate terms have included *developmental apraxia of speech* (DAS), *developmental verbal dyspraxia* (DVD), and *childhood apraxia of speech* (CAS), which currently is the preferred term. Similar to the research progression that is underway currently in the area of cluttering (e.g., van Zaalen-op't Hof, Wijnen,

& DeJonckere, 2009), Shriberg and colleagues (Shriberg, Aram, & Kwiatkowski, 1997a, 1997b, 1997c) conducted a series of studies in which they compared speech-language characteristics of children who had been diagnosed with developmental apraxia to those of children who had been diagnosed with delayed speech sound development. These studies and others have allowed for cross-validation of (a) the characteristics that are included within authoritative definitions of DAS, (b) the diagnostic labels that speech-language pathologists assign, and (c) the actual speech production deficits that children exhibit. From this research, Shriberg et al. (1997c) concluded that there might be subtypes of developmental apraxia, one of which is characterized by impaired stress assignment.[1] The possibility of cluttering subtypes has appeared in the research literature on cluttering, as well (St. Louis et al., 2007).

Characteristics of Cluttered Speech

A wide range of symptoms has been associated with cluttered speech. The primary characteristics of cluttered speech are reviewed in this section.

Fluency Characteristics

Most speakers who clutter show impairment in one or more dimensions of speech fluency. In this section, speech continuity, rate, rhythm, effort, naturalness, talkative-

---

[1]Incidentally, Shriberg et al. (1997b) noted anecdotally that a few of the children in their studies who were diagnosed with developmental apraxia exhibited fast rushes of speech that resembled cluttered speech. Developmental or childhood apraxia has been mentioned in the cluttering literature as a disorder that coincides with cluttering.

ness, and stability are discussed in relation to cluttered speech.

Continuity

Continuity refers to the connectedness of speech. Disfluency is the primary source of continuity interruption among most speakers who clutter. Although excessive disfluency in speech was not mentioned in Weiss's (1964) definition of cluttering, it is featured as a diagnostic marker of cluttering in several contemporary definitions (i.e., St. Louis, Raphael, Myers, & Bakker,, 2003; St. Louis et al., 2007). The current view is that speakers who clutter exhibit a disfluency pattern that is distinct from the one seen in speakers who stutter. That is, unlike developmental stuttering, wherein repetitions, prolongations, and blocks usually are the predominant type of disfluency, speakers who clutter tend to produce interjections, revisions, and "false starts" (i.e., abandoned segments of speech) more often than other types of disfluency, and the frequency of these disfluency types may be greater than what is observed in the general population. Accordingly, the disfluency pattern seen in speakers who clutter is, in a sense, the inverse of the pattern seen in speakers who stutter, which results in cluttered speech sounding distinctly different from stuttered speech. The expected disfluency profiles for speakers who clutter and speakers who stutter are illustrated in Figure 8–1.

Similar to cases of stuttering, the frequency of speech disfluency in speakers who clutter seems to vary across tasks. For example, van Zaalen-op't Hof et al. (2009) found that, among speakers who cluttered, the combined frequency for interjections, revisions, hesitations, and other "nonstutter-like" disfluency types

was about six to eight times greater than the combined frequency of "stutter-like" disfluencies such as part-word repetitions and prolongations during a monologue task and a story retelling task but similar during an oral reading task. Overall, in the van Zaalen-op't Hof et al. (2009) study, 75% of the speakers who cluttered produced at least three times as many of the "nonstutter-like" disfluencies as they did "stutter-like" disfluency.

Several authors (e.g., Myers & St. Louis, 1996; Preus, 1996) have noted the tendency for speakers who clutter to produce "maze-like" disfluency. As noted in Chapter 3, authors have used the term "maze behavior" in different ways. In some cases, it is used as synonym of any type of disfluency that a speaker produces and, in other cases, it refers to instances of linguistically based disfluency. In this text, the term *maze* is used in a restricted sense; that is, to signify disfluent segments that feature multiple and varied unsuccessful attempts to execute an utterance. Such disfluent segments will have a convoluted or complex quality. When evaluating speakers who clutter, a clinician might see "maze-like" disfluent segments of the sort shown below in Examples 8–1 and 8–2.

Example 8–1: | *He- his f-, no wait, um the m- um* | *my brother decided to hire my father.*

Example 8–2: | *um well, you know like- it's like- it's the gov- um* | *it's one of those patronage deals.*

Notice that the disfluent segments in Examples 8–1 and 8–2 lack the elements of part-word repetition, sound prolongation, and blocking that characterize stuttered speech and instead consist solely of editing terms and speech attempts that are

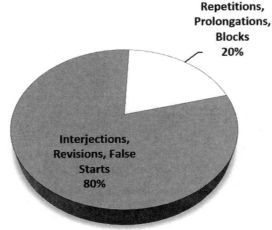

Figure 8-1A
Speaker who Clutters

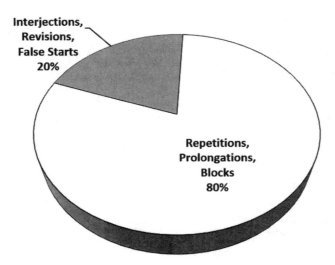

Figure 8-1B
Speaker who Stutters

Figure 8–1. Pie charts showing typical ratios of *nonstutter-like disfluency* types such as interjections, revisions, and false starts to *stutter-like disfluency* types such as part- and whole-word repetitions, sound prolongations, and blocks. **A.** Shows this ratio for speakers who clutter. **B.** Shows it for speakers who stutter. As indicated, most of the disfluencies for a speaker who clutters consist of interjections, revisions, and false starts (80% in this hypothetical case), and disfluency types that involve repeating, prolonging, and blocking make up the remainder. The inverse pattern occurs with most speakers who stutter. In this hypothetical case, 20% of all disfluencies consist of interjections, revisions, and false starts, and 80% involve repeating, prolonging, and blocking.

either abandoned ("false starts") or subsequently revised. This pattern of disfluency conveys a sense of disorganized or impaired linguistic formulation, characterizations that are included in some definitions of cluttering (e.g., Daly, 1992; Weiss, 1964). The maze-like disfluencies of cluttered speech also may contain elements of stutter-like disfluency (e.g., part-word repetition, sound prolongation); however, in cases of so-called "pure" cluttering, the interjections, revisions, and false starts generally will be the most prominent types of disfluency.

In contrast with the information discussed above, Daly and Burnett (1999, p. 232) stated that excessive repetitions of syllables, words, and phrases also are characteristic of cluttered speech and that some of the repetitions may feature numerous iterations. Although such a disfluency pattern might seem more characteristic of stuttering, Daly and Burnett (1999) claimed that the repetitions in cluttered speech differ from those seen in stuttered speech in the following ways: (1) repetitions in cluttered speech are not effortful, but those in stuttered speech are; (2) repetitions in cluttered speech usually span longer linguistic units (e.g., phrase and word repetitions) than those in stuttered speech (part-word repetitions); (3) repetitions in cluttered speech reflect difficulty in word retrieval or sentence formulation, whereas repetitions in stuttering do not; and (4) speakers who clutter generally are unconcerned about these lengthy repetitions, while speakers who stutter are concerned. Based on data from recent group-based studies of cluttering (e.g., van Zaalen-op't Hof et al., 2009), it seems that disfluency patterns like the one noted by Daly and Burnett (1999) are not common in cases of pure cluttering. Also,

given that people who stutter produce *all* types of repetition more frequently than typical speakers do (Ambrose & Yairi, 1999) and that scientists lack a reliable means of determining the source of specific instances of disfluency, it is probably premature to attribute multiple-iteration repetitions to either cluttering- or stuttering-related etiology.

The possibility of lengthy repetitions in cluttered speech raises the question of whether a speaker can exhibit both cluttering and stuttering concurrently. This issue is discussed in the next section.

Co-Occurrence of Cluttering and Stuttering

It is possible for a speaker to exhibit both stutter-like *and* clutter-like disfluency. In such cases, the speaker will exhibit markers of stuttering (i.e., excessive frequency of at least one of the primary forms of stutter-like disfluency) as well as markers of cluttering (i.e., excessive frequency of interjections, revisions, and false starts and/or any of the other symptoms of cluttered speech). As noted earlier in this section, these disfluency types can occur in clusters, a pattern that results in convoluted, maze-like interruptions in speech continuity. A maze-like disfluency that features both stutter-like and clutter-like disfluency is shown at the onset of the sentence in Example 8–3. A second, maze-like disfluency consisting of clutter-like disfluency precedes the word *hire*. Disfluent segments in speakers who clutter are not always convoluted or maze-like in nature, however. Note, for instance, that the sentence in Example 8–3 also contains two "simple" disfluent segments (an interjection preceding *my*, a part-word repetition in conjunction with *father*).

Example 8–3: | *H-He- his f- fa- fath-, no wait, um the um m- m- m-* | *my brother decided to* | *um well he, it's kind of- well* | *hire* | *um* | *my* | *f-* | *father.*

Disfluency Frequency in Speakers Who Clutter

As with developmental stuttering, disfluency frequency can vary considerably across speakers who clutter. In fact, if one adopts a rate-based definition of cluttering like the one proposed by St. Louis et al. (2007), it is possible for a speaker to be diagnosed with cluttering without exhibiting an excessive amount of disfluency. An example of the latter scenario is illustrated in Williams and Wener's (1996) study of an adult male who exhibited accelerated articulation rate, poor intelligibility, and poor cohesion during narration as primary symptoms of cluttering. The speaker's speech continuity, in contrast, fell into the normal range during conversation, with only 2 disfluencies per 100 words. A similar amount of disfluency was reported for the speaker during oral reading. In the latter context, however, the speaker blinked his eyes in conjunction with sound prolongations and syllable repetitions, a behavior consistent with stuttered speech. So, although disfluency frequency was within normal limits, other qualitative features of disfluency were indicative of fluency impairment.

Group-level disfluency data for speakers with developmental stuttering have been reported in hundreds, if not thousands, of published studies. From this research, it is known that the combined frequency of disfluent segments that feature repeating, prolonging, and blocking can range from as little as 1 or 2 disfluencies per 100 syllables to as many as 30 or 40 per 100 syllables. Unfortunately, to date, there have been no comparable large-scale, group studies to provide insight into how the disfluency frequency scores of speakers who clutter are distributed. Consequently, it is unclear at present whether speakers who clutter follow a pattern similar to that of speakers who stutter, wherein most cases exhibit either mildly or moderately elevated disfluency frequency, and a minority of cases exhibit severely elevated disfluency frequency.

Published case studies are a potential source of insight into how disfluency frequency is distributed in the population of speakers who clutter. Unfortunately, the case study literature on cluttering yields only a limited understanding of disfluency patterns. In some case reports, quantitative data are entirely absent and disfluency is described only as "excessive." When quantitative disfluency data are reported, one or more of the following limitations are commonly present: (1) data are not reported for specific disfluency types; (2) data are reported as the number of observed disfluencies rather than as the number of disfluencies per 100 syllables or words; (3) data are reported only in terms of "percentage of syllables stuttered," and (4) data are not compared to a control speaker. These issues make it challenging to gauge the severity of a given participant's disfluency and difficult to determine whether the disfluency patterns reflect the effects of stuttering or cluttering.

The disfluency data from four of the case-based publications in the *Journal of Fluency Disorders* (1996, Volume 21, Numbers 3 and 4) special issue on cluttering are presented in Table 8–2. Although disfluency frequency values were not provided for individual disfluency types in three of the four studies, and one of the

Table 8–2. Disfluency Frequency Results From Case Studies of Speakers Who Clutter

Study	Cases	Disfluency Data
Myers & St. Louis (1996)	12-year-old male	• Total disfluency = 8 per 100 syllables; 75% of total were interjections, revisions, or unfinished words.
	11-year-old male	• Total disfluency = 4 per 100 syllables; 71% of total were interjections, revisions, or unfinished words.
Lees, Boyle, & Woolfson (1996)	15-year-old male	• Reading: 9 per 100 syllables, including interjections and whole- and part-word repetitions. • Conversation: 10 per 100 syllables, including interjections, whole- and part-word repetitions, and revisions.
Williams & Wener (1996)	Young adult male	• Reading: 4 per 100 words, including prolongations, single-syllable repetitions, interjections, and multisyllable repetitions. • Conversation: 2 per 100 words, including prolongations, single-syllable repetitions, and interjections.
Teigland (1996)	3 adolescents who clutter; 3 matched controls	• Cluttering speakers produced three times as many revisions of grammatical errors as the speakers who did not clutter. • Speaking turns with grammatically based disfluency: cluttering: 19%, control: 7% .

studies (Teigland, 1996) reported only the observed numbers of disfluency, it still is possible to get a general sense for the severity of these cases.

As shown in Table 8–2, the overall disfluency frequencies reported by Lees, Boyle, & Woolfson, (1996) and Williams and Wener (1996) are not excessive in relation to normative data on fluency from typical speakers. To the extent that the participants' disfluencies stem from cluttering, this perhaps is an expected outcome. In other words, if clutter-like disfluencies are indeed mainly symptomatic of syntactic problems (see van Zaalen-op't Hof & DeJonckere, 2010), the location of disfluency in speakers who clutter should be biased toward the contexts in which syntactic planning occurs (i.e., utterance initiation, clause initiation). If so, the total number of disfluencies in a particular speech sample should be more strongly associated with the number of utterances or clauses within the sample than it is with smaller linguistic units such as phonological words. This prediction requires investigation. Although the disfluency frequency for a speaker who clutters may not be particularly high in any absolute sense, it still is possible for a speaker who clutters to be perceived as atypically disfluent if many of the speaker's disfluent segments are maze-like in nature.

Some speakers who clutter are excessively disfluent, however. In Figure 8–2, we present an excerpt from a transcript of cluttered speech that an adult speaker produced. When reading the transcript, it soon should become apparent that the speaker is highly disfluent. It also is evident that many of the disfluent segments are complex (i.e., maze-like) in form,

Line	Utterance	Disfluent segments	Syllables
1	|it's like she doesn't make a co-| **she probably doesn't make a lot of money but...**	1	13
2	|It's like it's prob- it's sort of- like you know| **it's** |like| **something that she loves.**	2	6
3	|Like at lea-| **she acts like she loves it.**	1	6
4	|She doesn't- she doesn't- like the- she- I mean| **Sorry, but this is the first time that I'm sharing this story.**	1	15
5	**So** |it's like har-| **I need a** |s-|**second to think about it!**	2	11
6	**But** |it's like- well- see- | **her husband acts like he doesn't want the clothing store.**	1	14
7	**But** |it's like- it's something that- and she's jus-| **it's kind of** |her best- the- | **her dream job.**	2	7
8	**I mean** |it's like- it's like she's- like| **the lady loves vintage clothing.**	1	10
9	**And it's interesting that** |like I- I kind of- it's like she- It's like she doesn't ev-| **she doesn't arrange clothing by sizes.**	1	16
10	|She does it very crea- like categorizes- | **I think she arranges it by** |pause| **color.**	2	10
11	**Or** |like by- I thi- she-| **she organizes** |it-| **some by fabric.**	2	10
12	**So she displays it really** |in her bes-| **in her own special way.**	1	13
Totals		17	131
Adjusted frequency (disfluencies per 100 syllables)		= (17/131) *100 = 12.98	

Figure 8–2. An excerpt from a transcript of a narrative by a speaker who clutters. The story deals with the speaker's trip to a second-hand clothing store. The core content of each utterance is shown in bold text and disfluent segments are shown in unbolded text. Disfluency frequency (12.98 disfluent segments per 100 syllables) is moderately high in a quantitative sense, but speech nonetheless sounds very disfluent because of the many lengthy, maze-like disfluent segments. Most of the disfluent segments consist of clustered interjections (particularly "like"), stereotypical phrases (particularly "it's like"), plus words or parts of words that subsequently are revised or abandoned. In addition to the disfluencies, the speaker's rate sounded excessively fast.

and they mostly consist of interjections along with bits of speech that are either abandoned or subsequently revised. The transcript does not the capture the fact that the speaker also was perceived to talk very rapidly.

Rate

Cluttered speech often is perceived as sounding excessively fast, rapid, rushed, or hurried (St. Louis & Hinzman, 1986; St. Louis, Myers, Faragasso, Townsend, &

Gallaher, 2004).[2] This seems to be a long-standing observation about the disorder, as each of the six definitions listed in Table 8–1 mention rate disturbance. In recent years, rate disturbance has emerged as a cardinal symptom of cluttered speech (see Table 8–1). In three of the definitions for cluttering that St. Louis and colleagues developed (St. Louis et al., 2003; St. Louis et al., 2007; St. Louis & Schulte, 2011), rate disturbance is characterized as the primary or essential characteristic of cluttered speech.

Speaking rate can be quantified in several ways. One commonly reported measure of speaking rate is *articulation rate*; that is, the number of linguistic units (syllables or words) a speaker produces per unit of time (seconds or minutes) during stretches of perceptibly fluent speech. Articulation rate typically is measured by dividing the number of syllables or words produced within fluent utterances by the time taken to produce those utterances. The fact that cluttered speech is commonly perceived to be excessively fast might lead one to assume that speakers who clutter exhibit abnormally high articulation rates during all sorts of speaking tasks or that they exhibit some extraordinary capacity to articulate rapidly. Research does not support either prediction.

Consider, for example, the results from Bakker, Myers, Raphael, and St. Louis (2011), who compared articulation rate patterns across three speaker groups: (1) adult females with typical fluency (control); (2) adult females who cluttered; and (3) adult females with exceptionally rapid speech but no cluttering. Group articulation rates were compared across four tasks:

diadochokinesis (DDK), recitation of nursery rhymes, oral reading, and sentence repetition; and across four rate conditions. During the DDK, nursery rhyme, and oral reading tasks, the researchers asked the participants to speak at a "comfortable" rate, a maximum rate, and a "maximum 2" rate. During the maximum 2 condition, participants attempted to exceed their initial attempt at a maximum rate. The main findings from the study with regard to rate were as follows:

- Both the cluttering group and the exceptionally rapid group spoke faster than the control speakers when using a "comfortable rate" during the oral reading and nursery rhyme recitation tasks. (Oral reading task: Cluttering = 7.59 syll/s; Control = 6.26 syll/s. Rhyme recitation task: Cluttering = 6.01 syll/s; Control = 5.60 syll/s.)
- Both the cluttering group and the exceptionally rapid group spoke faster than the control speakers when attempting to match the experimenters' "slow rate" during sentence imitation. (Cluttering = 0.89 syll/s faster than the experimenter's model; Control = 0.45 syll/s faster than the experimenter's model.)
- There were no differences across the groups during DDK production or during either of the maximum rate conditions in the oral reading and nursery rhyme recitation tasks.

Bakker et al. (2011) attributed the lack of group differences in the maximum rate

---

[2]In early writings on cluttering, authors often used the term *tachylalia* to describe excessively fast speech such as that seen in cluttering.

conditions to physiological constraints; that is, the speech articulation system can move only so fast. The group differences during oral reading and rhyme recitation were apparent only when the speakers used their customary rates. Thus, it may be that the speech production system is "tuned' differently across individuals such that some speakers (namely, speakers who clutter) gravitate toward faster articulation rates than others. In this view, when one's habitual rate is tuned at an excessively fast setting, other facets of speech, such as speech intelligibility and speech fluency, may be affected adversely (Alm, 2011; Bakker et al., 2011).

Bakker et al. (2011) did not report effect size data for the statistically significant rate differences; however, based on the summary statistics they reported, it is possible to compute Cohen's (1988) d statistic, which reflects the difference between two groups in terms of standard deviation units. Effects sizes for comparisons between the cluttering and control groups were as follows: oral reading: $d = 1.46$, nursery rhyme recitation: $d = 0.47$, and sentence imitation: $d = 1.24$. These values indicate that the magnitude of the rate difference between speakers who clutter and control speakers was very large during oral reading and sentence imitation and moderate during nursery rhyme recitation. Of course, one would expect at least *some* difference between groups in rate, because rate was one of the factors that the researchers used to define the groups. Nonetheless, the effect size analysis shows that these are not trivial differences in rate but meaningful ones in both a statistical and practical sense. Bakker et al. (2011) remarked that the lack of rate differences across the groups during the DDK tasks supports the notion that rate disturbance in cluttering is most apparent—and perhaps only apparent—during tasks that require linguistic formulation.

A final point worth mentioning is that none of the tasks in the Bakker et al. (2011) study examined rate production during *spontaneously* formulated connected speech. Some authors (e.g., van Zaalen-op't Hof & DeJonckere, 2010) have suggested that the symptoms of cluttered speech are more apparent during tasks that require spontaneous formulation of linguistic information than they are during tasks such as reading or rhyme recitation, wherein linguistic content is provided for the speaker. If this is so, then one would expect the rate differences between typical speakers and speakers who clutter to be greater during spontaneous conversation than they were in the tasks used in the Bakker et al. (2011) study. This possibility can be examined using results from van Zaalen-op't Hof et al., 2009).

Van Zaalen-op't Hof et al. (2009) compared speakers who cluttered, speakers who stuttered, and speakers with both cluttering and stuttering on several variables (including articulation rate) during monologue, oral reading, and story retelling tasks. Among the speakers who cluttered, articulation rate was faster during monologue than reading, although only moderately so (the effect size we computed was $d = 0.67$). As expected, articulation rate for speakers who cluttered was significantly faster than that of speakers who stuttered but only during the monologue, a task in which self-formulation demands were presumably greater than in the other tasks. Overall, the articulation rates for 56% of speakers who cluttered were more than 1 standard deviation above the average articulation rate for all of the participants in the study.

Several authors (e.g., Daly & Burnett, 1999; St. Louis et al., 2007; Weiss, 1964) have identified atypical variability in articulation rate as another key symptom of cluttered speech. The main pattern is for the speaker to accelerate articulation rate in a way that is atypical or unexpected within the context of the spoken utterance. At such times, speech is perceived as containing bursts of rapid speech. We will discuss articulation variability further in the following section on rhythm and again in a later section on speech sound articulation. In addition, some authors (e.g., Weiss, 1964) have mentioned *festination* (the tendency to articulate at a faster and faster rate the longer one talks) as a symptom of cluttering, as well.

Rhythm

The construct of rhythm falls under speech prosody. In disorders such as stuttering and cluttering, speech rhythm can be affected by several factors, including the frequency of disfluency within an utterance, the duration of those disfluencies, and aspects of utterance timing such as pause frequency and duration and segment and syllable duration. Controlled, empirical data on the speech rhythm in speakers who clutter are limited, however.

As noted, many experts have listed *maze behavior* as a symptom of cluttered speech. We have argued in this text that the term is most appropriately used in reference to instances of structurally complex or convoluted disfluency, particularly those disfluent segments that feature multiple consecutive false starts, revisions, and interjections (see Examples 8–1 and 8–2). To date, there is little information on the duration of such disfluencies during cluttered speech, but based on orthographic transcription alone, one can surmise that a maze-like disfluency is likely to last considerably longer than,

say, a single-iteration word repetition (e.g., |*we-*|*we*) or a simple interjection (e.g., *uh*). Thus, maze-like disfluencies are likely to disrupt speech rhythm noticeably, particularly when a speaker produces them often.

Several authorities on cluttering include pause abnormalities as a symptom of cluttered speech (e.g., Daly & Burnett, 1999; St. Louis et al., 2007; Van Riper, 1982). Some observations are that the pauses within running speech are too brief, absent, or misaligned with the syntactic or semantic properties of an utterance (St. Louis et al., 2007). Other authorities (e.g., Daly & Burnett, 1999) stated that inappropriately long pauses ("silent gaps") also may be present in cluttered speech and that they are associated with impaired word retrieval or sentence formulation. Recently, van Zaalen-op't Hof et al. (2009) found support for the claim of minimal pausing during cluttered speech in a study of speech samples from 42 speakers who cluttered. Interestingly, however, neither van Zaalen-op't Hof et al. (2009) nor any of the authors cited in Table 8–2 reported seeing excessively long pauses in the samples they analyzed. This suggests that if excessively long pauses (hesitations) are observed in speakers who clutter, they are present in only a minority of cases and are less commonly observed than very brief pauses are. The latter point is supported by the observation that many of the treatment-related publications for cluttering (Daly, 2010; Daly & Burnett, 1999; Logan, 2010) discuss the utility of teaching speakers who clutter to pause more frequently than they customarily do and to lengthen pause duration. Obviously, there is need for additional empirical investigation of pause behavior in speakers who clutter. Issues that warrant study include the following: (a) the percentage of cluttering speakers who exhibit pause abnormalities, (b) the frequency with which speakers who clutter typically produce atypical pauses, and (c) whether excessively short pauses are more common than excessively long pauses or misplaced pauses.

Speech rhythm also can be influenced by variations in articulation rate. Van Zaalen-op't Hof et al. (2009) examined rate variability in speakers who clutter by measuring articulation rate in five fluent utterances that each contained at least 10 syllables. Variability was defined as the difference between fastest and slowest articulation rates across the five sentences. Based on this definition of variability, there was no difference in rate variability across speakers who cluttered, speakers who stuttered, and speakers who cluttered and stuttered. In the cluttering literature, rate variations typically are described in terms of "spurts" or "bursts" of rapid speech within a spoken utterance. Thus, additional research is needed to assess rate patterns across intra-utterance linguistic units (e.g., phrases, phonological words). With the latter method, a researcher would compare articulation rate patterns for phonological phrases or phonological words in speakers who clutter against those of typical speakers.

Effort

Speech-related effort has not been studied extensively with speakers who clutter. Effortful speech is, of course, a commonly reported characteristic of stuttered speech. The general finding is that speakers who stutter sometimes sound or appear as if they are exerting excessive physical effort when talking (Bloodstein & Bernstein Ratner, 2008). Behaviors that drive this perception include the presence of extraneous body movements while talking, tremor in speech-related musculature during speech, and irregularities in speech breathing patterns during utterance production. Speakers who stutter commonly report that the act of speaking (or, at least, the act of attempting to speak fluently) is mentally effortful as well (Ingham et al., 2009). This perception perhaps is indicative of the speaker's attempts to regulate or monitor speech production or to conceal the symptoms of fluency impairment from listeners.

In contrast to the pattern seen with stuttering, information from case reports and authoritative accounts suggest that physically tense instances of disfluency are not commonly observed in speakers who clutter, nor are overt signs that the speaker is fearful of speaking (Daly & Burnett, 1999). This may stem from the fact that speakers who clutter seem to have little self-awareness of their moment-to-moment communication difficulties. It seems logical that a speaker first must have awareness of his or her communication impairment before he or she will actively attempt to compensate for it or conceal it. Compensation and concealment each require action and attention to implement, and in that sense, they are effortful.

Cluttered speech sometimes is characterized by convoluted or maze-like disfluency. Disfluent segments of this sort may convey a sense that the speaker is struggling to execute a spoken utterance and, thus, is expending excessive effort when talking. Perception of speech-related effort at such moments requires investigation. It also is possible that speakers who clutter display subtle markers of self-awareness during cluttered utterances (e.g., overactivation of the autonomic nervous system). This possibility has not been well studied in speakers who clutter, either, but it might provide additional insights into whether speakers who clutter are "aware" of their communication difficulties.

Naturalness

Nearly all of the research on speech naturalness comes from studies of people who stutter, and most of that research concerns the perceived quality of posttreatment speech patterns (i.e., the extent to which the "treated speech" of speakers who stutter sounds like that of typical speakers). Results from such studies indicate that the posttreatment speech of speakers who stutter is sometimes assigned less favorable naturalness ratings than comparable speech samples from speakers with typical fluency are (Ingham, Martin, Haroldson, Onslow, & Leney, 1985; Martin, Haroldson, & Triden, 1984).

There has been little systematic research to date on treatment outcomes with speakers who clutter, let alone the naturalness of their posttreatment speech. Thus, the status of posttreatment speech naturalness among speakers who clutter is unclear. Because of the overlap in treatments for stuttering and cluttering, one could imagine that people who clutter would exhibit many of the same naturalness limitations that are found in people who stutter (see, for example, Reichel, 2010). This issue needs to be studied. St. Louis et al. (2004) examined listeners' perceptual ratings of cluttered speech samples that came from two speakers. Listeners rated both the naturalness and rate attributes of the cluttered samples less favorably than they rated the language, articulation, and disfluency attributes. In one sense, this is not surprising because naturalness ratings seem to be correlated with other dimensions of speech production (Chakraborty & Logan, 2013; Hodgman & Logan, 2013). Thus, there is a need

for comparisons between pre- and posttreatment samples of speakers who clutter, who then are compared to control speakers.

Talkativeness

Talkativeness encompasses variables such as verbal participation, message coherence, and communicative flexibility. With regard to verbal participation, clinical authorities seem to be in agreement that speakers who clutter are prone to talking excessively (Daly, 1993; Scaler Scott, 2011; Ward, 2006; Weiss, 1964). This is in contrast to the profile for speakers who stutter, in whom verbal output usually is either typical or less-than-typical due to the speaker's desire to conceal his or her fluency impairment from others. Speakers who clutter also are prone to exhibiting difficulty with organizing information, particularly within narrative contexts, while speakers who stutter typically do not display difficulty in this area (Daly, 1993; Scaler Scott, 2011; Ward, 2006; Weiss, 1964).

Among those cluttering speakers who do exhibit disorganized thought expression, additional research is needed to determine the nature and extent of the organizational difficulties. Application of standard discourse analysis procedures to cluttered speech samples would be an important first step to address this gap in the research literature.

Stability in Speech-Language Performance

As with some other aspects of cluttered speech, relatively little is known about the extent to which cluttering symptoms vary over time, across tasks, or across situations. Based on our clinical experience, it seems that cluttering-related variables such as disfluency frequency, articulation rate, language organization, speech intelligibility, and so forth vary relatively little from day to day. Thus, a speaker who exhibits moderately fast speech at an initial evaluation is likely to exhibit moderately fast speech at a follow-up evaluation one week later. However, as noted earlier in this chapter, cluttering symptoms do seem to fluctuate across speaking tasks. For instance, nonmeaningful utterances such as those in a DDK battery are less likely to show evidence of cluttering than meaningful utterances during narration and sentence production are (Bakker et al., 2011).

Additional research is needed to determine the extent to which cluttering symptoms show situational variability (e.g., speaking with a friend *vs.* speaking with an authority figure). It has been suggested that the symptoms of cluttering are most apparent when a speaker is relaxed or comfortable (Daly & Burnett, 1999; Weiss, 1964). At such times, the speaker's self-monitoring of speech production is presumed to be either minimal or absent. Additional research is needed to validate this observation and to quantify the extent to which performance varies, both when a speaker is instructed to attend to speech production and when a speaker talks in his or her customary way. It also seems important to determine whether situational variability among speakers who clutter is manifested in a similar manner and to a similar extent as it is in speakers who stutter.

Speech Articulation Characteristics

Impairment in articulation also is a commonly reported characteristic of cluttered speech. Deficits may be apparent in at least two aspects of speech sound production. The first type of production deficit affects the timing of speech sound segments. This deficit is said to be manifest in the form of *excessive coarticulation*. The second type of production deficit involves the accuracy with which specific phonemes are produced. Both types of articulation-based problems are discussed further in this section of the chapter.

Coarticulation

The term *coarticulation* refers to the extent to which the articulatory movements associated with contiguous phonemes overlap with one another during speech production (Behrman, 2007). Although coarticulation most often is conceptualized as an aspect of speech articulation, some authors (e.g., Starkweather, 1987) have discussed coarticulation within the context of speech fluency as well. Either way, coarticulation is a suprasegmental construct—one that deals with the timing patterns of speech gestures.

Contemporary definitions of cluttering (e.g., St. Louis et al., 2007) identify excessively coarticulated speech as a core symptom of the disorder. Some authors (e.g., Daly & Burnett, 1999) have used the term "telescoped speech" to describe this phenomenon. Just as the segments of a telescope tube are nested so that they can slide into one another and decrease the overall length of the instrument, the gestural postures associated with contiguous speech sounds can overlap to varying degrees. It is thought that in many speakers who clutter the gestural postures for speech sound segment sometimes overlap too much (St. Louis et al., 2007). Although the speaker may be producing the appropriate consonants and vowel sequences, the temporal characteristics of the sound segments—or, more specifically, the temporal characteristics of the transitions between the sound segments—are atypical. Experts are in general agreement that the coarticulation difficulties of speakers who clutter are especially apparent during production of multisyllable words (Bakker et al., 2011; and see Examples 8–4 and 8–5 below).

An excerpt from a speech sample in an adult who demonstrated this type of speech is shown in Figure 8–3. In the sample, perceptibly rapid (and presumably coarticulated) speech occurs regularly and it usually spans entire phrases or clauses. During the underlined portions of the sample, speech sounded as if it was being said in bursts or spurts, a pattern that many authors have documented in conjunction with cluttering (e.g., Daly & Burnett, 1999; St. Louis et al., 2007). At these times, the speaker's intelligibility was reduced, sometimes to the point of becoming unintelligible. Other authors report similar patterns. For example, in a study of three teenagers who cluttered, Teigland (1996) reported that 18% of their speaking turns during a direction-giving task contained rapidly accelerating bursts of speech, and 8% of their speaking turns contained "barely interpretable or uninterpretable articulation" (versus 0% and 2% in control cases).

1. I've had a problem for a long time |uh| enunciating and having people clearly understand what I'm trying to say.

2. |uh um| some of the worst problems are |uh| when I'm saying my major.

3. No one hardly ever understands xx xx xx.

4. And I just can't get it out so they understand xx xx xx, which gets discouraging.

5. And |uh- w- a-| I'm taking a class in xx xx xx xx, and I sometimes have to present projects.

6. And when I'm up in front of the class talking, |uh| I have no problem being comfortable.

7. The problems are when I'm thinking the same time as I'm talking and not xx xx xx xx xx.

8. But if they ask me something that I don't know, I xx xx xx xx and my speech gets worse.

Figure 8–3. An excerpt of cluttered speech from an adult who produced what was perceived as spurts of very rapid speech (indicated by underlined words). At such times, speech intelligibility was, at best, marginal, possibly because speech sound segments were coarticulated excessively or articulated incompletely. In some stretches of the sample, speech articulation was fully unintelligible. (Each *xx* represents one unintelligible syllable.) The speaker's comments throughout the sample suggest some self-awareness of speech difficulty.

Many clinical authorities have noted that speakers who clutter are prone to reducing or deleting syllables within multisyllable words, a speech pattern that also results in the perception of "compressed" or "hurried" speech. St. Louis et al. (2007) offered the following examples to illustrate this phenomenon:

Example 8–4: Target *explanation* → [ɛkspleɪʃən];

Example 8–5: Target *inability* → [ɪnbɪəti].

The error in the word *explanation* is interesting in that the speaker fuses the two word-medial syllables. That is, the target form (i.e., [spləneɪ]), which features one unstressed and one stressed syllable, is merged into one new, stressed syllable (i.e., [spleɪ]), which includes constituents from the two original syllables. In contrast, the error on the target word *inability* features deletion of one unstressed syllable (i.e., [ə]) and reduction of another unstressed syllable (i.e., /lə/ → [ə]). Errors like these and the ones in Figure 8–3 point to phonological problems that extend beyond the boundary of a syllable. Whatever the source for these errors may be, the resulting speech is not indicative of systematic difficulty in saying specific sounds. Rather, it seems to reflect a nonsystematic problem with encoding the segmental and/or metrical forms of occasional phonological words. Alm (2011) proposed that the atypical coarticulation seen in speakers who clutter results from impairment at the speech planning level when the durations of consonant and vowel segments are specified.

As suggested above, if speech coarticulation and syllable realization are suffi-ciently aberrant, speech intelligibility can be compromised. Deficits in speech intelligibility are routinely mentioned in discussions of cluttered speech, and this bolsters the idea that cluttering is a disorder that affects both fluency and articulation. Group-level data are needed on matters such as the average percentage of unintelligible words among speakers who clutter and the extent to which unintelligible segments of speech correspond to phonological word boundaries. The relationship between articulation rate and speech sound coarticulation needs to be explored further, as well. It is conceivable that the speech sounds within a syllable can be coarticulated excessively, yet the overall duration of the syllable remains relatively normal. Such a pattern may result in a speech sample perceived as being spoken in "hurried" or "rushed" manner, while the measured articulation rate for the sample remains roughly within normal limits (St. Louis et al., 2007).

Phonemic Development

Information about the early stages of speech-language development in speakers who clutter is very limited. Some authors (e.g., Daly & Burnett, 1999; Weiss, 1964) have included developmental delay in phonemic development among the symptoms of cluttered speech. In this view, speakers who clutter are considered prone to exhibit systematic error patterns (substitutions, omissions, additions, distortions) of the sort that are seen in children with developmental speech sound disorders. Daly and Burnett (1999) characterized the speech sound production of speakers who clutter as "baby talk" but elsewhere in their chapter they suggested that speech sound production difficulties are most commonly associated with /r/, /l/, and sibilant production.

Systematic sound production errors are not mentioned in contemporary definitions of cluttering, and there is very little clinical data about the early articulation development of speakers who clutter. (In the adolescent and adult speakers who clutter who we have seen in our clinical practice, the majority has *not* displayed systematic difficulty in producing specific phonemes, phoneme sequences, or phoneme classes accurately. Nonsystematic difficulties in articulatory timing that results in poor intelligibility, however, have been noted in many of the speakers.) Thus, for now, it probably is best to regard systematic speech sound production problems as one of several speech-language impairments that a speaker *may* exhibit concomitantly with cluttering but also to realize that many speakers who clutter do not seem to have such difficulties.

Syntax and Discourse Characteristics

Various language-related difficulties have been linked to cluttered speech. Among these include difficulties with syntactic complexity and completeness, problems with linguistic cohesion, conciseness, and organization during connected discourse, as well as problems with pragmatic aspects of communication such as topic maintenance and the ability to recognize and repair unsuccessful communication attempts (Daly & Burnett, 1999; St. Louis, Hinzman, & Hull, 1985; Teigland, 1996; Ward, 2006).

Many authorities (e.g., Ward, 2011; van Zaalen-op't Hof & DeJonckere, 2010) regard the disfluency types that typify clut-

tered speech (i.e., interjections, revisions, false starts) as symptomatic of language formulation difficulties. The disfluent speech from the sample shown in Figure 8–2 is consistent with this notion, as many of the disfluent segments involved message reformulation, and there is little evidence elsewhere of stutter-like speech.

Epidemiological Considerations

Incidence and Prevalence

In contrast to the research on stuttering, little is known about the incidence and prevalence of cluttering at a population level. Until such research takes place, one can gain only a rough sense of how common cluttering is by considering results from a handful of small-sample epidemiological studies and by examining data on the occurrence of cluttering in relation to stuttering.

Several authors have reported diagnostic classification statistics for patients with fluency concerns. This approach provides information about matters such as whether cluttering is less common than stuttering and how often the two disorders co-occur. In most reports (Daly, 1993; Freund, 1952; Howell & Davis, 2011; Preus, 1992), cases of pure stuttering have outnumbered cases of cluttering-stuttering and cases of pure cluttering. The reported ratios of stuttering-only cases to cases with cluttering-only and/or cluttering-stuttering are quite variable, however, ranging from a low of 1.2:1 (Daly, 1993) to a high of 4.6:1 (Howell & Davis, 2011). To complicate matters further, Weiss (1964) reported an opposite pattern; that is, that cases of cluttering-stuttering were about twice as common as cases of pure stuttering and pure cluttering.

Howell and Davis (2011) conducted a methodologically rigorous study of cluttering epidemiology. They presented four judges who were experienced in fluency analysis with a series of speech samples that came from children that Howell and Davis had evaluated previously for fluency concerns. Two speech samples were available for each of the 96 children. One sample was recorded at approximately age 10, and the other was recorded at approximately age 14. Howell and Davis provided the judges with criteria for identifying cluttering (i.e., evidence of fast speech, evidence of poor/disorganized thinking, evidence of short attention span such as topic shifts), and then asked the judges to assign each of the speech samples into one of four categories (i.e., *only stuttering*; *only cluttering*; *stuttering and cluttering (with more stuttering than cluttering)*; *stuttering and cluttering (with more cluttering than stuttering)*). Howell and Davis then validated the judges' classifications by presenting the speech samples that a majority of judges had labeled *only cluttering* or *stuttering and cluttering* to two authorities on cluttering. Howell and Davis retained the speech samples that both authorities had labeled as *cluttering* for further analysis.

Overall, 12% (23/192) of all speech samples in the Howell and Davis (2011) study were labeled as cluttered. Among the 96 participants with fluency concerns, 18% (17/96) had at least one sample that met the criteria for cluttering, and the remainder (82%) met criteria for *only stuttering*. Only 6 of the 96 participants (6.25%) presented cluttered speech during both of their speech samples, and of

these cases, all of the cluttered samples came from the "age 10" assessments. Thus, there were no newly developed cases of cluttering during early adolescence, and some cases of cluttering at age 10 had resolved or improved substantially by age 14. Findings from this study suggest that cluttering is indeed less common than stuttering, with the ratio being about 4.6 cases of *only stuttering* for every 1 case of either *only cluttering* or *stuttering and cluttering*. On this basis, the observed occurrence of cluttering is somewhat less than that reported in several older sources (e.g., Preus (as cited in Daly, 1986; Freund, 1952; Weiss, 1964).

Onset and Developmental Course

Data regarding the age of onset for cluttering are limited, in part because of the apparently low incidence of pure cluttering. Some sources (e.g., Diedrich, 1984) contend that the onset of cluttering occurs much later than that of stuttering, while others (e.g., Van Riper, 1971; Weiss, 1964) suggest that cluttering can transform into stuttering, a scenario which would put cluttering onset earlier than stuttering onset. However, in Howell and Davis' (2011) recent study of 17 children who cluttered, the average age of reported onset for cases of stuttering (~49.5 months) was similar to that of the children who cluttered and the children who cluttered and stuttered (~53 months). The researchers' longitudinal assessments of fluency outcomes for the children who cluttered showed that 29% (5/17) normalized fluency by age 14, while the remainder (71%) persisted with cluttered speech. Reports on treatment outcomes with speakers who clutter are mixed, with some sources reporting poor outcomes but several others reporting improved performance (St. Louis, 1996; St. Louis et al., 2007). Such reports suggest that improved communicative functioning is possible for cases that do not necessarily "recover" from cluttering via unassisted means.

Van Riper (1982) described four developmental tracks or pathways for stuttering that were based on analysis of 300 clinical records from patients with impaired fluency. One of the four tracks (Track II) was composed of speakers who exhibited "hurried and irregular" repetitions of whole words, along with "more abortive beginnings, more revisions, (and) more revisions" than cases of classic stuttering. Individuals classified as Track II also exhibited unorganized speech and frequent articulation errors but minimal frustration about and self-awareness of their communication difficulties. Van Riper summarized his discussion of the Track II category by saying that the speech pattern "is the early cluttering-like speech delineated by Weiss (1964)." However, other aspects of Van Riper's Track II category (e.g., long series of unstoppable syllable and word repetitions accompanied by yelps and shouts, the presence of "avoidance tricks," failure to improve fluency when slowing speech) are not consistent with contemporary views on cluttered speech. Thus, Van Riper's Track II diagnostic category perhaps is most applicable to cases in which both cluttering and other fluency difficulties are present. Howell and Davis' (2011) longitudinal investigation of children's impaired fluency revealed that cases of cluttered speech can transform into stuttered speech over time—a pattern noted in several earlier sources (e.g., Van Riper, 1971; Weiss, 1964). However, according to Howell and Davis (2011), this pattern is uncommon (i.e., less than

30% of the cluttering cases in their study demonstrated it).

Gender and Familial Patterns

Like stuttering, cluttering seems to affect males more often than females. Howell and Davis (2011) reported that 88% of their participants who either cluttered or cluttered and stuttered were male, versus approximately 81% of the participants who only stuttered. The male-to-female ratio for cluttering in Howell and Davis' (2011) study is similar to that reported by St. Louis (1996) for the series of case studies within the *Journal of Fluency Disorders'* special issue on cluttering (i.e., 86% male to 14% female). That said, in one recent study of cluttered speech (Bakker et al., 2011), all of the participants who cluttered were female!

With regard to familial patterns, Weiss (1964, p. 50) concluded, "We have found that hereditary is a basic factor in cluttering." He continued (p. 51), "In virtually every case (of cluttering), we discover that at least one other member of the family has had a speech disorder." Weiss's conclusion was based, in part, on data such as that from Freund (1952), who reported that more than 90% of cluttering cases had a positive family history of speech-language impairment. More recent accounts differ from this view, however. For example, in St. Louis' (1996) summary of data from the *Journal of Fluency Disorders'* special issue on cluttering, only 7 of 18 (39%) speakers who cluttered had a positive family history of articulation or language disorders. Howell and Davis (2011) reported that 47% (8/17) of their participants who cluttered had a positive family history of impaired fluency. The latter statistics suggest that the role of hereditary factors in cluttering may be subtler and perhaps more complex than it was originally thought to be. Overall, the genetics of cluttering are not understood nearly as well as the genetics of stuttering, and there is a need for additional research into this aspect of the disorder (Drayna, 2011).

Co-Occurring Disorders

Based on clinical observation, it appears that clutter-like speech often occurs in the context of other disorders. The list of disorders that have been linked with cluttering is lengthy. Some disorders that co-occur with cluttering affect oral expression and were discussed earlier in this chapter (i.e., stuttering, impaired pragmatic functioning, impaired syntax/discourse formulation, atypical articulation performance). In this section, we review some other disorders that are said to co-occur often with cluttering.

Learning Disability

According to the National Center for Learning Disabilities (NCLD, 2014), a learning disability is "a distinct and unexplained gap between a person's level of expected achievement and their performance" in tasks involving listening, speaking, reading, writing, reasoning, or mathematical abilities. As a result of this discrepancy, the individual's achievement level is not commensurate with his or her chronological age. The term learning disability encompasses a range of disorders or subtypes. These include: *dyslexia* (which affects reading, writing, and spelling); *dyscalculia* (which affects mathematic functioning); *dysgraphia* (which affects written expression, handwriting, and spelling); as well as visual and auditory processing disorders and attention-deficit/hyperactivity disorder (ADHD).

According to the NCLD (2014), the etiology of learning disabilities is unknown; however, central nervous system dysfunction is assumed to be present. Hereditary factors appear to be a predisposing factor for some cases. It also is possible that exposure to teratogenic agents (e.g., a virus, drugs, chemicals) may affect neurodevelopment in ways that result in learning disabilities. Peripheral sensory deficits (e.g., hearing loss, vision loss) and intellectual disability (mental retardation) may be present in individuals who have a learning disability; however, by definition, these conditions are not a primary cause of learning disabilities. Social and cultural differences and/or economic disadvantages may be present as well; however, by definition, these characteristics are not a cause of the learning disability.

Learning disabilities seemed to assume a relatively prominent role in older views on cluttering (Weiss, 1964); however, St. Louis et al. (2007) noted that many individuals who clutter do not present concomitant learning disabilities. Learning disabilities that affect reading are not regarded as being caused principally by visual-perceptual processing deficits but instead by primary deficits in language deficits (St. Louis et al., 2007). As noted earlier in this chapter, an assortment of oral language deficits has been noted in speakers who clutter. It is unclear whether the etiology for these oral language deficits overlaps with those for the reading and writing deficits present in learning disabilities.

Attention Deficit/ Hyperactivity Disorder

Attention deficit/hyperactivity disorder (ADHD) is characterized by evidence of inattention and hyperactivity or impulsivity that is present before age 7, observed across different settings, and leads to disability in social, academic, or occupational functioning (National Institute of Mental Health [NIH], 2014). St. Louis et al. (2007) briefly reviewed reports from several authors who described symptoms consistent with attention deficit/hyperactivity disorder among speakers who clutter. St. Louis et al. (2007) cautioned, however, that controlled, empirical data regarding the extent to which the two disorders overlap is limited and that, in their experience, cluttering is not present in most people who meet definitional criteria for ADHD.

Auditory Processing Disorder

Disordered processing in the central auditory system also has been mentioned as a condition that co-occurs with cluttering. For example, Daly and Cantrell (2006) discussed the use of Daly's Checklist for Possible Cluttering in the development of clinical goals in a case study of a child who cluttered. The child was rated and scored somewhat below age expectations in the area of auditory comprehension, which was defined as difficulty in comprehending directions and being an "impatient" listener. Although rating-based measures of individual cases shed light on the type of difficulty speakers who clutter might exhibit in auditory processing, they offer a limited perspective on functioning in this domain.

To date, there has been relatively little scientific study with regard to auditory system functioning in speakers who clutter. Molt (1996) compared the performance of three individuals who cluttered with performance from three typical speakers on several measures of central auditory processing as well as electrophysiological functioning (i.e., auditory evoked potentials). In contrast with the noncluttering speakers, all three of the speakers who cluttered performed atypically on at least two of the four tests of central auditory processing that were administered. In addition, each of the three speakers who cluttered showed abnormalities in auditory evoked potentials, particularly over the frontal lobe region. The speakers who clutter also presented with attention deficit disorder; thus, it was difficult to determine the extent to which the participants' performance on the various tasks were associated with cluttering.

More recently, Howell and Davis (2011) reported data on several measures of auditory functioning in a group of 96 children with impaired fluency. Participants with cluttered speech ($n = 17$) did not differ from participants with stuttered speech in terms of their history of otitis media with effusion (OME) or pure-tone thresholds under three masking conditions.

Autism Spectrum Disorders

Symptoms of cluttering have been identified in the speech of some individuals with Asperger syndrome. Characteristics of Asperger syndrome include impaired functioning in social interaction, behavioral patterns that are restricted or repetitive, and significant occupational and social disability (Scaler Scott, 2008). Unlike autism, however, there is an absence of clinically significant cognitive or language impairment. Scaler Scott (2011) summarized findings from her 2008 dissertation in which she examined the speech characteristics of 12 children with Asperger syndrome and found that 3 of them met definitional criteria for either cluttering or cluttering-stuttering. A main characteristic of cluttering in the three children was speech rate that was perceived as rapid or irregular. Scaler Scott (2011) also discussed evidence of excessive coarticulation and atypical pause patterns among individuals with autism spectrum disorder.

Etiology of Cluttering

Early Views on Etiology

In his classic text on cluttering, Weiss (1964) offered what was, at the time, the most extensive exploration of cluttering etiology. At the time he published his textbook, understanding of the neurological and psycholinguistic bases of normal and disordered speech production was much more limited than the current knowledge bases in these areas. Thus, his views on etiology must be interpreted with the context of how speech-language functioning was understood at the time.

Weiss (1964) viewed cluttering as a hereditary disorder. Although data on the epidemiology of cluttering were very limited in the 1960s (and still are today), he noted that many of the clients he treated for clutter-like concerns reported having other family members, including parents, who spoke similarly. Weiss (1964) noted that although people who clutter do not present with frank signs of neurological impairment, the disorder nonetheless has an "organic flavor." He noted that a speaker who clutters often can alleviate the symptoms of cluttering by focusing attention on the speech production process, and when a speaker does not attend to how he or she talks, the symptoms worsen. Such a profile, he claimed, is more consistent with an organically based disorder than it is with a psychologically based disorder. Ultimately, Weiss said that cluttering most

accurately is conceptualized as an "inborn weakness" in the ability to communicate, and, as such, it falls along a continuum that ranges from normal fluency at one end to complete dysfunction at the other end.

In Weiss's (1964) view, cluttering was a manifestation of *central language imbalance*. Weiss (p. 9) defined central language imbalance as a deficiency in a speaker's "sense of harmony in language functions," and he stated that this condition could give rise to a host of problems, including delayed speech, disorders of reading and writing, disorders in musicality, and, of course, cluttering. He proposed that the extent of central language imbalance varied from person to person.

Weiss (1964, pp. 7–14) readily acknowledged that the underlying mechanisms of his central language imbalance hypothesis could not be studied with the technology of his era. Consequently, he offered several possibilities about what the source of a central language imbalance might be. These included the following:

- *Dysfunction in the striatum* (a region of the basal ganglia) that results from microscopic lesions.
- *Neurodevelopmental immaturity,* which is characterized by an extended period of neuroplasticity.
- *Dysfunction in cortical regions that are involved in speech planning and regulation.* Weiss cited data showing that electrical stimulation of the thalamus results in acceleration of speech rate and that electrical stimulation of Brodmann's area 6 (the premotor and supplementary motor areas) on the mesial surface of the brain elicited repetitions in speech.
- *A deficit in the ability to utilize proprioceptive feedback from*

articulatory structures and/or auditory feedback during ongoing speech.

In some respects, Weiss's (1964) ideas about the etiology of cluttering and fluency impairment, in general, were remarkably prescient, as subsequent research has provided support for the roles of neurodevelopment, basal ganglia functioning, proprioception, and auditory feedback in the attainment of normally fluent speech and in the symptoms of stuttered speech.

Contemporary Views on Etiology

Etiological models for cluttering received little attention between 1964 and 2000. Since then, however, several revised views of cluttering etiological models have been proposed.

Alm's Neurological Perspective

Impaired neurological functioning has been implicated in cluttering for some time. For instance, Luchsinger and Landolt (cited in Weiss, 1964) reported electroencephalographic (EEG) abnormalities in "almost 100 percent of their . . . cluttering sample." In this vein, Alm (2011) proposed a hypothetical neurological framework for explaining cluttered speech. Alm argued that although the core of cluttered speech appears to be fast and dysrhythmic speech, the disorder more accurately is viewed as a constellation of symptoms. That is, there are numerous symptoms of cluttering, but few clients present all of the possible symptoms.

In Alm's (2011) model, the core symptoms of cluttering implicate dysfunction in the medial wall of left frontal lobe. Alm noted that the medial wall of the left frontal lobe has been linked to the motivation to speak, sentence planning (especially aspects of syntax and phonology), execution of sequential motor activities, and monitoring of speech output. Cluttered speech is characterized by deficits in each of those aspects of performance. In Alm's model, areas within the region that have particular relevance to cluttering include the following:

- *Anterior cingulate cortex* (ACC): Alm (2011) stated that this area has an executive function (e.g., it is associated with the initiation of voluntary movements as well as willful attention and error monitoring). He noted that the ACC is involved in volitional control, including the suppression of behavior, making decisions under conditions of uncertainty, and the maintenance of willful attention for tasks such as error monitoring; and it has been implicated as an area of dysfunction in cases of attention deficit disorder. Consistent with these functions, Alm noted that the ACC receives input from a variety of areas, including the limbic, motor, and auditory systems. Accordingly, Alm characterized the ACC as a "hub" or an integration center.
- *Supplementary motor area* (SMA): In Alm's (2011) model, the SMA is viewed as an "assembly center," as it is associated with retrieving linguistic information from lateral regions of the left temporal and frontal lobes as well as controlling the timing of articulation through inputs from the basal ganglia and cerebellum and monitoring

utterance production through input from the auditory cortex. Alm noted that, like the ACC, the SMA has affective, cognitive, and motor divisions.

- *Presupplementary motor area*: Alm noted that the preSMA has been linked with aspects of phrase assembly such as word selection, word form selection, and word sequencing. It also has been linked to speech error detection.
- *Basal ganglia*: The basal ganglia have a variety of functions, but with regard to cluttered speech, Alm (2011) emphasized the role of this region in word selection and regulation of speech timing.

Alm (2011) proposed that the symptoms of cluttering are consistent with dysfunction (i.e., hyperactivation, dysregulation) of the medial wall of the frontal lobe that occurs secondary to a lack of inhibitory input to this region from the basal ganglia due to a hyperactive dopamine system. In other words, many of the key symptoms of cluttering (i.e., excessive drive to talk, disrupted message sequencing, mistimed message delivery, and a reduced ability to sustain attention and monitor performance) are consistent with the presence of excessive amounts of the neurotransmitter dopamine (i.e., a *hyperdopaminergic state*). This hypothesis leads to the question of why a hyperdopaminergic state exists. Researchers have not yet offered possible answers to that question in relation to cluttering, and it remains to be seen whether disease or genetic variation might lead to neurodevelopmental problems in the dopamine system. Nonetheless, models such as the one that Alm developed offer a use-

ful roadmap that others can use to guide future research efforts.

Motor Control Considerations

As indicated in the preceding section, contemporary models of cluttered speech assign a central role to the motor system. Data on the speech motor performance of speakers who clutter are limited. Ward (2011) summarized findings from a study that he recently had completed in which five speakers who cluttered exhibited significantly shorter voice onset times than normally fluent speakers and speakers who stutter did during specific CV sequences within conversational speech. This finding is consistent with the notion of coarticulation anomalies in cluttered speech. There were no differences across the groups in vowel duration, however.

Hartinger and Moosehammer (2009) examined the spatiotemporal characteristics of articulatory movements in three speakers who clutter. They detected evidence of speech motor control deficits in the speakers who clutter during the articulation of multisyllable words. In the study, the speakers who cluttered exhibited greater variability in the amplitude and duration of tongue blade movements, as well as reduced range of movement. Ward (2011) noted the similarities between the motor performance of these speakers who clutter and speakers with Parkinson's disease. A final point that warrants discussion: The cluttering literature is replete with claims that speakers who clutter exhibit more clumsiness and motor coordination difficulties than noncluttering speakers do. The support for this claim is largely anecdotal, however, and requires further assessment before considering it an etiological model of cluttering.

Ward's Motor Speech Processing Perspective

Ward (2011) discussed a multifactor model of cluttering that is consistent with Alm's (2011) view on the nature of cluttering. Ward's model includes four potential points of impairment that could account for cluttering symptoms.

1. *Linguistic planning:* Inclusion of this component in a model of cluttering is based on the substantial number of cluttering speakers with deficits in pragmatics and syntactic formulation.
2. *Motor planning:* Inclusion of this component is based on the nonsystematic speech sound sequencing errors that some speakers who clutter exhibit.
3. *Speech motor programming:* Inclusion of this component in Ward's model of cluttering is based on the substantial number of cluttering speakers who show imprecision in the execution of speech movements.
4. *Speech motor execution:* Inclusion of this component in Ward's model of cluttering is based on the similarities that exist between cluttered speech and speech patterns seen in some forms of dysarthria (particularly the hypokinetic dysarthria that is associated with Parkinson's disease).

Summary

Cluttering has long been recognized as a disorder that negatively impacts verbal communication. Although cluttering is customarily categorized as a fluency disorder; in some cases (and some would argue *many* cases), it arguably could be classified instead as an articulation or language disorder, or perhaps as a syndrome that affects fluency, articulation, language, as well as motor functioning and cognitive processes such as self-monitoring and attention.

The many and varied symptoms that are associated with the disorder have complicated efforts to generate a standard definition for cluttering. The lack of a standard definition in combination with the disorder's relatively low incidence may explain why the research base for cluttering is more limited than that for stuttering and many other communication disorders. Much of what is known about cluttering comes from anecdotal clinical data and case reports, retrospective caseload analyses, and authoritative assertions. In recent years, authorities on cluttering have increasingly emphasized the need to conduct group-level studies that feature either carefully matched groups (e.g., cluttering versus typical fluency) or randomized assignment of participants to experimental and control groups.

The fluency characteristics of cluttered speech have been reasonably well detailed. It is widely agreed that the disfluency types seen in cluttering differ from those seen in stuttering. Although disfluency frequency in cluttered speech may not be high in a numerical sense, speech still can sound very disfluent because of the tendency for speakers who clutter to produce lengthy, maze-like disfluencies. Stuttering and cluttering sometimes coexist, and when they do, a speaker's disfluency pattern can be expected to feature disfluency types that typify both disorders. Excessive articulation rate has emerged in recent years as a primary (and to some authors, *obligatory*) symptom for diagnosing cluttering. Bursts of especially rapid sounding speech have been linked to overly coarticulated speech sound production and during such stretches of speech, speech intelligibility often is reduced. The continuity and rate qualities of cluttered speech disrupt speech rhythm and naturalness. Concomitant difficulties in language, particularly syntax and pragmatics, can lead to problems in message formulation and organization. A counter position to the "cluttering-as-rate-disorder" is that cluttering fundamentally is a type of language impairment.

Epidemiological data on cluttering are limited, but it appears that the disorder is less common than stuttering and that, when cluttering is present, it is not uncommon for it to co-occur with stuttering rather than presenting in a "pure" form. There is even limited evidence that the two disorders sometimes may unfold consecutively, such that clutter-like speech during childhood transforms into stutter-like speech by adolescence (Howell & Davis, 2011; Van Riper, 1971).

Many aspects of cluttering are understudied, but one area that is in particular need of research is the effect that cluttering has on the quality of life. To date, there are few first-hand personal and caregiver accounts that describe the effects of cluttering-associated disability on daily life (e.g., Dewey, 2010; Wong, 2010). These reports suggest that the effects of the disorder are significant particularly when combined with the effects of whatever coexisting disorders a person might have (e.g., learning disability, ADHD). In other sections of this text, we discuss issues related to assessment and treatment with people who clutter. Clearly, there is plenty of work left to do with regard to advancing the understanding of cluttering from both a basic science and a rehabilitation science perspective.

9

Other Patterns of Disfluency

The focus in the preceding chapters has been on well-known fluency problems; that is, stuttering and cluttering. The focus in the present chapter is on disfluency patterns that are associated with other clinical populations. For the most part, these disfluency patterns are distinct from those seen in stuttering and cluttering. Many of the fluency-related behaviors discussed in this chapter occur in conjunction with some other developmental impairment that adversely affects language, speech, and/or cognitive functioning. As such, the fluency difficulties discussed in this chapter often are not the client's most pressing concern.

Fluency and Developmental Language Impairment

The first issue to be discussed concerns the fluency patterns that are observed in conjunction with developmental language impairments that are observed in some children. Several researchers have examined this issue in school-aged children, and a few have examined it with preschool-aged children. In these studies, researchers have used many terms to describe children's language difficulties, including the following: *delayed language* (Merits-Patterson & Reed, 1981); *language learning disability* (MacLachlan & Chapman, 1988; Scott & Windsor, 2000); *specific language impairment* (Guo, Tomblin, & Samelson, 2008), and *specific expressive language impairment* (Boscolo, Bernstein Ratner, & Rescorla, 2002). A common inclusion criterion across all of the studies is that the research participants have scored significantly below age-level expectations on at least one and, usually, several formal measures of language performance. In most studies, analysis of speech fluency has addressed the frequency and types of disfluency that speakers produce. In some studies, however, researchers have examined variables related to verbal output.

Frequency and Types of Disfluency in Developmental Language Impairment

Although findings from the research literature have been mixed, the overall pattern of results suggests that children with developmental language impairment are, on average, less fluent than children who exhibit typically developing language. This is not to say that children with language disorders routinely stutter or clutter, but they do appear to lack the relatively seamless continuity of speech production that children with proficient language skills exhibit.

Effects of Language Impairment on Fluency Performance

MacLachlan and Chapman (1988) examined fluency characteristics in a group of seven children with language learning disability (LLD) during both conversation and narration. The children in the LLD group were 9- to 11-years old, with normal nonverbal intelligence. Each of the children exhibited deficits in more than one aspect of language-related functioning. Deficit areas included language comprehension, language production, word retrieval, reading, verbal reasoning, and auditory memory. The fluency performance of the LLD children was compared to the fluency performance of seven chronologically age-matched controls and seven language age-matched controls. The groups were compared on the frequency with which they produced four types of disfluency: (1) *stalls* (i.e., interjections and part-word, whole-word, and phrase repetition); (2) *repairs* (i.e., revisions of syntactic, semantic, and phonologic errors); (3) *abandoned* utterances; and (4) *other* types of disfluency. MacLachlan and Chapman hypothesized that the LLD group would exhibit higher levels of disfluency in narration than in conversation because narration features more complex syntax and greater organizational requirements than conversation does, and during narration, speakers are less able to draw upon discourse support from a speaking partner than they are during conversation.

MacLachlan and Chapman (1988) found significant differences in the frequency with which the children produced stalls and repairs. Overall, all children were more disfluent during narration than during conversation, and disfluency frequency increased as a function of utterance length. Unlike the two control groups, the LLD children showed a trend toward a proportionally greater difference in disfluency frequency during conversation than during narration. In addition, the ratio of interjections to repetitions in the LLD group was significantly greater than it was in the language age-matched control group. Thus, when LLD children "stalled" in speech, they did so through the use of interjection more often than the younger, language age-matched controls did. MacLachlan and Chapman originally reported disfluency data in terms of disfluencies per utterance and data were subdivided according to utterance length. Because of this, it is not possible to compare their disfluency frequency data to those from most studies in the fluency disorders literature. Still, it is possible to approximate the "per 100 words" disfluency frequency based on the information they presented. It appears that during conversation, the combined frequency of stalls and repairs for the LLD group was between 3.00 and 6.00 per 100 words, depending on the utterance length. During conversation, however, the combined frequency of stalls and repairs for the LLD group was between 8.60 and 11.50 per 100 words, again depending on the utterance length. The disfluency frequency scores for the LLD group during narration were about 70% to 90% greater than those in the two control groups. Given the small sample size in the study and variations in disfluency across participants within groups, these frequency scores should be interpreted cautiously.

In several other studies, researchers have examined fluency performance in speakers with specific language impairment. Children in the latter studies presented deficits in communication that were limited to language usage, particularly expressive language usage. Boscolo et al. (2002) examined fluency performance during a basic narrative task with 22 pairs of 9-year-old children. In each of the pairs, one of the children had a history of specific expressive language impairment and the other had a typical language development history. The children with a history of expressive language impairment produced narratives that were significantly less complex in structure than the narratives from the typical children. The researchers also compared the groups on total disfluency frequency, the frequency of "stutter-like disfluency" (defined in the study as part-word repetitions, sound prolongations, blocks, and "tension pauses"), and the frequency of "normal disfluency" (defined as whole-word and phrase repetitions, revisions, and interjections). The children in the language-impaired group produced significantly more total disfluency and significantly more stutter-like disfluency than children with typical language development did. The observed disfluency frequencies for both groups were relatively low for both groups, however (for total disfluencies: the control group produced 3.3 disfluencies per 100 words and the language-impaired group produced 4.56 disfluencies per 100 words; for stutter-like disfluencies: the control group

produced 0.33 disfluencies per 100 words and the language-impaired group produced 0.76 disfluencies per 100 words). Boscolo et al. suggested that the greater disfluency in the children with a history of expressive language impairment might be evidence of "persistent subtle difficulty with language formulation."

In a another study of school-aged children, Guo et al. (2008) examined fluency performance in 60 fourth-grade children: 20 children with specific language impairment (SLI), 20 typically developing children who were matched to the SLI children by chronological age (CA-matched), and 20 typically developing children who were matched to the SLI children by language age (LA-matched). Guo et al. compared the groups on the number and duration of silent pauses produced and also on the frequency of what they termed "vocal hesitation rates." The latter consisted of familiar disfluency types such as filled pauses (e.g., "um"), interjections (e.g., "well"), whole-word repetitions, part-word repetitions, and revisions. The findings revealed that the children with SLI produced more total fluency disruptions than the children who were matched for chronological age but not more than the children who were matched for language age—a finding that supports the idea that disfluency in language-disordered children is related to the process of linguistic formulation. There were no significant differences among the groups in the frequency of vocal hesitations, and the total frequency of disfluency for all three groups was relatively modest (i.e., 4 per 100 words for the CA-matched group, and 5 per 100 words for both the SLI group and the LA-matched group).

Guo et al. (2008) also examined four categories of silent pauses, which were defined by duration; that is, 250 to 500 ms, 500 to 1000 ms, 1000 to 2000 ms, and greater than 2000 ms. The SLI group differed from the CA-matched control group only in the frequency of 500 to 1000 ms pauses. Also, the SLI group was much more likely to produce speech disruptions at the start of syntactic phrases than the CA-matched group was. The two groups did not, however, differ in the frequency with which they produced silent pauses before words, clauses, or sentences. For all three groups in their study, the 500 to 1000 ms silent pauses occurred most often and pauses more than 2000 ms occurred least often. Guo et al. again interpreted these results as supporting the idea that, with SLI, a child's speech disruptions are related to his or her language ability. The relatively high frequency of intermediate-length pausing in the SLI group and the positioning of these pauses at the start of phrases were posited to be symptomatic of a deficit in activating syntactic frames and/or associated lexical items.

Fluency and Language Therapy

Merits-Patterson and Reed (1981) examined fluency performance in 27 children who were between 4 and 6 years old. Nine of the children had been diagnosed with language delay, as evidenced by low scores on formal tests of language development, and were enrolled in language therapy. Another nine children similarly had been diagnosed with language delay but had not yet commenced language therapy. The remaining nine children had normal language functioning and served as a control group. Merits-Patterson and Reed elicited speech samples from the children using a combination of picture description and play-based conversation. Analysis of the speech samples revealed that the language-delayed children who were receiving therapy were significantly more disfluent (6.6 total disfluencies per 100 words) than both the language-delayed children who were not receiving therapy (3.08 total disfluencies per 100 words) and the control group (3.36 total disfluencies per 100 words). Additional analysis showed that the language-delayed children who were receiving therapy produced significantly more whole- and part-word repetitions than the other two groups did. Merits-Patterson and Reed suggested that the elevated disfluency frequency in the language therapy group might have reflected the children's incomplete mastery of recently learned linguistic forms or, possibly, "communicative pressures" that arise during language therapy activities.

Disfluency Subtypes in Children With Language Impairment

Hall, Yamashita, and Aram (1993) examined the fluency performance of 60 preschool-aged children (mean age = 4;5) who had developmental language disorders. Each of the children showed a discrepancy of at least one standard deviation between their nonverbal intelligence score and their global language functioning score. Analysis of group data revealed the presence of a subgroup of 10 children who produced substantially more disfluency than the remaining 50 children in the group. While the "typical fluency" subgroup of 50 children produced only 3.59 disfluencies per 100 words, the "high disfluency" subgroup produced an average of 14.39 disfluencies per 100 syllables. Although most of the disfluency in the high disfluency subgroup was "nonstutter-like" in nature, the average number of stutter-like disfluencies in the high disfluency subgroup (4.59 per 100 words) was substantially higher than that seen among both typically developing children and the typical fluency subgroup of language-impaired children. Post hoc analysis showed that the high disfluency subgroup was significantly older than the other children in the study and that they also scored significantly higher on formal tests of receptive and expressive vocabulary. Given the small sample size in the high disfluency subgroup, the findings should be viewed cautiously, but they are suggestive of a link between children's language competence and their speech fluency.

Rispoli's (2003) study of speech disfluency in typically developing children provides additional support for a link between a child's fluency and the types of syntactic forms he or she is attempting to produce. Rispoli analyzed data from children who ranged from 22 to 48 months old. He found a moderate, positive correlation between a child's level of grammatical development and frequency of sentence revisions. More specifically, he found that as children's grammatical proficiency increased, they attempted to say increasingly complicated utterances, and when doing so, the frequency with which they produced revisions increased as well. Disfluency types that involved "stalling" (e.g., interjecting, repeating) were not significantly correlated with grammatical development and thus were viewed as arising from the formulation or production of a specific utterance, rather than the child's background level of language proficiency.

Hall (1999) compared the number and nature of speech fluency disruptions in two groups of children with SLI. One group of children presented with only SLI; the other group presented with SLI plus disordered phonology (DP). In this study, the total frequency of disfluency for the two groups was comparable (10.00 per 100 words for the SLI-only group and 12.22 per 100 words for the SLI+DP group. Children in the SLI+DP group did, however, exhibit about twice as much variation in the total frequency of disfluencies they produced as the children in the SLI-only group did. In addition, when subcategories of disfluency were examined, children in the SLI+DP group exhibited a significantly greater frequency of "stutter-like disfluency" than children in the SLI-only group did (i.e., 3.11 per 100 words versus 0.33 per 100 words, respectively). As with total disfluency frequency, the frequency of stutter-like disfluency was more variable in the SLI+DP group than it was in the SLI-only group.

Role of Language Learning and Acquisition

As noted earlier, Boscolo et al. (2002) studied fluency patterns in typically developing children and children with specific language impairment. The two groups did not differ in their frequency of "normal disfluency" types (typical group: 3.3 per 100 words; SLI group: 3.8 per 100 words), and analysis of the frequency for individual disfluency types failed to differentiate the groups, as well. There were some subtle differences between the groups, however. For example, 78% of the children in the SLI group produced one or more stutter-like disfluency (versus 52% of the children in the typical language group). The frequency of stutter-like disfluency was quite low for both groups (0.76 per 100 words for the children in the SLI group, 0.33 per 100 words for the typical group) but still significantly different in a statistical sense. Although the SLI group produced more stutter-like disfluency than the typical group, none of the children in the group were judged to exhibit developmental stuttering. Given the absence of excessive physical tension during the stutter-like disfluency, Boscolo et al. speculated that these disfluency types were associated with processes related to language formulation.

Other researchers (e.g., Prelock & Panagos, 1989) have documented fluency differences between language-impaired children and typically developing children during production of sentences of varying syntactic complexity. Similar to findings with children who stutter (e.g., Bernstein Ratner & Sih, 1987; Logan & Conture, 1997), language-impaired children show a disproportionate increase in disfluency frequency relative to typically developing children during production of grammatically complex sentences. In a study of four Spanish-speaking "disphasic" children who ranged from 6;0 to 8;10 in age, Navarro-Ruiz and Rallo-Fabra (2001) reported findings that were consistent with those from English-speaking, language-impaired children: The children produced more disfluency during narration than conversation, and they demonstrated greater use of stutter-like disfluency such as word repetition. In addition, the language-impaired children in the study were less likely to repair language errors and more likely to completely abandon utterances than the normally functioning children were.

Fluency as a Measure of Reading Performance

The main focus in this textbook is on speech fluency during spontaneously formulated language contexts such as conversation and narration. Another speaking context that warrants consideration, however, is reading. In the fluency disorders literature, data on fluency during reading deal primarily with the continuity or rate with which a person with a fluency disorder reads a printed passage aloud. The speaker's performance during passage reading then is compared to that of a nonfluency-impaired speaker. Such an approach is appropriate for use with proficient readers; however, it does not account for fluency-related difficulties that a reader might exhibit as part of learning to read or reading-related difficulties that result from having a reading impairment that is independent of a disorder of speech fluency such as stuttering or cluttering. Thus, the notion of fluency within the context of normal reading development and reading disability are discussed within the present section.

Defining Reading Fluency

In the reading arena, the notion of fluency has been defined as "freedom from word identification problems that might hinder comprehension" (Harris & Hodges, 1995, p. 85). Fluency has come to be a primary construct in the measurement of children's reading proficiency (Breznitz, 2006; Hasbrouck & Tindal, 2006; Pikulski & Chard, 2005; Rasinski, 2012). The notion of fluency in reading has evolved steadily during the past 30 to 40 years. Perfetti

(1985) discussed fluency as the product of a reader's decoding accuracy, reading rate, and comprehension level for the text. Chall (1983) linked reading fluency to a child's developing proficiency with word decoding and automaticity in word recognition. In this view, children learn to read words accurately and, with practice, develop the ability to recognize words automatically; that is, without having to implement word decoding skills. Eventually, a proficient reader comes to process printed words as orthographic units; that is, as integrated visual units.

Professionals who work in the area of reading make a distinction between reading fluency and reading comprehension. In other words, the ability to read quickly does not necessarily equate with the ability to understand what one is reading (Rasinski, 2012). Reading comprehension is the primary functional outcome that beginning readers seek to attain; however, researchers have found a link between reading fluency and reading comprehension (Hasbrouck & Tindal, 2006). In current models of reading performance, the ability to recognize printed words in a rapid, accurate manner is essential to attaining comprehension, as it allows the reader to attend to the meaning of what is being read rather than to deciphering what the words are (Nathan & Stanovich, 1991; Rasinski, 2012). Several experts have described reading fluency as a bridge between word recognition accuracy and comprehension (Pikulski & Chard, 2005; Rasinski, 2012).

Reading Development

The development of reading often is described as a staged process. Ehri (1995) described a developmental sequence characterized by four primary phases:

1. *Pre-alphabetic phase:* a child at this level does not yet show letter-to-sound correspondence but does demonstrate the ability to link graphic symbols such as the logo for a restaurant to the name of the restaurant;

2. *Partial alphabetic phase:* a child at this level realizes that printed letters are related to spoken speech sounds and uses some of the letters within a printed word (usually the first and the last letters) to generate a prediction for what the word might be;

3. *Fully alphabetic phase:* a child at this level has a well-developed understanding of letter-to-sound correspondence and uses that skill to decode novel words through sound blending. The process of grapheme-to-phoneme mapping results in the development of "sight words"—letter sequences that the child recognizes instantly. A child's growing repertoire of sight words assists with decoding words that are spelled irregularly and with handling the "many-to-one" mapping that is characteristic of many alphabet systems. (For example, in English, the letter "c" can be linked to [s] or [k], depending on the word in which it occurs.); and

4. *Consolidated alphabetic phase:* At this stage, the reader can recognize whole-word sequences instantly. In addition, common multiletter sequences such as those associated with bound morphological affixes (e.g., *-ing, -tion*) and orthographic minimal pairs (e.g., *hat, bat, sat*) are recognized as a single unit. The act of processing letter sequences in chunks of this sort

presumably reduces the reader's processing load and allows for allocation of attentional resources toward processing the meaning of a text. At this point, the reader essentially has attained automaticity and has access to advanced decoding strategies for dealing with novel words.

Chall (1983) stated that, for most children, reading fluency is attained at approximately grade 2 or 3, which is around the time that they make the transition from "learning to read" to "reading to learn."

Approaches to Assessing Reading Fluency

Reading Rate

A basic approach to documenting a reader's fluency is to compute the number of words that are read per unit of time. This approach is analogous to the computation of speech rate during tasks that incorporate spoken oral language. Two main measures can be made (Rathvon, 2004):

- *Words read per minute.* This approach entails the computation of the number of words read per minute. It is computed by dividing the total number of words in the passage by the time in seconds taken to read the passage, and then multiplying by 60. (In studies with speakers who stutter, this is the approach that most researchers have used.)
- *Words read correctly per minute.* This approach entails the computation of the number of words read correctly per minute. In the context of reading assessment,

the number of words read correctly per minute is regarded as the more meaningful of the two rate measures because of its strong correlation with reading comprehension (Hasbrouck & Tindal, 2006). It is computed by dividing the total number of correctly read words in the passage by the time in seconds taken to read the passage, and then multiplying by 60. (This is approach is widely used in educational settings to document the skills of developing readers.)

Rate-based measures often are computed using a *curriculum-based assessment* (CBM) model in which several graded reading passages from a local school curriculum are used as materials. The child's reading rate is determined by averaging performance across two or more reading passages. The reading passages are analogous to topic- or situation-based speech samples that are used to assess speech fluency during conversation or narration.

Hasbrouck and Tindal (2006) published national norms for oral reading fluency (Table 9–1). The oral reading rates are reported in terms of *words correct per minute,* and they span grades 1 through 8. The norms are based on methods associated with curriculum-based assessment, wherein a child reads an unfamiliar passage aloud for one minute. The examiner records the total number of words that the child has read and then subtracts the number of words read incorrectly from that total. This yields the number of words correct per minute. As shown in Table 9–1, percentile ranks are reported at three points in the academic year (fall, winter, spring) and consist of oral reading fluency rates that correspond to the

Table 9–1. Hasbrouck and Tindal's (2006) Oral Reading Fluency Norms, Presented by Grade-Level and Time of Academic Year

Grade	Percentile	Fall WCPM	Winter WCPM	Spring WCPM
1	90		81	111
	75		47	82
	50		23	53
	25	—	12	28
	10		6	15
	SD		32	39
	Count		16,950	19,434
2	90	106	125	142
	75	79	100	117
	50	51	72	89
	25	25	42	61
	10	11	18	31
	SD	37	41	42
	Count	15,896	18,229	20,128
3	90	128	146	162
	75	99	120	137
	50	71	92	107
	25	44	62	78
	10	21	36	48
	SD	40	43	44
	Count	16,988	17,383	18,372
4	90	145	166	180
	75	119	139	152
	50	94	112	123
	25	68	87	98
	10	45	61	72
	SD	40	41	43
	Count	16,523	14,572	16,269
5	90	166	182	194
	75	139	156	168
	50	110	127	139
	25	85	99	109
	10	61	74	83
	SD	45	44	45
	Count	16,212	13,331	15,292
6	90	177	195	204
	75	153	167	177
	50	127	140	150
	25	98	111	122
	10	68	82	93
	SD	42	45	44
	Count	10,520	9,218	11,290

continues

Table 9–1. *continued*

Grade	Percentile	Fall WCPM	Winter WCPM	Spring WCPM
7	90	180	192	202
	75	156	165	177
	50	128	136	150
	25	102	109	123
	10	79	88	98
	SD	40	43	41
	Count	6,482	4,058	5,998
8	90	185	199	199
	75	161	173	177
	50	133	146	151
	25	106	115	124
	10	77	84	97
	SD	43	45	41
	Count	5,546	3,496	5,335

Note. WCPM = words read correctly per minute; *SD* = standard deviation; *Count* = number of student scores.

Source: The Reading Teacher by International Reading Association; Oral reading fluency norms: A valuable assessment tool for reading teachers, J. Hasbrouck & G. A. Tindal, Vol. 59, No. 7, 2006. Reproduced with permission of INTERNATIONAL READING ASSOCIATION in the format Republish in a book via Copyright Clearance Center.

10th, 25th, 50th, 75th, and 90th percentiles for each point in the academic year across the grade levels. As indicated in the "count" rows of Table 9–1, the data are based on large samples of readers at each interval. The norming sample included children from all ability levels and 23 American states. Hasbrouck and Tindal state that the oral reading fluency measure is useful as a screening tool to identify children who may need additional or individualized reading instruction and as a diagnostic tool for determination of a student's instructional reading level. When combined with other assessment instruments, the oral reading fluency data also can be used to diagnose reading disability and to document changes in reading performance over time.

Another means of computing reading rate is through an approach called Repeated Reading (Samuels, 1979). With this approach, a student is timed while reading a passage aloud. If the student's reading rate is below a predetermined criterion (e.g., 85 words per minute), he or she is directed to practice rereading the passage silently either with or without the benefit of listening to an audio recording of the passage. The student then repeats the oral reading assessment and, if the criterion still is not met, he or she completes the silent rereading/practice process again and continues doing so until the criterion is met. Samuels (1979) demonstrated that such an approach is effective at increasing reading rate and decreasing errors in word recognition. As such, it is effective at measuring the changes that a struggling reader can realize after practicing a passage multiple times.

There is an assortment of standardized tests and formalized procedures for assessing reading fluency in kindergarten through elementary-school-aged children. A complete listing of these assessment procedures is beyond the scope of this chapter; however, examples of two such instruments are provided below:

- *Fox in a Box* (CTB/McGraw-Hill, 2014). This assessment tool can be used for students in Grades 1 and 2. Fluency assessment is conducted using graded passages, which the child reads aloud. The child's performance is evaluated on a 3-point, criterion-referenced scale. Other portions of the tool examine phonemic awareness, phonics, vocabulary, and reading comprehension.
- *Gray Oral Reading Tests-5* (GORT-5; Wiederholt & Bryant, 2012). This assessment tool is normed on children ages 6;0 to 23;11. Thus, it is appropriate for students at elementary school through college levels. Fluency assessment is conducted using graded passages, which the examinee reads aloud. The examinee's performance is evaluated in terms of rate and accuracy, and these data are used to generate a reading fluency score.

Multidimensional Rubrics of Reading Fluency

Several holistic scoring rubrics have been developed to document reading development. One such scale is the *Oral Reading Fluency Scale* (National Center for Education Statistics, 2002). As shown in Table 9–2, this scale features a four-part classification in which fluency is rated on the basis of prosody, vocal expression, word accuracy, and correction of reading errors.

A second example of a holistic scoring rubric for reading development is the

Table 9–2. The *Oral Reading Fluency Scale* (National Center for Education Statistics, 2002)

Level	Characteristics
4	Reads primarily in larger, meaningful phrase groups. Although some regressions, repetitions, and deviations from text may be present, those do not appear to detract from the overall structure of the story. Preservation of the author's syntax is consistent. Some or most of the story is read with expressive interpretation.
3	Reads primarily in three- or four-word phrase groups. Some smaller groupings may be present. However, the majority of phrasing seems appropriate and preserves the syntax of the author. Little or no expressive interpretation is present.
2	Reads primarily in two-word phrases with some three- or four-word groupings. Some word-by-word reading may be present. Word groupings may seem awkward and unrelated to the larger context of sentence or passage.
1	Reads primarily word by word. Occasional two- or three-word phrases may occur, but these are infrequent and/or they do not preserve meaningful syntax.

Note: The scale captures developmental aspects of a child's reading through descriptions of phrasing, accuracy, and vocal expression. Levels 1 and 2 correspond to "Nonfluent" oral reading; Levels 3 and 4 correspond to "Fluent" oral reading.

Source: U.S. Department of Education, Institute of Education Sciences, National Center for Education Statistics, National Assessment of Educational Progress (NAEP), 2002 Oral Reading Study.

Multidimensional Fluency Scale (Zutell & Rasinski, 1991). The scale utilizes a three-part model of reading fluency: *phrasing*, *smoothness*, and *pace*. Each of these dimensions is rated on a 4-point scale, and the scale points for each dimension are accompanied by descriptive criteria. Zutell and Rasinski reported high interjudge reliability for the scale, and the overall score for the scale is moderately correlated with scores on standardized reading assessments at grades 3 and 5 (Walker, Mokhtari, & Sargent, 2006).

Fluency in Impaired Readers

There are several factors that contribute to the development of reading fluency. Included among these are the following: (1) the proportion of words in text that the reader is able to recognize by sight, (2) individual variations in the speed with which sight words are processed, (3) the speed with which the reader is able to use decoding processes to identify novel words, (4) the reader's ability to use linguistic context in facilitating word identification, and (5) the speed with which the reader can access word meanings (Chard, Pikulski, & McDonagh, 2006). Poor readers take longer to recognize printed words than typically developing readers do and must be exposed to printed words for a longer amount of time than typical readers in order to recognize them by sight (Breznitz, 2006). Other background language skills such as the size of the reader's receptive lexicon, and his or her knowledge of syntactic rules and skills in phonological awareness, pragmatics, and cognitive processing (e.g., memory, attention) play a role in reading fluency as well.

A child's reading performance can be affected by the difficulty of the text that he or she attempts to read. Traditionally, experts in reading (e.g., Gickling & Armstrong, 1978) have identified three reading levels in this regard. *Frustration level* is characterized by word identification accuracy below 93%. At this level, reading is likely to proceed at a slow rate and comprehension is likely to be poor. *Instructional level* features a word identification accuracy of 93% to 97%. With accuracy levels in this range, the reader can benefit from instruction but should demonstrate adequate comprehension nonetheless. Lastly, an *independent level* of reading is characterized by word identification accuracy of 98% or greater. With accuracy levels in this range, the reader should be able to read without assistance and demonstrate excellent comprehension. Children spend more time on task when reading at instructional level than they do when reading at either frustration level or independent level (Gickling & Armstron, 1978; Treptow, Burns, & McComas, 2007); thus, it is is worthwhile to match developing readers with texts that are appropriate in terms of their difficulty.

Children's reading-based errors often lead to disfluency that mostly is similar in form to the disfluency that occurs in conversational speech. In the general population, the source of disfluency in oral reading often can be traced to difficulty that the reader is having in deciphering specific printed words or, perhaps, in generating a prosodic structure that accurately reflects the prosodic phrasing that is conveyed through punctuation in the printed text. Zutell and Rasinski (1991) noted the following types of disfluency during the oral reading of nonfluency-impaired children: pauses, hesitations, false starts, repetitions, "sound-outs," and multiple attempts at restarting a word or portion of a sentence. With the exception of sound-outs, wherein a reader purposively breaks a word into its phonemic constituents, each of these disfluency forms is noted in conversational speech. In reading-based assessments with speakers who stutter, the challenge is to separate disfluent events that reflect reading errors from those that reflect the speech production problems that underlie stuttering. This can be challenging to do when the surface characteristics of the child's reading- and stuttering-based disfluencies are similar.

Fluency and Intellectual Disability

A number of researchers have studied the speech fluency performance of individuals with intellectual disability. According to the American Association on Intellectual and Developmental Disabilities (AAIDD, 2013), *intellectual disability* is characterized by "significant limitations both in intellectual functioning (reasoning, learning, problem solving) and in adaptive behavior, which covers a range of everyday social and practical skills." Onset of the disability occurs before the age of 18 years. The AAIDD indicates that the term intellectual disability encompasses the "same population of individuals who were diagnosed previously with mental retardation" and that "every individual who is or was eligible for a diagnosis of mental retardation is eligible for a diagnosis of intellectual disability." In a clinical context, the notion of intellectual disability is defined in terms of performance on intelligence tests (i.e., intelligence quotient or IQ) as well as adaptive functioning in the areas of conceptual skills (e.g., language and literacy, time and money concepts), social skills (e.g., interpersonal skills, gullibility), and practical skills (occupational skills, personal care). Individuals with intellectual disability typically have significant limitations in both intellectual functioning and adaptive functioning.

The research literature on fluency performance in individuals with intellectual disability spans many decades. Bloodstein and Bernstein Ratner (2008) reviewed results from 15 studies that were published between 1912 and 1978. Consistent with societal policies of that era, most of the studies reported on individuals who lived in institutional settings. Thus, the sample sizes were generally large, often exceeding 200. One purpose in many of these studies was to determine the prevalence of stuttering among individuals with intellectual disability. Data in this regard were quite variable, with many researchers reporting prevalence rates in the 1% to 3% range (e.g., Chapman & Cooper, 1973; Sheehan, Martyn, & Kilburn, 1968), but others reporting prevalence rates of 10% or more (e.g., Schlanger & Gottsleben, 1957). Cooper (1986) reviewed many of these same studies and concluded that stuttering severity tended to worsen with an individual's degree of intellectual disability.

Another issue of interest concerns the extent to which the stutter-like patterns observed among individuals with intellectual disability are consistent with those observed in cases of developmental stuttering. Bonfanti and Culatta (1977) noted that many of the participants in their study were severely disfluent and that repetition tended to be the predominant type of disfluency. Many of the participants seemed aware that they stuttered but not particularly concerned about it, as evidenced by a relative lack of word substitution, word avoidance, and other symptoms that would suggest attempts to cope with impaired fluency. Other research has demonstrated that individuals with intellectual disability exhibit improvement in speech fluency when asked to say the same utterance several times in succession (a process often termed "adaptation"), but they are less likely than speakers who stutter to report expectancy for upcoming stuttering-related disfluency (Chapman & Cooper, 1973).

Naremore and Dever (1975) examined language and fluency characteristics of spoken narratives produced by a group of children who had intellectual impairment (IQ scores ranged from 74 to 84, and in the parlance of that era, they were described as "educable mentally retarded") and two comparison groups of typically developing children—one of which was matched for mental age and the other for chronological age. Analysis of the children's language performance indicated that normally developing children produced significantly more elaboration of subject and verb phrase constituents and greater use of subordination in sentence construction than the children in the intellectual disability group did. With regard to fluency, the children with intellectual disability showed a disfluency profile that was characterized by a higher frequency of repetition in comparison to the children in the control groups. The children in the control groups, however, exhibited a higher frequency of filled pauses (interjections) and false starts (revisions) than the children with intellectual impairment did.

Disfluency and Genetic Syndromes

Disfluency in Individuals With Down Syndrome

Fluency characteristics of individuals with Down syndrome have been studied since at least the 1950s. The reported prevalence rates for stuttering among people with Down syndrome are greater than 30% in several studies (Gottsleben, 1955; Preus, 1972; Schlanger & Gottsleben, 1957). Thus, stutter-like speech seems to be more common among people who have Down syndrome than it is among the general population. Rohovsky (cited in Kent & Vorperian, 2013). Reported that the prevalence of stuttering among individuals living in institutions was considerably higher that it was among individuals not living in institutions.

Some researchers have reported very high prevalence rates for cluttering among people with Down syndrome. For example, Preus (1972) found that nearly 32% of the participants with Down syndrome in the study met criteria for cluttering. More recently, Van Borsel and Vandermeulen (2008) assessed for the presence of cluttering using the *Predictive Cluttering Inventory* (PCI; Daly & Burnett, 1999) and found that nearly 80% of the participants with Down syndrome met the PCI's criterion for "possible cluttering."

Several of the classic types of disfluency have been noted to occur at relatively high frequencies in individuals with Down syndrome (Otto & Yairi, 1974; Preus, 1990). The extent to which individuals with Down syndrome use compensatory and associated behaviors (e.g., avoidance, rhythmic movements to facilitate fluency) has not been studied extensively. Preus (1990) reported that about 30% of the individuals with Down syndrome exhibit such behaviors Otto and Yairi (1974) reported that individuals with Down syndrome produced significantly more part-word repetitions, dysrhythmic phonations (e.g., sound prolongation), and physically tense disfluencies than fluent controls did. In contrast, the fluent controls produced significantly more interjections than the individuals with Down syndrome did. The overall disfluency frequency scores (i.e., total disfluency) for the two groups were not significantly different, however (Down syndrome group: $M = 8.78$, $SD = 5.72$; Control group: $M = 6.48$, $SD = 2.14$). As in cases of developmental stuttering, disfluencies involving repetitions, prolongations, and blocks were the predominate type observed in the Down syndrome group.

Several authorities have questioned whether the repetitions and prolongations that individuals with Down syndrome produce truly are similar to those seen in people who stutter. For instance, Lebrun and Van Borsel (1990) described a 17-year-old girl with Down syndrome who showed deficits in both language comprehension and production, along with distortions, substitutions, and omissions of phonemes. The girl also exhibited stutter-like disfluency (sound prolongations, blocks, and phrase, word, syllable, and sound repetitions). Overall, 15.5% of her words were spoken disfluently. However, of these disfluencies, 19% involved repetition of word-final sounds, and 32% involved repetition of word-initial sounds. The word-final repetitions were limited to voiceless stops and fricatives. Some of the repetitions featured a brief pause between iterations of the affected consonant. A disfluency pattern on this sort is not typical of developmental stuttering.

Stansfield (1995) reported on four adult speakers who had a history of "learning difficulties," "mental handicap," and/or Down syndrome as well as the presence of word-final disfluency. Across the four cases, disfluency frequency ranged from 6% to 19% of words. All four cases also exhibited impaired articulation or phonology (two with mild impairment, two with severe impairment). For these cases, the word-final repetition constituted a minority of the disfluencies produced—ranging from 8% to 33% of their total disfluencies. For three of the four cases, word-final rep-

etition constituted more than 20% of all the disfluencies the speaker produced.

Many studies of speech disfluency in individuals with intellectual disability have focused on people with Down syndrome. Thus, the variable prevalence rates for stuttering in studies of people with intellectual disability may, in part, reflect the extent to which people with Down syndrome were represented in the sample.

Kent and Vorperian (2013) published a comprehensive review of the literature that deals with speech characteristics associated with Down syndrome. Specific aspects of speech included in the review were articulation, phonology, voice, prosody, intelligibility, and fluency. The authors concluded that, at a group level, people with Down syndrome have difficulties in all of these domains and that at an individual level, it is not uncommon for a person to show impairment in multiple domains. In light of this, Kent and Vorperian (2013, p. 189) stated that individuals with Down syndrome face "serious challenges in spoken communication, which may substantially interfere with their participation in social, educational, and vocational activities."

Disfluency in Other Genetic Syndromes

Van Borsel and Tetnowski (2007) summarized the extant literature on the fluency difficulties associated with several genetic syndromes. Brief summaries of their reviews for three of these syndromes are presented below.

Fragile X Syndrome

According to Van Borsel and Tetnowski (2007), fragile X syndrome is the second leading cause of mental retardation after Down syndrome. Van Borsel and Tetnowski's review suggested that stutter-like disfluency occurs more often among people with fragile X syndrome than it does in the general population, but less so than it does among people with Down syndrome. The reported symptom presentation in fragile X syndrome shares some similarities to developmental stuttering in terms of the types of disfluency produced most often; however, in some reports, these disfluencies diverge from those seen in developmental stuttering (e.g., disfluency in sentence-final positions). The average frequency with which stutter-like disfluency occurs among individuals with fragile X syndrome seems to fall roughly in the range of 3 to 5 per 100 words, which is greater than that seen in the general population, but when compared to developmental stuttering, it is consistent with mild fluency impairment.

Prader-Willi Syndrome

Excessive disfluency has been reported in several studies of individuals with Prader-Willi syndrome. In several studies, the disfluency types that are less characteristic of stuttering (e.g., interjections, revisions) seem to be predominate; however, stutter-like disfluency (e.g., repetitions, prolongations) are routinely noted as well. Defloor, Van Borsel, and Curts (2000) reported that all 15 participants in their study exhibited excessive disfluency, with interjections comprising more than half of the total number of disfluencies produced. The participants were most disfluent during conversation and monologue and much less disfluent during tasks involving stimulus repetition and automatic speech. With regard to disfluency types, repetitions constituted about 30% of all disfluencies, and prolongations, blocks, and broken words constituted about 5% of all disfluencies.

Tourette Syndrome

According to the National Institute of Neurological Disorders and Stroke (NINDS, 2014), Tourette syndrome is "a neurological disorder characterized by repetitive, stereotyped, involuntary movements and vocalizations called tics." Research findings support the idea that Tourette syndrome is a heritable disorder. The NINDS states that the most recent models point toward a complex inheritance pattern involving several or perhaps many genes. Van Borsel and Tetnowski (2007) noted that stuttering often is mentioned as one of many behavioral concomitants associated with Tourette syndrome; however, they stated that much of the older research literature is difficult to interpret due to inconsistent terminology for disfluency analyses and/or poorly specified research methodologies.

More recent research has failed to support the idea that people with Tourette syndrome are prone to stuttering, as stutter-like disfluency constitutes a minority of all disfluency types produced (e.g., Van Borsel, Goethals, & Vanryckeghem, 2004; Van Borsel & Vanryckeghem, 2000). Consistent with this, stutter-like speech is not mentioned as a characteristic of Tourette syndrome on the NINDS' most recent "fact sheet" for the disorder. Evidence of excessive production of other types of disfluency has been noted, however (De Nil, Sasisekaran, Van Lieshout, & Sandor, 2005). In addition, Van Borsel and Tetnowski noted that several researchers have reported the presence of unusual sentence-final repetitions in some individuals with Tourette syndrome.

Uncommon Disfluency Patterns

Palilalia and the Repetition of Utterance Final Words

Palilalia is a speech disorder that is characterized by compulsive repetition of a sentence, phrase, or word (Duffy, 1995). Unlike developmental stuttering, the reiterations in palilalic speech typically are produced at the end of an utterance (e.g., *She likes to play tennis, play tennis, play tennis, play tennis*). The successive reiterations that characterize palilalic speech are produced often, but not always, with increasing rate and decreasing loudness (Kent & LaPointe, 1982), and they are more common during spontaneously generated speech than they are during rote or serial speech (LaPointe & Horner, 1981). Although patients generally are aware of and sometimes bothered by the reiterations, they typically do not appear to make an obvious effort to prevent their occurrence (Boller et al., 1973). Palilalia generally is considered to reflect bilateral basal ganglia dysfunction, and the disorder is reported most often in patients who have a history of postencephalitic Parkinson's disease, dementia, pseudobulbar palsy, and Tourette syndrome (Duffy, 1995; Williams, 1978). Palilalia has been noted in conjunction with idiopathic Parkinson's disease as well (Boller et al., 1973).

Boller et al. (1973) reported on a case of familial palilalia, in which both a mother and her son exhibited palilalic speech, as well as evidence of dementia, chorea (involuntary, purposeless movements), and "extensive intracerebral calcification." The mother exhibited excessive repetition of utterance-final linguistic elements and instances of "moving the mouth and tongue as though to speak but without producing any sound." X-ray images showed evidence of calcification in the basal ganglia, cerebellum, and cerebral gyri. Utterance-final repetition was observed during tasks that involved serial speech, such as counting and reciting the days of the week. Verbal output during conversation was quite limited. The woman's son exhibited more marked symptoms of palilalia, often repeating either an entire sentence or several of the final words from a sentence several times in succession. The reiterative speech fit the definitional criteria of palilalia in that speech rate tended to accelerate, and speech intensity tended to trail off. Palilalic reiterations also were noted during serial speech such that upon completing a recitation of the alphabet, the days of the week, or the months of the year, the man then restarted the series from the beginning. Palilalic reiterations were noted occasionally in writing, as well. Other deficits also were noted, including use of simplistic expressive language and limited verbal memory. The man exhibited calcification patterns similar to those seen in his mother. Boller et al. speculated that palilalic speech might be related to chorea. In other words, just as chorea reflects impairment in movement inhibition, palilalia seems to reflect impairment in speech inhibition.

LaPointe and Horner (1981) reported descriptive data for a 29-year-old male who showed symptoms of palilalic-like speech. The cause of the speech disturbance could not be determined definitively; however, the man had a history of barbiturate abuse, phenobarbital addiction was suspected, and a previous psychiatric evaluation had resulted in a tentative diagnosis of simple schizophrenia.

Overall, 38% of the man's running speech consisted of palilalic speech. The maximum number of reiterations in the palilalic repetitions varied across tasks: 28 reiterations during spontaneous conversation, 14 reiterations during picture description, and 6 reiterations during sentence reading. When explaining the meaning of the proverb "look before you leap," however, the speaker produced a total of 52 iterations during a single repetition. The mean number of iterations for these tasks, of course, was less than the maximum: 2.8 reiterations during spontaneous conversation, 3.1 reiterations during picture description, and 1.8 reiterations during sentence reading. Verbal formulation tasks like the proverb explanation evoked the longest repetitions—an average of 5.0 reiterations per trial.

Kent and LaPointe (1982) reexamined acoustic properties of data from LaPointe and Horner 's (1981) study and found that the reiterative speech did not conform to classic characteristics of palilalic speech. That is, upon examining the rate and loudness of the reiterations, they found that the reiterative segments of speech did not get progressively faster, and in fact, the last iteration in a series often had a longer duration than earlier ones. Similarly, the final iteration often was produced with greater intensity than the other ones. The authors concluded that the speech pattern might have been indicative of some reiterative speech problem other than palilalia and/or a variation of palilalia that resulted from neurological impairment other than that seen in most cases of palilalia.

Logan and Maren (1998) reported a case study of a 6-year-old child who presented both developmental stuttering and a form of whispered perseverative speech that was similar in some respects to palilalia. Case history information revealed that the child had begun stuttering at age 3. In the months leading up to the child's speech assessment at age 6, there was a progressive worsening of the stuttering along with the emergence of whispered repetitions of entire sentences (or significant portions thereof). During the speech evaluation at age 6, the child produced 9.6 speech disfluencies per 100 syllables of conversational speech, with part-word repetition, phrase repetition, and sound prolongation as the most common disfluency types, and results from the *Stuttering Severity Instrument (SSI-3)* (Riley, 1994) indicated "moderate" stuttering. Several instances of palilalic-like repetition were noted during the evaluation. The palilalic-like reiterations usually were verbatim whispered repetitions of entire utterances or large portions of utterances that the child initially had said with normal intensity, voicing, and rate. In addition, the child sometimes silently "mouthed" the articulatory movements associated with the just-completed utterances. Phonological development and other aspects of expressive and receptive language developmental were within normal limits. Results of a comprehensive neurodevelopmental assessment that was conducted elsewhere following the initial speech assessment indicated deficits in fine motor coordination but no evidence of other neurodevelopmental impairment.

The child's performance was monitored across a two-year period, in the context of a fluency treatment program. Data on the child's speech fluency at that time are summarized in Table 9–3. As shown in the table, palilalic-like repetitions occurred on about one-quarter of all utterances and when combined with the silent, mouthed repetitions, about one-third of

Table 9–3. Frequency of Palilalic-Like Repetitions, Mouthed Repetitions, and Stutter-Like Disfluency Across a 27-Month Span in a School-Aged Child (from Logan & Maren, 1998)

	Observation Point					
	1	**2**	**3**	**4**	**5**	**6**
Behavior	**Initial evaluation**	**+6 months**	**+12 months**	**+18 months**	**+24 months**	**+27 months**
Palilalic-like repetitions	25	16	9	4	<1	0
Mouthed repetitions	6	4	9	4	<1	0
Stutter-like disfluency	6.14	3.56	9.98	9.64	3.74	1.24

Note. Stutter-like disfluency is reported as number of disfluencies per 100 syllables. The other two behaviors are reported as percentage of utterances containing the behavior.

all utterances featured repetition of final portions of an utterance. The palilalic-like speech and mouthed repetitions fluctuated in frequency during the year following the initial speech evaluation, after which they declined steadily until they eventually seemed to resolve. The role of treatment in the resolution of these behaviors was unclear, as the child showed very little awareness of when the palilalic-like behaviors occurred. The frequency of the palilalic-like speech decreased steadily during the course of the observations despite an increase in stuttering frequency during the middle stages of the treatment program, and it occurred with equal frequency following fluent and stuttered utterances. Stuttering-related disfluency was never observed during the course of the palilalic-like repetitions. During the course of the study, palilalic-like repetitions reiterated an average of 72% of the syllables spoken in the original utterance, and for 90% of the instances of sentence-final repetition, the original utterance was repeated only once.

Repetition of Word-Final Sounds and Syllable Rimes

There are scattered reports in the fluency literature of speakers who produce repetition of word-final sounds and/or syllable rimes. Six published reports on this phenomenon are summarized in this section.

Rudmin (1984)

Rudmin (1984) reported the presence of word-final repetitions in a longitudinal case study of his daughter. The girl exhibited repetition of word-final voiceless stop consonants from age 16 to 29 months. After the word-final repetition resolved, the girl exhibited sound prolongation on liquid and glide consonants for about 4 months, after which the latter disfluency type resolved.

Mowrer (1987)

Mowrer (1987) reported on a case of final consonant repetition in a 2-year-old boy.

Like many 2-year-olds, the boy exhibited the phonological pattern termed *final consonant deletion*, and the boy's mother reported that she had attempted to teach him to produce word-final consonants by emphasizing and demonstrating them in her speech. The boy often imitated his mother's models of word-final consonants and sometimes repeated the final consonants several times, with added aspiration, in an apparently intentional manner. In the months following the mother's attempt to address the final consonant deletion, however, the frequency of the boy's final consonant repetition increased markedly and no longer appeared to be under the child's volitional control. After several unsuccessful attempts to help her son stop the final consonant repetition, the mother sought the assistance of a speech-language pathologist, which resulted in Mowrer's case study. Mowrer consulted with the family on several occasions during a one-year period.

At the initial evaluation, the boy produced 3.28 final consonant repetitions per 100 syllables. The next most frequent disfluency type, interjection, occurred only 1.31 times per 100 syllables, and the frequencies for other disfluency types were less than this and within normal frequency expectations. The boy also exhibited noticeable aspiration on many of the word-final stop consonants that were not repeated. During the course of the 12-month study, the frequency of word-final consonants gradually diminished and eventually resolved. Following the initial speech assessment, Mowrer provided the child's parents and caregiver informational material on how to reduce environmental demands that might negatively impact the child's fluency. The extent to which this information led to the changes in the child's word-final repetition was unclear.

Camarata (1989)

Camarata (1989) documented word-final repetition of voiceless stop consonants (i.e., /p/, /t/, /k/) in a preschool-aged boy. The repetitions were first noted at age 2;1 but seemed to resolve after about one month and did not return in the child's speech as of age 3;5. Other than the word-final repetition, the child's communication development appeared to be within normal limits, and the child showed no evidence of stuttering. The boy exhibited several phonological patterns that are common at age 2, including *final devoicing* and *stopping*. Thus, when the child encountered a word that featured a word-final voiced consonant, he routinely devoiced the consonant (e.g., "tub" was pronounced as [tʌp]), and when the child encountered words that featured a voiced word-final fricative, the child devoiced it and then substituted a stop sound (e.g., "buzz" was pronounced as [bʌt]). Interestingly, words that featured devoicing of a voiced final consonant *never* featured word-final repetition. The word-final repetition only occurred on words that naturally featured voiceless word-final sounds. Thus, "but" and "bus" were produced as [bʌt- t], however, "buzz" was produced as [bʌt].

On this basis, Camarata (1989) hypothesized that the boy's final consonant repetition was phonologically motivated; that is, it was used to prevent homonymy. In other words, without the use of final consonant repetition, minimal pairs such as "beat" and "bead" would have sounded the same in the child's speech. The use of final consonant repetition enabled the boy to contrast the two words. The child's repetition pattern always contained two iterations of the target consonant (e.g., pet- t). Camarata noted that double consonant use has been documented in some languages, where it serves a phonemic function. Camarata also argued that Mowrer's (1987) case of final consonant repetition was likely phonological in nature as well, because the repetition patterns in the two studies shared many similarities.

Lebrun and Van Borsel (1990)

Lebrun and Van Borsel (1990) reported word-final repetition of stops, fricatives, and /r/ in an 8-year-old boy. The boy also presented with a rapid articulation rate, "numerous phrase, word, syllable, and sound repetitions," and some sound prolongations. The final sound repetition almost always consisted of reiteration of the final sound in the word, although on a few occasions the final two sounds in a word were reiterated. During reading, the word-final repetitions occurred on 8.25% of words. The frequency of word-final repetition remained constant in all but the middle trial of an adaptation task in which the child read a passage five times in succession. Thus, the frequency of word-final repetition did not clearly improve with repeated practice across the adaptation trials, as it would be expected to do with stuttered speech. In conversational speech, 16% of the boy's words featured disfluency, but there was only one instance of word-final repetition in the 320-word sample, which translates to an adjusted frequency of 0.31 word-final repetitions per 100 words during conversation.

McAllister and Kingston (2005)

McAllister and Kingston (2005) reported on word-final, part-word repetition during conversation, reading, and sentence repetition in two school-aged boys. In each case, the repetition pattern featured reiteration of some portion of the rime from the final syllable of the word. The frequency of these disfluencies was relatively low for each child, with both boys producing roughly 3 per 100 words. The repetitions occurred on content words and function words. The first child (age 8;0) had a history of phonological disorder and stuttering, each of which had resolved by age 6;8. Shortly thereafter, at age 7;4, word-final, part-word repetitions emerged in the child's speech. The second child began to produce word-final, part-word repetitions at age 5;11, and the behavior still was present at age 7;6 (when the study was completed). The boy's older brother reportedly had exhibited similar repetitions from age 5 to age 9. McAllister and Kingston reported that the word-final, part-word repetitions obeyed the following phonological constraints.

- *Child 1* exhibited repetition of the last syllabic nucleus of the final word, plus any consonants that were in the coda. For instance, "army" would have featured repetition of the word-final vowel /i/ and "poke" would have featured repetition of the vowel /o/ plus the /k/ from the coda (i.e., [ok]).
- *Child 2* exhibited repetition of the last syllabic element in a word, unless the word contained a diphthong, in which case the off-glide of the diphthong was repeated along with any consonants that were in the coda. For instance, "army" would have featured repetition of the word-final vowel /i/; but the word "then" would have featured repetition of the word-final /n/, and the word "light" would have featured

repetition of the off-glide [ɪ] along with the final consonant (e.g., "light" was produced as [laɪtɪt]).

McAllister and Kingston (2005) proposed both motoric (e.g., a type of compulsive action, a symptom of palilalia) and psycholinguistic (e.g., a symptom of sentence planning problems) explanations for these disfluencies. They also questioned whether repetitions such as these, when produced infrequently, should be regarded as evidence of a communication disorder.

Cosyns and Colleagues (2010)

Cosyns and colleagues (Cosyns, Mortier, Janssens, Saharan, Stevens, & Van Borsel, 2010) reported on instances of word-final disfluency in 21 adults with neurofibromatosis type 1. Neurofibromatosis type 1 is a genetically based disorder that is characterized by a cluster of symptoms including characteristic changes in skin color (café-au-lait spots), freckling in the underarm and groin regions, and benign tumors that grow on or under the skin, often in nerves along spinal cord or along nerves in other parts of the body. Cosyns et al. reported relatively high mean disfluency frequencies for the participants in their study during conversation and monologue task (11% and 9%, respectively), with several of the participants exhibiting 16 or more total disfluencies per 100 words. Disfluency frequency during conversation and monologue was significantly greater than it was during oral readings, stimulus repetition, and automatic speech, each of which featured a total disfluency frequency of about 3%. The frequency of interjections was higher than that of all the other disfluency types with the exception of revisions. In turn, revisions were produced at a higher frequency than the

classic stuttering-related disfluency types (repetitions, prolongations).

The mean frequency for SLDs was relatively low (1.82 per 100 words), and 19 of the 22 participants produced fewer than 3 stutter-like disfluencies per 100 words. In contrast with developmental stuttering, the participants with neurofibromatosis type 1 produced stutter-like disfluency more often during word-initial and word-final positions than they did during word-medial positions. There was no effect for sentence position or grammatical class on distribution of stutter-like disfluency, and the participants showed no evidence of speech-related struggle when repeating or prolonging. Some participants presented complications of the central nervous system as a result of tumor growth. However, the disfluency levels of these individuals were similar to those of participants who did not exhibit central nervous system complications. Cosyns et al. (2010) did not find evidence that the individuals with neurofibromatosis type 1 routinely presented stutter-like speech. Instead, they found that the disfluency pattern in this population was more similar to that of individuals with fragile X syndrome, Prader-Willi syndrome, and Tourette syndrome.

Disfluency and Autism Spectrum Disorders

During the past decade, there has been growing interest among speech-language pathologists in studying fluency functioning in the context of autism spectrum disorders. The research literature in this area is emerging and consists of many case-based reports and some small group descriptive studies. Scaler Scott (2011) summarized past research on disfluency patterns associated with autism spectrum disorders and reported the occurrence of both classic types of disfluency (e.g., repetitions, interjections, prolongations, revision) and uncommon forms of disfluency such as repetition of word-final sounds and mid-vowel interruptions (sometimes termed "broken words"). According to Scaler Scott, characterizations of speaking rate have been mixed in past research —excessively fast in some studies, excessively slow in others, and excessively variable in still others.

Scaler Scott (2011) also summarized results of her 2008 dissertation that involved 12 children with Asperger syndrome and 12 typically functioning controls. Overall, 8 of the 12 children met criteria for a diagnosis of stuttering, although in all cases, severity fell into either the very mild or mild range. Nonetheless, in most of these cases, disfluency types such as revision and interjection tended to predominate. Scaler Scott also reported that the children exhibited "tense pauses" between word boundaries but indicated that it was unclear whether these behaviors were indicative of stuttered speech. In addition, 3 of the children with Asperger syndrome met definitional criteria for cluttering and/or cluttering-stuttering.

Other authors have reported the presence of uncommon disfluency types in children with Asperger syndrome. For example, Sissken (2006) added the disfluency categories "final part-word repetition" and "mid-syllable insertion" to her disfluency classification system when reporting on two cases of Asperger syndrome (one aged 7 years and the other aged 17 years). The 17-year-old case exhibited a disfluency profile in which 90% of the disfluencies were not characteristic of typical developmental stuttering. Final part-word repetitions and mid-syllable insertions (e.g. "see-hee" for the word "see") were the most common types of disfluency (50% and 30% of the total, respectively). The 7-year-old case showed a similar profile: 50% of the disfluencies were not characteristic of typical developmental stuttering, with mid-syllable insertions constituting 33% of the total disfluencies and final part-word repetitions constituting 25% of the total.

Plexico, Cleary, McAlpine, and Plumb (2010) reported disfluency characteristics of 8 children with autism spectrum disorders. As with other researchers, they observed a mix of disfluency forms including common types such as part- and whole-word repetition, sound prolongation, interjection, and revision, along with uncommon types like those that Sissken (2006) reported. Overall, the total mean disfluency frequency for the 8 children was relatively low (about 4.5 per 100 syllables) and, unlike Sissken's (2006) report, uncommon disfluency types such as repetition of word-final sounds were the least common, occurring with a frequency of about 0.4 per 100 syllables.

Summary

This chapter dealt with patterns of disfluency in clinical populations other than stuttering and cluttering. Disfluency patterns associated with various developmental language impairments were reviewed first. Children with language learning disorders seem to be less fluent than children with typical language skills, and they seem to produce a significant amount of stutter-like frequency. Overall, however, the combined frequency of these stutter-like disfluencies is less than that seen in most children who stutter and generally not sufficiently aberrant in quality or quantity to warrant a diagnosis of stuttering. Some researchers have speculated that the part-word repetitions and sound prolongations seen in children with language impairment may arise for reasons other than those in children who stutter.

The next topic in the chapter concerned fluency in oral reading. The concept of reading fluency was contrasted with that of fluency during oral speech, and basic methods for assessing reading fluency were introduced. In general, children may demonstrate difficulties in reading fluency for one or more of the following reasons: (1) typical developmental limitations associated with reading acquisition; (2) limitations associated with impairment in the ability to read; and (3) impairment in the ability to speak fluently. Challenges in differentiating disfluencies associated with reading disability from those associated with speech-based fluency impairments like stuttering were discussed.

The remainder of the chapter dealt with fluency impairment in other clinical populations, including intellectual impairment, Down syndrome, fragile X syndrome, Tourette syndrome, and autism spectrum disorders. Of these populations, individuals with Down syndrome seem to be the most at risk for experiencing significant disability in speech fluency. The prevalence of stuttering among individuals with Down syndrome seems to be much greater than it is among the general population and, when combined with elevated risks for other types of communication difficulty, creates the potential for multiple communication challenges. The chapter concluded with an overview of several uncommon types of disfluency. Some of the latter behaviors involve compulsive forms of repetition in which a speaker seems to have difficulty with terminating an utterance. As a consequence, linguistic units at the end of the utterance are repeated. This type of fluency difficulty seems to be quite different from that seen in developmental stuttering, wherein the speaker has difficulty moving an utterance forward to its completion. Atypical forms of disfluency have been noted in conjunction with a range of conditions, including autism spectrum disorders and Parkinson's disease and, in some cases, behaviors that appear to be atypical disfluency actually may be a symptom of processes related to phonological development.

SECTION
III

Clinical Assessment

10

Fluency Assessment: Basic Concepts and Data Collection Methods

In this section of the text, we discuss issues related to the assessment of speech fluency, particularly as it pertains to disordered speech. We use the term *assessment* in a broad sense, conceiving of it as a process that includes: (a) describing how a person functions in a particular domain; (b) determining why the person functions as he or she does; and (c) developing an action plan that will enable the person to function better than he or she currently does. In this textbook, the domain of primary interest is, of course, speech fluency. In this chapter, the focus primarily is on presenting a conceptual framework for fluency assessment and reviewing tools and techniques that clinicians can use to collect data about fluency functioning. In Chapter 11, specific methods for analyzing fluency data are discussed and, in Chapter 12, issues related to data interpretation are discussed in relation to diagnosing fluency disorders, estimating a patient's prognosis,

and making recommendations for future action. Together, these assessment activities form a platform upon which one can build effective treatment programs.

A Framework for Assessment

Assessment Phases

As suggested above, fluency assessment is a structured and systematic part of clinical practice. It includes three main phases, which are outlined briefly in this section.

Data Collection

Assessment begins with the collection of data. A variety of data collection methods are available—everything from clinician-designed tasks to published, norm-referenced tests.

Although it is not necessary to use every possible means of data collection during every fluency assessment, it is not unusual for a clinician to use multiple data collection methods during a single fluency assessment.

Data Analysis

After a clinician collects data about the client's functioning, he or she must analyze it. Data analysis leads to quantitative and qualitative descriptions of how a client functions. Such data can be used to describe functioning across the various dimensions of fluency. Analyzed data also can be used to describe functioning in terms of specific tasks and actions that a client performs. This approach leads to an understanding of the nature and types of fluency difficulties the client has.

Data Interpretation

The third phase of assessment is data interpretation. In this segment of assessment, the clinician integrates all available data to arrive at global decisions or impressions about the client. Included under the heading of data interpretation are issues related to diagnosis and prognosis, as well as the recommendation of actions that should follow the assessment. With some cases, the data interpretation phase is straightforward; that is, the nature of the client's fluency problem is clear and steps for future action are obvious to both the clinician and the client. In other cases, it is challenging—it may be difficult to determine whether the person has a disorder, and even when it does seem that the person has a disorder, it still may be difficult to determine whether the implementation of formal treatment is the best course of action to recommend. The complexities of data interpretation are discussed at greater length in Chapter 12.

Assessment Terminology

The discussion of fluency assessment begins with an overview of 13 assessment-related terms that are central to the World Health Organization's (WHO, 2001) *International Classification of Functioning, Disability, and Health* (abbreviated as ICF). The ICF is a clinical tool that speech-language pathologists and other health care providers can use to generate comprehensive descriptions of people's health status. Within the ICF framework, the ability to speak fluently is regarded as an aspect of a person's overall health. Several authors (e.g., Logan, 2005; Yaruss, 1998; Yaruss & Quesal, 2004) have discussed the applicability of the ICF instrument to the assessment and treatment of fluency disorders. The use of ICF terminology provides clinicians with a common language for clinical assessment, which, in turn, promotes accurate and precise communication among clinicians. The terms also provide an excellent starting point for understanding principles of fluency assessment, and they lead directly into the goals of fluency assessment.

Functioning, Performance, and Capacity

Each of the three terms discussed in this section deals with activities that an individual does. The term *functioning* is the broadest of the three. It refers to the structure of an individual's body (i.e., anatomy) and the way in which body structures function (i.e., physiology). It also encompasses how an individual performs across daily activities, including the manner in which he or she engages in the activities. In the ICF framework, the notion of functioning is intended to emphasize *what a person does*, rather than what a person does not do. Many behavioral and instrumental measures are available to help clinicians describe a person's fluency functioning. Several of these tools are discussed later in this chapter and in the following chapter.

The term *performance* pertains to how a person behaves or acts within his or her current environment. The concepts of performance and functioning are similar in that both deal with a person's actions within daily activities. Performance is a narrower concept than functioning, however, as it does not include matters related to body structure and function. Nearly all of the tools that clinicians commonly use in fluency assessment describe patient performance. When assessing fluency, it is important to remember that a person's within-clinic performance can be markedly different from his or her beyond-clinic performance. Consequently, it is critical to assess how a person performs across a range of daily activities.

The term *capacity* refers to "the highest probable level of functioning that a person may reach" within a uniform or standard environment (WHO, 2001, p. 20). Clinical assessments of speech fluency typically occur in a relatively uniform or standard environment; thus, a person's capacity for speech fluency often is defined in terms of the speaker's "within-clinic speech." Many people with impaired fluency report that their fluency during clinical interactions is substantially better than it is during less controlled "real world" settings.

Activities and Activity Limitations

The term *activity* refers to the tasks or actions that a person performs. In the context of fluency assessment, it is important to determine the types of communication activities a patient performs. Most people exhibit a unique profile of communication activities. Some activities, like conversation, are common to nearly everyone. However, other activities (e.g., lecturing, arguing a court case) are performed by only some people. To complicate matters further, any particular activity can assume an almost limitless number of permutations. For example, conversations can vary in terms of the number of participants, the level of familiarity between the participants, the physical proximity of the participants, the amount of background noise, the complexity of the topic, and the underlying communicative purpose. Thus, it is important to gain insight into how a patient performs across a variety of activities. It also is important to determine the relative importance of an activity for a person. For instance, a person may rarely engage in an activity like reciting wedding vows yet consider it crucial to perform well when it does occur.

According to the WHO (2001), the term activity has a positive connotation. That is, it refers to the tasks and actions that a person *does,* regardless of how well those tasks and actions are performed. The term *activity limitation*, in contrast, refers to problems or difficulties that a person has when performing an activity. Thus, the concept of activity limitation has a negative connotation. In other words, it refers to how a client's performance falls short when compared to the performance of other speakers. As such, activity limitations can contribute to disability and are viewed as a symptom of impairment. Within the context of fluency assessment, a clinician will compare the person who is undergoing assessment to people who do not have impaired fluency. It is common for speakers with impaired fluency to exhibit situational difficulties; that is, no limitation when performing one activity but marked limitations when performing another activity. Consequently, it is important to collect information about performance across a variety of activities when assessing fluency.

Participation and Participation Restrictions

The term *participation* refers to the extent to which a person engages in an activity. Participation refers to a person's degree of engagement in life activities. The concept includes the number of activities in which a person is engaged as well as the extent to which the person is engaged in a particular activity. For example, one person might participate verbally during only a handful of daily activities but when the person is engaged in those activities, he or she talks extensively. In contrast, another person might participate verbally in many daily activities but say very little during most of those activities. Within the fluency dimension framework that we outlined in Chapter 1, the notion of participation is an aspect of talkativeness. Similar to the concept of activity, participation has a positive connotation: It refers to what a person *does,* regardless of how it compares to the participation patterns of other people.

In the context of fluency assessment, the term *participation restriction* refers to limitations in a person's involvement in verbal communication. As with activity limitations, participation restrictions are determined by comparing an individual's participation patterns against the participation patterns of normally functioning individuals. As such, they can contribute to disability and be viewed as a symptom of impairment. Participation restrictions can dissociate from activity limitations. For example, a person might speak very disfluently in a particular activity yet engage in that activity often and extensively. A range of factors, including personal attributes (e.g., temperament) and environmental factors (e.g., teasing from a listener), potentially can affect a speaker's verbal participation.

Impairment and Disability

The term *impairment* refers to structural or functional differences in a person's body. In the ICF framework, impairment is defined as a *deviation* or *limitation* in body structure or body function. Most of the fluency disorders that we discuss in this text are linked to deviations in neuroanatomy and/or neurophysiology.

In the ICF framework, the term *disability* has a broad meaning. It refers to the impairments, activity limitations, and participation restrictions that an individual exhibits. The term *disability* conveys what a person *does not do*, rather than what a person *does*. As such, disability essentially is the inverse of functioning. Disabilities are defined in reference to how a person *without* a specific health condition such as stuttering or cluttering would function in a particular activity.

Environmental and Personal Factors

The WHO defines *environmental factors* as the "physical, social, and attitudinal (context) in which people live and conduct their lives" (p. 12). The concept is broad: It includes not only physical features of the world but also societal roles, attitudes, values, social systems and services, as well as policies, rules, and laws. Of course, the typical clinician has little control over societal-level environmental factors. However, the typical clinician often is able to alter a host of immediate environmental factors that affect a patient's functioning (e.g., how a classroom teacher responds to a student's disfluent speech) if it appears that they aggravate the effects of a child's fluency impairment.

The term *personal factor*, in contrast, refers to intrinsic characteristics such as a person's age, gender, religion, and social status as well as a person's feelings, attitudes, and beliefs toward fluency impairment and others' reactions to it. Personal factors can affect a person's functioning. For example, a teenage boy who stutters may develop feelings of shame because of his fluency disability, and the shame (a personal factor) may cause the boy to avoid participation during class discussions (a self-imposed participation restriction).

Facilitators and Barriers

Facilitators are features of the environment that improve a person's functioning and, in doing so, reduce disability. Within the context of fluency impairment, facilitators can be either intrinsic to the speaker (e.g., a client deliberately speaks at a particular articulation rate) or extrinsic to the speaker (e.g., a conversational partner refrains from interrupting the client).

Barriers, in contrast, are aspects of the environment that limit or hinder a person's functioning and, in doing so, either create or exacerbate disability. Examples of barriers include the lack of an anti-bullying program at an elementary school and a client's lack of reliable transportation to a treatment center.

From Assessment Concepts to Assessment Goals

The assessment-related terms that we outlined in the previous section provide a conceptual platform for evaluating clients who have fluency concerns, and they lead directly into questions that are important to answer in assessment. The basic questions to be addressed in fluency assessment are outlined in Figure 10–1. As shown, there are four broad questions to be answered: (1) How does the speaker function?, (2) Is there evidence of disability?, (3) How does context affect functioning and disability?, and (4) What should happen next? The main goal in assessment is to generate answers to each of the four questions. In this section, we discuss this process in more detail.

Goal 1: Describe How the Client Currently Functions

Fluency Functioning

The first goal in fluency assessment is to describe the client's fluency functioning. The WHO (2001) defines *functioning* broadly, which means that a clinician may need to assemble a range of data to address this goal completely. Data that fall under the heading of functioning include fluency-related details about speech production, such as disfluency frequency, disfluency duration, speech rate, speech effort, and speech naturalness. Also included is information about

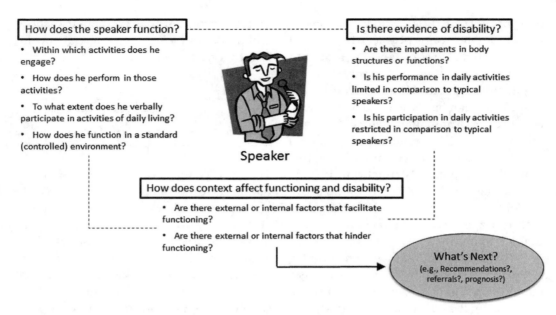

Figure 10–1. The relationship between the ICF (WHO, 2001) concepts and the primary goals of fluency assessment. As shown, four primary goals to address in assessment are (1) describe how the speaker currently functions; (2) describe any disability that is present; (3) describe how context affects functioning; and (4) provide recommendations for future actions. Answers to the questions in these areas provide a platform for treatment.

the kinds of *activities* within which the client engages and the manner in which fluency *performance* in those activities is expressed. The notion of *participation* falls under the concept of functioning, too. Here, the focus is on the depth and the breadth of the client's verbal engagement in daily activities. As noted earlier in the chapter, participation is distinctly different from disfluency. That is, a person with impaired fluency can speak in a highly disfluent manner during a certain situation yet still participate as fully as a person with typical fluency does.

The notion of *capacity* also comes under functioning. Here, the focus is on determining the client's highest or best level of fluency. Usually, such fluency occurs within a structured or controlled setting, such as a clinical visit. Speakers can exhibit marked differences in perfor-

mance between clinic and "real world" contexts. Thus, determination of a client's fluency capacity helps the clinician and the client set expectations, at least in the near term, for how well the client is capable of performing.

Functioning in Other Communication-Related Domains

Fluency impairment sometimes co-occurs with difficulties in other communication-related domains. Thus, fluency functioning may not be the only aspect of communication that warrants attention. Clinicians should be alert for signs of other impairments that limit communication and potentially exacerbate the effects of fluency impairment.

In one comprehensive survey of school-based speech-language pathologists (SLPs) across 10 American states (Arndt & Healey, 2001), 44% of 467 children who were being treated for stuttering also met their state's criteria for phonological and/or language disorder, and another 23% of the children were "suspected" of having impairment in one or both areas. Brazell and Logan (2001) conducted a similar survey of SLPs within the state of Florida and reported results that were very similar to those of Arndt and Healey.

Fluency difficulties also can co-occur with an assortment of neurological conditions (e.g., Parkinson's disease). In all such cases, a clinician must consider the fluency difficulties of the client within the broader context of the client's other disabilities, such as those in memory, attention, or language.

Goal 2: Describe the Client's Current Areas of Disability

As noted above, the WHO (2001) defines *disability* in terms of the impairments, activity limitations, and participation restrictions that an individual exhibits. On a surface level, the impairment that most people with fluency disorders exhibit is the inability to speak with the same degree of fluency as typical speakers. Thus, a main goal of fluency assessment is to identify the presence of fluency-related disability and then to describe its nature and severity. One of the main challenges in fluency assessment is to capture how a client performs in speaking activities outside of the therapy room context. The performance differences within and beyond the clinic can be dramatic, and it is critical that the clinician has an accurate grasp of the extent of the client's fluency limitations in everyday life.

A clinician may find it equally challenging to describe the extent to which a client participates in beyond-clinic speaking activities. It is common for clients to report that they speak relatively fluently during one activity or another but, at the same time, to say that they do not speak *at all* in many other activities due to concern about disclosing their impaired speech to others. Self-imposed participation restrictions sometimes can be profound—and lead a person to be quite isolated from others. Therefore, it is critical that the clinician get a sense for not only when the client *talks* but also when the client *does not talk*.

Participation restrictions sometimes originate with other people. Often, participation restrictions of this sort are subtle. For example, during a lunchtime conversation among classmates, a boy with impaired fluency might find that the classmates direct fewer comments toward him than they do toward the other children. At other times, the externally based participation restrictions can be remarkably blatant. For example, a college student who stutters might be met with overtly discouraging or derisive comments from peers when he seeks a leadership role within a university club. Restrictions of the latter sort obviously go beyond verbal participation to affect the person's overall desire to belong to the club.

Goal 3: Determine How Context Affects the Client's Performance

The Role of Personal Factors

Personal factors include things such as age, gender, personal values, coping styles —elements that constitute the backdrop for a client's life activities. One can include the client's attitudes, beliefs, and feelings about communication and fluency impairment under the heading of personal factors, as well. It is critical to evaluate this realm of a client's life given the impact that it can have on how a client reacts to and copes with fluency impairment and responds to treatment. In some cases, a client's attitudes, feelings, and/or beliefs about his or her fluency impairment deviate so far from the norm that they constitute a form of impairment in and of themselves. Examples of the latter include disorders such as depression and social phobia, which sometimes co-occur with fluency impairment (Blumgart, Tran, & Craig, 2010a; Miller & Watson, 1992). In such cases, the client's attitudes, feelings, thoughts, and beliefs go beyond a mere "backdrop to functioning" and become an aspect of functioning.

The Role of Environmental Factors

The environment within which a client lives can affect the expression of his or her fluency impairment. Thus, it is important to describe the extent to which a client's environment facilitates or hinders fluency performance. Areas of consideration under environmental factors include things such as the quality of the relationships that the client has with other people, the attitudes that other people have toward the client's communicative disability, and the verbal and nonverbal reactions that others exhibit when a client speaks disfluently. Each of these things has the potential to facilitate or hinder the client's fluency functioning. Also included under the heading of environmental factors are issues that relate to institutional policies that are in place within the client's school or work setting. For instance, a school system's policy on bullying can be critical in shaping the type of speaking environment within which a person with impaired fluency performs. With adults, a corporation's procedures for adhering to disability laws can affect the nature of the job performance evaluations a client receives.

Goal 4: Interpret Data to Make Recommendations

The process of fluency assessment culminates with data interpretation and the formulation of recommended "next steps." In most cases, analysis of clinical data will enable the clinician to arrive at a diagnosis (i.e., classification) of the type of fluency impairment that a client exhibits and a determination as to whether treatment is necessary, and if so, which type of treatment would be most appropriate. Consideration of information about the client's current levels of functioning and disability and contextual factors also may enable the clinician to estimate the likelihood that the client will improve (i.e., prognosis).

A Basic Protocol for Fluency Assessment

Having outlined some basic assessment goals, we now turn our attention to the concept of an assessment protocol. It is customary practice to organize speech-language assessments around an assessment protocol. A protocol is a plan or menu of activities that the clinician is likely to conduct. Use of a protocol helps to ensure that the clinician addresses each of the important aspects of client functioning and limits the occurrence of inadvertently overlooking areas of potential importance. It also facilitates the clinician's ability to make comparisons between one client and another and, within a client, to compare performance at different points in time.

In Figure 10–2, the basic components of a fluency assessment protocol are outlined. As shown, the components are grouped under the assessment phase with which they are associated.

In the remainder of the chapter, the focus primarily is on the details associated with data collection. Issues related to data analysis and data interpretation are addressed in subsequent chapters. Clinicians can use a range of approaches to collect data during a fluency assessment. As a rule, it is helpful to use a variety of data collection methods. The actual methods that one uses in assessment will vary according to factors such as the age of

the client, his or her specific symptoms, whether the assessment represents an initial appraisal of the person's functioning or a reassessment, the setting in which the assessment takes place, and the amount of time available for assessment. Each of the methods is described in more detail below.

Collecting Data: The Case History Form

The case history form is a data collection tool that the client or caregiver completes prior to the assessment. The information on the completed case history form enables the clinician to develop an assessment protocol that is uniquely suited to the client's concerns. The case history form is a flexible instrument; that is, the

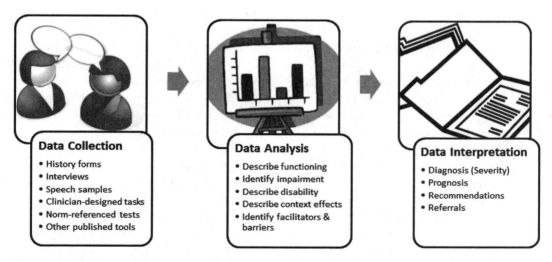

Figure 10–2. Basic components of a protocol for assessment of speech fluency. Assessment begins with data collection. Clinicians typically use a variety of methods to collect information about the client's functioning in fluency and, often, in other aspects of communication. The data then are analyzed to yield quantitative and qualitative descriptions of the client's fluency across the various fluency dimensions. Analyzed data yield descriptions of the kinds of activities the client performs, patterns of verbal participation, the influence of context on fluency, and so forth. In the third stage of assessment, analyzed data are integrated and interpreted.

clinician can adapt its content as necessary for use with specific age groups, clinical populations, or clients. Ideally, the clinician will send the case history form to the client well in advance of the assessment appointment. This provides the client with ample time to review personal records while completing the form and with the opportunity to acquire supplemental medical or educational records that may be relevant to the client's fluency concerns.

Formats for the case history form vary, but most contain the following sections:

- A statement of the client's primary concerns or complaints;
- Details about the client's fluency concerns, including circumstances surrounding symptom onset, past and current symptoms, and impact on daily activities and general quality of life;
- Medical history, including a list of medications the client currently takes;
- Developmental history, including information about the client's speech-language development and changes in fluency over time;
- Educational/occupational history, including information about the impact of fluency on the client's performance in school or work settings;
- Functioning in other domains that are relevant to speech fluency (e.g., expressive and receptive language, speech sound production, attention, memory);
- Presence of concomitant illnesses, disorders, diseases, or conditions;
- Outcomes from previous speech-language services (e.g., past assessments, past treatments);

- Family history of communication disorders or difficulties (or other relevant diseases or disorders);
- Social context, including a list of individuals with whom the client regularly talks (e.g., family members, friends, coworkers) and information about how fluency varies across those contexts; and
- Goals and aspirations, particularly with regard to the complaint behavior(s) and communicative functioning.

Collecting Data: Oral Interviews

Clinicians often begin assessment sessions by conducting an oral interview with either the client or the client's caregiver. The format for the oral interview is flexible. Usually, the clinician builds the interview around a set of standard open-ended prompts (e.g., *Tell me about . . .*). In most cases, the clinician will supplement these general prompts with specific questions and requests. The content of follow-up questions will vary from case to case, depending on what the client or caregiver has said in response to the general prompts. With some cases and in some settings, the clinician also may interview other people (e.g., teachers, counselors, psychologists, previous clinicians). Clinicians always should obtain appropriate consents from the client and/or caregivers prior to interviewing such individuals.

Oral interview questions/requests often fall into subcategories that mirror the ones found on a case history form. Although the focus for the oral interview often is on the complaint behavior, portions of the interview may address other topics, including issues from the case history form that the client answered either unclearly or incompletely. Oral interviews often conclude with inquiries about the client's communication-related goals and interest in enrolling in treatment should the clinician recommend it.

Table 10–1 contains a list of oral interview prompts that pertain to fluency performance. Such prompts are appropriate to present to adolescent and adult clients. Preschool- and early-elementary-aged clients generally are less able to construct meaningful responses to queries like those in Table 10–1. Thus, in such cases, a primary caregiver should serve as the informant. Many children in the 8- to 12-year-old range are quite capable of describing the basic aspects of their

Table 10–1. Prompts to Use During an Oral Interview to Elicit Information About Fluency Concerns

Prompts	
1. Tell me what brings you here today. How can we assist you?	11. Have the things you learned in therapy helped you to communicate better?
2. When did you first notice your fluency problem? What symptoms occurred?	12. How do you cope with your disfluent speech? Do you avoid words or speaking situations to hide disfluency?
3. How did your fluency problem start? What do you believe caused it?	13. Does anyone else in your family have difficulty speaking fluently or with other aspects of communication?
4. What was your speech like when the problem first began, and how has it changed since then?	14. Do you ever discuss your speech difficulties with others? What do you say? Does it help to discuss it?
5. Right now, is your speech better or worse than usual, or about the same?	15. How do you react to your fluency difficulties? Describe your feelings, attitudes, or thoughts about it.
6. How does your speech problem affect your daily life? Does it limit you? If so, how?	16. How do other people react to your fluency difficulties? Do people react negatively or positively?
7. Describe your fluency difficulties. What does your speech sound like? What do think about or feel when you have problems speaking fluently?	17. What do you hope to accomplish in speech therapy? How long do you think it will take?
8. In a list of your life problems, where does your fluency rank? At the top, the middle, or the bottom of the list?	18. Is there anything else that you would like to mention or discuss?
9. Tell me about any prior evaluations or treatment that you have received.	19. Additional follow-up questions, as needed.
10. What things seem to help you to speak fluently? What hinders you?	

Note. The prompts in this table are oriented toward adolescent and adult clients. The prompts should be paraphrased and/or modified before being used with children.

fluency-related experiences. Thus, with such cases, it is useful to interview both the child and the caregiver. Of course, the range of questions that a child will be able to answer generally is much narrower than that for an adult.

The prompts presented in the table are merely a starting point for obtaining information about the client's fluency experiences and concerns. In most cases, the clinician will need to supplement the prompts in Table 10–1 with additional prompts, in order to obtain a complete and accurate account of the client's experience. When clinicians interview children, they should reword the questions into language that is meaningful to the child. Additional examples of fluency-related questions to pose during an oral interview can be found in Conture (2001), Logan (2009), and Manning (2010).

Collecting Data: Speech Samples

Speech samples constitute the core source of data for most fluency assessments (ASHA, 1995). As noted above, people with impaired fluency often exhibit considerable variability in fluency performance across settings and tasks, and they may exhibit variability over time as well (Ingham & Riley, 1998; Yaruss, 1997). Thus, to obtain an accurate picture of the client's fluency, clinicians should elicit a range of speech samples.

Speech samples can assume many forms: structured or unstructured; spontaneous or rehearsed; scripted or spontaneous; formal or informal; and so forth. Each approach has its advantages and disadvantages and, consequently, each has its place

in fluency assessment. A *formal elicitation approach* involves the use of standard materials and methods. Thus, variables such as instructions, speaking topic, reading passages, and conversational partners are fixed or controlled. Although formal elicitation is most closely associated with published, norm-referenced instruments, a clinician can administer a self-designed speech sample task in a standard way, as well.

A standard method of speech sample elicitation allows for both *within-subject* and *between-subject* comparisons. With the within-subject approach, the clinician compares a client's performance at two or more points in time (e.g., $Time_1$ versus $Time_2$). Such an approach is useful when the clinician seeks to determine the client's *baseline* (i.e., pretreatment) level of functioning or the client's response to treatment by comparing pre- and post-treatment performance (Ingham & Riley, 1998). The use of a common elicitation method enables the clinician to make valid comparisons between the repeated measurements. The use of standard speech sample elicitation methods leads to valid between-subject comparisons as well. For instance, a clinician can compare the performance of two clients on a caseload (i.e., $Client_A$ versus $Client_B$) and, more importantly, compare a client's performance to that of a comparison group (e.g., *people with normal fluency* or *other people who stutter*). The latter types of comparisons are integral to the diagnosis of fluency impairment and the determination of impairment severity.

Informal elicitation methods, in contrast, incorporate materials or procedures that are not standardized. As such, the materials, instructions, and speaking topics that the clinician uses vary from sample to sample. The clinician's elicitation methods may differ from those of other clinicians as well. Informal elicitation methods are best suited for obtaining samples of speech in naturalistic (i.e., real-world) settings, where neither the clinician nor the client has much control over how the speaking activity transpires. Although informal elicitation methods can yield important information about a client's performance, the lack of a replicable speech elicitation method limits the clinician's ability to compare the client's performance to that of other speakers or to how the client has performed in similar situations at other times.

In the remainder of this section, the characteristics of several common formats for speech sample elicitation are discussed. These formats for sampling are outlined in Figure 10–3. As shown, the sampling formats are organized into three broad categories: clinician-designed tasks, norm-referenced tasks, and other published tasks. Several options for speech sampling exist within each category, and each is discussed in some detail below.

Clinician-Designed Tasks

Clinician-designed tasks can be either informal or formal in nature. As discussed above, the use of formal (i.e., standardized) elicitation procedures facilitates comparisons of data both within and between clients. Therefore, it is recommended that the primary speech samples used within a fluency assessment follow a standard elicitation method.

Options for Speech Sampling	**Clinician-designed tasks:**
	- Conversation, narration, oral reading
	- Sentence production, rote speech, singing
	- Fluency enhancing conditions, trial use of treatment strategies
	Norm-referenced tasks:
	- *Stuttering Severity Instrument-4* (SSI-4)
	-*Test of Childhood Stuttering* (TOCS)
	- *Controlled Oral Word Association Test* (COWAT) [verbal fluency]
	Other published tasks:
	-Informal application of tasks from certain tests that are normed for something other than fluency
	-E.g., Tests of speech sound production, expressive language

Figure 10–3. Options for speech sampling in fluency assessment. Clinicians can implement self-designed tasks in either a systematic (standard) or nonsystematic (informal) manner. Norm-referenced tasks are published instruments that utilize standard administration and data analysis procedures. The category of "Other published tasks" is reserved for tasks that utilize a standard administration procedure but lack norms, and for procedures that utilize a standard administration procedure but are normed for something other than fluency. Clinicians can assess speech from the latter tasks informally.

Conversational Samples

Speech-language pathologists routinely use conversation as a context for speech sampling during fluency assessment (ASHA, 1995; Williams, Darley, & Spriestersbach, 1978). Such conversations usually are *dyadic* in structure, meaning that they involve only two communicators. In clinical settings, client-clinician and client-caregiver dyads are most common. When assessing children, it is useful, when possible, to observe client-sibling conversations. The latter context sometimes features a higher rate of fluency stressors (e.g., verbal interruptions, verbal conflict) than the child-adult interactions do (Logan, 2003a). As such, it may provide insight into how the child performs under relatively demanding conditions.

Contemporary authorities recommend eliciting conversational samples that contain 300 to 500 syllables (e.g., Conture, 2001; Manning, 2010). With adolescents and adults, samples of this length usually take only a few minutes to complete. With young children, recalcitrant clients, or clients with severely impaired fluency, speech sample elicitation can take considerably longer, however. Some researchers have examined the effect of sample length on disfluency results. For example, Sawyer and Yairi (2006) examined differences in preschooler's disfluency frequency for various 300-syllable subsections of a 1200-syllable sample. They reported that, on average, the preschooler's disfluency frequency increased during the latter stages of the sample (e.g., the children produced more disfluency during syllables 900 to 1200 than they did during syllables 1 to 300). In a follow-up study, Sawyer, Chon, and Ambrose (2008) found that preschoolers tended to use more complicated utterances in the late

stages of the interactions than they did in the early stages. Based on this finding, the authors attributed the variation in the preschooler's disfluency to demands associated with utterance production. They hypothesized that children become increasingly at ease as the speech sample progresses and, thus, more talkative.

In a similarly designed study with adult speakers, Logan and Haj-Tas (2007) found no difference in disfluency frequency across 300-syllable subsections of speech samples that contained at least 1800 syllables. They concluded that, with adults, a clinician could obtain essentially the same information about disfluency frequency from a 300-syllable sample as he or she could from an 1800-syllable sample. Of course, disfluency frequency is not the only behavior of interest in a fluency assessment, and fluency patterns can vary from day to day. Thus, as a rule, the longer a clinician observes a client, the more likely he or she is to obtain a valid measure of the client's functioning.

Conversation is, by its nature, a dynamic activity. As discussed above, however, it is useful for clinicians to introduce at least some standardization to the conversational samples they elicit. Although it is unrealistic and undesirable to control exactly what the client says, there are several aspects of the conversational sample that can be at least partially controlled. With interactions that include children, for example, the clinician can standardize the toys that he or she introduces to facilitate conversation. With adolescent and adult clients, the clinician can base the interaction around a standard set of prompts such as the ones described above in the section on oral interviews. Methods like these increase the similarity of the speaking context across clients.

When assessing child-caregiver interactions, the clinician also can provide the child's caregiver with guidance on how to interact with the child. Some caregivers may be eager to "get the child to talk" in speech sampling contexts. This leads them to pepper the child with questions, most of which are designed to elicit a single bit of information; for example, *What are you holding?* (a dog); *What color is it?* (Black); *Do you like it?* (Yep); *How many animals are here?* (Three). Although the caregivers mean well, such questions invariably elicit very short, linguistically simple utterances. Because children produce short, simple utterances more fluently than they produce long complex utterances (Bernstein Ratner & Sih, 1987; Gaines, Runyan, & Meyers, 1991; Logan & Conture, 1995, 1997; and see Zackheim & Conture, 2003, for a review), a sample that consists mostly of 1- to 3-word utterances is almost guaranteed to yield an inflated estimate of the child's fluency functioning. For this reason, we routinely encourage caregivers to allow the child to take the lead in conversation and, rather than presenting a series of narrowly focused questions to the child, they instead should spend time narrating either their own actions or the child's actions (e.g., *I'm driving the car. You're putting lots of animals in the barn!*). Such remarks generally lead to a wider variety of utterances from the child: short and long utterances, simple and complex utterances, responses and assertions, and consequently, a more representative sample of how the child speaks.

Clinicians can gain insight into the effects of utterance complexity on conversational fluency by systematically altering the types of requests they present to clients (Logan & Caruso, 1997). As noted above, closed-ended requests tend to evoke short, simple responses and, often, fluent speech as well. In contrast, open-ended requests (e.g., *Tell me how it looks.*)

and simple assertions (e.g., *I like the blue one best.*) tend to evoke relatively long, complex utterances, along with disfluent speech (Logan, 2003a; Sawyer et al., 2008; Weiss & Zebrowski, 1992). To summarize, if the clinician's goal is to assess a child's fluency performance during relatively low-demand discourse, he or she can spend a portion of the conversation presenting the child with a series of closed-ended requests that are likely to elicit narrow bits of information. Alternately, if the goal is to assess the child's performance during high-demand discourse, a clinician can spend a segment of the conversation presenting open-ended requests or assertions to the child. We illustrate the process of eliciting various types of utterances further in Figure 10–4. As shown in the figure, the adult's utterances tend to shape the complexity of the child's utterances. Factors such as topic familiarity, audience size, and time demands can affect fluency performance during conversation as well. These issues are addressed under the topic of fluency stressors later in the chapter.

A variation of the face-to-face conversational sample is the telephone-based conversation. Many people who stutter report that it especially is difficult for them to talk fluently during telephone conversations. The reasons for this are not entirely clear, but one obvious difference between telephone and face-to-face interactions is the access that the conversationalists have to visual information about their partner's actions. The lack of visual cues during telephone conversations can make it difficult for a person to recognize instances of disfluency in the partner's speech, particularly when the disfluency involves fixed articulatory postures and a cessation of audible speech. At such times, the person who is assuming the listener role may misinterpret the silence

Line	Clinician utterance	Child utterance
1	Look at these!	
2	Lots of toys!	
3	What is this?	
4		A lion
5	Yes. What sound does he make?	
6		{makes growling sound}
7	Does he run fast or slow?	
8		Fast.
9	What's that called?	
10		An elephant.
11	Yes, and what's this?	
12		A trunk.
13	Elephants are really big.	
14	I saw one at the zoo.	
15		|I- I- I-| I saw one too |and-| and |it- it-|it picked up a tree |with-| with its trunk.
16	Elephants are kind of scary.	
17		|No but-| No |but-| but elephants are kind of nice.

Figure 10–4. Segment of a transcribed conversation between a clinician and a preschool-aged child. Clinicians can influence the length and complexity of children's utterances by attending to the types of utterances they produce during conversation. The clinician presents narrowly focused requests for information on lines 3, 5, 7, 9, and 11 of the transcript. The child responds to each of these requests appropriately, and, in each case, the utterance is very short and fluent. The clinician's general comments on lines 14 and 16 elicit relatively long and complex comments from the child. On line 16, the clinician presents information with which the child is likely to disagree. The child's comments on lines 15 and 17 contain more words, greater syntactic complexity, and more disfluency than the utterances on lines 4, 8, 10, and 12.

as the end of the speaker's conversational turn and then interrupt the speaker. It also is common for the listener to think that the telephone connection has been disconnected or that some other kind of technical difficulty has arisen. Such misinterpretations can lead to inquiries about whether the partner remains on the telephone (e.g., *Hello? Hello? Are you there? Hello?*), to comment about the quality of the connection (e.g., *I think something is wrong with your phone*) or, worse yet, to hang up. Such actions often exacerbate the fluency difficulties of people who stutter.

When assessing fluency in adolescent and adult clients, it is useful to ask them to make at least one telephone call. The call can consist of an inquiry to a local business regarding the cost or availability of some item or service. Although telephone conversations are much briefer than face-to-face conversations, they provide a way to introduce fluency stressors that are more authentic and intense than those tend to occur in clinical settings.

Narrative Samples

Another common speech elicitation task used during fluency assessment is *narration*. A narrative essentially is a monologue, during which the speaker talks at some length on a particular topic or theme. Authorities often classify narratives according to the type of information conveyed within them and the way in which they are elicited (Gillam & Pearson, 2004). Heath (1982), for example, used a four-part classification system to describe narratives:

- *Recounts*, which are prompted verbal reports of past factual events;
- *Accounts,* which are unprompted verbal reports of past events;
- *Eventcasts*, which are descriptions of ongoing activities; and
- *Fictional stories*, which involve descriptions of imaginary characters and events.

Narratives tend to elicit relatively complex sentence forms. As such, they can be more demanding to produce fluently than conversational speech. Byrd, Logan, and Gillam (2012) found that school-aged children who stutter demonstrated higher frequencies of repetitions and prolongations during a narrative task than they did during a structured conversation task. Some types of narratives are more challenging for speakers to produce than others are. For instance, children speak more fluently when the objects that they are speaking about are immediately present than they do when the objects are removed from view (Trautman, Healey, & Norris, 2001). Factors such as topic familiarity, audience size, and time demands can affect fluency performance during narration as well. We discuss these issues further under the topic of contextual factors later in the chapter.

Informal narrative elicitation tasks are relatively simple to design. A common approach is to ask a client to talk about one or more topics for a set length of time (ASHA, 1995; Riley, 2009). In our experience, 2 to 3 minutes is an appropriate length of time. Examples of topic prompts that are likely to elicit substantial samples of speech with adolescents and adults include the following:

- Describe the plot of a favorite movie, television show, or book;
- Describe a pleasant (or unpleasant) experience;
- Describe a memorable trip, adventure, or vacation;
- Describe the rules, strategy, and challenges associated with a favorite video game;
- Describe the routines, duties, and/or challenges associated with school or work;
- Propose a solution to a societal problem;
- Express an opinion about some current, controversial topic; and
- Explain a particular group's stance on some current, controversial topic.

Many clients, adults included, find it challenging to talk continuously for more than a few minutes. Thus, before the client begins the narrative, it helps to remind him or her of the objective (i.e., continuous talking for *x* minutes) and to explain that the objective will be easier to meet if the client attempts to provide a highly detailed account of the topic. The clinician may find it necessary to issue general prompts (e.g., *Tell me more about ____*) when the client appears poised to finish the narrative prematurely.

Another option is to elicit fictional narratives. With this type of narrative, the clinician typically provides the speaker with a structure or framework around which to base the story. Many researchers have used wordless picture books to elicit fictional narratives from children. The clinician prompts the child to look through the book first to obtain the gist of the story. The clinician then instructs the child to construct a story that goes along with the picture sequence. Another option is for the clinician to model a fictional narrative for a child using a picture sequence and then prompt the child to retell the story. Children in the 9- to 11-year-old range produce longer and more structurally complex narratives when retelling a clinician's narrative than they do when generating a fictional narrative from scratch in response to a story prompt such as "Once upon a time, two boys wandered into a deep dark cave . . . " (Merritt & Liles, 1989).

Bilingual clients may report that their fluency difficulties are more severe in one language than in the other. In such cases, it often is useful to elicit narratives from the client in both English and the other language. Although the second language may be one that the clinician does not speak, the clinician nonetheless may still be able to recognize evidence of fluency impairment as the client speaks (Ginther, Dimova, & Yang, 2010; Van Borsel & de Britto Pereira, 2005). It is not appropriate to base diagnostic decisions entirely on analysis of an unfamiliar language, however, as research shows that clinicians arrive at more accurate and detailed diagnoses of fluency impairment when speech samples are presented in their native language as opposed to a language they do not speak (Van Borsel & Medeiros de Britto Pereira, 2005).

Oral Reading Samples

If the client is able to read independently, samples of oral reading are useful to elicit. Oral reading differs from narration and conversation in several ways. One main difference is that the content of what the reader can say is constrained by the printed text. For some clients, this seems to enhance fluency—perhaps because it places fewer demands on the language formulation system. For other clients, however, oral reading elicits much more disfluency than either narration or conversation—perhaps because the client is no longer able to use compensatory strategies such as word substitution, word-order transposition, and circumlocution in response to impending disfluency.

Any reading passage that is consistent with the client's reading level is appropriate to use. The clinician simply provides the client with the passage and asks him or her to read it aloud. Suitable passages exist in magazines, newspapers, books, and so forth. As we will discuss in the section on norm-referenced tasks, passages from formal, published tests are available, as well. Such tests typically contain a series of passages that differ in reading difficulty. This property makes it easier for the clinician to select an appropriate passage for the client.

Reading samples typically are elicited by having the client read aloud alone (i.e., solo reading). A variation of this method is to use *choral reading*, wherein the clinician and the client read the passage aloud in unison. People who stutter usually exhibit much less disfluency during choral speaking conditions than they do in solo speaking conditions, and they perceive speech production as being much less effortful as well (Andrews, Howie, Dozsa, & Guitar, 1982; Ingham, Warner, Byrd, & Cotton, 2006). Although the stuttering-related behaviors may not be completely eliminated in speech under choral reading, the change in a client's performance often is quite impressive (Stager & Ludlow (1998). Choral reading offers other potential benefits during assessment, as well. For example, in cases where a client exhibits extremely disfluent speech, choral reading provides a way for the clinician to help the client finish an oral reading passage that the client otherwise might be inclined to abandon. In addition, we have found that the fluency enhancement that occurs during choral reading often prompts the client to initiate discussion about the variable nature of fluency in disorders such as stuttering.

Sentence Production Tasks

Sentence production tasks allow clinicians to examine the effects of syntactic, prosodic, and phonologic structure on speech fluency. Sentence production tasks have two primary forms: *sentence imitation* and *sentence generation*. With a sentence imitation task, the clinician says a sentence aloud and then asks the client to repeat it, verbatim. The sentence stimuli typically vary in difficulty according to the number or nature of syllables, words, syntactic forms, and stress patterns they contain. Sentence imitation is similar to oral reading in that the clinician provides the client with what he or she must say, and the client is obligated to say it. Given these constraints, a sentence imitation task is another potentially useful method to identify clients who rely on circumlocution, word substitution, and the like to attain fluent-sounding speech.

In Table 10–2, we provide examples of some of the sentence types that researchers have elicited in disfluency research.

Table 10–2. Utterance Types, Listed by Approximate Syntactic Difficulty and Impact on Disfluency

Syntactic Difficulty	Utterance Type	Example	Disfluency Impact
Very low[a]	Single word	Green.	Very low
	Phrase	After school.	
Low	Simple active affirmative declarative	The boy threw the little ball.	Low
	Negative	The boy didn't throw the ball.	
	Question with auxiliary inversion	Did the boy throw the ball?	
Moderate	Passive	The ball was thrown by the boy.	Moderate
	Dative	The boy threw the dog a ball.	
High	Center-embedded relative clause	The ball that the boy threw was new.	High
	Left-branching adverbial clause	When the boy threw the ball, the dog ran.	
	Adjunct (subordinate) clause	The boy patted his dog after throwing the ball.	

[a]Single-word utterances and phrases often occur in response to questions. For example, when presented the question, "What color is your new shirt?," the speaker responds "Green." The response is *elliptical*, meaning that the speaker has deleted linguistic content that he or she shares with the communication partner (in this example, "My shirt is . . . ").

As shown in the table, the relative difficulty of a sentence's syntax is associated with the likelihood for disfluency to occur within it. Bernstein Ratner and Sih (1987) examined the effect of various syntactic forms—including some of the forms shown in Table 10–2—on children's fluency within the context of a sentence imitation task. They presented 10 different sentence forms, which varied in developmental difficulty, to children. Results of the study showed that late-emerging syntactic forms evoked significantly more disfluency from children than the early-emerging forms did, and syntactic complexity affected the fluency of children who stutter more than it did the fluency of typical children. Others (e.g., Gordon & Luper, 1989; Gordon, Luper, & Peterson, 1986) have used similar approaches with children and reported similar effects using a narrower range of syntactic forms. Note in Table 10–2 that when an utterance consists of only a single word or a phrase (nonsentence forms), the impact on fluency usually is minimal; that is, speakers tend to produce such utterances very fluently.

Several researchers have examined whether syntactic complexity effects persist beyond childhood. For example, Logan (2001) presented blocks of sentences to adolescents and adults who stutter. The participants read, memorized, and then reproduced the target sentences a short time later within the context of a reaction time task. The sentences differed in terms of the syntactic structure of the subject noun phrase, such that ostensibly simple subject forms (e.g., Determiner + Noun) were contrasted with complex subject forms (e.g., Determiner + Noun + Relative Clause). In contrast to previous research with children, however, the syntactically complex sentence forms elicited no more disfluency than did the relatively simple sentence forms.

Tsiamtsiouris and Cairns (2013) used a wider variety of sentences than the ones in Logan (2001) within a prepared sentence context and did report an increase in adults' disfluency in sentences with high syntactic complexity. More specifically, sentences containing relative clauses in the subject noun phrase and sentences containing left-branching subordinate clauses evoked more disfluency in adults than contrasting sentences that featured simpler syntax. Examples of both of these complex sentence types are shown below.

Example 10–1:

The applicant <u>the man liked</u> got the new position of supervisor with the school. (Relative clause [underlined text] in a subject noun phrase)

<u>*Due to the snowstorm and high gusty winds,*</u> *the superintendent closed the school.* (Left-branching subordinate clause [underlined text])

Taken together, the results from such studies suggest that syntactic structure contributes to variations in speech fluency. A clinician can adapt sentences such as these in fluency assessment to examine the effect of linguistic complexity on fluency.

Effects of other language-related variables on fluency can be assessed using sentence-level tasks, as well. For example, Klouda and Cooper (1988) examined the effect of contrastive stress on the frequency and location of stuttering-related disfluency within a set of experimental sentences. They asked participants to read a target sentence silently. Each target sentence was followed by one of three focusing questions. The focusing questions obligated the participants to place primary stress on certain nouns within the sentences. After reading the focusing question, the participants then read the target sentence aloud. The researchers found a significant relationship between the word that carried primary stress within a sentence and the occurrence of stuttered speech. Thus, a task like this seems to be a straightforward way to elicit information about the effect of stress assignment on speech fluency. An example of the focusing questions and target sentence stimuli that Klouda and Cooper used appears below:

- Target sentence: <u>Maryann</u> picked the gift that <u>Priscilla</u> sent to her <u>grandfather</u>. (Candidate words for stress focus are underlined.)
  - Focusing question 1: *Did Maryann or Nancy pick the gift that Priscilla sent to her grandfather?* (Resulting place of stress focus = *Maryann*);
  - Focusing question 2: *Did Maryann pick the gift that Priscilla or Beth sent to her grandfather?* (Resulting place of stress focus = *Priscilla*); and
  - Focusing question 3: *Did Maryann pick the gift that Priscilla sent to her sister, or the one sent to her grandfather?* (Resulting place of stress focus = *grandfather*).

Other permutations of the *sentence generation* task exist as well. Another commonly used approach incorporates modeling of desired syntactic forms. That is, the clinician presents a model sentence to a client and then asks the client to generate a new sentence that features the same syntactic form as the clinician's model but different content words. An example of the modeled sentence method appears in Figure 10–5. The approach is an effective

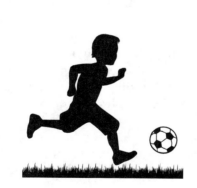
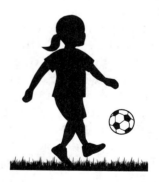

Clinician's Model:
The boy kicks a soccer ball when he runs.

Client's Target Response:
The girl kicks a soccer ball when she walks.

Figure 10–5. Example of stimuli used in a modeled sentence task. The clinician produces a model sentence by describing the picture on the left. The clinician then asks the client to describe the picture on the right using the syntactic form of the modeled sentence (e.g., "Make your sentence like the one I just said"). The clinician can vary the syntactic form of the modeled sentences so that some sentence targets are more difficult than others are. With children, syntactically complex sentences usually elicit more disfluency than syntactically simple sentences do.

way to elicit information about fluency performance in syntactic contexts that the client may produce only occasionally during spontaneous speech.

Introducing Fluency Stressors Into Sampling Tasks

There is value in attempting to incorporate real-world fluency stressors into clinic-based speech samples. The goal behind fluency stressor introduction is not to traumatize a speaker or to completely impede his or her ability to communicate. Rather, it is to simulate the types of speaking challenges that a speaker faces in daily life and, in doing so, to obtain a clear picture of the extent to which a client's fluency varies.

Yaruss (1997) analyzed children's disfluency frequency across a variety of speaking tasks and found that a "pressured conversation" task elicited significantly more disfluency from the children than other speech elicitation contexts did. In the study, the pressured-speech context featured a clinician who spoke rapidly and interrupted children at a greater-than-typical frequency—behaviors that resulted in the children talking faster as well. As noted above, linguistic complexity is another stressor that tends to elicit disfluency, particularly with children (Logan & Caruso, 1997). Clinicians can influence a client's utterance complexity during conversation by presenting open-ended queries (e.g., *Tell me about . . .*)— request types that tend to elicit replies that contain relatively many syllables and grammatical units.

Kully and Langevin (1999) identified several other variables that clinicians can manipulate to make a speaking task more or less demanding for a client to produce fluently. Included on their list are the following:

- *Amount of cueing support.* In this context, the term *cue* refers to clinician-based reminders for the client to talk in a particular way (e.g., slower, with more frequent pauses). Clients tend to talk more fluently when provided with ample clinician cues and less fluently when talking without clinician cue support.

- *Amount of feedback.* In this context, the notion of feedback refers to the clinician's evaluative statements about the client's speech fluency and/or use of fluency management techniques (e.g., *Good!, That sounds right.*).

- *Physical setting.* Clients often report that certain environmental settings aggravate their fluency difficulties. Such settings vary across clients, so it is best to first ask the client to rank which settings are relatively difficult and which are relatively easy to speak fluently within. One commonly reported environmental stressor is audience size—many speakers with impaired fluency produce more disfluency when speaking to a large audience than they do when speaking with one person.

In our experience, it is challenging for clinicians to replicate the subtleties of the day-to-day fluency stressors that clients encounter in real-world settings. It also is challenging for clinicians to deliver fluency stressors in a systematic or controlled way from one client to the next. Thus, clinicians are advised to rehearse the fluency stressors that they intend to introduce and to develop an implementation plan that specifies how and when the stressors will be delivered within various sampling tasks.

Other Sampling Conditions

There are several other informal sampling tasks that a clinician may wish to consider using. These are described in this section.

Sampling Rote Speech and Other Performative Acts

Rote speech entails the production of well-rehearsed, fixed content. Examples of rote speech include the following: counting from 1 to 20, saying a familiar prayer or poem, reciting the *Pledge of Allegiance*, listing the letters of the alphabet, and naming the days of the week or the months of the year. Tasks of this sort allow the clinician to examine fluency in contexts that, from a pragmatic perspective, are *performative* in nature (see Fey, 1986). That is, the speaker accomplishes a communicative act merely by saying whatever it is he or she says. With such speech acts, there is no communicative "give and take" as there is in conversation, and some of the tasks (e.g., counting, alphabet recitation) are organized in a serial manner rather than in accordance with syntactic rules. The speaker's language formulation load presumably is relatively low during rote speaking tasks because the message essentially is "prepackaged" in memory.

Elicitation of rote speech normally takes very little time. Generally, speakers with typical fluency will have no difficulty performing these activities fluently. Many speakers with developmental stuttering and cluttering will exhibit relatively little disfluency during rote speaking tasks, as well. Thus, when a speaker does exhibit symptoms of fluency impairment in this context, it is unusual and, in a sense, an indication of the breadth of the person's disability. Speakers with acquired stuttering are more apt to exhibit significant disfluency during rote speech than speakers with developmental stuttering are (Market, Montague, Jr., Buffalo, & Drummond, 1990). This pattern perhaps is indicative of the nature or scope of the client's fluency impairment. The fixed content within such tasks also is useful for identifying speakers who conceal their stuttering from others using word substitution and other compensatory strategies.

Singing is another sampling context that clinicians sometimes include in fluency assessment (Andrews et al., 1982). In our experience, clients with developmental stuttering rarely, if ever, exhibit disfluency while singing. Simple, familiar songs such as "Happy Birthday" or "Row, Row, Row Your Boat" are suitable for this activity. Results from neuroimaging studies suggest that the neural activation patterns associated with performance singing are distinct from those associated with propositional speech (Bella & Berkowska, 2009; Jeffries, Fritz, & Braun, 2003; Özdemir, Norton, & Schlaug, 2006; Zarate, 2013), with singing involving (among other things) a greater degree of bilateral to right-lateralized cortical activation than speech in some studies. The unique neural activation pattern that typifies singing, then, may help to explain the dissociation in fluency performance that speakers who stutter usually exhibit between talking and singing.

Trial Use of Fluency Management Strategies

Before the assessment ends, it is useful to spend a few minutes assessing the effects of common fluency management strategies on the client's fluency performance (ASHA, 1995). Activities like these sometimes are termed "trial therapy." With this activity, the clinician gains insight into issues such as which types of speech modification have the greatest initial impact on the client's performance and how the client reacts to various potential treatment approaches. Most behaviorally based fluency management strategies require conscious effort to employ: Clients must attend to their speech-related movements on a moment-to-moment basis. Speaking in this manner can feel quite unnatural at first. Thus, it is important to understand how the client perceives these regulated forms of speech and to provide the client with a chance to voice any reservations that he or she may have about these speaking modes prior to commencing treatment. See Table 10–3 for examples of speech modifications that a clinician can introduce as part of a trial therapy sequence.

The speaking styles shown in Table 10–3 mirror the fluency management techniques that many speech-language pathologists commonly use in therapy. The first approach, "talking as smoothly as possible," provides insight into the client's capacity for fluent speech and the effect of attentional focus on speech fluency. The second approach, "tallying disfluency," provides insight into a client's ability to self-monitor disfluency from moment to moment. The remaining approaches involve alterations in speech timing and/ or tension, and many of them often result in immediate and substantial reduction in disfluency frequency—at least within a clinical setting (Andrews et al., 1982).

Eliciting Speech Under Fluency-Inducing Conditions

Research with speakers who stutter has revealed that certain speaking conditions tend to reliably induce speech that is much more fluent than it is during ordinary speaking conditions. Such conditions have been variably termed *fluency-inducing conditions* or *fluency-enhancing contexts.* Data from speech that is produced under fluency-inducing conditions provide additional insight into a client's fluency variability and, possibly, his or her suitability for certain treatment strategies. Some authors (e.g., Seery, 2005) have used fluency-inducing conditions for forensic purposes to determine whether an individual truly is stuttering or, instead, merely pretending to do so (i.e., *malingering*). If a client does not show substantial fluency improvement under these conditions, it would provide partial support for the hypothesis that the stuttering is not authentic.

In a study of three adults who stuttered, Andrews et al. (1982) examined the effects of 15 conditions that others previously had determined to have fluency-inducing properties. In their study, 7 of the 15 tested conditions resulted in greater than 90% reduction in stuttering frequency for the participants. We already have discussed 4 of the 7 conditions in the previous sections (*singing* [under performative speech]; *slowing, prolonged speech,* and *syllable-timed speech* [under trial use of fluency management strategies]). In this section, we focus on the methods associated with the three remaining contexts from Andrews et al.'s study, each of which also was associated with marked reduction in stuttering frequency:

1. *Chorus reading:* The participants read a passage aloud in unison with two members of the research team;
2. *Shadowing:* The researchers presented the participants with a recording of a speaker who was reading a passage aloud and asked the participants to repeat back what the speaker said as the speaker talked; and

Table 10–3. Speaking Patterns to Assess When Conducting "Trial Intervention" With a Client

Speaking Pattern	Instructions	Model
Increasing attention to speech articulation	"Pay attention to how you are speaking. Try to talk as smoothly as possible, without any disfluency."	None.
Self-monitoring of disfluency	"For next minute, put a tick mark on the paper each time your speech is disfluent. Continue to talk as you make the tick mark."	Demonstrate several sentences that contain (deliberate) instances of disfluency. Make a tick mark on the paper after each one.
Reducing speaking rate by producing longer, more frequent pauses	"For the next minute, slow your speech by inserting more pauses and making the pauses last a bit longer than usual."	Demonstrate several sentences that feature substantial pauses (i.e., ~250 ms) at most phrase boundaries (e.g., *"In the morning [pause] I am going [pause] to the gym. And then [pause] . . . I am coming home."*
Stopping and then restarting a disfluent word	"For the next minute, stop yourself during or immediately after disfluency. Then say the disfluent word or disfluent part of the sentence again in a slower, more relaxed way."	Demonstrate examples of (deliberate) disfluency that is similar to the client's disfluency. Stop during or after disfluency and then redo the word with controlled or less severe stuttering.
Reducing articulation rate by increasing syllable duration	"For the next minute, try talking while using a slow, drawn-out style of speech. Make each syllable you say last about __ seconds."	Demonstrate several sentences at a rate of ~1 syllable per second. Maintain the intonational contour throughout each of the sentences and blend syllables seamlessly. Use a timer to monitor syllable duration.
Regulating speech timing by focusing on speech rhythm.	"During the next minute, focus on the rhythm of your speech as you talk. Try to put more of a 'beat' into the syllables you say."	Demonstrate several sentences in which the stressed syllables in each utterance are said more emphatically and syllable duration is less variable.

3. *Response contingent stimulation:* Participants spoken in narrative fashion and the researchers presented them with a signal to stop speaking for 10 seconds after each instance of stuttering.

Each of these three conditions are straightforward to administer during a fluency assessment. As will be explained in Chapters 13 and 14, clinicians have researched response contingent stimulation extensively as a treatment for stuttering and to a lesser extent for cluttering. Neither choral speech nor shadowing has been studied extensively as stand-alone treatments for fluency impairment; however, both techniques may be used incidentally as part of some other behavioral treatment. For example, if a client exhibits difficulty maintaining a target speech rate independently during the early stages of treatment, the clinician then might offer the client temporary support by asking the client to shadow or talk in unison with his or her speech until the client demonstrates the ability to produce the target rate consistently.

We conclude this section with a brief discussion of one other fluency-inducing context—*adaptation*. In the literature on stuttering, the term *adaptation* refers to the tendency for speakers to produce progressively fewer instances of disfluency with each successive reading of a passage (Williams et al., 1978). To measure adaptation, the clinician presents a client with a printed passage and asks him or her to read it aloud. When the client finishes reading the passage, the clinician promptly asks the client to read it aloud again. This process is repeated until the client has read the passage aloud several times in succession. Disfluency (or stuttering) frequency is computed for each rendition of the passage. The extent of improvement (i.e., adaptation) in speech fluency then is computed using the following formula:

$$\% \text{ of Adaptation} = \frac{(SW \text{ in Reading } 1 - SW \text{ in final Reading})}{SW \text{ in Reading } 1} \times 100$$

Note: SW = number of stuttered words

So, for a client who exhibited 25 stuttered words during the first reading of a passage and 10 stuttered words during the fifth reading, the adaptation score would be 60%. For some clients, the fluency improvement associated with adaptation may be less than that in conditions such as choral reading or prolonged speech. None-theless, data from the task still can be of use by providing insight into the extent to which the client's fluency performance improves as a function of motor rehearsal.

Collecting Data: Speech Samples From Norm-Referenced Tests

An alternative to clinician-designed speech sampling tasks is the use of norm-referenced fluency assessment instruments. Such instruments are considered "formal" because they feature standardized methods for eliciting speech samples and norms for typical fluency performance. At present, surprisingly few published assessment instruments feature both standardized speech sample elicitation tasks and normative data on fluency performance. We summarize the primary instruments in Table 10–4 and discuss them below.

The *Stuttering Severity Instrument–Fourth Edition (SSI-4)*

The *Stuttering Severity Instrument–Fourth Edition* (SSI-4; Riley, 2009) was first published in 1972 and currently is in its fourth edition. Both clinicians and researchers have used the SSI widely. As suggested by its title, the instrument is designed to

Table 10–4. Characteristics of Published Tests That Feature Standardized Speech Sample Elicitation Methods and Age-Based Norms for Fluency Performance

Test	Purpose	Sampling Tasks	Norms Reference Group	Age
SSI-4 (Riley, 2009)	Rating stuttering severity	Oral reading	PWS	Preschool to adult
		Conversation[a]	PWS	
TOCS (Gillam et al., 2009)	Diagnosing stuttering, rating stuttering severity	Rapid picture naming	TS, PWS	Children 4 to 12 years old
		Modeled Sentences	TS, PWS	
		Structured Conversation[a]	TS, PWS	
		Narration	TS, PWS	
COWAT (Benton et al., 1994)	Diagnosing deficits in categorical naming	Word generation	TS	Adults

Note. SSI-4 = Stuttering Severity Instrument–Fourth Edition; *TOCS* = Test of Childhood Stuttering; *COWAT* = Controlled Oral Word Association Test; *PWS* = people who stutter; *TS* = typical speakers.
[a] Examiner-directed conversation is recommended or described in test manual.

assist clinicians with rating the severity with which a person stutters. The SSI-4 does not include norm reference data from speakers with typical fluency; thus, it is not a diagnostic test, per se. The test does include fluency-related norms that are based on speakers who stutter, however, and these data provide a sense of how a particular speaker compares to other people who stutter. Two primary types of speech samples are elicited: oral reading and spontaneous speaking.

The oral reading task on the SSI-4 fits the definition of a standardized task more closely than the conversational task does. The SSI-4 contains 10 unique reading passages (two each at the 3rd grade, 5th grade, and 7th grade reading levels, and four at the adult reading level). The passages vary in length from 157 syllables to 378 syllables, and the clinician asks the client to read a passage of appropriate dif-

ficulty aloud. (Children who read at a second grade level or under do not attempt the reading task.) The use of common reading passages across clients facilitates comparisons both within and between individuals.

- For the speaking task, the SSI-4 contains four line-drawn pictures that the clinician can use to elicit speech from young children. Two pictures feature events that are "silly" or improbable (e.g., a flying a pig, goats on the roof of a barn), and two pictures feature action-oriented scenes. The examiner is instructed to make remarks as necessary to prompt the child to talk about the pictures. Based on wording in the manual, it appears that use of the picture-based elicitation procedure is optional, however. With older clients, the examiner engages the client in conversation about topics such as school, jobs, television shows, or movies. With younger children, examiners are instructed to elicit at least two conversations, which should take place on separate days. Examiners also are encouraged to have parents record the child's speech at home so that speech can be sampled in a naturalistic setting. Telephone samples are encouraged with clients who are old enough to complete the reading passage. At all ages, examiners are instructed to include "normal conversational pressures" through "questions, comments, and mild disagreements." The SSI-4 manual does not specify how frequently or intensively the examiner should introduce these pressures.

The examiner scores the SSI-4 by computing the percent of syllables stuttered during the reading and/or speaking tasks. Stuttering is not defined in the SSI-4; however, test norms for the SSI-4 appear to be carried over from the previous edition of the test (i.e., the SSI-3), wherein stuttering was defined as "repetitions or prolongations of sounds or syllables (including silent prolongations)" (Riley, 1994, p. 4). The stuttering frequency scores then are converted to a weighted "task score" using a conversion table that is included with the test and combined with weighted scores for stuttering duration and the appearance of concomitant behaviors. The overall weighted score then is compared with scores from other people who stutter to yield a

severity rating that can range from "very mild" to "very severe."

The *Test of Childhood Stuttering (TOCS)*

The *Test of Childhood Stuttering* (*TOCS*; Gillam, Logan, & Pearson, 2009) is a norm-referenced assessment tool for stuttering. The test is intended for children aged 4 to 12 years. The test is normed on children with typical fluency and children who stutter. Procedures for informal fluency analysis are included as well. The norm-referenced section of the test consists of the *Speech Fluency Measure* (which is discussed here) and the *Observational Rating Scales* (which is discussed later in this chapter, in the section on rating scales). The Speech Fluency Measure on the TOCS contains four speaking tasks:

- The first task is *Rapid Picture Naming*. For this task, children are asked to name pictures of 40 common objects as rapidly as possible. The examiner uses a stopwatch to time how long it takes the child to name the pictures. The examiner's request for rapid naming and the use of the stopwatch are designed to introduce time pressure into a task. Time pressure often has more of a debilitating effect on speakers with fluency impairment than it does on typically fluent speakers. Thus, the relatively simple task of naming pictures becomes more challenging for some speakers with the introduction of time pressure.
- The second task is *Modeled Sentences*. The structure of this task is identical to the format presented in the example of clinician-devised

modeled sentence production (see Figure 10–5). Nineteen sentences are elicited. The syntax within the sentences ranges from simple declarative forms (e.g., *The kids are taking a nap.*) to left branching adverbial clauses (e.g., *When the boy got mustard on his face, the girls laughed*). Variations in syntax are designed to stress speech production in ways that are likely to elicit symptoms of fluency impairment.

- The third task is *Structured Conversation*. This task is based on a sequence of pictures, which tell the story of an encounter between three children and two alien creatures. The examiner presents the child with 32 requests for information (4 per picture), most of which are open-ended questions or commands that are designed to elicit multiword utterances. Children with impaired fluency often find multiword utterances more challenging than word- or phrase-level utterances to produce fluently.

- The fourth task is *Narration*. This task utilizes the pictures from the Structured Conversation task. The examiner asks the child to use the pictures to construct a narrative about the story events. The child's responses from the Structured Conversation task form the basis for the narrative content. For many children who stutter, the Narration task elicits the highest levels of disfluency on the test (Byrd, Logan, & Gillam, 2012).

The examiner scores the TOCS by summing the number of responses that contain part- and whole-word repetitions and/or prolonged or "blocked" sounds. For the Rapid Picture Naming task, each word is scored for the presence or absence of disfluency. For the other speaking tasks, disfluency scoring is restricted to the presence or absence of disfluency within the first three words of each response. A child's total disfluency frequency score then is compared to norm-referenced data from children with typical fluency and other children who stutter.

Elicitation Tasks From Norm-Referenced Tests of Verbal Fluency

The construct of *verbal fluency* has been studied largely in relation to lexical retrieval. It typically is defined in terms of the number of unique words a person can generate within a specific category during a fixed amount of time. Thus, from a clinical standpoint, verbal fluency assessment focuses on the patient's verbal output (an aspect of talkativeness) more than the number or type of disfluencies that are produced. Although verbal fluency assessment can be used in any fluency assessment, it is most suitable to use when neurological disease or disorder and concomitant language impairment is present or suspected. With some cases, it may provide insight into how a client's fluency "holds up" under time pressure.

The *Controlled Oral Word Association Test* (COWAT; Benton, Hamsher, & Sivan, 1994) is described as a test of verbal fluency. Speakers are asked to produce as many words as possible that begin with a specific letter of the alphabet. Speakers are allotted one minute per letter to generate the words. Traditionally, the task has been organized around the letters *F*, *A*, and *S*. Alternate letter sets (i.e., *C*, *F*, and *L*; *P*, *R*, and *W*) have been used more recently, however (Rosset al., 2005). The examiner scores the test by summing the number of total words that the speaker produces across the three letters, and the score total then is compared against a reference score for typical adults.

The COWAT is sensitive particularly to frontal lobe dysfunction (Benton et al., 1994). Success on the task is thought to depend on both the speaker's semantic store of words and the ability to search the semantic store effectively in order to access and retrieve words (Chertkow & Bub, 1990). A variety of patient populations, including people with Parkinson's disease, schizophrenia, and Alzheimer's disease, tend to score poorly on the test; however, the nature of the performance difficulties varies across clinical populations (Ross et al., 2005). It is possible for people with one type of fluency disorder to score well on the COWAT and another type to score poorly.

The Word Associations subtest is part of the *Clinical Evaluation of Language Fundamentals–Fourth Edition* (CELF-4; Semel, Wiig, & Secord, 2003). The CELF-4 is used to assess functioning in receptive language, expressive language, and working memory. It is appropriate for use with individuals aged 5 to 21 years. The Word Associations task is similar to the COWAT (described above), in that the examiner asks the test-taker to name as many words as possible within 1 minute. Rather than letter names, however, the examiner provides the test-taker with a semantic category. Three categories are presented: (1) animals; (2) foods people eat; and (3) jobs or occupations that people do. The total number of words generated across the three categories is compared against an age-based criterion score. Like the COWAT, the Word Associations subtest can be expected to provide information about a speaker's verbal output and

lexical retrieval strategies more than the number or types of disfluency produced.

Speech Samples From Other Formal Tests

Clinicians also can describe fluency informally using the speech samples that result from any number of standardized tests of expressive language or speech sound production that are being administered to assess other aspects of a client's functioning. In Table 10–5, we provide examples of several such tests. The tasks for the first three tests listed in Table 10–5 (TOLD-P:4, CELF-4, TNL) feature norms for aspects of communication other than fluency. In our experience, each of these tasks or subtests is reliable at eliciting isolated sentences and/or consecutive sentences, some of which may feature relatively advanced syntax. As such, the tasks provide a context for stressing the speech production system in ways that potentially induce disfluency. This may provide useful information about fluency performance with clients who are suspected of having impaired fluency but exhibit little or no disfluency during casual conversation.

The *Goldman-Fristoe Test of Articulation-2* (GFTA-2; Goldman & Fristoe, 2000), like other tests of speech sound production, elicits single-word responses through picture labeling. Because single-word responses normally have a high likelihood of being spoken fluently, the presence of disfluency types such as part-word repetition or sound prolongation during the task is highly unusual among typical speakers and even relatively uncommon among people with impaired fluency. Assessment of speech sound production is a routine component in clinical evaluations of children's speech. Thus, it is not

Table 10–5. Examples of Published Tasks and Subtests That Feature Standardized Speech Sample Elicitation Methods but Are Normed for Aspects of Language or Speech Sound Production

Test	Age	Task or Subtest	
		Name	**Description**
Test of Language Development-Primary 4th Edition (TOLD-P:4)[a]	4 to 9	Relational Vocabulary	Describing similarities in word meanings
		Oral Vocabulary	Defining word meanings
		Sentence Imitation	Repeating sentences
Clinical Evaluation of Language Fundamentals–4th Edition (CELF-4)[b]	5 to 21	Recalling Sentences	Repeating sentences
		Formulated Sentences	Generating sentences
		Word Classes	Describing relationships between word meanings
		Understanding Spoken Paragraphs	Responding to requests for information
Test of Narrative Language (TNL)[c]	5 to 12	Narration	Retelling stories when given (a) no picture cues, (b) a single picture, and (c) a sequence of pictures
Goldman-Fristoe Test of Articulation–2 (GFTA-2)[d]	2 to 22	Sounds-in-Words	Naming pictures
		Sounds-in-Sentences	Story retelling
Apraxia Battery for Adults-2nd Edition (ABA-2)[e]	—	Diadochokinetic Rate	Rapid, sequenced repetition of 1-, 2-, and 3-syllable targets
		Utterance Time for Polysyllabic Words	Time taken to initiate naming of pictured object following stimulus presentation
Boston Diagnostic Aphasia Examination–3rd Edition[f]	—	Conversational and Expository Speech	Simple social responses, free conversation, picture description, narrative discourse
		Oral Expression	Saying automatized word sequences (e.g., counting); reciting of nursery rhymes; repeating words, phrases, and sentences
Western Aphasia Battery–Revised (WAB-R)[g]	—	Spontaneous Speech	Structured conversation elicitation, picture description
		Word Fluency	Generating words within a semantic category
		Repetition	Repeating words, phrases, and sentences

Note. Dashes indicate that test scoring is not age dependent.

[a]Newcomer and Hammill (2008); [b]Semel, Wiig, and Secord (2003); [c]Gillam and Pearson (2004); [d]Goldman and Fristoe (2000); [e]Dabul (2000); [f]Goodglass et al. (2000); [g]Kertesz (2006).

uncommon for a child with suspected fluency problems to complete a test such as the GFTA-2 during an initial evaluation. When a client exhibits symptoms of fluency impairment on single-word elicitation tasks such as the Sounds-in-Words subtest of the GFTA-2, it provides the clinician with insight into the breadth and depth of the client's disability as well as the types of stimuli that he or she may find challenging during the early stages of treatment.

For adults who present with fluency concerns secondary to acquired neurologic disorders such as aphasia, options for standardized speech sample elicitation include the conversational and expository speech tasks from the *Boston Diagnostic Aphasia Examination–Third Edition* (BDAE-3; Goodglass, Kaplan, & Barresi, 2000) and the spontaneous speech, word generation, and repetition tasks from the *Western Aphasia Battery–Revised* (WAB-R; Kertesz, 2006). The BDAE-3 features several recommended conversational topics as well as pictures (e.g., picture sequences in a cartoon-strip format and the well-known "cookie theft" scene), which are used to elicit narrative-style speech. The BDAE-3 also includes a protocol for eliciting automatized speech (e.g., counting, reciting the days of the week) and repetition of words, phrases, and sentences.

The WAB-R (Kertesz, 2006) features structured conversation and narrative elicitation tasks as well as a repetition task and a word generation task that is similar to both the COWAT and the Word Associations subtest on the CELF-4. The speech samples elicited from the *Apraxia Battery for Adults–Second Edition* (ABA-2; Dabul, 2000) consist of syllable- and word-level responses, some of which are produced under time constraints. The time pressure and multisyllable sequences on these tasks may make it challenging for some clients to speak fluently. The test also features tasks with connected speech (i.e., picture description, oral reading, and counting to 30 [forward and backward]). As with the BDAE-3 and the WAB-R, the disfluency characteristics of speech produced during administration of the ABA-2 can be analyzed informally.

Collecting Data: Rating Scales

Rating scales offer another means of collecting data about fluency functioning. Most of the rating scales used in fluency assessment provide information about a client's current functioning in speech fluency and associated domains such as quality of life and communication-related attitudes, feelings, and emotions. In most cases, the rating scales capture a time-frame that extends beyond an immediate situation; for example, "speech during the past month" or "speech in recent weeks." Most of the fluency-related rating scales entail *self-evaluation*. That is, the client assesses his or her own performance or experiences. With some ratings scales, someone other than the client (e.g., a parent, a teacher, a clinician) rates the client's functioning.

Published Rating Scales Specific to Developmental Stuttering

Most of the fluency-related rating scales in the speech-language pathology literature are oriented toward the assessment of developmental stuttering. This means that the content of such scales primarily pertains to the symptoms and experiences that are associated with the disorder. For this reason, we will discuss the stuttering-specific scales separately from rating scales that are applicable to other disorders or broader segments of the population.

In Table 10–6, we present an overview of rating scales that pertain to the assessment of developmental stuttering. The instruments in the top portion of Table 10–6 are oriented toward adults and college-aged students. The instruments in the mid-section of the table are oriented toward children, and those at the bottom of the table are useful for all ages. As indicated in the table, many of the instruments feature comparison or reference data (albeit, sometimes to a limited extent). Such data enable clinicians to determine how a particular client's performance compares to that of other people. Assessment instruments that lack such data do not allow for such comparisons. Still, they are potentially useful for use in evaluating pre- versus posttreatment performance within a single client.

Franic and Bothe (2008) evaluated the psychometric properties of 10 stuttering-related instruments (including several of the ones presented in Table 10–6) on criteria such as presence of a conceptual model, reliability, validity, interpretability, depth of content, administrative burden, and versatility. They identified several limitations with the instruments they reviewed, including the following: lack of a comprehensive conceptual model as a basis for the instruments, limited reliability and validity, and lack of comprehensive normative data.

Formal, Stuttering-Related Scales for Use With Adults

Nine stuttering-relating rating instruments that are designed for use with adult clients are presented in the top section of Table 10–6. Of the nine instruments, seven feature some type of reference data from speakers who stutter and, in four cases, typical speakers, as well. Such data are useful in interpreting the performance of individual clients.

In first row of the adult section of Table 10–6 is the the *Behavior Assessment Battery for Adults Who Stutter* (BAB-Adults) which is a collective term for three related rating scales described by Brutten (1975). Two of the rating scales are based on a list of 51 common speaking situations. With the *Speech Situation Checklist–Emotional Reaction* (SSC-ER) scale, the client provides ratings of the amount of anxiety that he or she experiences during each of the 51 situations. On the *Speech Situation Checklist–Speech Disruption* (SSC-SD) scale, the client rerates the same situations in terms of the amount of speech disruption experienced within each. Ratings such as these provide information about the client's perceptions of speech fluency and his or her speech-related feelings and emotions. With the third component of the BAB-A, the *Behavior Checklist* (BCL), the client reviews a list of potential coping strategies that accompany stuttering, and then marks the list to indicate which of them he or she uses when stuttered speech is expected. Hanson, Gronhovd, and Rice (1981) conducted an analysis of items on the SSC-ER scale to determine which scale items best discriminated between responses of speakers who stuttered and speakers who did not. They identified a subset of 21 SSC items that attained adequate discriminative power,

Table 10–6. Examples of Published Rating Scales Used in the Assessment of Developmental Stuttering

Instrument	Items	Responses	Norms/ Comparison Group
	Rating Scales for Adults		
Behavior Assessment Battery (Adults)[a]	Three subscales. Client rates 51 speech situations in terms of his/her (1) emotional reactions and (2) extent of speech disruption. Client also indicates (3) the coping behaviors he/she uses when anticipating stuttering.	51 items each on Emotional Reaction and Speech Disruption Checklists; 5 pt. labeled rating scales	Comparison data are available in for speakers of several languages.
Perceptions of Stuttering Inventory (PSI)[b]	Client reports whether various indicators of speech-related struggle, avoidance, and expectancy of stuttering are currently present when speaking.	60 items (20 each related to struggle, avoidance, and expectancy); binary ratings: present/absent	None
S24 Scale[c]	Client indicates his/her agreement with statements about various communication behaviors, beliefs, and feelings.	24 items; true/false responses	39 S; 25 NS
Self-Efficacy Scaling for Adult Stutterers (SESAS)[d]	Client rates speaking situations in terms of self-confidence for entering and maintaining fluency in each.	50 situations; 10 pt. labeled rating scales	20 S; 20 NS
Shortened Speech Situation Checklist–Emotional Reactions (S-SSC-ER)[e]	Client rates 21 situations (from long version of Speech Situation Checklist [see Behavior Assessment Battery (Adults)] for extent of negative emotions (e.g., anxiety, fear, tension).	21 items; 5 pt. labeled rating scales	33 S; 32 NS
Stutterer's Speech Situation Rating Sheet (SSRS)[f]	Client rates 40 speaking scenarios for (1) frequency of avoidance, (2) amount of enjoyment in participation, (3) severity of stuttering, and (4) frequency of stuttering.	160 distinct ratings (40 scenarios x 4 rating dimensions); 5 pt. labeled rating scales, one for each dimension	95 S
Subjective Screening of Stuttering (SSS)[g]	Client rates his/her stuttering severity, locus of control, and use of speech-related avoidance.	9 items; 9 pt. labeled rating scales	16 S
Wright & Ayres Stuttering Self-Rating Profile (WASSP)[h]	Clients rates the severity of their stuttering-related behaviors; use of avoidance strategies; thoughts/feelings about stuttering; and consequences of stuttering.	24 items; 7 pt. labeled rating scales	32 S

Instrument	Items	Responses	Norms/Comparison Group
Rating Scales for Children and Adolescents			
Behavior Assessment Battery for School-Aged Children Who Stutter (BAB-Children)[i]	Client rates various speech situations for emotional reactions and extent of speech disruption. Client also indicates the types of coping behaviors he/she uses when anticipating stuttering and provides ratings of speech-related attitudes (CAT).	50 items each on Emotional Reaction and Speech Disruption Checklists with 5 pt. labeled rating scales; 50 items on Behavior Checklist, yes/no response; 33 items on CAT, true/false response	(Ages 6 to 15)
Communication Attitude Test-Revised (CAT-R)[j]	Children rate 18 statements concerning their communication behaviors and attitudes toward talking.	Self-ratings, true/false response	70 S, 271 NS (ages 7 to 14)
Self-Efficacy for Adolescents Scale (SEA-Scale)[k]	Client rates speaking situations in terms of self-confidence for entering and maintaining fluency in each.	100 situations; 10 pt. labeled rating scales	45 S; 45 NS
TOCS: Observational Rating Scales (ORS)[l]	Parents, teachers, and/or clinicians rate the frequency with which a child produces various disfluency behaviors and experiences various negative consequences of disfluency.	18 items (9 on Speech Behaviors Scale; 9 on Disfluency-Related Consequences); 4 pt. labeled rating scales	123 S; 173 NS
Rating Scales for Children, Adolescents, and Adults			
Overall Assessment of the Speaker's Experience of Stuttering (Child, Teen, Adult Versions)[m]	Client completes a multi-item rating instrument that provides information about the impact of stuttering and rates the impact of stuttering on a person's life.	Self-ratings using 5 pt. labeled rating scales	Child version (ages 7 to 12); teen version (ages 13 to 17); adults 18 to 78
SSI-4: Clinical Use of Self-Reports (CUSR)[n]	People who stutter rate their perceived stuttering severity, locus of control, and extent of avoidance during face-to-face and telephone interactions.	13 items; 9 pt. labeled rating scales	None

Note: S = person who stutters; *NS* = person who does not stutter.

[a] Brutten (1975); [b] Woolf (1967); [c] Andrews and Cutler (1974); [d] Ornstein and Manning (1985); [e] Hanson, Gronhovd, and Rice (1981); [f] Shumak (1955); [g] Riley, Riley, and Maguire (2004); [h] Wright and Ayre (2000); [i] Brutten and Vanryckeghem (2007); [j] De Nil & Brutten (1991); [k] Ornstein and Manning (1985); [l] Gillam, Logan, and Pearson (2009); [m] Yaruss and Quesal (2006); [n] Riley (2009).

which then were compiled into a new instrument, the Shortened SSC. Hanson et al.'s shortened version of the SSC correctly classified the fluency status (stuttering, nonstuttering) of 93% of the people in a 29-person pool. These instruments are in some ways similar to the *Stutterer's Speech Situation Rating Sheet* (Shumak, 1955), which is an older instrument that entails reiterative ratings of speech situations. In the latter case, the client rates 40 speaking scenarios for the amount of avoidance, stuttering frequency and severity, and participatory enjoyment.

The *Perceptions of Stuttering Inventory* (PSI; Woolf, 1967) is another self-report instrument. With the PSI, a client evaluates 60 statements that describe behaviors that are plausibly associated with stuttering. Item response is binary; that is, the client indicates whether or not the described behaviors are characteristic of his or her speech at the time of scale completion. Twenty of the statements on the PSI describe manifestations of stuttering-related *struggle*; 20 describe manifestations of stuttering-related *avoidance*; and 20 describe manifestations of the *expectation* of stuttering. Subscale scores are summed and can range from 0 to 20.

Rating instruments like the *S24* scale (Andrews & Cutler, 1974) and the *Self-Efficacy Scaling for Adult Stutterers* (SESAS; Ornstein & Manning, 1985) differ from the instruments mentioned above in that they make no mention of stuttering-specific behaviors. Rather, the content in each of the instruments is relevant to both speakers who stutter and speakers who do not stutter. The S24 Scale requires the client to make a true/false response to 24 statements (e.g., *I often ask questions in group discussions*). A client's responses can be compared to data from adults who stutter and adults with typical fluency.

With the SESAS, the client uses a scale rating to indicate how likely he or she would be to enter 50 speaking situations (e.g., *order a pizza over the phone),* and, then, how likely he or she would be to speak without any symptoms of stuttering in those same situations. Such ratings are thought to provide information about *self-efficacy*; that is, an individual's confidence in his or her ability to engage in a behavior or attain a particular outcome.

The *Subjective Screening of Stuttering* (SSS; Riley, Riley, & Maguire, 2004) is a relatively new, concise instrument that, like several other instruments, is designed to assess a speaker's self-perceptions of stuttering severity and avoidance. In addition, the SSS features several items that examine the construct of *locus of control,* which concerns the extent to which an individual considers various life-events to be either self-determined or, conversely, the product of external factors (e.g., luck, other's actions). Speakers with an internal locus of control might be more apt to exhibit greater mastery over stuttering management than speakers with an external locus of control. There is some evidence to support that idea (Craig & Andrews, 1985); however, others have not found locus of control scores to be predictive of treatment outcomes (e.g., De Nil & Kroll, 1995).

Other instruments published during the past decade include the *Wright and Ayre Stuttering Self-Rating Profile* (WASSP; Wright & Ayre, 2000) and the *Overall Assessment of the Speaker's Experience of Stuttering* (OASES, Yaruss & Quesal, 2006). Each of these instruments incorporates concepts from the *International Classification of Functioning, Disability, and Health* (ICF; WHO, 2001). The OASES is the lengthier of the two instruments, featuring 100 distinct scale items that are spread across four broad categories (general information, reactions to stuttering, communication in daily settings, and quality of life). Translations of the test are available in Spanish and Dutch. The 24-item WASSP contains subsections that deal with stuttering-related behaviors, thoughts, feelings, and avoidance behaviors, as well as penalties or disadvantages that result from stuttering, and its reference data include adolescents.

Formal, Stuttering-Related Scales for Use With Children

The *Behavior Assessment Battery for School-aged Children Who Stutter* (Brutten & Vanryckeghem, 2007), like its counterpart the BAB-Adult, is composed of several distinct rating instruments. The *Speech Situation Checklists* (SSC) are designed to capture children's perceptions of their emotional reactions and speech disruption during various speaking contexts. The *Behavior Checklist* (BCL) provides a means of capturing a child's self-report on the methods they use to cope with disfluent speech. Finally, the *Communication Attitude Test* (CAT) uses a binary response format to capture children's beliefs about their communication ability and others' reaction to it. The SSC instruments, the BCL, and the CAT are normed in several languages for children ages 6 to 15. A fifth instrument, the KiddyCAT, is normed on preschool- to kindergarten-aged children to provide information about communication-related attitudes and beliefs.

The *Test of Childhood Stuttering* (TOCS; Gillam et al., 2009) features an *Observational Rating Scales* component, which serves as a complement to the four speech elicitation tasks that are incorporated in the test's *Speech Fluency Measure*. It is normed on children ages 4 to 12.

Two rating scales are included. The first one, the Speech Fluency Rating Scale, features nine items that pertain to various forms of disfluency behavior, while the second one, the Disfluency-Related Consequences Scale features nine items that pertain to the child's and others' reactions to the disfluent speech. Unlike the other instruments reviewed in this section, a parent, a teacher, or the clinician completes the scales. As such, they yield speaker-independent data about how a client performs beyond the clinical setting. Finally, the Self-Efficacy for Adolescents Scale (SEA-Scale; Manning, 1994; also see Manning, 2010) is a counterpart to the SESAS, described above, and is designed to collect data about self-efficacy in children and adolescents.

Child and teen versions of the OASES (Yaruss & Quesal, 2006) are available as well. The general purpose and organization for these versions of the OASES are similar to that of the adult version, which was described in the preceding section.

Multiage Scales for Stuttering

The Stuttering Severity Instrument-4 (SSI-4; Riley, 2009) features a self-report rating scale called the *Clinical Use of Self-Reports* (CUSR), which captures information about stuttering severity, locus of control, and stuttering-related avoidance during four types of face-to-face interactions (i.e., with a close friend, a parent, a stranger, and an authority figure) and during telephone conversations. The CUSR is similar in structure to the SSS instrument described in the section on adult assessment. Norms are not provided for the task, so it is best suited for making "within-subject" comparisons such as pretreatment versus posttreatment. The SSI-4 includes three additional 9-point rating scales, which clients can use to rate speech naturalness, satisfaction with treatment, and impressions of how they think other people would rate their stuttering.

Informal rating scales also can be used to rate stuttering severity. O'Brian, Packman, and Onslow (2004a) described a 9-point rating scale (1 = no stuttering; 9 = extremely severe stuttering) that adults who stutter can use to self-rate their stuttering severity upon completion of a speaking task. O'Brian et al. found that 9 of the 10 participants' self-ratings of stuttering severity were comparable to a speech-language pathologist's ratings. They also found that the participants' ratings were reliable, as demonstrated by a comparison between their initial ratings and ratings that they made six months later using a recorded version of the sample upon which the initial ratings were made.

Others (Logan, Byrd, Mazzocchi, & Gillam, 2011; O'Brian, Packman, Onslow, & O'Brian, 2004b; Yairi & Ambrose, 1999) have used similar scales to obtain clinician—and/or parent-based ratings of stuttering severity and have reported both acceptable levels of reliability and adequate correspondence between rating scale values and traditional syllable-based measures of disfluency (e.g., percent of syllables stuttered). Yairi and Ambrose's (1999, p. 1100) informal tool (the *Parent Severity Scale*) ranged from 0 to 7, with 0 defined as "normally fluent," 1 as "borderline," 2 as "mild," 3 as "mild-to-moderate," 4 as "moderate," 5 as "moderate to severe," 6 as "severe," and 7 as "very severe."

Several authors (e.g., Berry & Silverman, 1972; Schiavetti, Sacco, Metz, & Sitler, 1983) have suggested that a rating technique called *direct magnitude estimation* is preferable to the use of equal-appearing interval scales when rating stuttering severity across multiple speech samples

(e.g., samples from several speakers). This is because severe cases of stuttering are likely to exhibit many more symptoms than mild cases, which is likely to cause a listener's perceptions of stuttering severity to grow in an unequal fashion (Schiavetti et al., 1983). Thus, the degree of severity difference between cases that are rated as, say, "7" and "8" on a 9-point equal interval scale (where high numbers correspond to more severe stuttering) is likely to be wider than that of cases that are rated as "2" and "3" on the scale. (Research results [e.g., Berry & Silverman, 1972; Schiavetti et al., 1983] show that this does indeed happen!) Direct magnitude estimation addresses this measurement problem by requiring the rater to link his or her severity ratings to a fixed reference point. See Figure 10–6 for an illustration of how direct magnitude estimation is accomplished (see also Stevens, 1975).

Schiavetti et al. (1983) studied two methods of direct magnitude estimation for use with stuttering severity ratings:

- *Approach 1:* The researchers presented a "standard sample" of speech. The sample was from a speaker whose stuttering frequency was near the average frequency for a group of 20 speakers who stuttered. Raters were told to assign the standard sample a value of 10 and to "scale the stuttering severity of the other speakers relative to the standard" (p. 570).
- *Approach 2:* The raters were told to rate the first sample of speech using any number they desired, and then to rate the second sample as desired in relation to the first sample. Each subsequent sample then was rated proportionately to reflect the magnitude of scaled

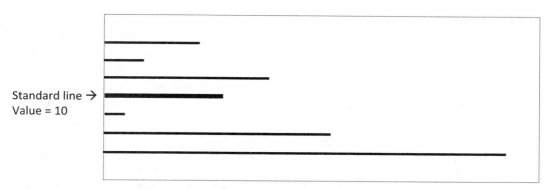

Figure 10–6. Illustration of the type of training task a researcher might use to introduce the concept of direct magnitude estimation to research participants. This figure is derived from Schiavetti et al.'s (1983) written description of the training task they used in a study of stuttering severity ratings. In one condition, the middle line was termed the "standard" and its length was arbitrarily assigned a value of 10. In another condition, participants assigned their own standard value. Participants then rated the remaining lines in relation to the value of the standard. After practicing the use of direct magnitude estimation with lines, participants then applied it to the rating of samples of stuttered speech.

differences between the previous ratings.

Both proved to be acceptable and easy-to-implement methods of rating stuttering severity.

Assessing Temperament, Anxiety, and Self-Concept

To identify contextual factors that influence fluency performance, it can be useful to assess constructs such as temperament, anxiety, and self-concept.

Instruments for Assessing Temperament

Several researchers have examined the temperamental characteristics of children who stutter using scale-based rating instruments (e.g., Anderson, Pellowski, Conture, & Kelly, 2003; Johnson, Walden, Conture, & Karrass, 2010; Schwenk, Con-

ture, & Walden, 2007). Although temperament is not a specific dimension of fluency, clinicians may find that information about this construct is useful to consider when designing and implementing treatment plans, particularly with regard to how a client might respond within certain environmental contexts. Examples of temperament scales used in stuttering-related research (and suitable for clinical application during assessment) include the following:

- *Behavioral Style Questionnaire* (BSQ; McDevitt & Carey, 1978). The BSQ is used with children ages 3 to 7. The instrument contains 100 items, which are used to collect information across several dimensions of temperament (activity level, adaptability, approaching behavior, mood quality [positive or negative], distractibility, attention span/ persistence, sensory threshold, and rhythmicity of physiological functions (e.g., sleep cycles, hunger cycles).

- The BSQ is part of a larger collection of questionnaires, the *Carey Temperament Scales* (CTS; Carey & McDevitt 1995). The CTS features five distinct questionnaires, including the BSQ, which are designed to assess temperament at different stages of the life span. The other questionnaires included in the CTS are the *Early Infancy Temperament Questionnaire* (EITQ), which is used with infants aged 1 to 4 months; the *Revised Infant Temperament Questionnaire* (RITQ, which is used with infants aged 4 to 11 months; the *Toddler Temperament Scale* (TTS), which is used with children aged 1 to 3 years; and the *Middle Childhood Temperament Questionnaire* (MCTQ), which is used with children aged 8 to 12 years.
- *Taylor-Johnson Temperament Analysis* (TJTA; Taylor & Morrison, 1996). The client rates 180 items on bipolar scales in which each end of the scale is labeled with oppositional terms (e.g., dominant–submissive). The instrument assesses 18 personality dimensions and can be used with adolescents and adults.

Instruments for Assessing Anxiety, Self-Concept, and Self-Efficacy

Some people with impaired fluency find verbal communication to be anxiety provoking. Sources for the anxiety include the negative consequences that are associated with an unpredictable speech production system (i.e., sometimes the person speaks very fluently, and sometimes very disfluently) and uncertain listener reactions (e.g., some listeners react to disfluent speech in supportive ways, and others react in unsupportive ways). Assessment in this area can provide the clinician with information about the pervasiveness of a client's anxiety and the extent to which it seems to impact dimensions of fluency such as continuity, effort, and talkativeness. Examples of anxiety and self-concept scales used in stuttering-related research (and suitable for clinical application during assessment) include the following:

- The *State-Trait Anxiety Inventory* (STAI; Spielberger, Gorsuch, Lushene, Vagg, & Jacobs, 1983) is a 40-item instrument that is designed to diagnose anxiety disorders. Adult respondents use a 4-point rating scale to indicate the frequency with which they experience various feelings associated with the presence or absence of anxiety. The construct of state anxiety refers to context-specific emotion (e.g., how a person feels now), while trait anxiety refers to one's tendency to experience anxiety in general.
- The *Revised Children's Manifest Anxiety Scale* (RCMAS; Reynolds & Richmond, 1985) is a self-report instrument that is suitable for ages 6 to 19 years. Test items address physiological symptoms of anxiety (e.g., sweaty hands), worry, oversensitivity (e.g., easily hurt feelings), and social concerns (e.g., feeling alone).
- The *Endler Multidimensional Anxiety Scales-Trait* (EMAS-T; Endler, Edwards, Vitelli, & Parker, 1989) is a 60-item inventory suitable for adults, and respondents

use a 5-point scale to rate how often they experience various feelings that are associated with the presence or absence of anxiety in situations that involve social evaluation, physical danger, novel or unusual events, and daily routines.

- The *Locus of Control of Behavior* scale (LCB; Craig, Franklin, & Andrews, 1984) is a 17-item instrument upon which respondents indicate their strength of agreement regarding "statements about how various topics affect (one's) personal beliefs." The scale is intended to capture the extent to which a person considers daily events to be a result of his or her behavior. A person who views himself/herself as "in charge" of events (i.e., an *internal locus of control*) is thought to be more likely to maintain newly learned treatment behaviors than a person with an *external locus of control*. Craig et al. (1984) presented data from adults who stuttered that supported that hypothesis. The LCB scale features comparison data from university students, nurses, people who stutter, and people with agoraphobia.

Instruments for Use With Cluttering

Daly and Cantrell (2006) described the Predictive Cluttering Inventory (PCI), a a tool that Daly developed for use in the assessment and identification of cluttering. The scale items were derived from input that Daly and Cantrell solicited from 60 fluency experts regarding the cluttering symptoms that they had observed. The PCI features 33 items, which are organized into four domains (pragmatics, language, cognition, and speech motor) and rated on a 7-point scale. Van Zaalen-op't Hof, Wijnen, and DeJonckere (2009) conducted a study of the PCI to validate its use as a diagnostic tool. They found that the scale in its original form correctly identified only a small percentage of individuals who had been independently diagnosed with cluttering by speech-language pathologists. Through their analysis of the PCI, they identified a core set of six items that significantly identified speakers who clutter. These items pertained to the following characteristics: irregular speech rate, rapid rate, trailing off of vocal intensity during an utterance, lack of anxiety or concern about speaking patterns, excessive disfluencies and stuttering, and disorganized language. On this basis, they proposed that the PCI could be shortened considerably—a process that would increase the instrument's sensitivity in identifying cluttering.

Bakker (2010) developed the *Cluttering Assessment Program*, which is a computer-based tool that features a visual analog rating scale for measuring rate, articulation, and language performance in speakers who clutter. It also contains a module that a clinician can use to compute the frequency of clutter-like speech within a speech sample. The program is available for free download on the Internet.

Open-Ended, Written Responses

Written, open-ended response tasks offer an alternative to oral interviews and rating scales for collecting information about a client's attitudes, feelings, beliefs, and experiences concerning fluency-related disability.

Prompts to Elicit Written Narratives

A clinician presents the client with a prompt and allots the client time to respond. An example of this approach to data collection is illustrated in the following box. As can be seen, the adult client generates a relatively detailed summary of the thoughts, feelings, and beliefs that occur just prior to making a telephone call. A clinician can use this information as a basis for developing treatment goals that address the client's stuttering-related reactions and coping strategies.

What do think about, feel, or envision before making a phone call? (Please write your response below.)

Before a phone call, I picture myself having trouble speaking, especially when the person first answers the phone. I can see myself trying to calm down so that I can use my fluency techniques. I can see the person I'm calling trying to decide if it's a prank call when he doesn't hear anything. The person is drumming his fingers on the table like, "Hurry up, hurry up."

When I get stuck, the person will start filling in words for me and then I'll get stuck even harder and longer. I try not to think about stuttering, but I can't think of anything else. Sometimes, I substitute a word in place of a word I'm about to stutter on, and sometimes, I just won't make the call and will go to the store so that I can talk with the person face-to-face.

The boxed text is an example of an open-ended written response that describes stuttering-related thoughts, feelings, and beliefs associated with making a telephone call. The adult client demonstrated highly fluent speech during clinic-based conversations but continued to demonstrate moderate stuttering when making telephone calls. Prompts can be adjusted to elicit information about a client's fluency difficulties in other contexts.

Clinician-Devised Worksheets

Informal paper-pencil tasks and worksheets are another useful option for collecting data about a client's fluency-related experiences. Chmela and Reardon (2001) published a workbook that contains numerous child-friendly activities that are designed to elicit information about stuttering-related attitudes and emotions. An example of a worksheet from the book that is designed to elicit information about a child's worries is presented in Figure 10–7. In our experience, children are more likely to reveal their thoughts on fluency disability in activities like these than they are during oral interview situations.

A variety of other informal published materials are available through publishers that specialize in clinical materials. Examples include practical clinical guidebooks such as *The Source for Stuttering* (Reardon & Yaruss, 2004) and *The Child and Adolescent Stuttering Treatment and Activity Resource Guide* (Ramig & Dodge, 2005), both of which contain a host of informal, practice-ready forms and data collection tools that are suitable for distribution to clients, parents, and teachers. Materials such as these can be a helpful supplement to the various tests and norm-referenced rating instruments discussed earlier in this chapter in the data collection process.

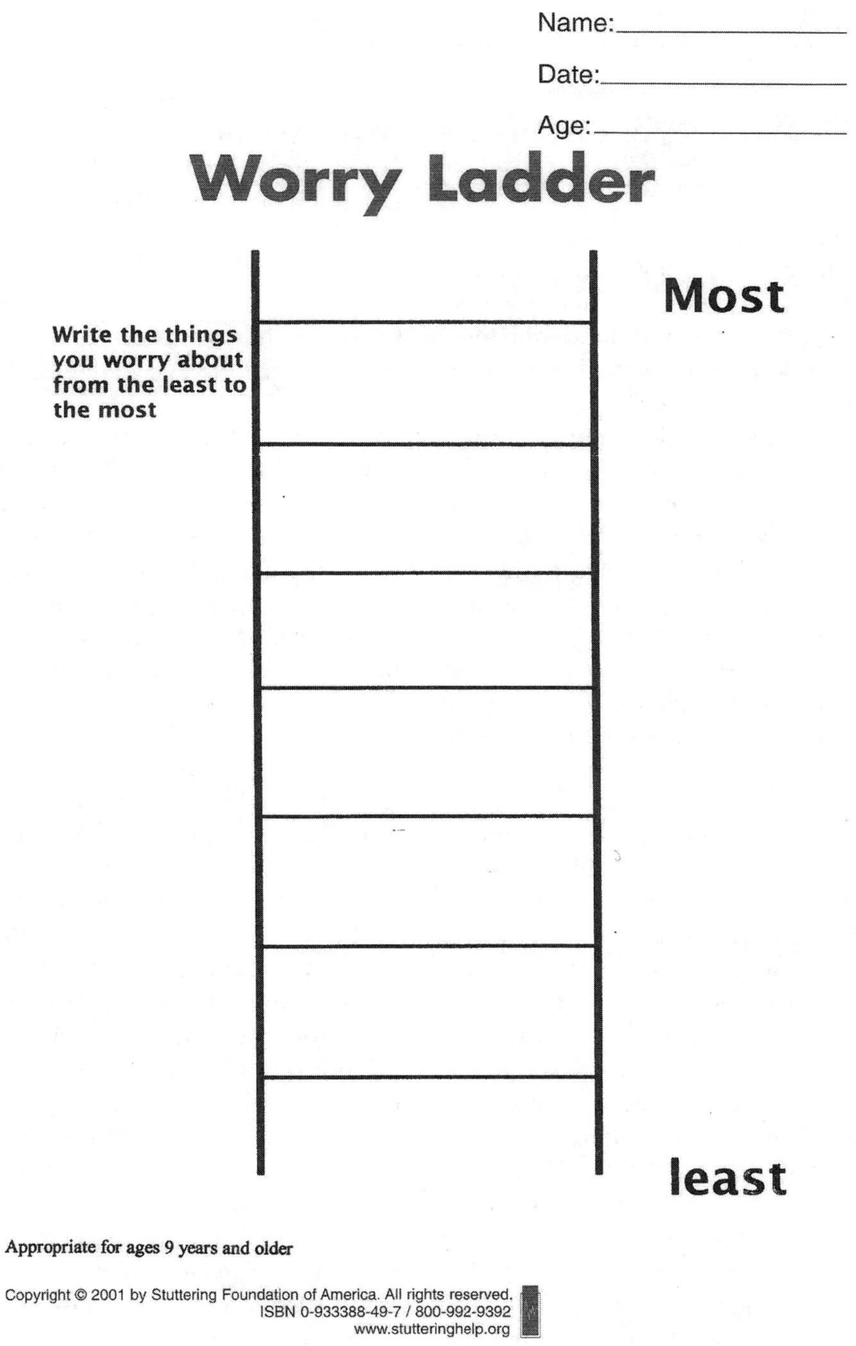

Name:_____

Date:_____

Age:_____

Worry Ladder

Most

Write the things
you worry about
from the least to
the most

least

Appropriate for ages 9 years and older

Figure 10–7. Example of a "Worry Ladder" worksheet for eliciting information about children's daily concerns. The clinician asks a child to rank the things that concern him or her most. The activity provides the clinician with insight into how fluency disability fits within the broader context of a child's life. The "Worry Ladder" is from *"The School-Aged Child Who Stutters: Working Effectively With Attitudes and Emotions,* by K. A. Chmela and N. Reardon, 2001. Memphis, TN: Stuttering Foundation of America. Reprinted with permission. Copyright 2014 by the Stuttering Foundation of America. 800-992-9392; http://www.stutteringhelp.org

Designing Assessment Protocols

A *protocol* is a set of specific rules or procedures that one follows when doing a task. Within the context of fluency assessment, a protocol is a list of standard clinical activities that a clinician will implement when evaluating a specific client, such as a person with suspected fluency impairment. Protocols create consistency in the assessment process, and consistency enables a clinician to make valid comparisons between a client's performances at two or more points in time and also to make valid comparisons between clients.

Although the use of an assessment protocol implies a rigid approach to clinical assessment, this is not necessarily so. Factors such as a client's age or background history will influence the specific activities that a clinician selects from the menu of possibilities. Generally speaking, the more data collection activities a clinician has on a protocol, the more he or she will know about a client. However, more tasks are not always better, as each data collection procedure takes time to complete. Thus, the goal is to administer enough tasks to obtain an accurate determination of the client's fluency functioning but not so many tasks that it becomes impractical to implement the protocol.

In Figure 10–8, we present a worksheet that one can use to develop data collection activities for use in a fluency assessment. The worksheet features the various tasks and instruments that we discussed in this chapter. Of course, a clinician never would administer all of the activities listed in Figure 10–8 within a single assessment, and the tasks and instruments presented in Figure 10–8 are not an exhaustive list of all possible options. Rather, the clinician would use what is known about the client's age and complaint behaviors to formulate a data collection protocol that is tailored to fit the client's profile.

Summary

The primary focus of the chapter was on data collection methods for fluency assessment. Under this broad heading, three main topics were discussed: (1) a framework for fluency assessment, (2) fundamental assessment concepts, and (3) specific methods that clinicians can use to collect data about fluency functioning. The chapter began with an overview of the phases of assessment. Data collection is the first step in the assessment process, and it leads naturally to data analysis and data interpretation, topics that are the focus of the following two chapters.

The chapter began with an overview of 13 terms associated with the WHO's (2001) ICF model. These terms offer clinicians a comprehensive conceptual framework for examining what clients are and are not doing with regard to fluency and the factors that influence fluency performance. These terms provided the backdrop for the main portion of the chapter, which dealt with data collection methods. Methods for collecting background information about a client were reviewed (e.g., case history forms, oral interviews), along with an assortment of formal and informal options that exist for eliciting speech samples. The notion of strategic speech sampling was explored in the context of speech elicitation tasks. Strategic sampling involves not only the use of varied talking tasks but also the introduction of fluency stressors as well. Such an approach

Data collection area	Approach	Options/Examples
Background information, history, concerns	Data collection form Oral interview	• *Case History Form* • Relevant questions from Table 10-1 • Additional questions as necessary
Speech samples	Clinician-devised elicitation tasks Tests with stuttering-related norms Tests with verbal fluency norms Tests normed in areas other than fluency	• Conversation • Narration • Oral reading • Sentence production • Rote speech, Singing • Trial therapy • Fluency inducing conditions • *SSI-4* (conversation, narrative) [M] • *TOCS* (conversation, narration, rapid naming, modeled sentences) [C] • *COWAT* [A] • *CELF-Word associations* [C] • *GFTA-2* [M]; *ABA-2* [A] • *TOLD-P:4* [C]; *BDAE-3* [A] • *TNL* [C]; *WAB-R* [A]
Self- or Other-ratings of fluency-related functioning and disability	Instruments to measure perceptions of stuttering experiences (see Table 10-6)	• *BAB-A* [M] / *BAB-C* [C]; *SSS* [A] • *PSI* [A]; *WASSP* [A] • *S24* [AT]; *CAT-R* [C] • *SESAS, SEA* [AT]; *TOCS-ORS* [C] • *Shortened SSC-ER* [A]; *SSI-4-CUSR* [M] • *SSRS* [A]; *OASES* [M] • Informal writing prompts
Self-ratings about other aspects of functioning and disability	Instruments to measure perceptions of areas such as temperament, anxiety, self-concept and self-efficacy	• *CTS* [M]; *STAI* [A] • *TJTA* [AT]; *RSES* [TC] • *EMAS* [A]; *RCMAS* [TC] • *LCB* [A]
Other areas of communication-related concern	Tests and procedures to evaluate other aspects speech, language, hearing, cognition, feeding swallowing	• Expressive/receptive language • Articulation • Voice & resonance • Cognition • Hearing • Social aspects of communication • Swallowing • Communication modalities

Note: Letters in square brackets correspond to age range for an instrument: [A] = adult, [T] = teen, [C] = child, [M] = multi-age. Italicized letters indicate test names. Complete names of each test are presented in the text. Tests and rating scales noted in the table are examples and not meant to be an exhaustive list.

Figure 10–8. Worksheet for designing a data collection protocol. A clinician uses the client's age and preassessment information about the client's areas of concern to select appropriate data collection activities. Other areas may require assessment as well (i.e., verbal fluency, temperament, motor skills, and other aspects of speech, language, and communication).

will increase the likelihood of capturing how the client's fluency varies in real-life settings. Although it is not necessary to implement every speech elicitation task with every client, observation of the client across a range of talking tasks increases the likelihood of capturing the "highs" and "lows" of a client's fluency, which, in turn, improves the accuracy of diagnosis and judgments about the severity of disability. With disorders such as cluttering, where impairment in language, fluency, *and* speech intelligibility are common, it often will be necessary to implement sampling tasks that elicit these types of problems.

Rating-based approaches to fluency assessment were discussed at some length. Although existing rating instruments have limitations (Franic & Bothe, 2008), they still remain an efficient means of obtaining information about aspects of fluency performance that are not practical or possible to observe in a clinical setting. Rating scales can be a primary source of information about a client's participation patterns across speaking contexts and his or her attitudes, thoughts, and feelings about speaking and communication disability. In our experience, the latter variables play a critical role in determining how a client responds to treatment, and the more information one has about such factors, the better.

The chapter concluded with examples of informal data collection tools. The open-ended nature of such tasks makes them an attractive choice for collecting information about narrow or client-specific issues. When "home-made" tools such as these are administered prior to and following treatment, they offer yet another source of information about treatment effects.

11

Analyzing Speech Samples

In this chapter, we focus on some primary methods for analyzing the fluency characteristics of speech samples. In many respects, speech samples are the most important source of clinical data in a fluency assessment. Speech samples afford clinicians the opportunity to hear, first hand, how a client sounds while talking. Without such information, the clinician is left to rely on the client's self-reports and/or the observations of other people such as caregivers and teachers. Although these individuals may offer useful information about the client's fluency concerns, it is possible that at least some of the information they provide is incomplete, inaccurate, or distorted. Thus, speech sample analysis is an essential assessment activity for the differential diagnoses of fluency disorders and the measurement of behavioral changes and treatment outcomes. Although our main focus is on analyses that quantify fluency, we briefly review some qualitative approaches to speech sample analysis, as well. Most of the analyses that we discuss are ones that can be performed readily in any work setting, without the need to access expensive or highly specialized equipment. The data that a clinician obtains from these analyses are integral to the act of diagnosing fluency disorders, describing disorder severity, and formulating plans for treatment.

Analyzing Speech Continuity

Perhaps the most common types of speech sample analyses are those that pertain to continuity. As noted in previous chapters, continuity refers to the connectedness of spoken utterances or, more specifically, the extent to which the sounds, syllables, and words within an utterance are articulated seamlessly. Analysis of speech continuity begins with the elicitation of one or more speech samples. (See Chapter 10 for a discussion of speech sample options and elicitation methods.) To quantify speech continuity, the clinician needs to count both the amount of speech and the number continuity disruptions the client has produced. These counts typically are based on a transcription of what the speaker has said. We discuss several options for transcription in the next section.

Speech Sample Transcription

A transcript is a written record that captures essential details about a speech sample, and it serves as the basis for many of the analyses discussed in this chapter. The clinician has two main decisions to make regarding the transcription method (Figure 11–1). The first decision pertains to when transcription should take place. The options are to create the transcription (a) as the client is talking during the assessment (i.e., *real-time* or *online transcription*) or, instead, (b) while listening to a recording of the client some time after the assessment takes place. Online transcription is time efficient, but it can be challenging to do if a speaker is highly disfluent, talks rapidly, or produces many sentences in succession. The issue is that the transcriber—even one who is relatively experienced at real-time transcription—can find it difficult to keep pace with all that is happening in the client's speech. Also, the clinician's focus on the transcription process can potentially disrupt his or her rapport with the client and limit his or her ability to observe other aspects of the client's behavior. Thus, those who are new to developing fluency transcripts are advised to begin by working from an audio recording of the client's speech. This *off-line* approach to transcription makes it possible to listen to complex or rapid segments of a speech sample repeatedly and to recheck one's analysis for completeness and accuracy.

The second decision pertains to how much detail the transcription should con-

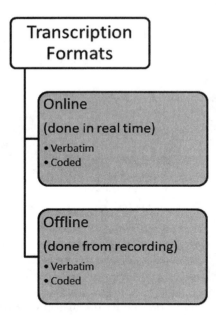

Figure 11–1. Options for speech sample transcription when analyzing fluency. Online transcripts are created in real time; that is, as a client is speaking. Off-line transcripts, in contrast, are developed some time after speech sample elicitation takes place and are created by replaying a recording of the speech sample. Online transcription is more time efficient than off-line transcription, but it can be challenging to do accurately with clients who speak rapidly or produce many behaviorally complex disfluencies. Verbatim transcripts are word-for-word accounts of what a client says. Coded transcripts capture some aspects of what a client has said (e.g., number of words spoken) but not others (e.g., the content of the spoken words). As such, coded transcripts tend to be quicker and easier to develop than verbatim transcripts.

tain. The options are to create a verbatim record of all that the client says, or, instead, to create a transcription that is based on codes that capture only those aspects of the speech sample most relevant to fluency analysis. *Verbatim transcription* entails documenting the content of a speaker's target utterances and any associated disfluent speech. Thus, it is a record of what the client has said and how he or she has said it. Such transcripts are useful in cases where the clinician wishes to analyze both the client's fluency and language performance. They, however, can be challenging to create in real time and time consuming to create when working from an audio recording. *Coded transcription*, in contrast, is designed to document how much a speaker has said as well as where, how, and how often disfluency has occurred. Several authors have discussed the utility of coded transcription in fluency analysis (e.g., Conture, 2001; Gillam, Logan, & Pearson, 2009; Riley, 1994, 2009; Yaruss, Max, Newman, & Campbell, 1998), Coded transcription differs from verbatim transcription in that it does not capture the content of what the speaker has said. As such, it generally is less time

consuming to create and more feasible to construct in real time. The transcript, however, would not be in a format that allows for a thorough analysis of language performance.

An excerpt of a speech sample that was analyzed via verbatim transcription is shown in Figure 11–2. The same speech sample then is reanalyzed in two different coded formats in Figure 11–3. The methods shown in these figures are just some of the possible formats that a clinician can use for data transcription.

Determining Sample Size and Disfluency Frequency

Analysis of speech continuity is rooted in the quantification of sample size and disfluency frequency. As noted earlier in

Line #	Utterance	Syllables	Disfluencies	PWR	REV
1	We |fou- fou-|found Linda's wallet.	6	1	1	0
2	Under the |bu-|blue notebook.	6	1	0	1
3	Nothing was missing.	5	0	0	0
4	Yeah, I think so.	4	0	0	0
5	|Ne-|next time |he-|she will put it here.	7	2	1	1
Sums		28	4	2	2

Figure 11–2. An excerpt from a verbatim transcript of a speech sample. The transcript was developed using Microsoft® Excel, a spreadsheet program. In each of the transcribed utterances, disfluent speech is separated from the target utterance using vertical lines, and both the number of syllables within the target utterance and the number of disfluencies within the spoken utterance are tallied. Instances of disfluency also can be classified by type, if desired. Only two types of disfluency exist in this transcript: part-word repetition (PWR) and revision (REV). Additional columns can be added to the spreadsheet as needed to document the occurrence of other types of disfluency or other variables of interest. In clinical assessment of conversational speech, the transcribed samples normally will feature at least 300 to 500 syllables.

		1	2	3	4	5	6	7	8	9	10	Sum
1	F	- (We)	- (found)	- (Lin)	- (da's)	- (wa)	-/ (llet)	-	-	-	-	10
1	D		PWR								REV	1
2	F	-	-/	-	-	-	-	-/	-	-	-	10
2	D											0
3	F	-/	-	-	-	-	-	-	-/			8
3	D		PWR		REV							2

A

	1	2	3	4	5	6	7	8	9	10	Sum
1	- (We)	PWR (found)	- (Lin)	- (da's)	- (wa)	-/ (llet)	-	-	-	REV	10
2	-	-/	-	-	-	-	-/	-	-	-	10
3	-/	PWR	-	REV	-	-	-	-/			8

B

Figure 11–3. This figure shows coded transcriptions that are based on the verbatim speech sample in Figure 11–2. In this figure, data are coded on a grid in two ways. In Version **A**, the syllables from the target utterances in Figure 11–2 are represented with a dash and entered in the rows labeled "F" (fluent). (The content of the first utterance from the sample in Figure 11–2, "We found Linda's wallet," is entered into the grid to illustrate the relationship between linguistic content and codes.) Coding proceeds from left to right until 10 codes have been entered and then continues at the left margin of the next row. In Version **A**, disfluency that precedes or occurs during the course of a target syllable is coded beneath the affected syllable, in the rows labeled "D" (disfluent). Target syllables and disfluencies are summed for each row in the far right column. The code "PWR" refers to part-word repetition; REV refers to revision. In Version **B**, the fluent and disfluent rows are combined such that a disfluency code is entered into the cell associated with a target syllable that either contains or is preceded by disfluency. The transcribed utterance from line 1 of the transcript in Figure 11–2 ("We found Linda's wallet") is again entered in the cells to illustrate the relationship between the codes and the actual utterance content. Slashes indicate utterance boundaries.

this text, disfluency involves a break in the execution of a target utterance. Thus, a fundamental component in the analysis of continuity is to separate disfluent segments of speech from target utterances. Another way to think of the target utterance is this: How would a particular utterance sound if all evidence of disfluency (e.g., repeating, prolonging, interjecting, and revising) was removed? Quantification of sample size is based on the speaker's target utterance. The main objective is to count the number of syllables or words within each of the target utterances within the speech sample and then sum the utterance counts to obtain the total number of syllables or words across all target utterances in the speech sample. With this approach, speech within disfluent segments is regarded as unproductive and thus is not included in the count of syllables or words that are used to determine the sample size.

For utterances that are executed without any disfluency, the target utterance is equal to whatever actually has been spoken. This concept is illustrated in the example below:

Example 11–1:

Spoken utterance: *Chris is driving to the beach.*

Target utterance: *Chris is driving to the beach.*

In disfluent utterances, however, the target utterance consists of those words that remain within the utterance boundary when all instances of disfluency are excluded. This concept is illustrated in the example below:

Example 11–2:

Spoken utterance: *Chris- um Chris is dr- driving um to the beach.*

Spoken utterance with disfluency boundaries marked: *|Chris- um| Chris is |dr-| driving |um| to the beach.*

Target utterance: *Chris is driving to the beach.*

The spoken utterance shown in Example 11–2 contains three disfluencies: one that involves repetition of the word *Chris*; one that involves repetition of *dr* (the syllable onset in the syllable *drive*), and one that involves the use of the editing term *um* between the words *driving* and *to*. The number of syllables within the target utterance for Examples 11–1 and 11–2 equals 7.

Selecting a Disfluency Labeling System

The creation of speech sample transcription naturally leads to the labeling of disfluent segments. Many researchers have employed descriptive labels that capture the salient characteristics of disfluency. In Chapter 3, we introduced several of the many disfluency labeling systems that researchers have employed, and we discussed some of the shortcomings associated with existing methods. One main shortcoming is that none of the existing labeling systems seems capable of capturing the full range of behavioral variation that occurs in disfluent speech. This situation can lead to several problems, the most important of which is the overcounting of disfluent segments within an utterance. Still, if a comprehensive labeling system did exist, it likely would include so many categories that it would be unwieldy to use.

Beyond this, it is unclear whether the ability to assign a unique label to each and every structural variant of disfluency offers any particular advantages in terms of understanding the nature or treatment of fluency impairment. Thus, disfluency labeling becomes a matter of the clinician deciding how much detail is needed to describe a client's fluency performance adequately at a particular point in time. Highly detailed disfluency labels are most useful during comprehensive assessment such as the initial evaluation or the post-treatment evaluation. At such times, documentation of specific types of disfluency may guide diagnosis and allow for analysis of how particular facets of a client's fluency change over time. Such detail may not be necessary at other times, such as when a clinician is measuring how well a client has performed during a treatment activity. At such times, it may be necessary to record only how much disfluency occurred. Specific details about the types of disfluency produced many not be useful in such contexts, especially if the client produces a fairly narrow range of stuttering-related disfluency.

Computing and Reporting Summary Statistics

After generating a transcript that captures the client's fluency and labeling the types of disfluency the client has produced, the clinician is in a position to compute some basic statistics that quantify the client's fluency performance. Such statistics are useful in diagnosing fluency disorders, determining the severity of impairment, and evaluating treatment outcomes.

Syllable- and Word-Based Frequency Measures

Summary statistics for speech continuity usually are computed by dividing the number of disfluencies observed in the sample by the number of linguistic units within the sample. Such an approach yields a *sample-size-adjusted frequency*, which allows for valid comparisons between speech samples that differ in the number of linguistic units they contain. The computational formulas for two common disfluency-related statistics are presented below.

$$\text{Disfluencies per 100 syllables} =$$
$$\frac{\text{Total number of disfluencies produced}}{\text{Total number of syllables produced}} \times 100$$

$$\text{Disfluencies per words} =$$
$$\frac{\text{Total number of disfluencies produced}}{\text{Total number of words produced}} \times 100$$

In Figure 11–4, we present an example of how the formulas are used to generate summary statistics that are related to disfluency frequency.

From a mathematical standpoint, the wording "disfluencies per 100 syllables" (see Figure 11–4) is equivalent to *percent of syllables disfluent*. We prefer to use the wording *per 100 syllables* when reporting data because it allows for the possibility that disfluency can occur either "before" (e.g., |*Um Marg-*| *Jonelle bought a scooter*) or "on" (e.g., |*J-*| *Jonelle bought a scooter*) a specific target syllable. The *percent of syllables disfluent* wording, to our way of thinking, creates the impression that disfluency always occurs *on* a particular syllable, which is not necessarily true. Rather, disfluency at one point in an utterance can be associated with planning difficulties that exist further ahead in the developing utterance.

When reporting data in terms of word-based sample sizes, we again prefer the per *100 words* designation to *percent of words*. This time, however, the main reason is that the two measures are not always mathematically equivalent. We explain this further in the following example.

Example 11–3:

Target utterance: *Denali National Park is in Alaska.*

Spoken utterance: |*De-*|*De* |*na-*|*nali National Park is in* |*A-*| *A* |*la-*|*laska.*

The target utterance contains 6 words. There are two disfluencies during *Denali* and two more during *Alaska.* Thus, two words have at least one instance of disfluency within them (2 disfluent words), and the utterance contains a total of four disfluencies. The *percent of words* disfluent is computed as follows: (2 disfluent words/6 target words) × 100 = 33.33. In contrast, the *number of disfluencies per 100 words* = (4 disfluencies/6 target words) × 100 =

A. Summary Table Sample size: Syllables = _457_ Words = 402

Disfluency Type	Observed Frequency	Adjusted frequency (*disfluencies per 100 syllables*)	Adjusted frequency (*disfluencies per 100 words*)
Part-word repetition	6	(6/457) x 100 = 1.31	(6/402) x 100 = 1.49
Whole-word repetition	3	(3/457) x 100 = 0.66	(3/402) x 100 = 0.75
Multiword repetition	5	(5/457) x 100 = 1.09	(5/402) x 100 = 1.24
Sound Prolongation	19	(19/457) x 100 = 4.16	(19/402) x 100 = 4.73
Interjection	8	(8/457) x 100 = 1.75	(8/402) x 100 = 1.99
Revision	4	(4/457) x 100 = 0.88	(4/402) x 100 = 1.00
Pause	12	(12/457) x 100 = 2.63	(12/402) x 100 = 2.99
Total	57	(57/457) x 100 = 12.48100	(57/402) x 100 = 14.18

B. Summary statistics

Disfluencies per 100 syllables:	(57 / 457) × 100 = 12.48
Disfluencies per 100 words:	(57 / 402) × 100 = 14.18
Repetitions and prolongations per 100 syllables:	(1.31 + 0.66 + 1.09 + 4.16) = 7.22
Percent of all disfluency that features repetition or prolongation:	((6 + 3 + 5+ 19) / 57) × 100 = 58

Figure 11–4. Computational examples of two measures of disfluency frequency for a speech sample that contained 457 syllables. Disfluencies were labeled during transcription, and the number of each type of disfluency observed in the speech sample was tallied to yield the numbers in the "Observed Frequency" column. The number of observed disfluencies for each type of disfluency was divided by the sample size, which in this case was measured in both the number of syllables and the number of words within the target utterances, to yield sample-size-adjusted frequencies of disfluency: the number of disfluencies per 100 syllables, and per 100 words. With this adjustment, the disfluency frequency values can be compared to values that are derived from speech samples of other lengths.

66.66. Although both statistics are potentially relevant to describing a person's fluency performance, we would argue that the *number of disfluencies per 100 words* approach represents the speaker's performance more precisely than the *percent of words* approach does.

Utterance-Based Frequency Measures

Instead of coding individual syllables or words, one can code longer linguistic units, such as entire utterances, for disfluency. This yields disfluency metrics such as *percent of disfluent utterances*. With an utterance-based analysis, the clinician codes an entire utterance as either "disfluent" or "fluent," depending on whether the utterance contains disfluency or not. This is illustrated in Examples 11–4 to 11–6 below.

Example 11–4: *The weather is very humid this time of year.* [Code = fluent]

Example 11–5: *The |w-|weather is very humid this time of year.* [Code = disfluent]

Example 11–6: *The |w-|weather is |v-|very humid this |t-|time of year.* [Code = disfluent]

The coding of entire utterances, as opposed to individual syllables or words, substantially reduces the number of tally marks that a clinician must make during data analysis. For example, the target utterance in Examples 11–4 to 11–6 above contains 12 syllables and 9 words, each of which would need to be documented with a unique code in a traditional approach to transcription. In the utterance-based analysis, however, a single code can capture the entire utterance. The reduced coding burden associated with the utterance-based analysis makes it more feasible for a clinician to analyze a client's fluency performance in real time during an assessment or treatment session.

It is obvious that, in cases where a speaker routinely produces several disfluencies per utterance, the *per utterance* disfluency metric is less precise than either the *per 100 syllables* or the *per 100 words* approaches. This is because utterances that contain multiple instances of disfluency (see Example 11–6) are coded in the same way as utterances that contain only one instance of disfluency (see Example 11–5). Still, there are research studies (e.g., Bernstein Ratner & Sih, 1987) that have used utterance-based disfluency analyses and found them to be sensitive enough to discriminate between speakers who stutter and speakers who do not stutter. So, this type of analysis has utility for certain types of clients—particularly those mild to moderate cases of fluency impairment where the speaker generally produces only one instance of disfluency

per utterance. The *per utterance* measure also may be suitable for use during certain treatment activities in which the clinician decides that a "rough estimate" of fluency performance is sufficiently precise. If greater precision is needed, another option is to use a three-part utterance classification system: *utterances with no disfluency*, *utterances with one disfluency*, and *utterances with more than one disfluency*. One could then compute the frequency with each of these utterance types occurs within a speech sample.

Estimating Per Syllable Frequency With Strategic Analyses

Recently, some authors (e.g., Gillam et al., 2009; Logan & Gillam, 2006) have described the use of disfluency frequency metrics that are based on analysis of specific portions of an utterance—an approach that might be termed *strategic analysis*. This approach exploits the well-known tendency for disfluencies, particularly those that children produce, to coincide with the onset of utterances. In other words, speech disfluency is more likely to occur near the start of the utterance than in the middle or end portions of an utterance. Thus, with strategic analysis, one focuses the analysis primarily on utterance-initial contexts—the context that is most likely to feature disfluency.

This approach is implemented in the *Test of Childhood Stuttering* (TOCS; Gillam et al., 2009). With the TOCS scoring procedure, an utterance receives a score of 1 if it features one or more instance of part- or whole-word repetition or sound prolongation/blocking *during the course of the first three words*. Utterances that contain both categories of disfluency within the first three words receive a score of 2. Utterances with no repeating, prolonging or blocking in the first three words receive a score of 0. This scoring approach is illustrated in the examples below:

> Example 11–7: |*Tha- Tha-*|*That* |*d-*|*dog was barking really loud* [TOCS score = 1]

> Example 11–8: |*Tha-*|*That dog* |*www*|*was barking really loud* [TOCS score = 2]

> Example 11–9: *I still think he is* |*fr-*|*friendly* [TOCS score = 0]

Note that the first three words of an utterance are scored as a single unit for the presence or absence of select disfluency categories—but not for how many of those disfluencies have occurred during the first three words. Thus, the utterance in Example 11–7 receives a score of "1" even though the speaker produced part-word repetitions in conjunction with the first and second words. The utterance in Example 11–8 receives a score of "2" because it contains an instance of repeating and an instance of prolonging during the course of the first three words.[1] The utterance in Example 11–9, in contrast, is scored as "0" because the part-word repetition associated with *friendly* occurs after the first three words (*I*, *still*, and *think*) of the target utterance.

Technically, the disfluency metric that is incorporated in this portion of the TOCS is the *number of utterances with repeating, prolonging, or blocking within the first three words of an utterance*. The phrase admittedly is a bit cumbersome to say, but data show that the measure yields a very good estimate of the frequency score one would obtain by analyzing all words in an utterance for presence of part-word repetition, whole-word repetition, sound prolongation, and physically tense blocks. These correlational analyses yield equations that enable a clinician to convert the disfluency scores that result from analysis of utterance-initial fluency into traditional *per 100 words* scores. Logan and Gillam (2006) reported correlations of greater than .85 for both children who stutter and children with typical fluency in comparisons of the *all words* and *first three words* disfluency analyses (Figure 11–5). Approaches such as this appear to offer a way to assess disfluency frequency in an easy-to-implement manner during live, clinical settings. Research on this approach is ongoing.

Time-Based Frequency Measures

A less common measurement approach is to report disfluency frequency in terms of disfluencies per unit of speaking time. With time-based frequency measures, the clinician's job is to determine how many disfluencies a speaker produces within a specific period. The most commonly reported statistic in this category is *number of disfluencies per minute*, and it usually is calculated using the following formula:

$$Disfluencies\ per\ minute = \frac{Total\ number\ of\ disfluencies\ produced}{Total\ seconds\ spent\ talking} \times 60$$

The *disfluencies per minute* metric is best suited for tasks such as narration and oral reading, both of which involve

---

[1]As described in the TOCS test manual (Gillam et al., 2009) prolongations and physically tense blocks are scored separately from part- and whole-word repetitions in order to capture the dimension of physical tension in addition to continuity. Many of the prolongations/blocks that speakers who stutter produce are characterized by excessive physical tension.

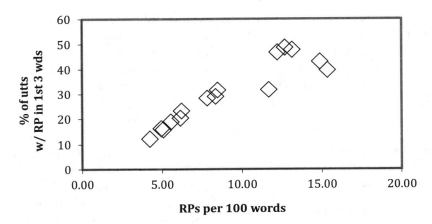

Figure 11–5. Relationships between a traditional disfluency metric (number of disfluencies per 100 words) and an alternative disfluency metric in which an utterance receives one point if one or more of target disfluency types occurs within the first 3 words of an utterance. Data are based on conversational utterances, 3 words or longer in length that preschool-aged children who stutter produced. Target disfluencies are those that typify stuttered speech (i.e., part- and whole-word repetitions, sound prolongations, RPs). From *A comparison of two sampling approaches in fluency analysis,* by K. J. Logan and R. B. Gillam, November 2006. Poster presented at the annual convention of the American Speech-Language-Hearing Association, Miami, FL [Unpublished material].

relatively long stretches of uninterrupted speech. Assuming that the speech is indeed uninterrupted, the clinician needs only to perform two timings: the starting time and stopping time. We have used time-based disfluency measures most often during narrative tasks that are done as part of treatment-related practice activities. In such activities, the client is asked to implement a particular strategy or behavioral change for a set amount of time (e.g., *Talk for one minute about the classes you are taking this semester, and while doing so, practice using your disfluency management strategy*). During the timed interval, the clinician notes the number of disfluencies produced and, perhaps, other facets of disfluency, such as disfluency type.

Time-based disfluency measures are cumbersome to use in conversational set-

tings, particularly when the client's utterances are relatively short and sandwiched between another speaker's utterances. In conversations of the latter sort, the clinician will need to start and stop the timing device many times, and because it can be difficult to predict when the client will start or stop a speaking turn, the potential for imprecise utterance timings seems great, particularly when the timings are made as the client is speaking.

Computer-Assisted Approaches to Determining Disfluency Frequency

The *Stuttering Severity Instrument–4* (SSI-4; Riley, 2009) features a software tool—the *Computerized Scoring of Stuttering Severity* (CSSS-2.0, Bakker & Riley, 2009)—that can be used to measure disfluency (or stuttering) frequency in either real time (i.e., as a speaker is talking) or while listening to playback of an audio recording. To measure disfluency frequency with this tool, the clinician listens to a running sample of speech and depresses a specific computer key each time a syllable within a target utterance is produced. A second, separate key is depressed each time an instance of disfluency (or stuttering) occurs. The software automatically tallies the total number of disfluencies (or stuttering instances) and the total number of target syllables to compute the number of disfluencies (or stutters) produced per 100 syllables.

The *Stuttering Measurement System* (SMS; Ingham, Ingham, Moglia, & Kilgo, n.d.) is a program that has been available for download via a website at the University of California, Santa Barbara. The program can be used for measuring stuttering frequency (i.e., percent of syllables stuttered) and speech naturalness. The software is accompanied by a detailed training manual (Ingham & Ingham, 2011) that provides users with information on how to develop their competence at conducting these measurements.

Some software programs that are designed primarily for analysis of language performance can be used for generating statistics about disfluency types, as well. One such program is *Systematic Analysis of Language Transcripts* (SALT; Miller, Chapman, & Nockerts, 1998). With this program, the clinician must generate a written transcript of what a speaker has said. Disfluent speech ("mazes" in the parlance of the SALT manual) is coded within the transcripts by putting parentheses around disfluent segments of speech (e.g., *(He) He went home.*) Using this and other transcription conventions, the pro-

gram can recognize and tally instances of part-word, whole-word, and multiword repetitions, as well as filled pauses (i.e., interjections). If additional specificity in disfluency description is needed, the program allows for the use of descriptive codes after any word. The descriptive codes are placed within square brackets and are automatically tallied during data analysis, as well. See Figure 11–6 for an example of disfluency coding on a SALT transcript.

Another option is to use the coding conventions and data analysis tools associated with the *Child Language Data Exchange System* (CHILDES; MacWhinney, 1995). The CHILDES system features explicit coding conventions for developing transcriptions of language samples (Codes for Human Analysis of Transcripts [CHAT]) and an open-access, Web-based repository of transcripts that clinicians have developed using the transcription convention. The computer software associated with the system, Computerized Language Analysis (CLAN), executes automated analyses of language samples as well. Bernstein Ratner, Rooney, and MacWhinney (1996) provided a tutorial of how the system can be used to code and compute the frequency of specific disfluency-related behaviors. They developed a set of straightforward, keyboard-based codes for various types of disfluency. For example, prolonged sounds are coded by entering a colon after the sound that features atypical duration ("sssssun" $\rightarrow$ *s:un*). The transcription development approach in CHILDES is conceptually similar to the one employed in the SALT environment and, as with SALT, it allows for analysis of various aspects of language form, content, and use, as well as automatic computation of both the frequency and types of disfluency a speaker produces.

```
+ [BeginMS]
+ 5:54
C {1} three kid/s are make/ing a snowman.
C {2} (the boy) the boy[phrep] is paint/ing the shoe/s.
C {3} three kid/s are fish/ing.
C {4} two kid/s are wash/ing the car.
C {5} the girl is get/ing out of the car.
C {6} three kid/s are run/ing.
C {7} (the) the[wwr] kid/s are have/ing a rest .
C {8} is the boy brush/ing (her) his[rev] hair?
C {9} (is the) is the[phrep] dog pull/ing the girl?
C {10} (i*) is[pwr] the girl clean/ing the bathtub?
C {11} are the two children brush/ing their teeth?
C {12} is the boy catch/ing the ball?

Note. C = child
```

Figure 11–6. Excerpt from a transcript that was developed using the language analysis software Systematic Analysis of Language Transcripts (SALT, Miller, et al., 1998). A child who stutters produced these sentences while completing the Modeled Sentences task from the Test of Childhood Stuttering (Gillam et al., 2009). Disfluent speech is enclosed within parentheses. Disfluency types are coded in square brackets, and bound morpheme boundaries are coded with slashes. The "C" at the left margin of each line indicates that the child produced the utterances. Examiner utterances (not transcribed here) would be coded with "E." Analytic scripts in the program can calculate statistics such as mean length of utterance, total number of words, and total number of disfluencies.

Analyzing Speaking Rate

Speaking rate is another dimension of fluency that warrants assessment in clinical settings. Rate-based measures provide information about the speed at which a speaker communicates information. Highly disfluent speakers usually will take more time than highly fluent speakers to communicate the same amount of information. This is because disfluent behaviors such as pausing, interjecting, repeating, and prolonging speech sounds consume time that otherwise would be spent in productive communication. Two primary rate-related measures have been reported in the fluency disorders literature: *articulation rate* and *speech rate*. We describe each of them in this section.

Articulation Rate

Articulation rate is defined as the number of linguistic units (usually syllables or words) that a speaker produces per unit of time during fluent stretches of speech (Logan, Byrd, Mazzocchi, & Gillam, 2011). The measure provides information about how quickly a speaker communicates when the speech continuity is uninterrupted.

As indicated below, the computation of articulation rate is straightforward. The first step is to identify samples of fluent speech to be analyzed. With speakers who exhibit relatively little disfluency, the analysis usually is based on a corpus of randomly selected fluent utterances. In conversational samples, it is advisable to exclude 1- and 2-word utterances from the analysis because utterances of this length are common and often feature stereotypical content (e.g., *Yeah, No*). There is a risk that such utterances could be oversampled, a situation that might yield a distorted account of a speaker's articulation rate.

If a speaker produces very few utterances that are entirely fluent, it may be necessary to base the analysis on another unit of fluent speech, which is termed a *run*. Researchers define the term *run* as a string of consecutive syllables (usually at least 4 or 5) that are spoken without interruption. A run may constitute an entire utterance, but it also can consist of something less than an utterance.[2] Examples of runs that consist of at least 5 consecutive fluent syllables are shown in Example 11–10. Run boundaries are indicated by the underlined words; disfluency boundaries are marked with vertical lines.

Example 11–10:

a. <u>We met for brunch at the new restaurant</u>. (This run consists of 10 consecutive fluent syllables and spans an entire utterance.)

b. We |m-|met for |b-|brunch <u>at the new restaurant</u>. (This run consists of 6 consecutive fluent syllables and spans a complete prepositional phrase.)

To our knowledge, there is not a clear consensus concerning the minimum number of utterances or runs that must be analyzed to yield a valid estimate of articulation rate. In clinic practice and research activities, rate statistics for conversational data typically are based on a minimum of 10 fluent utterances or runs, although in some rate-related studies, the number of analyzed utterances is much greater than 10 (e.g., Kelly & Conture, 1992; Logan et al., 2011; Logan, Roberts, Pretto, & Morey, 2002; Meyers & Freeman, 1985).

Computing Articulation Rate

The procedure for computing articulation rate from a conversational or oral reading sample is as follows:

1. Elicit a sample of speech from the speaker. Make an audio or video recording of the sample.
2. Randomly select at least 10 fluent utterances from the sample. (With highly disfluent speakers, randomly select 10 fluent runs.)
3. Tally the amount of speech (i.e., syllables or words) in each of the utterances (or runs). Syllable (or word) tallies are based on the target utterance. Speech produced during disfluent segments is excluded from the tally.
4. Sum the number of syllables (or words) that are spoken in each utterance (or

---

[2]Many disfluencies are positioned at or near the onset of either utterances or clauses within utterances. Thus, when run-based analyses of articulation rate are used with highly disfluent speakers, there is a risk of oversampling the "tail end" of utterances. This potentially is problematic because articulation rate is not uniform throughout the course of an utterance (Starkweather, 1987). Rather, there is a tendency for speakers to articulate relatively quickly near the start of utterances and then to gradually decrease articulation rate when approaching an utterance's end. Thus, analysis of noninitial runs may yield articulation rates that are slower than articulation rates that are based on all parts of an utterance.

run) to obtain the total number of syllables (or words) in the sample.

5. Measure the duration of each selected utterance (or run). For each utterance (or run), begin timing at the start of the first word within the utterance (or run). End timing at the end of the last word within the utterance (or run). Timings can be made using a stopwatch; however, measurements that are obtained from computer-based speech imaging tools, such as a digital sound spectrogram, are likely to be more accurate.[3]

6. Obtain the total speaking time by summing the amount of time taken to say all of the utterances (or runs).

7. Use the following formula to compute articulation rate in syllables per second:

Articulation rate =

$$\frac{Total\ syllables\ spoken\ in}{fluent\ utterances\ (or\ runs)}{Total\ seconds\ spent\ talking}$$

8. Use the following formula to compute articulation rate in syllables per minute:

Articulation rate =

$$\frac{Total\ syllables\ spoken\ in}{fluent\ utterances\ (or\ runs)}{Total\ seconds\ spent\ talking} \times 60$$

9. To obtain word-based articulation rates, substitute word counts for syllable counts in the formulas shown in steps 7 and 8 above.

Speech Rate

Speech rate is defined as the number of linguistic units (usually syllables or words) that a speaker produces per unit of time. It differs from articulation rate in that both fluent and disfluent utterances are considered for analysis. Thus, speech rate yields information about a speaker's customary rate of communication. Speech rate is a superior measure to articulation rate for documenting treatment outcomes. This is because the speech rate measure captures information about the speaker's speed of articulatory movement as well as the number and duration of disfluencies the speaker produces.

Computing Speech Rate

Speech rate measurement is very similar to articulation rate measurement. The procedure for computing speech rate within a conversational sample is as follows:

1. Elicit a sample of speech from the person who is being assessed. Make an audio or video recording of the sample.

2. Randomly select a subset of utterances from the sample for the speech rate analysis. As in the articulation rate analysis, it is advisable to exclude 1- and 2-word utterances. We suggest that the analysis be based on a minimum of 10 to 15 utterances. The use of random sampling should result in both fluent and disfluent utterances being selected for the analysis. The ratio between the two utterance types

---

[3]A spectrogram is an image of the acoustic characteristics of a speech signal (Orlikoff & Baken, 1993). Contemporary spectrograms are generated using computer-based applications. Some spectrographic images appear in this chapter (see Figures 11–9 and 11–10). On the spectrogram, the *x*-axis denotes time, the *y*-axis denotes frequency, and the darkness of the vertical striations denotes intensity. In fluency analysis, spectrograms are useful for obtaining precise temporal measurements of utterances, syllables, pauses, and other units of interest.

should approximate that of the full sample if the utterances are selected randomly.

3. Tally the amount of speech produced by counting the number of syllables (or words) in each of the utterances. Syllable (or word) tallies are based on the target utterance. Exclude syllables (or words) that occur within disfluency boundaries from the tally.

4. Sum the number of syllables (or words) that are spoken in each utterance to obtain the total number of syllables (or words) in the sample.

5. Measure the duration of each selected utterance. For each utterance, begin timing at the start of the utterance, including any speech that is part of utterance-initial disfluency. Stop the timing at the end of the last word within the utterance. Timing can be done using a stopwatch; however, measurements that are obtained from computer-based speech imaging tools, such as a digital spectrogram, are likely to be more accurate.

6. Compute the total speaking time by summing the amount of time taken to say all of the selected utterances.

7. Use the following formula to compute speech rate in syllables per second:

$$Speech\ rate = \frac{Total\ syllables\ spoken\ in\ utterances}{Total\ seconds\ spent\ talking}$$

8. Use the following formula to compute speech rate in syllables per minute:

$$Speech\ rate = \frac{Total\ syllables\ spoken\ in\ utterances}{Total\ seconds\ spent\ talking} \times 60$$

9. To obtain word-based speech rates, substitute word counts for syllable counts in the formulas shown in steps 7 and 8 above.

An example of a speech rate analysis, based on 15 utterances produced by a child during the Modeled Sentences subtest of the *Test of Childhood Stuttering* (Gillam et al., 2009), is presented in Figure 11–7.

Computation of speech rate within tasks such oral reading and narration generally is much more straightforward than it is within conversational tasks. During oral reading and narration, the speech sample is comprised of a string of consecutive utterances. Thus, rather than having to time each utterance individually, as is required for conversational samples, the clinician measures only the amount of time elapsed from the beginning to the end of the reading passage or narrative. Speech rate then is computed by dividing the total time spent talking into the total number of syllables (or words) in the oral passage or target utterances within the narrative. Articulation rate during these tasks is computed using the same method if the speaker produces no disfluency. However, if the speaker produces disfluency, the clinician will need to analyze individual sentences (or runs) using the method described for conversational speech, earlier in this section.

Speech Initiation Time

For speech samples that consist of either word or sentence responses, one also can analyze the promptness with which a client initiates a response. Analyses of this sort provide information about a speaker's speech-based reaction time after being

Line	Utterance	Words	Sylls	Time (in sec)
1	|Th-|Three kids are making a snowman.	6	8	2.93
2	The boy is polishing the shoes.	6	8	2.75
3	|t-t-|Two kids are washing the car.	6	7	2.83
4	The kids are taking naps.	5	6	2.34
5	|Is the girl-| is the dog |um| pulling the girl?	6	7	3.44
6	Is the girl cleaning the tub?	6	7	2.93
7	Are the children |brush-|brushing their teeth?	6	8	3.09
8	Is the boy giving the girl some ice_cream?	8	10	3.11
9	The girl is getting off the boat.	7	8	2.65
10	The boat has |um| a flag on it.	7	7	2.74
11	The vegetables are on top of the table.	7	11	3.32
12	The children are riding on the train.	7	9	3.12
13	|when- when the- um| When the dog barked at the cat, the cat got very scared.	12	13	3.47
14	When the boy |was-| did a handstand the girls clapped.	9	10	3.25
15	When the boy paid his |mmm-| money he got |i-|ice-cream.	9	11	3.51
	Sums	107	130	45.48

- *Syllables per second* = (130/45.48) = <u>2.86</u>; *Syllables per minute* = 2.86 × 60 = <u>172</u>
- *Words per second* = (107/45.48) = <u>2.35</u>; *Words per minute* = 2.35 × 60 = <u>141</u>

Figure 11–7. Analysis of speech rate based on 15 responses from the Modeled Sentences task of the *Test of Childhood Stuttering* (Gillam et al., 2009). Word and syllable (Sylls) counts are based on analysis of target utterances; thus, they exclude speech from disfluent segments. Utterance timings were determined using a computer-based spectrogram.

given a signal to talk or "go," and, when combined with disfluency analyses, the speaker's ability to attain smooth, fluent speech in time-constrained conditions. In the fluency disorders literature, a variety of terms are used to characterize the measure. In this text, we will refer to it as *speech initiation time* (SIT). The "talk" (or "go") signal usually is something exter-

nal to the speaker such as the conclusion of a speaking partner's utterance, a tone that a computer generates, the beep of a voice mail system, and so forth. There are many practical advantages to being able to initiate speech promptly. Examples include things such as obtaining a speaking turn during a conversation, getting the attention of a busy waiter at a restaurant, and delivering the punch line of a joke at a moment that yields maximum comedic effect. Time constrained speaking tasks such as these can be challenging for speakers with impaired fluency to initiate as quickly as unimpaired speakers do (Bloodstein & Bernstein Ratner, 2008).

SIT is not routinely included in clinical assessment protocols; however, it has been measured extensively in research settings, where it serves as an index of language and/or motor functioning (Logan, 2001). In experimental settings, SIT has been assessed in several ways. An example of an assessment approach that might appear in a research study is shown in Figure 11–8A, along with a second, more practical example (Figure 11–8B) of how reaction time applies to a common activity such as answering the telephone.

In the first example from Figure 11–8, both the "get ready" and the "go" signals are presented via audio signals. Visual signals (e.g., pictures, symbols, typed words) would be acceptable, too. The speaker's responses are recorded, and the resulting recordings are analyzed using an acoustic waveform or spectrographic image to determine speech initiation time. In the approach shown in Figure 11–8, SIT is

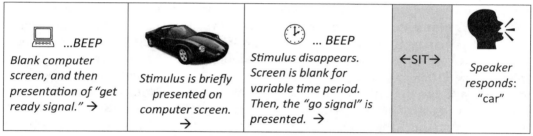

A

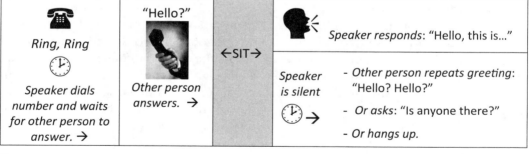

B

Figure 11–8. Examples of methods used to measure speech initiation time (SIT). In Example **A**, the speaker is instructed to name pictured stimuli as soon as possible after being given a signal to "go." The naming trial proceeds through a five-stage sequence, which provides information about the speaker's capacity for initiating speech promptly. In this case, SIT is the time elapsed between the presentation of the "go" signal and initiation of the word "car." Example **B** shows the event sequence associated with initiating a telephone call. After the other person answers and greets the speaker with "hello," the speaker has a relatively short time window in which to initiate speech. If the speaker does not initiate speech within a socially acceptable time frame, the other person may repeat the greeting, may ask if the speaker is actually there, or hang up.

defined as the amount of time elapsed between the presentation of the "go" stimulus and the initiation of the speaker's response. In Example A, the target response is the name of the pictured object; however, sentences can be elicited, as well. Computer-based tasks such as this transpire in a highly controlled setting and, as such, are likely to provide information about a speaker's *capacity* for initiating speech promptly.

In contrast, activities in which the client answers a ringing telephone or initiates a conversation after another person answers a ringing telephone provide information about a speaker's performance in authentic, time-constrained environments. With such activities, the speaker's initial challenge is to initiate speech before the telephone partner either (a) questions whether the speaker is actually there (e.g., *Hello? . . . Hello?*) or (b) hangs up. By measuring the average amount of elapsed time between the signal to begin speaking and the client's attempt to begin speaking, the clinician can gain insight into the client's current response patterns. It may be that a client is attempting to initiate speech at a pace that is incompatible with his or her current capacity to do so. In such cases, the therapeutic strategy might involve encouraging the client to take *more time* when initiating speech production in time-constrained contexts.

Rate Deviations

The term *rate deviation* refers to a transient fluctuation in articulation rate during a particular stretch of speech. Listeners judge the stretch of speech as inappropriately fast or slow in relation to the rate of the surrounding speech. Deviations in articulation rate often are regarded as a primary or common symptom of clut-

tered speech (St. Louis, Myers, Bakker, & Raphael, 2007). The main pattern of rate deviation in cluttering is that bursts of excessively fast-sounding speech occur within the context of speech that otherwise seems to be articulated at a normal rate. In the context of cluttering, the affected segments of speech typically are relatively short—spanning either a single phonological word or phonological phrase. Sometimes, the bursts of speech are unintelligible to the listener. Some speakers who stutter manifest the opposite pattern—brief stretches of unusually slow articulatory rate. The latter rate pattern may represent a compensatory response to the anticipation of fluency disruption on an upcoming syllable. Either way, if rate deviations occur with any consistency during a speech sample, it is worth documenting their frequency. In clinic settings, judgments of rate deviation can be made subjectively. The clinician and perhaps the speaker or a caregiver listens to a speech sample and marks segments of speech that they perceive as being unusually fast or slow in relation to the surrounding speech. The length of each marked segment can be computed in syllables, words, or phonological words and then summed across the entire sample. From these data, a clinician can compute the percent of linguistic units within the sample that feature deviant rate as well as the total number of rate deviation episodes within the sample.

Analyzing Rhythm

As discussed in Chapter 1, *rhythm* is an aspect of prosody that arises from variations in the duration of syllables, segments, and pauses during a spoken utterance. So, in a sense, speech rhythm is a manifestation of the time course in which the linguistic units within an utterance unfold. English is regarded as a stress-timed language, with utterances divided into strings of syllables called stress groups, each of which consists of a stressed syllable and one or more unstressed syllables (Hixon, Weismer, & Hoit, 2008). Research shows that within an utterance, or even across a stretch of contiguous utterances, the duration of these stress groups is roughly equivalent, even though the individual stress groups may contain different numbers of syllables (Lehiste, 1973). In large part, speech rhythm seems to reflect the effects of prosodic planning, though the biomechanical properties of the speech production system may play some role in influencing events such as the duration of specific speech sound segments within certain phonetic contexts (Behrman, 2007; Selkirk, 1984).

The presence of disfluency within an utterance can disrupt the rhythm of an utterance by distorting the expected or typical time course of an utterance. Segment durations can change; pause durations can change as well; and with these changes, the predictable distribution of stressed syllables is altered as well. As such, disfluent utterances generally are perceived as being *dysrhythmic*. A speaker who exhibits frequent disfluency is likely to be regarded as speaking less rhythmically than a speaker who exhibits infrequent disfluency. In this section, we discuss two quantitative analyses that pertain to speech rhythm. The first involves the measurement of disfluency duration; that is, the length of time that a speaker's disfluencies last. Disfluency duration has been used as an indicator of stuttering severity (e.g., Gillam et al., 2009; Riley, 2009), and it has been proposed as measure of speaker's overall communicative productivity (Starkweather, Gottwald, & Halfond, 1990). It is reasonable to assume

that lengthy disfluencies disrupt the perceived rhythm of an utterance more so than brief disfluencies do. The second analysis involves the structural components within repetitions, particularly the number of attempts a speaker makes at repairing an utterance and the temporal patterns associated with those attempts.

Measuring Disfluency Duration

Measurement of disfluency duration involves identifying and then timing the portions of an utterance that are extraneous to the target or core utterance. The analysis is relatively straightforward to do after a digitized image of a speech signal such as a spectrogram has been created. The method for measuring disfluency duration is as follows:

1. Record a sample of speech from the client and then randomly select a pool of disfluencies (10 to 20 usually will suffice) from the speech sample for analysis. Depending on the clinician's goals for the analysis, the selected disfluencies either can be drawn from all of the disfluency types that the client produces or restricted to certain types of disfluencies. For example, clinicians with an interest in stuttering usually will restrict the disfluency duration analysis to repetitions and prolongations—disfluency types that are most characteristic of stuttered speech (Logan et al., 2011; Throneburg & Yairi, 1994). In contrast, clinicians with an interest in cluttering might restrict their analysis to the disfluency types that are most characteristic of that disorder (e.g., interjections, revisions, or structurally complex "mazes").

2. Create digital images for each of the disfluent utterances using speech analysis software that is capable of creating amplitude waveforms or spectrograms.

3. Using the procedures outlined in Table 11–1, identify the boundaries of each instance of disfluency. Place the cursor of the speech analysis software at the leftmost edge of the first disfluent segment that is to be measured. Note the time code on the computer screen that is associated with the cursor placement. Time codes can be reported in either seconds or milliseconds.

4. Place the cursor of the speech analysis software at the rightmost edge of the disfluent segment. Again, note the time code associated with the cursor placement.

5. Subtract the time code obtained in Step 3 from the time code obtained in Step 4. The difference between these two time codes is the disfluency duration.

6. Repeat this process for each of the other randomly selected disfluencies that are to be analyzed.

7. Sum the durations for each of the measured disfluencies. This yields the total duration for all of the measured disfluencies. Divide the total duration by the total number of disfluencies measured to obtain the average duration for all of the disfluencies. Average durations can be computed for specific categories of disfluency, if desired.

The process of measuring disfluency duration is illustrated in Figure 11–9. The spectrogram in Figure 11–9 shows an excerpt from a disfluent utterance. As shown in the figure, the computer software allows for marking the boundaries of the disfluent segment (i.e., speech that is superfluous to the target utterance)

and for indicating its duration. Disfluency duration may be reported either in milliseconds (e.g., 1330 ms) or in seconds (e.g., 1.330 s).

Alternately, disfluency duration can be measured using software tools such as *Computerized Scoring of Stuttering Severity* (CSSS-2.0, Bakker & Riley, 2009), which is a component of the *Stuttering Severity Instrument–4* (SSI-4; Riley, 2009), or the *Stuttering Measurement System* (SMS; Ingham et al., n.d.). With both programs, disfluency duration is measured by depressing a specific computer key at the onset of a perceived disfluency (or instance of stuttering) and releasing the key at the offset of the disfluency (or stuttering event). Measurement accuracy in these cases is tied to the clinician's ability to recognize and promptly activate the timing device at the onset and offset of the behavior of interest (Bakker & Riley, 2009). Thus, when a clinician uses either a stopwatch or a button-press function on a computer system, it is advisable to practice the technique extensively. Some researchers also adopt the practice of timing each behavior of interest multiple times and then taking the average of the timings as the duration for the speech event (e.g., Pindzola, Jenkins, & Lokken, 1989; Sturm & Seery, 2007). This approach presumably reduces the measurement error that is associated with the use of manually controlled timing devices.

Analyzing Repetition Structure: Counting Unsuccessful Attempts

Another approach to analyzing speech rhythm involves the study of structural components within repetitions. The general focus is on the number of attempts a

Table 11–1. Determining Disfluency Boundaries Within a Spoken Utterance

Spoken Utterance[a]	Disfluency Label	Boundaries
Riley| cha- cha- |chased the lizard.	Part-word repetition	*Left edge:* Point within the original utterance to which the speaker retraces after interrupting speech (i.e., after *Riley*). *Right edge:* Start of successful repair (i.e., *chased*).
Riley|chased$_1$- |chased$_2$ the lizard.	Whole-word repetition	*Left edge:* Point within the original utterance to which the speaker retraces after interrupting speech (i.e., after *Riley*). *Right edge:* Start of successful repair (i.e., onset of *chased$_2$*).
|Riley$_1$ chased-| Riley$_2$ chased the lizard.	Multiword ("phrase") repetition	*Left edge:* Point within the original utterance to which the speaker retraces after interrupting speech (i.e., onset of utterance). *Right edge:* Start of successful repair (i.e., onset of *Riley$_2$*).
Riley|ch→|ased the lizard.	Sound prolongation	*Left edge:* End of word preceding the start of the prolonged sound (i.e., after *Riley*). *Right edge:* Start of the speech segments that follow the prolonged sound (i.e., the syllable rime [eɪst].
Riley| *silence* |chased the lizard.	Pause	*Left edge:* Point within the original utterance where speech is interrupted (i.e., after *Riley*). *Right edge:* Start of successful repair (i.e., onset of *chased*).
Riley| um |chased the lizard.	Interjection	*Left edge:* Point within the original utterance where speech is interrupted (i.e., after *Riley*). *Right edge:* Start of successful repair (i.e., onset of *chased*).
Riley| ray- |chased the lizard.	Revision	*Left edge*: Point within the original utterance to which the speaker retraces after interrupting speech (i.e., after *Riley*). *Right edge:* Start of successful repair (i.e., onset of *chased*).
Riley|p- paced-| chased the lizard.	Revision with embedded part-word repetition	*Left edge:* Furthest point within the original utterance to which the speaker retraces after interrupting speech (i.e., after *Riley*). *Right edge:* Start of successful repair (i.e., onset of *chased*).

Note: Target utterance is *Riley chased the lizard.*

[a]Dashes in this column represent moments of interruption. The arrow (→) indicates prolonged duration.

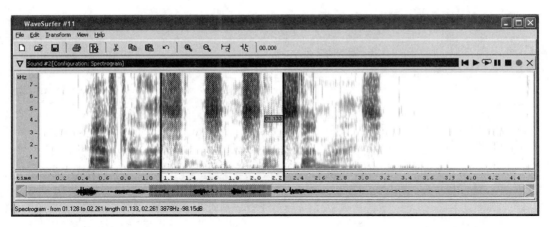

Figure 11–9. Spectrographic image of the phrase *after the s- s- s- sunrise.* The disfluency boundaries were identified using criteria described in Table 11–1 and marked on the spectrogram by clicking the cursor at the left-most edge of the part-word repetition and then by dragging it to the right-most edge. Upon doing so, the computer program automatically reported the duration of the marked area. This disfluency lasts approximately 1.33 seconds. The spectrogram was created using the Wavesurfer software program (Sjölander & Beskow, 2006). Bold vertical lines were superimposed on the original cursor markers to enhance the clarity of the disfluency boundaries in the figure.

speaker makes at producing a particular syllable or word for the purpose of advancing the target utterance. As described in Chapter 4, three main methods have been implemented in the fluency disorders literature for the study of repetition structure:

- Counting the *total number of attempts* a speaker makes at producing a target syllable or word,
- Counting the *number of unsuccessful attempts* a speaker makes at producing a target syllable or word, and
- Counting the *number of initiations needed to repair* an interruption in production of a target syllable or word.

The distinction among the three approaches is illustrated in Example 11–11 below, where attempts at producing the

syllable *Matt* are underlined (there are four total attempts), unsuccessful attempts at producing *Matt* are marked with the superscript "U" and numbered to indicate their sequential position (there are three unsuccessful attempts), and repair initiations are marked with the superscript "R" and numbered to indicate their sequential position (there are three repair initiations). The same notational pattern would apply to repetitions of whole words and phrases. As noted in Example 11–11, analysis of the number of repair initiations and unsuccessful attempts yields the same answer (three, in this case), and the number of total attempts (four, in this case) is always one greater than those counts.

Example 11–11: $\underline{M^{U1}\text{-}\ M\text{-}^{U2/R1}\ M\text{-}^{U3/R2}}$ $\underline{Matt^{R3}}$ *flew home.*

Any of the three methods is acceptable to use in clinical practice, provided the clinician employs the same approach when comparing data within a client. The method that we outline below is focused on counting the unsuccessful attempts at a syllable or word. Similar methods would be used when basing the analysis on repair initiations or total attempts at the target.

1. Elicit a sample of speech from the client. If possible, make an audio or video recording of the sample and base the analysis on it.
2. Randomly select a sample of repetitions for analysis. If desired, sampling can be restricted to a subcategory of repetition such as part-word repetition. We suggest that the analysis be based on a minimum of 10 to 15 repetitions.
3. Count the number of unsuccessful attempts at producing the target syllable/word in each of the selected repetitions.
4. Sum the number of unsuccessful attempts across all of the selected repetitions.
5. Divide the total number of unsuccessful attempts across all analyzed repetitions by the total number of analyzed repetitions. This yields the average number of unsuccessful attempts during repetition.

Additional examples of part-word, whole-word, and phrase repetition are presented below to illustrate the concept further. Unsuccessful attempts at advancing the utterance beyond the point of interruption are marked with superscript "U" and numbered to indicate their sequential position.

Example 11–12: *Kay^{U1}- Kay^{U2}-Kayla moved to New Jersey.*
(2 unsuccessful attempts)

Example 11–13: *Bal^{U1}- bal^{U2}- b^{U3}-Baltimore won the game.*
(3 unsuccessful attempts)

Example 11–14: *Trey decided^{U1}-decided to hire three cashiers.*
(1 unsuccessful attempt)

Example 11–15: *Can we^{U1}- Can we^{U2}- Can we get candy?*
(2 unsuccessful attempts)

Structural analyses such as this provide insight into a speaker's ability to repair problems in speech production and the depth or severity of the person's disability. Unfortunately, it is not possible at present to say with precision *why* some disfluencies feature multiple unsuccessful repair attempts, and others feature only one.

Analyzing Repetition Structure: Temporal Patterns

A second way to describe speech rhythm is to examine rhythmic patterns during disfluencies that involve repetition. The main goal is to distinguish between those repetitions that preserve the rhythm of fluent speech that precedes the disfluency and those that do not (Pindzola & White, 1986; Van Riper, 1982). Repetitions of the latter sort would sound choppy, uneven, or irregular to a listener.

Scale-Based Approaches

Pindzola and White (1986) described a two-category rating approach to analyzing repetitions of young children who stutter. The clinician judges the repetitions of a child as being either "slow/normal; evenly paced," which corresponds to nondisordered fluency performance, or "fast, perhaps irregular," which corresponds to "abnormal fluency performance" (in this case, stuttering). One easily could expand on Pindzola and White's (1986) approach by using a multipoint, Likert-type rating scale that features terms such as "Highly rhythmic" and "Highly dysrhythmic" at each end point. In this way, the clinician could assess changes in the rhythmicity of a client's repetitions at various stages of treatment.

Measuring the Duration of Disfluency Components

Yairi and colleagues (Throneburg & Yairi, 1994; Yairi & Hall, 1993) compared the temporal characteristics of part- and whole-word repetitions produced by children who stuttered and children who did not stutter. The two groups of children were compared in terms of the duration of repeated units during their disfluencies as well as the silent intervals (i.e., the editing phases) between the repeated units. In both studies, the researchers found that children who stuttered spent less time within the editing phase (i.e., less time being silent) than the children who did not stutter. That is, the editing phases of children who stuttered lasted for fewer milliseconds, and they occupied a significantly smaller proportion of the overall disfluency duration in comparison to children who did not stutter. Disfluencies with this sort of temporal pattern are likely to be perceived as "rushed" or "hurried" by a listener and thus would sound dysrhythmic in relation to surrounding syllables of fluent speech. Based on this finding, the researchers concluded that children who stutter tend to produce repetitions at a significantly faster rate than children who do not stutter.

In the Throneburg and Yairi (1994) study, the mean duration for the silent interval within single-unit, part-word repetitions among the children who did not stutter was about three times longer than it was for the children who stuttered (i.e., 418 ms versus 136 ms, respectively). A similar disparity was noted between the groups for single-unit, whole-word repetitions. In two-unit repetitions, the first silent interval was longer than the second for both groups; however, children who stuttered once again exhibited shorter silent periods than children who did not stutter. Interestingly, the children who did not stutter showed much greater between-subject variability in the absolute duration of silent periods than the children who stuttered. Thus, the children who stuttered tended to utilize a more constrained timing pattern for their repetitions in comparison to the children who did not stutter. Further analysis of the data showed that a child's diagnostic classification (i.e., stuttering versus nonstuttering) could be predicted on the basis of the editing phase within repetitions with 72% to 87% accuracy, depending on the disfluency type analyzed. The editing phase (i.e., silent period) within single-unit, whole-word repetitions had the best predictive value of a child's diagnostic status. Examples of excerpts from two phrases, each with multi-iteration, part-word repetitions of [s] within the phrase *after the sunrise*, are shown in Figure 11–10.

Analyzing Effort

The construct of effort in speech production has been measured both subjectively and objectively in relation to physical and mental activity.

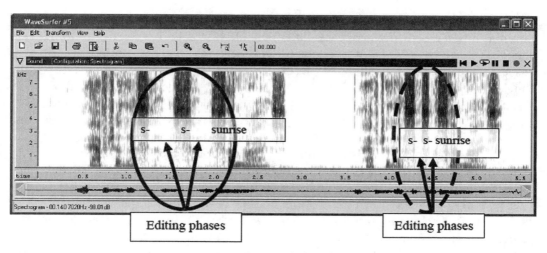

Figure 11–10. In this figure, excerpts from two phrases, each with multi-iteration, part-word repetitions of [s] within the phrase *after the s- s- sunrise*, are shown. The rhythmic structure of the repetition in the phrase on the left (solid-line oval) is the sort that likely would be observed in a child who does not stutter. It features relatively long silent periods (i.e., editing phases) between iterations of [s]. About 55% of the total disfluency duration is spent in editing. The rhythmic structure of the repetition on the right (dashed oval) is of the sort that would be observed in a child who stutters. It features relatively short silent periods (i.e., editing phases) between iterations of [s], and a smaller proportion of the total disfluency duration (about 44% in this case) is spent in editing. The spectrogram was created using the Wavesurfer software program (Sjölander & Beskow, 2006).

Subjective Ratings

Subjective ratings of effort are straightforward to do: A rater is presented with a sample of speech and attempts to quantify his or her perception of the amount of effort being expended. Ratings may be based on samples of connected speech such as a one-minute period of speech (e.g., Ingham, Warner, Byrd, & Cotton, 2006; Ingham et al., 2009) or on specific fluency-related events such as instances of disfluency (Weber & Smith, 1990). The ratings can be performed either by the speaker (e.g., Ingham et al., 2006) or by a listener (e.g., Young, 1981). Such ratings often are made on a multipoint, Likert-style rating scale. In the fluency disorders literature, such scales typically feature either 7 or 9 points, which are spaced at equal intervals. The scale end points typically are labeled with contrasting terms such as "very effortless" and "very effortful" or "least severe" and "very severe" (e.g., Ingham et al., 2006; Ingham et al., 2009; Weber & Smith, 1990).

Physical Measures

The notion of effort also can be assessed using measures of aerodynamic events, speech physiology, speech kinematics, and so forth. Objective assessment of variables that correspond to the notion of effort typically requires the use of specialized equipment, some of which is likely to be found only in research laboratories.

Thus, in this section, we focus our discussion mainly on electromyography, as it is plausible that the equipment needed for this measure might be available in both educational and medical work sites.

Electromyography

Electromyography (EMG) is a clinical tool that provides information about the electrical activity that is present within a muscle. EMG provides information about the health of muscles and the neurons that innervate them. Use of EMG in the area of fluency dates back to the 1930s, when Travis (1934) examined the nature of action potentials in bilaterally paired speech muscles in speakers who stuttered. There are two main types of EMG: *intramuscular* and *surface*. We discuss each type below.

Intramuscular EMG requires the insertion of an electrode into muscle tissue via either a hypodermic needle or hooked insertion (Behrman, 2007). The electrode is capable of detecting electrical activity within specific regions of a muscle when the muscle is at rest and when the muscle is active. Resting muscles typically feature very little electrical activity. Contracted muscles, in contrast, feature greater levels of electrical activity, and activity increases as a function of how much contraction is present.

Intramuscular EMG has been used to document effort in a range of research studies involving people who stutter (e.g., Freeman & Ushijima, 1978; Guitar, Guitar, Neilson, O'Dwyer, & Andrews, 1988; Smith, Denny, Shaffer, Kelly, & Hirano, 1996). Given the invasive nature of the procedure, the need for anesthetization, and the potential for discomfort, intramuscular EMG is much more likely to be used in research activities than it is in clinical activities such as a treatment program.

Surface EMG, in contrast, is performed by affixing disk-like electrodes to the skin in locations that correspond to particular muscles. As with intramuscular EMG, the surface electrodes collect data about electrophysiological events within particular muscles; however, it typically offers less sensitive assessment of specific muscles in comparison to intramuscular EMG. Because surface EMG is less invasive than intramuscular EMG, it is more apt to be used in clinic-based fluency intervention activities and in basic research and treatment studies with children (e.g., Conture, Colton, & Gleason, 1988; Kelly, Smith, & Goffman, 1995). Indeed, a number of research studies have been conducted to examine the effects of EMG-based biofeedback at reducing stuttering frequency. In such studies, the surface EMG instrument is configured to provide auditory or visual feedback (e.g., a tone, a color) that changes, proportionately, in response to changes in the amplitude of the EMG signal. The speaker attempts to alter muscle activity utilizing the auditory or visual feedback about muscle activity.

The effect of surface EMG feedback on speech fluency has been examined in numerous studies. Most applications within the area of fluency disorders have focused on developmental stuttering (e.g., Craig & Cleary, 1982; Craig et al., 1996; Guitar, 1975; Hancock et al., 1998; Hanna, Wilfling, & McNeill, 1975). Results from those studies indicate that speakers can reduce stuttering frequency significantly when provided with feedback about the activity level in speech-related muscles.

Use of Associated or Compensatory Behaviors

A final analysis to discuss under the heading of effort concerns the use of *associ-*

ated or *compensatory* behaviors. In the fluency disorders literature, such behaviors also have been termed *secondary* behaviors, *concomitant* behaviors, and *physical concomitants*. The main point is that these are behaviors that coincide with disfluency and related speech behaviors that are symptomatic of stuttered speech. These behaviors are more common among speakers who stutter than they are among speakers who clutter. Individuals in the latter group often exhibit limited awareness of their fluency-related difficulties, and this may explain the limited use of compensatory behaviors. The behaviors discussed in this section by no means are an exhaustive list of the types of associated or compensatory behaviors that a clinician might encounter in speakers who have impaired fluency, but the discussion here hopefully provides a sense of the range of behaviors one can expect to see and some insight into their nature and functional role in speech production.

Indicators of Excessive Tension and Speech-Related "Struggle"

Some speakers with impaired fluency show signs of excessive effort during speech production. Excessive effort perhaps is most noticeable during moments of disfluency, where it sometimes is manifested as tremor. Excessive tension during disfluency appears to be an emergent aspect of stuttered speech: Older children who stutter are more likely to exhibit tremor-like oscillations in their speech musculature while talking than younger children are (Kelly et al., 1995). Thus, tremor may be a reaction to or a means of coping with interrupted speech continuity. In our experience, the most obvious signs of excessive effort occur in conjunction with disfluency that is characterized by

fixed articulatory postures. The tension is not the cause of the disfluency, per se but it likely does contribute to the duration of the disfluency and the production of fixed, inaudible articulatory postures. For example, highly contracted laryngeal muscles are incompatible with vocal fold vibration and, hence, with phonation.

The appearance of excessive physical tension can be coded on a speech sample transcript. A clinician can indicate which syllables or words are affected, and if desired, perceptions of the degree of tension the speaker exhibits can be recorded on a rating scale. Another option is to document which muscles or regions of the speech production system appear to be most affected (e.g., abdominal, chest/upper torso, larynx and neck, tongue and lips) and the manner in which they are affected (e.g., rapid, audible or uneven inhalation). Additional notes about the aspects of speech most affected (e.g., speech breathing, phonation, articulation) can be added as well. Certain phonatory behaviors are indicative of excessive tension. We mentioned cessation of phonation above. Sometimes, speakers who stutter exhibit abrupt, upward shifts in vocal pitch as they release fixed laryngeal postures associated with "inaudible prolongation" of vowel sounds.

Extraneous Movements or Speech Sounds

Some speakers who stutter exhibit what have been termed *extraneous* movements in conjunction with speech. Some of these behaviors are rhythmical in nature (e.g., tapping of a finger, a foot, the jaw) and appear to be designed to facilitate speech fluency. Some speakers will exhibit the rhythmical movement prior to initiation of an utterance. In such cases, the speaker typically will attempt to time the occurrence of vocal tract constriction with the end of a tap cycle (e.g., a speaker attempts to time lip approximation for the [p] in "Paul" with the time at which his or her finger strikes the table top). Some of these compensatory movements can be quite subtle such that the clinician is unable to detect their usage. For example, a speaker might time a vocal tract constriction with an eye-blink. For this reason, it is prudent to ask a client about whether he or she uses such strategies to facilitate fluency, even in cases where the behaviors are not observed during an assessment.

Other speakers who stutter may use nonspeech vocalizations to facilitate the initiation of a spoken utterance. Examples of this include the use of a prolonged [m] or the interjection "um" prior to the first word of an utterance. Less commonly, a speaker deliberately will substitute one speech sound for another, in an attempt to increase the likelihood of being able to initiate a particular word. For example, a person may initiate words that ordinarily begin with [h] by using a bilabial voiceless fricative. In some cases, it may be difficult to discern why the speaker is using such vocalizations or sound substitutions. If this is the case, it is best to ask the client about it directly.

Attempts to Minimize or Conceal the Effects of Fluency Impairment

Fluency disruption and the listeners' reactions associated to it can be emotionally painful for clients. This seems especially true for speakers who stutter. Some speakers will go to great lengths to mask the symptoms of their impaired fluency from others. Clinicians should be alert to behaviors such as the following while observing clients:

- Use of sound or word substitution;
- Intentionally transposing word order so that words upon which disfluency are anticipated are moved toward the end of an utterance;
- Pretending to have forgotten what one had planned to say, pretending not to know an answer; and
- Adopting alternate patterns of speaking, such as use of a foreign accent or speaking in a whisper.

Analyzing Naturalness

As indicated in Chapter 1, speech naturalness has become an increasingly common construct to assess with speakers who stutter, particularly within the context of treatment outcomes (Ingham & Riley, 1998). The construct typically is left undefined for raters and is measured using a 7- or 9-point, equal-interval scale. In many studies of speech naturalness with speakers who stutter, the low end of the scale (i.e., 1) has been labeled as "highly natural" and the high end of the scale (i.e., 9) as "highly unnatural." The *Stuttering Severity Instrument* (SSI-4; Riley, 2009) features informal examiner- and client-based assessments of naturalness, which are based on a 9-point scale.

Naturalness seems to be a multidimensional construct that includes elements of continuity and rhythm (Martin, Haroldson, & Triden, 1984), rate (Logan et al., 2002), as well as effort (Hodgeman & Logan, 2013; Ingham et al., 2006). A rater typically is presented with an excerpt of the client's speech. After listening to the sample, the rater then assigns a subjective rating to it. In clinical settings, such ratings can be assigned either during an assessment or in conjunction with treatment activities. In the latter case, the clinician provides the client with regular feedback about his or her speech naturalness as the client attempts to use the fluency management strategy. The speaker's goal is to produce speech that sounds like the speech of an unimpaired speaker. Research has shown that when a clinician provides a client with this type of feedback, clients can make the necessary adjustments to bring their speech naturalness levels into the range of typical speakers (Ingham, Martin, Haroldson, Onslow, & Leney, 1985; Ingham, Sato, Finn, & Belknap, 2001).

Analyzing Talkativeness

In Chapter 1, we described how the term *talkativeness* can be used in a broad sense to capture the four fluency dimensions that Fillmore (1979) outlined: (1) *verbal output/participation*; (2) *succinctness*; (3) *situational flexibility*; and (4) *communicative creativity*. In the remainder of this section, we discuss several straightforward ways that clinicians can analyze speech samples to obtain information about functioning in these areas.

Verbal Output

Talkativeness most commonly is conceived of in terms of *verbal output*. Verbal output refers to how much a speaker says, and it is a fundamental indicator of communicative competence. At first glance, it

might seem that verbal output should be evaluated within a "more-is-better" framework, and to a certain extent, that is true. However, as studies of speakers who clutter indicate, excessive verbal output sometimes can actually hinder communication by impeding the clear, fluent, and orderly development of conversational topics.

Analysis of verbal output has been employed with a range of clinical populations. It has been used as a diagnostic marker for disorders such as schizophrenia, bipolar disorder, depression, dementia, and cluttering; as an indicator of personality style; and as a response variable in studies of drug effects on verbal behavior (Barch & Berenbaum, 1997; Wardle, Cederbaum, & de Wit, 2011). A range of factors can affect one's verbal output. Such factors should be taken into account when assessing this aspect of fluency. Included among these factors are the following:

- *Topic familiarity.* Individuals who have extensive experience with a subject are likely to have well-developed conceptual schemas for subject-related information and thus should be well positioned to generate a range of communicative intentions to share with others.
- *Linguistic proficiency.* Individuals who possess well-developed lexicons and who are adept at formulating linguistic codes are well positioned to formulate a range of utterances that allow expression of their communicative intentions.
- *Physical environment.* Physical characteristics of the communication environment (e.g., the presence of background noise, physical distance between communicators) can affect a speaker's verbal output.

- *Characteristics of communication partners.* The verbal behavior of conversational partners (e.g., their speaking rates, interruption patterns, relative social status) can affect a speaker's ability to obtain or maintain a conversational turn.
- *Social conventions.* Social conventions can affect verbal output as well. For example, when greeting a newly married couple in a receiving line following a wedding, it would be inappropriate for a speaker to tell a lengthy story and thus bog down the flow of the line for other wedding guests.
- *Personal factors.* Factors that are unique to a speaker, such as gender, temperament, and motivation, can influence verbal output as well.

Verbal output can be described in relation to language-, time-, and/or task-based units (see Leaper & Ayres, 2007; Leaper & Smith, 2004). These approaches are discussed below.

Language-Based Measures of Output

Numerous language-based approaches to measuring verbal output have been reported in the research literature (Leaper & Ayres, 2007; Leaper & Smith, 2004). With each of the approaches, the goal essentially is to quantify the *linguistic density* of a speaker's verbal output. This is accomplished by computing the number of linguistic units that are nested within other linguistic units. Examples of these measures include the following:

- *Number of syllables, words, morphemes, syntactic phrases, or clauses per utterance.* With this approach, talkativeness is defined in terms of how many linguistic units a speaker produces per utterance. The *number of syllables per utterance* accomplishes this from a phonologic perspective. The other measures do so from a (morpho)syntactic perspective. With each of these specific measures, a talkative speaker is one who produces relatively many linguistic units per utterance in comparison to other speakers.
- *Number of syllables, words, morphemes, syntactic phrases, or clauses per conversational turn.* This approach to measuring talkativeness is similar to the one described above. Here, the focus is on the linguistic density of a conversational turn. With each of these specific measures, a talkative speaker is one who produces relatively many linguistic units per turn in comparison to other speakers.

Computation of the statistics listed above is straightforward and can be accomplished using the following procedure.

1. Elicit a speech sample from the speaker.
2. Create a written transcript of the speaker's verbal output. When doing so, parse the transcript into either utterances or conversational turns. The analyses described here are well suited to be done in the context of coded transcription in real time.
3. Count the number of linguistic units (e.g., syllables, words, phrases, syntactic phrases, clauses) within each utterance or turn, and then sum across all utterances or turns to obtain the total

number of linguistic units produced in the sample.

4. Divide the total number of linguistic units produced in the sample by the total number of utterances or turns.

In clinical settings, it often is desirable to document changes in a speaker's verbal output over time. To do this, it is necessary to elicit the "before" and "after" speech samples in a controlled manner (i.e., using highly similar narrative prompts, conversational topics, or speaking tasks; using highly similar physical, environmental, or social settings).

Time-Based Measures of Output

Talkativeness also can be described in reference to time-based units. Examples of such measures include the following:

- *Time spent talking.* With this approach, the clinician uses a stopwatch or other similar timing device to record the amount of time a speaker talks during a particular task. Highly talkative speakers will have longer talking-time values than less talkative speakers will. Computation of time spent talking can be challenging to do in real time within conversational speech samples because of the need to record the duration of each of the speaker's utterances. When comparing time spent talking across speech samples, it is important to ensure that the client has had an equal opportunity to talk in each of the speech samples.
- *Linguistic units produced per time unit.* A variation of the method described above is to link the *time spent speaking* measure to a

linguistic unit, such as syllables or words. With this approach, a highly talkative speaker produces relatively more syllables or words per unit of time in comparison to other speakers. The resulting statistics (e.g., syllables per second, words per minute) were described above in the section on speaking rate. When used as an index of verbal output, the measure can be refined further by linking data to a particular task such as picture description, story retelling, classroom discussion, or casual conversation among peers. With this approach, a talkative speaker is one who produces relatively many linguistic units (e.g., syllables, words, and conversational turns) within a particular task that lasts for a prescribed length of time. A speaker's verbal output can be compared to other speakers or to his or her performance at another point in time.

Analyzing Verbal Participation

Verbal participation is regarded as a fundamental aspect of communicative functioning (World Health Organization, 2001). The notion of verbal participation is similar to that of verbal output, as it also conveys a sense of *situational involvement*. With verbal participation, the focus is on the number and variety of communication contexts in which a speaker is engaged and then, once the speaker is in a situation, the depth of that involvement. As noted in Chapter 10, measures of verbal participation are commonly included in self-rating instruments that are designed for speakers who stutter.

The self-rating instruments offer a good starting point for analyzing a client's verbal participation patterns. If necessary, however, a clinician can assess verbal participation further, using clinician-designed data collection tools that are tailored to client-specific speaking activities. The latter approach is based on the creation of an inventory of the actual communication activities in which the client is routinely engaged. Upon developing the inventory, the next step is to determine the nature of participation in each activity.

An inventory of a client's unique communication activities can be created through discussion with the client and/or or caregivers and, in school settings, teachers. Through further discussion, the clinician can collect additional information about such things as (a) the frequency with which a particular activity from the inventory occurs during a typical week and the length of time it typically lasts; (b) how often the client currently participates in each activity on the inventory; (c) how much the client usually says during those activities (i.e., verbal output); (d) the extent to which the client (or caregivers/teacher) considers it important for the client to participate in each activity; and (e) the extent to which the client (or caregiver/teacher) is satisfied with the client's current level of participation. Information such as this can be useful in determining treatment objectives and evaluating treatment outcomes.

Communicative Flexibility

Communicative flexibility refers to the ability to use speech for a range of purposes. With fluency disorders such as stuttering, this ability sometimes is diminished as a result of a client's reluctance to use speech in situational contexts that are likely to exacerbate the effects of fluency impairment. We can view *situations* in terms of both physical settings and communicative contexts. We discussed the assessment of fluency within physical settings in the previous section on participation. In this section, we focus on the functions that verbal communication serves. With some clients, there is value in analyzing speech samples with regard to the types of communicative functions a speaker expresses, as well as the frequency with which the intentions are expressed and the impact that they have on the client's fluency.

Fey (1986) described a *speech act analysis* that is well suited for analyzing the types of communicative functions a speaker expresses. Although Fey applied the analysis to children's language samples, it can be extended to examine speech communication and fluency behavior in fluency-impaired speakers as well. With the speech act analysis, clinicians classify the functions of a speaker's conversational utterances in two ways. The first, an *utterance level analysis,* describes the function of a particular utterance in relation to the utterance that immediately precedes it. At this level, utterances can be classified into one of four main categories: *assertive acts, responsive acts, imitations,* and *other.* Assertive acts are unsolicited, meaning that a speaker *initiates* verbal communication without being asked or obligated to do so by another person. Responsive acts, in contrast, are those verbal remarks that are solicited by another person. In other words, a conversational partner says or does something that obligates the speaker to respond (e.g., the partner asks a question such as, "What is your name?"), and the speaker can choose to respond verbally to this obligation. Imitative acts are utterances that simply copy the content of an utterance that a conversational partner has just produced. They tend to occur infrequently after the preschool years, although occasionally a listener might ask a speaker to repeat something he or she has said if the listener did not hear what the speaker said the first time. In our experience, many people who stutter report that "self-repetitions" such as this tend to induce stuttering-related disfluency. Other speech acts affect a client's disproportionately as well. Thus, it is helpful to collect information about this aspect of speech production during assessment.

In Table 11-2, we present a form that we developed to illustrate how a clinician can collect information about a client's speech act performance and its relationship to fluency. As shown, the form contains a series of questions that pertain to the client's performance when responding to others' requests and when initiating verbal communication with others. The client rates communicaton performance in terms of how often he or she chooses to engage in the situation and, once the client is in the situation, how much he or she says. The client rates his or her fluency as well. In reality, the relationship between fluency and speech acts is more complicated than it appears on this form. For example, a client may choose to say a little as possible in response to requests within a classroom setting but may generate long responses when conversing with a family member. Nonetheless, completion of a data collection form like the one Table 11–2 can provide a good starting point for discussing such information.

Analysis of Communicative Flexibility

A very basic analysis would be to compute the ratio of assertive acts to respon-

sive acts within a speech sample across a range of speech samples. Clients who, in Fey's (1986) terms, are *active communicators* would exhibit evidence of using both assertive and responsive acts regularly. Clients who present with a "speak only when requested to do so" communicative style would exhibit very few assertive communicative acts and very many responsive acts. Such a profile might be observed in a speaker who copes with stuttering by withdrawing from conversational participation as much as possible. At the other extreme are clients who produce mostly assertive acts and tend to ignore or barely address a partner's requests for information. Such a profile might be observed in some speakers who clutter. In the latter two cases, the goal would be to improve the speakers' communicative functioning by extending the types of speech acts that they routinely produce.

Additional analysis of a client's fluency performance during specific speech act types can yield useful information as well. As noted above, some speakers who stutter report that the symptoms of their fluency impairment are aggravated when they attempt to respond to requests for clarification (e.g., "What? I didn't hear you."). Often, a speaker can fulfill such requests by simply repeating whatever they just said. On the surface, this task seems simple. However, for speakers who stutter, it often results in considerable disfluency, perhaps because the social expectation is that a speaker will respond promptly. Hesitation in this context implies that the speaker has forgotten what he or she just said a few seconds ago! So, responding to requests for clarification often is a time-constrained context—a context within which many people who stutter speak disfluently. Even relatively slight hesitations in initiating the response will

Table 11–2. Form for Collecting Information About Speaking Performance During Various Speech Acts

Directions: Rate yourself in terms of how often you speak, how much you speak, and how fluently you speak in the following situations. **SPEECH SITUATIONS**	Performance Rating: [1 = *strongly disagree*; 5 = *strongly agree*]			
	I am satisfied with how often I choose to engage in this situation.	**I say as much as I would like to say in this situation.**	**I am satisfied with how fluently I speak when I do this.**	
Responding to Other People's Requests				
Requests you can answer in a word (e.g., *Do you like it?*)	1 2 3 4 5	1 2 3 4 5	1 2 3 4 5	
Requests you can answer in a few words (e.g. *Where did our dog go?*)	1 2 3 4 5	1 2 3 4 5	1 2 3 4 5	
Requests you can answer in a few sentences (e.g., *What do they have on their menu?*)	1 2 3 4 5	1 2 3 4 5	1 2 3 4 5	
Requests that you need many sentences to answer (e.g., *Tell me about your trip.*)	1 2 3 4 5	1 2 3 4 5	1 2 3 4 5	
Requests that require you to repeat what you said. (e.g., *What did you say? I did not hear you.*)	1 2 3 4 5	1 2 3 4 5	1 2 3 4 5	
Requests that require you to clarify what you said. (e.g., *What do you mean by that?*)	1 2 3 4 5	1 2 3 4 5	1 2 3 4 5	

Directions: Rate yourself in terms of how often you speak, how much you speak, and how fluently you speak in the following situations.

Performance Rating: [1 = *strongly disagree*; 5 = *strongly agree*]

SPEECH SITUATIONS

Initiating Communication with Other People

	I am satisfied with how often I choose to engage in this situation.	I say as much as I would like to say in this situation.	I am satisfied with how fluently I speak when I do this.
Requesting information from others (e.g., *Do you want to go to the gym later? Can you show me how this works?*)	1 2 3 4 5	1 2 3 4 5	1 2 3 4 5
Requesting others to repeat (e.g., *Can you repeat that?*)	1 2 3 4 5	1 2 3 4 5	1 2 3 4 5
Asking questions in order to keep a conversation going (e.g., *And what did you do next?*)	1 2 3 4 5	1 2 3 4 5	1 2 3 4 5
Requesting others to clarify what they said (e.g., *I don't get it. Can you explain it further?*)	1 2 3 4 5	1 2 3 4 5	1 2 3 4 5
Commenting on daily events (e.g., *My watch is broken.*)	1 2 3 4 5	1 2 3 4 5	1 2 3 4 5
Remarking on feelings (e.g., *I am tired of the situation.*)	1 2 3 4 5	1 2 3 4 5	1 2 3 4 5
Disagreeing with others (e.g., *That's not what happened . . .*)	1 2 3 4 5	1 2 3 4 5	1 2 3 4 5
Introducing yourself (e.g., *Hi, I'm ___ and I'm a student.*)	1 2 3 4 5	1 2 3 4 5	1 2 3 4 5
Telling entertaining stories or jokes (e.g., *Listen to what happened to me yesterday . . .*)	1 2 3 4 5	1 2 3 4 5	1 2 3 4 5

draw a reaction from the partner, and the partner's reaction can compound fluency difficulty. Other speech act types may pose fluency challenges for other reasons. For example, assertive acts tend to be more linguistically complex than responsive acts (Logan, 2003a), and complexity often is a trigger for fluency difficulty.

To summarize, by analyzing the relationship between a client's fluency and speech act usage, one can obtain information about the range of communicative intentions a speaker conveys and, perhaps, insight into whether a client might be actively avoiding certain types of communicative roles or functions. Speech act usage can vary widely across communicative tasks. This may be the reason that there are not norms, per se, regarding how often speakers should use certain speech acts. Still, informal analysis of utterance function patterns can provide insight into the communicative behaviors of speakers with impaired fluency.

Analyzing the Succinctness of Verbal Output

Succinctness refers to the ability to speak in a logically organized and semantically dense manner (Fillmore, 1979). As noted in Chapter 1, the notions of coherence and circumlocution are relevant to succinct communication. In this section, we discuss several straightforward strategies for assessing these areas.

Coherence

Coherence often is assessed through examination of topic maintenance. Difficulties in topic maintenance are observed in some speakers who clutter. Thus, the construct of coherence is particularly rel-

evant to that population. The key issues to consider when assessing coherence are the extent to which a speaker is able to do the following things: (a) produce conversational utterances that are semantically relevant to the topic that currently is under discussion, (b) terminate an ongoing topic before introducing a new topic, and (c) inform conversational partners that an upcoming utterance is about to diverge from a current topic (Mackenzie, 2000). Bliss, McCabe, and Miranda (1998) noted that relevant utterances are those that expand upon, continue, or contradict a theme within the current topic. Irrelevant utterances, in contrast, are those that are deemed tangential, vague, or ambiguous—in other words, whatever is being said is not clearly tied into the current theme or topic.

Coherence typically is assessed by labeling or rating specific utterances according to whether their content is semantically related to immediately preceding utterances. Utterance analysis can be either binary (i.e., relevant versus irrelevant) or scaled in terms of degree of relevance (e.g., Glosser & Deser, 1990; Mackenzie, 2000; Rogalski, Altmann, Plummer-D'Amato, Behrman, & Marsiske, 2010). Coherence can be specified further by assessing an utterance at a "global" level (Is the utterance relevant to the broad topic?) and at the "local" level (Is the utterance relevant to the utterance that immediately precedes it?). Speakers who fail to maintain conversational topics can affect the fluency of conversational exchanges, as their forays into unexpected or unrelated topics can trigger interruptions and requests for clarification from communication partners, as the partner attempts to steer communication back toward the original topic. Events such as these obviously disrupt the flow of verbal communication.

In Fey's (1986) speech act analysis, a clinician codes each of the utterances in a speech sample at the *discourse level*. With the discourse-level analysis, the focus is on how an utterance functions in relation to the conversational topic. As indicated in Table 11–2, utterances can introduce, maintain, or extend a topic. In clinical settings, a clinician would look for evidence that the client exhibits all three of the topic functions. Clients who cope with fluency impairment by withdrawing from verbal communication are likely to exhibit a discourse profile that features very few attempts to initiate conversation, relatively few attempts to extend conversation through the addition of new information, but a lot of utterances that simply maintain conversation through the use of relatively simple verbal acknowledgments ("uh-huh") and agreements ("yeah"). Therefore, in effect, the client who exhibits this pattern of discourse is allowing the communicator partner to control the content and structure of the conversation. The client is a relatively passive participant in communication, and with such cases, the goal would be to help the client become a more active communicator by initiating and extending conversation more often.

Circumlocution

Jourdain (2000, p. 185) defined *circumlocution* as the " . . . linguistic means by which speakers describe objects for which they lack precise terminology." We add that, in the context of disordered populations such as stuttering, the definition might be modified somewhat to add the notion of *a temporary or situational response to impairment in the speech production process*. In the latter sense, circumlocution can be considered as a repair strategy or compensatory response to impairment in the speech production process, and in the context of stuttering it is closely associated with concepts such as word avoidance and word substitution. Examples of circumlocution patterns that might be observed in stuttering include the following: the use of superordinate terms (e.g., "faculty member") for proper names (e.g., "Mrs. Morgan"); the use of synonyms (e.g., "frisky" for "energetic"), and the substitution of verbal descriptions, definitions, or examples for distinct words (e.g., "a big, flying dinosaur with long wings and a long tail" for "pterodactyl").

With typical speakers or speakers with limited proficiency in a language, the use of circumlocution often is linked to difficulties in lexical access or limitations in lexical representation (Jourdain, 2000). With disorders such as anomia, where lexical retrieval difficulties may be widespread and severe, circumlocution may even be encouraged as an adaptive response to impairment (Francis, Clark, & Humphreys, 2002). Further, frequency of circumlocution has been found to be positively associated with recovery of oral word production abilities in adults who experienced stroke (Cloutman, Newhart, Davis, Heidler-Gary, & Hillis, 2009). In contrast, with neurodegenerative diseases such as dementia, circumlocution frequency may be tracked over time, to serve as a marker of disease progression (Cuetos, Gonzalez-Nosti, & Martínez, 2005). With stuttering—where speakers often report knowing which word they want to say but being temporarily unable to produce the movements associated with the word—circumlocution more often may be a response to an impending problem in the formulation or execution of speech-related movement.

Quantifying Stuttered Speech

Stuttering Judgments in the Context of Fluency Assessment

The final fluency-related analysis that we discuss in this chapter pertains to *stuttering judgments*. Some readers may find it unusual that we have placed this topic near the end of our discussion on fluency assessment. After all, stuttering judgments are a staple of clinical assessment with speakers who stutter, and stuttering is the most common fluency impairment. Our decision to discuss stuttering judgments in this particular part of the chapter was quite intentional, however. We have positioned it here for two reasons. First, clinicians who are new to fluency analysis often confuse the act of disfluency analysis with the act of making stuttering judgments. They tend to see them as being interchangeable, but this is not so at all. This confusion may arise in part from the way in which stuttering currently is defined. Many contemporary definitions place great emphasis on the types of disfluency that speakers who stutter produce but less emphasis (or *no* emphasis) on other dimensions of fluency or other symptoms of the disorder. In any case, to promote this notion of separateness, we decided to put plenty of print space between the two topics.

Second, as we will see, the concept of stuttering judgment is broader than that of disfluency. That is, the identification of stuttered speech involves *multidimensional analysis* (Bloodstein & Bernstein Ratner, 2008; Einarsdóttir & Ingham, 2005; Schiavetti, Sacco, Metz, & Sitler, 1983). As

such, the act of making stuttering judgments usually incorporates more than one dimension of fluency, and in some instances, incorporates other aspects of speech (e.g., vocal pitch) and even non-speech behaviors. Disfluency analysis, on the other hand, deals principally with the issue of speech continuity. So, by placing our discussion of stuttering judgment *after* the discussion of the other fluency dimensions, it hopefully is apparent that each of the fluency dimensions has relevance to stuttering identification.

Measuring the Frequency of Stuttered Speech

Conventional Method

In contemporary clinical practice, the measurement of stuttered speech is accomplished through the following steps:

1. Identify places within the speech sample (e.g., syllables, words) wherein a speaker exhibits observable symptoms of the speech disorder known as stuttering (i.e., stuttered speech). This process involves marking the onset and offset of stuttering "events."

2. After the boundaries of stuttered speech have been identified, the clinician quantifies the size of the speech sample by counting the number of syllables (or words) in the speaker's target utterances. (Identification of the target utterances is accomplished using the same method that was described in the section on disfluency assessment.)

3. The clinician then counts the total number of syllables (or words) that either are characterized by or preceded by stuttered speech. Stuttering judgments largely are qualitative in

nature. The rater attempts to determine whether specific segments of speech are symptomatic of the speech disorder called stuttering. This process yields the number of stuttered syllables (or words) in the sample.

4. The observed number of stuttered syllables (or words) is divided by the total number of syllables (or words) in the target utterances within the speech sample and then multiplied by 100. This yields a stuttering frequency score that is adjusted for sample size: the *percent of syllables that contain or are preceded by stuttering*. (Most clinicians refer to this statistic as *percent of syllables stuttered*).

We illustrate this procedure in Example 11–16 below. In the example, stuttered speech is underlined and disfluency boundaries are marked with vertical lines.

Example 11–16: |Ma-|Manny took a quick^E trip to |um| Pittsburgh |last- | last Tuesday.

We created this example to illustrate some of the differences between the acts of stuttering judgment and disfluency analysis. Note that the sentence contains two "instances" of stuttering, only one of which is characterized by overt continuity interruption (i.e., the part-word repetition associated with *Manny*). The rater judged the word *quick* to be stuttered as well, even though speech continuity was not interrupted by disfluency. The superscript "E" after the word *quick* is a code for *excessive effort*. So, apparently the rater detected physical tension or struggle (e.g., a facial grimace) as the speaker produced this word and regarded it as evidence of stuttering. The final two disfluent segments in the utterance (i.e.,

um and *last*) were not judged as instances of stuttering. Apparently, the rater decided that the *um* reflected a speech production problem other than the kind that leads to stuttered speech. For example, the speaker may have had difficulty remembering where Manny went—a problem that would result in a delay in accessing the lexical item <Pittsburgh>. The rater apparently regarded the repetition of *last* similarly; that is, as a product of a speech production problem other than stuttering, such as difficulty in remembering when the trip occurred. The prosodic characteristics of the repetition and the speaker's nonverbal behavior during the disfluency may have influenced the rater's judgment about the word as well. So, in this example, not all instances of repetition are judged as instances of stuttering, and not all instances of stuttering involve overt continuity interruption.

From this example, we see that the identification of stuttered speech involves qualitative judgment. The rater must decide whether a specific speech pattern sounds or looks like a speech pattern that is symptomatic of the speech disorder called stuttering. The judgment is multidimensional in nature; that is, the rater considers factors that go beyond disfluency. We explore the multidimensional nature of stuttering judgment in the next section.

Stuttering Judgments and Fluency Dimensions

Stuttering identification is in some ways similar to the identification of sound prolongation, which we have discussed elsewhere in this text. In both cases, a clinician is charged with making a qualitative judgment about a speech event. With sound prolongation, the clinician must judge whether a specific speech sound is abnormally long. With stuttering instances, the clinician must judge whether a given point of speech is representative of the speech disorder known as stuttering. With both prolongation identification and stuttering identification, there are—to date—no listener-independent objective criteria that one can apply when attempting to decide whether a specific point in speech is or is not an exemplar of the behavior (Bloodstein & Bernstein Ratner, 2008). As such, the identification process is prone to error and disagreement.

In Figure 11–11, we present a schematic representation of the kinds of information a rater might consider when judging whether stuttered speech has occurred. In our model, a rater is hypothesized to use multiple dimensions of fluency to evaluate a spoken utterance. The specific factors that influence stuttering judgment for any specific sample of speech are likely to vary, and the rater may weigh these factors differently from one occasion to another and one speaker to another. Hypothesized factors that may affect decision-making include:

- Disfluency type: Repetitions and prolongations are more characteristic of stuttered speech than interjections, revisions, or pauses.

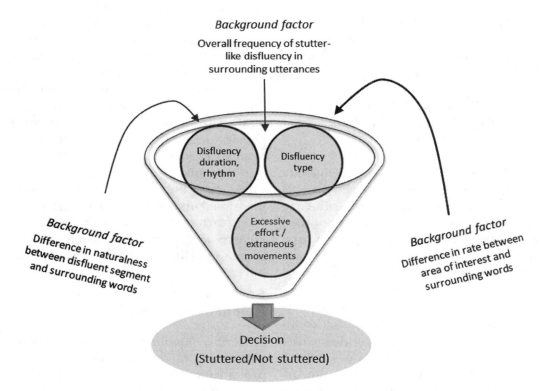

Figure 11–11. Model of the kinds of factors a rater might consider when making judgments about whether stuttering has occurred at a specific point within a speech sample. Immediate factors are those shown inside the funnel. Characteristics of fluency performance in surrounding speech (e.g., surrounding words, phrases, and sentences) also are likely to influence the decision that the rater makes about whether a specific speech segment is stuttered.

- Disfluency duration: Lengthy disfluencies are more apt to be judged as instances of stuttering than short disfluencies.
- Rhythm: Dysrhythmic or fast-paced repetitions are more characteristic of stuttered speech than rhythmic or slow-paced repetitions.
- Effort: Segments of speech that appear to be unusually effortful are more characteristic of stuttered speech than segments of speech with typical effort levels. Signs of unusual effort might include excessive muscle tension as well as extraneous movements of muscles or body parts not directly involved in speech production.
- In our experience, background characteristics may influence the decisions that a rater makes about specific instances of speech. For example, a disfluency such as |*He-*|*He went home* may be more apt to be judged as "stuttered" in:
  - A speaker who produces many other stutter-like behaviors than it would in a speaker who produces few such behaviors;
  - A speaker who exhibits a speech rate that is markedly slower than most typical speakers; and/or
  - A speaker who exhibits speech that sounds relatively unnatural in comparison to other speakers.

Limitations of the Conventional Method for Stuttering Assessment

Although the stuttering measurement procedure outlined in the preceding section may seem relatively straightforward to do, in clinical practice, it does not always turn out this way. Research has shown that both laypersons and experts struggle with identifying instances of stuttered speech reliably (Cordes & Ingham, 1994; Curlee, 1981; Ingham & Cordes, 1992; Kully & Boberg, 1988; MacDonald & Martin, 1973; Martin & Haroldson, 1981). One basic problem is that, within a particular speech sample, only a relatively small percentage of all the identified stuttering events may labeled as "stuttered" by a majority of raters. Put another way, in these research studies, the *point-by-point agreement* for whether or not stuttering has occurred at a particular location tends to be relatively low.

Fortunately, both experienced and inexperienced judges show improved reliability when they are asked to evaluate larger units of speech such as a spoken narrative, an entire utterance, or a four-second segment of speech for the presence of absence of stuttering (Armson, Jenson, Gallant, Kalinowski, & Fee, 1997; Ingham, Cordes, & Gow, 1993). Reliability also is improved when raters are asked to make global judgments about whether a particular speaker is or is not a person who stutters (Bloodstein & Bernstein Ratner, 2008). Also, although raters may not always agree on exactly where an instance of stuttering has occurred, their summary statistics (e.g., percent of syllables stuttered) tend to be similar (Curlee, 1981; Yaruss et al., 1998). Still, experienced raters tend to identify more instances of stuttering in comparison to inexperienced raters (Brundage, Bothe, Lengeling, & Evans, 2006); thus, it is important for clinicians who are new to the stuttering judgment process to be knowledgeable about the kinds of behaviors highly experienced clinicians identify as "stuttered." Training materials to assist with the process can be found along with the automated fluency analysis software that Ingham and colleagues developed (e.g., Ingham & Ingham, 2011; Ingham et al., n.d). Still, the challenges associated with defining stuttered speech and identifying exemplars of it reliably in speech samples have led Bloodstein and Bernstein Ratner (2008, p. 9) to conclude that, at present, stuttering is best defined as "whatever is perceived as stuttering by a reliable observer who has relatively good agreement with others."

Despite all of the attention that has been devoted to the reliability with which raters identify stuttering events, some authorities have questioned whether it is even accurate to think of stuttered speech as consisting of discreet events. The "event-based" view of stuttering can leave the impression that a speaker moves in and out of fluency impairment while talking. In this view, segments of speech that are produced smoothly and with typical rate, rhythm, and effort are regarded as "nonstuttered" (or, to some, "normal"), while segments of speech that feature marked disruption, dysrhythmic speech, excessive effort and so forth, are not. The work of Smith and colleagues, however, calls this view of stuttering into question. Their research has demonstrated, among other things, that markers of stuttering are present in speakers' speech breathing patterns and autonomic nervous system activation during segments of speech that precede continuity interruptions and, from an acoustic perspective, sound fluent (Denny & Smith, 1992; Smith & Kelly, 1997; Weber & Smith, 1990). In a series of more recent studies with adults who stutter, they have demonstrated that samples of speech that *sound normal* from an acoustic perspective actually *look disordered* when one examines patterns of spatial-temporal coordination in connected speech (e.g., Kleinow & Smith, 2000; Smith, Sadagopan, Walsh, & Weber-Fox, 2010). The main pattern is that speech-related movements of speakers who stutter during ostensibly "fluent" speech show much greater variability than those of nonstuttering speakers. Other researchers have reached similar conclusions based on other types of analyses (e.g., Armson & Kalinowski, 1994; Lickley, Hartsuiker, Corley, Russell, & Nelson, 2005). Research findings such as these suggest that, rather than viewing stuttered speech in terms of discrete instances, it perhaps is more accurate to think of stuttered speech as any speech that a person who stutters produces. In this view, the widely used practice of using acoustic data to make judgments about stuttered syllables yields only a partial picture of the fluency difficulties experienced by speakers who stutter (Smith & Kelly, 1997). With the analysis of "stuttered events," clinicians may be tagging only the most obvious or aberrant points of dysfunction in speech production. Meanwhile many other relevant, but more subtle, symptoms of impairment may be apparent at other points within an utterance. These subtle symptoms of stuttering may only be detectable when one uses instruments that are sufficiently sensitive and capable of evaluating aspects of speech production other than the acoustic signal.

Summary

The present chapter focused on clinical methods and tools that are used in the analysis of speech samples. Among the topics discussed were the following: approaches to speech sample transcription, quantifying and labeling disfluency within a speech sample, and computing summary statistics for disfluency frequency, disfluency duration, rate, and rhythm. Other topics included methods for assessing speaking effort, speech naturalness, talkativeness, participation, and the compensatory and associated behaviors that often accompany disfluency in impaired populations. Approaches for making judgments about stuttered speech were described as well. For these clinical analyses, implementation of standardized procedures is critical in order to attain acceptable levels of measurement reliability.

Clinical measures such as those outlined in this chapter are useful in creating rich descriptions of a client's fluency performance. Of course, not every measure described in the chapter will be applicable to all clients. As such, the information presented here constitutes an overview of the possible approaches one can implement. We return to these methods in the next chapter, where they are discussed within the context of (a) diagnosing fluency impairments, (b) measuring changes in fluency performance, and (c) assessing the impact of fluency impairment on quality of life.

12

Interpreting Data and Making Recommendations

Upon completing a fluency assessment, the next steps are to interpret the data, determine whether communication is impaired and, if it is, determine what type of impairment exists and what should be done about it. These actions set the stage for the specific goals and objectives that the clinician will recommend in order to help the client maximize his or her ability to communicate.

Diagnostic Classification of Fluency Impairment

Integration of assessment data leads naturally to diagnosis, which simply is a statement about the client's current status. The most familiar diagnostic labels for fluency impairment are *stuttering* and *cluttering*; however, there are several other conclusions that a clinician might reach about a client's status, including the possibility that the client is functioning in the normal range.

In Figure 12–1, a general classification system is presented for labeling various types of fluency outcomes. The classification system is modeled after one that Shriberg and colleagues developed to classify various patterns of speech sound development (Shriberg, Austin, Lewis, McSweeney, & Wilson, 2001; Shriberg & Kwiatkowski, 1982). The fluency classification system presented here is preliminary in its content and form.[1] Nonetheless, it should serve as a useful starting point for conceptualizing the types of fluency

[1]Shriberg et al. (1997) developed and systematically validated their classification system based on speech sound production data from more than 800 children and adults with normal and disordered speech. In contrast, the classification system presented here for fluency disorders is mainly based on published empirical data and authoritative reports from the fluency disorders literature concerning the range of cases that a clinician is likely to encounter. It also is influenced by our clinical experiences in assessing individuals who have fluency concerns. The classification system presented here is a first step in the development of a comprehensive classification scheme for fluency disorders. Systematic research of the sort that Shriberg et al. (1997) conducted is needed in order to validate the preliminary fluency disorders classification system described here.

1. Normal Fluency Functioning
    1.1. Normal fluency
    1.2. Normally developing fluency
    1.3. Normalized fluency
    1.4. Fluency difference
2. Developmental disorders that affect fluency
    2.1. Stuttering
    2.2. Cluttering
    2.3. (Stuttering –cluttering)
    2.4. Fluency disorders and atypical fluency that co-occur with other developmental disorders
    2.5. Other developmental fluency disorders
        2.5.1. Atypical disfluency types (with no co-occurring developmental disorders)
        2.5.2. Late-onset stuttering
3. Nondevelopmental disorders that affect fluency
    3.1. Acquired stuttering (in the context of…)
        3.1.1. Neurological trauma
        3.1.2. Neurodegenerative disease
        3.1.3. Drug use
        3.1.4. Other disorders that affect neurological functioning (e.g., migraine headache, epilepsy)
    3.2. Acquired cluttering
    3.3. Other acquired fluency disorders

Figure 12–1. A classification system for describing fluency functioning. The classification system is modeled after the classification system that Shriberg and colleagues developed for use with speech sound development (i.e., Shriberg et al., 1997; Shriberg & Kwiatkowski, 1982). In this figure, three general classifications are presented, each with several subtypes. Disorders are classified according to whether they occur in the context of developmental processes or not. *Stuttering-cluttering* appears in parentheses to indicate uncertainty about whether it is a distinct fluency disorder or two independent types of fluency impairment that co-occur in an individual.

performance profiles that exist and how they relate to one another.

As shown, there are three main categories for fluency performance patterns. One deals with *normal fluency functioning*, another deals with *developmental fluency disorders*, and another deals with *nondevelopmental fluency disorders*. Of course, the second and third categories could be subsumed under the broader heading of *fluency disorders*. The distinction between normal and disordered fluency refers to a speaker's *overall* or *net* fluency performance pattern; that is, the way in which a person functions on a day-

to-day basis, as opposed to how a person functions when saying a particular word or sentence.

As shown in Figure 12–1, there are four descriptive subtypes proposed under the heading of normal fluency functioning, five descriptive subtypes under the heading of developmental disorders, and three descriptive subtypes under the heading of nondevelopmental disorders. Some of the descriptive subtypes are specified further with etiologic descriptors. The subtypes of normal fluency functioning are discussed in some detail below. The main characteristics for each of the disordered or atypical types of fluency are reviewed briefly, as well. Detailed descriptions of the primary developmental and nondevelopmental fluency disorders are presented in the chapters that comprise Section II of this textbook.

Normal Fluency Functioning

The notion of normal fluency functioning is consistent with the concept of "typical fluency," a term that has been used in other chapters in this text. As shown in Figure 12–1, there are four descriptive subtypes under the heading of normal fluency functioning. A common feature of the four subtypes is the notion of proficient, unimpaired performance in speech fluency. Fluency functioning—normal or disordered—is defined in relation to the fluency dimensions that were outlined in Chapter 1. Thus, normal fluency functioning implies that a speaker's functioning in each of the various dimensions of fluency is normal, as well. Examples of the fluency profiles associated with clients who exhibit normal fluency functioning are outlined in Table 12–1. In the table, illustrative data are presented for various fluency-related behaviors across each of the four descriptive subtypes. As can be seen, there are many similarities across the four categories of normal functioning. This is expected because each subtype is an instance of normal or typical functioning.

Normal Fluency

Speakers who exhibit *normal fluency* are those who show no sign of impairment in speech continuity, rate, rhythm, effort, naturalness, or stability. In each of these fluency dimensions, the speaker functions in a manner that is similar to that of most speakers in the general population. Total disfluency frequency is relatively low, and those disfluent segments that are present involve pausing, interjecting, or revising. Rate, rhythm, and effort are within normal limits. In addition, the speaker reports no significant difficulties with or concerns about any aspect of speech fluency. (See Chapter 4 for additional details on normal patterns of functioning in the areas of continuity, rate, rhythm, effort, naturalness, and stability.) Further, the speaker's talkativeness shows no sign of limitation or impairment. The individual speaks as often and as fully as he or she desires; consistently accomplishes a variety of speech acts when conversing with others; and consistently presents information that listeners regard as being clear, succinct, and relevant to ongoing conversations. Although any speaker who meets these criteria can be classified as having "normal fluency functioning," the label perhaps is most confidently applied to those speakers who have passed the upper bounds for when the onset for developmental fluency impairment is likely to occur. For developmental stuttering, this occurs at roughly age 10 to 12 (Andrews, 1984), although more recent data suggest that a substantial percentage of the children who present with developmental stuttering will incur onset of the disorder before age 6 (Reilly et al., 2013; Yairi & Ambrose, 1999). Detailed data concerning the age-of-onset characteristics of cluttering are lacking. What data there are suggest that onset often takes place by early adolescence (Howell, 2011).

Normally Developing Fluency

The term *normally developing fluency* is appropriate for use with children who are roughly between the ages of 1 to 10

Table 12–1. Fluency Profiles of Hypothetical Clients With Normal Fluency Functioning

Variable	Fluency Subtype			
	Normal Fluency	**Normally Developing Fluency**	**Normalized Fluency**	**Fluency Difference**[a]
Client age	15;0	5;8	6;0	18;0
Disfluency frequency (all types) per 100 syllables	5.25	4.87	3.81	3.48/8.50
RPBs per 100 syllables	1.10	0.80	1.05	1.39/1.39
IRs per 100 syllables	4.15	4.07	2.76	2.09/7.11
Percentage of total = RPBs	21%	16%	28%	40%/16%
Most common disfluency type	Revision	Revision	Revision	Interjection
Mean # of iterations per PWR/MWR	1.02	1.01	1.07	1.05
Articulation rate	WNL	WNL	WNL	WNL
Speech rate	WNL	WNL	WNL	WNL/Slow
Repetition rhythm	Rhythmic	Rhythmic	Rhythmic	Rhythmic
Mean duration of RPBs	<1 s	<1 s	<1 s	<1 s
Speaking effort	WNL	WNL	WNL	WNL
Fluency-based activity limitations	None	None	None	None
Fluency-based participation restrictions	None	None	None	None
Client's expressed fluency-related concerns	None	None	None	None

Note: *RPBs* = repetitions, prolongations, and blocks; *IRs* = interjections and revisions; *PWR* = part word repetition, *MWR* = monosyllable word repetition; *WNL* = within normal limits; *Slow* = slower than normal rate.

[a]When two values appear in a cell, it illustrates how fluency data would change if overuse of *like* as a sociolectal difference is ignored (first value) or scored (second value) in a fluency analysis.

years. This is the time at which children are in the process of acquiring adult-like proficiency with the form, content, and use of language, as well as the speech-based gestural patterns that are used in language expression. This also is the time during which the primary developmental fluency disorder, stuttering, is most likely to emerge. So, although a child may be 5 years old and show no signs of stuttering, it is prudent to consider that child as exhibiting normally *developing* fluency, because he or she remains within the developmental window during which stuttering onset can occur.

Fluency performance seems to be particularly volatile for children who are between 2 and 3 years old (Colburn & Mysak, 1982a, 1982b; Wijnen, 1990; Yairi, 1981, 1982); thus, the notion of *developing fluency* is particularly apt for clients of that age. Between the ages of 2 and 3, some children exhibit as much as a three- to four-fold increase in disfluency frequency, driven primarily by more frequent use of revisions, phrase repetitions and, to a lesser extent, whole-word repetitions (Yairi, 1982). Such disfluencies seem to be particularly common within action-based utterances (e.g., *Agent + Action + Object*) and the use of emerging syntactic forms (Colburn & Mysak, 1982b).

The disfluency patterns observed in young children during the early stages of language acquisition are largely distinct from the ones seen in developmental stuttering (described in the next section). Thus, the spikes in disfluency that occur in children with normally developing fluency during childhood, and particularly during the preschool years, are not equivalent to those seen in developmental stuttering. Children's relatively abrupt increases in disfluency frequency during the preschool years may draw the attention of parents who are unaccustomed to hearing their child repeat or alter what is being said. In most children, however, the overall frequency of disfluency (i.e., combined, across all disfluency types) remains relatively modest. For example, Yairi (1981) reported that about half of all normally developing 2- to 3-year-old children in that study had 5 or fewer total disfluencies per 100 words, and 27 of 33 (82% of the total) had 10 or fewer total disfluencies per 100 words. Yairi (1982)

tracked changes in children's fluency development between the ages of 25 to 41 months and found an overall decrease in the frequency of total disfluency as children approached the upper age bounds for the study (i.e., 41 months). Also, the frequency of part-word repetitions, a disfluency type that characterizes stuttered speech, tended to decrease as the children aged, even during periods of the study when a child's total disfluency frequency was spiking. Disfluency spikes that occur in conjunction with the acquisition of language and associated speech motor patterns are classified as "normal" because many children in the general population exhibit them when they are in the midst of speech-language acquisition. Developmental stuttering, in contrast, is not classified as "normal" because that type of speech pattern is observed in only 3% to 5% of the general population. Because developmental stuttering is considered a *disorder*, it therefore is presumed to indicate an impaired or atypical speech production system. As such, it is not "normal" to be a person who stutters in either a statistical or neurodevelopmental sense.

There are occasional cases in which clinicians may have difficulty determining whether a child shows normally developing fluency. Such cases may show, for example, excessive repetition of words and, occasionally, parts of words but lack other markers of developmental stuttering such as prolonged or blocked speech sounds or excessively tense or lengthy disfluency, or they may show some signs of developmental stuttering during some clinic visits but none during others. Guitar (2006) suggests using the term *borderline stuttering* with such cases. Other potential terms include *possible developmental stuttering* or *marginal fluency development*. The latter terms capture the idea that speech fluency may not be developing normally, but further assessment is needed before a definitive conclusion can be reached.

To summarize, the term *normally developing fluency* captures those children who currently exhibit normal fluency (as described in the preceding section) but remain at risk for experiencing the transient spikes in speech disfluency that sometimes coincide with early syntactical, morphological, phonological, lexical, and/or speech articulation development. In addition, the child still is within the age range when the onset of stuttering and cluttering can occur. To reiterate, a child with normally developing fluency does *not* exhibit disfluency patterns that are consistent with a diagnosis of stuttering or cluttering (described below). Total disfluency frequency is relatively low, and most disfluent segments involve interjection or revision. Rate, rhythm, and effort are within normal limits, and there are no fluency-based activity limitations or participation restrictions.

Note that *normally developing fluency* is not an appropriate term to use for a child who currently exhibits stuttered speech but may recover from it at some time in the future. The latter type of client most appropriately would be labeled as "stuttering" for as long as the stuttered speech is present, and then relabeled as "normalized fluency" if the symptoms of stuttering have been absent for a substantial length of time (see *normalized fluency* below).

Normalized Fluency

The classification of *normalized fluency* is similar to that of normal fluency, in that the speaker exhibits typical functioning across all dimensions of fluency and reports no present difficulties or concerns

in any of these areas (see Table 12–1). Unlike normal fluency, however, the notion of normalized fluency implies that the speaker had experienced impaired or disordered fluency in the past but no longer does so. The notion of normalized fluency is consistent with the concept of "recovery from stuttering," in cases where the symptoms of stuttered speech resolve in such a way that the client's speech currently is indistinguishable from that of unimpaired speakers and has been that way for a significant length of time (see Yairi & Ambrose, 1992a, 1999, for examples). However, the notion of normalized fluency is not synonymous with broader definitions of "recovery" that encompass scenarios in which a speaker's exhibits improved fluency but continuing instances of atypical disfluency and ongoing self-identification as a "person with disordered fluency" (see Anderson & Felsenfeld, 2003; Finn, Howard, & Kubala, 2005; and Howell, 2011, for examples of such cases).

The classification of normalized fluency most confidently is applied in cases where a clinician has access to longitudinal data concerning a speaker's fluency. This approach enables the clinician to document that the speaker did indeed show symptoms of impaired fluency but now no longer does so. Even when longitudinal data are available, the classification of normalized fluency is complicated by the fact that, to date, there is no standard criterion for how long a speaker must exhibit typical fluency behavior before he or she can be regarded as having "normalized." Obviously, the longer the time frame is, the more confident one can be in the classification. Yairi and Ambrose (1999, p. 1103) set a criterion of one year of symptom-free speech before classifying preschoolers as having recovered from stuttering. Additional criteria that Yairi and

Ambrose used to determine fluency normalization were as follows:

- The clinician and parent both had general judgments that the child no longer stuttered;
- The clinician and parent both gave the child ratings of less than 1 on a 0 to 7 stuttering severity scale (0 = "normally fluent," 7 = "very severe stuttering");
- The child's combined frequency of part-word repetitions, monosyllable whole-word repetitions, and "dysrhythmic phonations" (e.g., prolongations, blocks) was less than 3 per 100 syllables; and
- Neither the clinician nor the parent mentioned stuttered speech in their reports on the child's speech for at least 12 months. (If either the clinician or parent identified even suspected indicators of stuttering such as unusual hesitancy in speech during the 12-month period, the child was reassigned to the persistent stuttering group.)

Finn, Ingham, Ambrose, and Yairi (1997) asked three types of judges (sophisticated, unsophisticated, and experienced) to analyze videotaped recordings of 10 children who met Yairi and Ambrose's (1999) criteria and 10 children who had never stuttered. The results indicated that the fluency patterns of the two groups of children were indistinguishable across all three types of judges. On this basis, it appeared that the children had truly normalized their speech fluency. Data from Yairi and Ambrose (1999) indicated that girls are more likely to normalize stuttered speech than boys.

The use of *normalized fluency* as a clinical descriptor also might be used with clients who report having fully recovered from fluency impairment that was present in the remote past. Retrospective reports on fluency functioning are prone to error, however, due to distortions or lapses in memory and the possibility that clients do not define disorders like stuttering and cluttering in the same way that clinicians do. Thus, use of the term "normalized fluency" as a descriptor for cases in which recovery reportedly occurred in the remote past should be done cautiously.

Finn and colleagues (Finn, 1996, 1997; Finn et al., 2005) reported on a multistep procedure for validating adolescent and adult speakers' reports of recovery from previous stuttering. The first step was to corroborate the speaker's claim of past stuttering by collecting data from someone who was familiar with the speaker's fluency patterns in both the past and present. The data collection process entailed the use of yes/no questions (i.e., Did the person ever have a speech problem? Did the person ever stutter? Is the person now a normally fluent speaker?). Finn and colleagues then asked participants to complete a speech behavior checklist, which included various characteristics of stuttered speech. The final step in the validation process involved a content analysis of the speaker's descriptions of stuttering and recovery from stuttering. The purpose of the content analysis was to validate the speaker's reports of stuttering and recovery from stuttering by noting the extent to which speakers mentioned themes that people who stutter commonly express when talking about the disorder (e.g., characteristic speech behaviors, associated behaviors, negative emotions about stuttering) and by documenting how their descriptions of recovery matched those from other people who stutter. Finn et al. (2005) found that these procedures were effective at identifying two types of fluency outcome: (1) speakers who reported they had recovered from stuttering and no longer had any tendency to stutter, and (2) speakers who reported they had recovered from stuttering yet continued to stutter on occasion. As suggested earlier in this section, the first group meets the criteria for normalized fluency more completely that the second group does. Finn et al. (2005) speculated that, for the second group, the sense of feeling recovered while still stuttering occasionally might reflect the fact that these speakers no longer view stuttering as a handicap.

Other researchers have used similar but less elaborate methods of validating speaker reports of past stuttering. For example, Cooper (1972) interviewed young adults who had reported having fully recovered from stuttering. Among other things, Cooper asked the participants to describe and to demonstrate how they used to stutter. He also asked them whether they currently anticipated stuttering on specific words or certain situations or used strategies such as word substitution in response to the expectation of stuttering. An affirmative response to any of the questions suggests that the individual's speech had not truly normalized.

Fluency Differences

The notion of communication *differences* has received substantial attention with regard to certain aspects of speech and language performance. For example, researchers have described variations in the phonologic, syntactic, and/or morphologic forms that speakers from different racial or ethnic groups and geographic regions use (Craig & Washington, 2004). In such contexts, the notion of a communication difference typically is contrasted with that of a communication disorder. A communication difference comes under the heading of normal functioning, whereas a communication disorder does not.

This leads to the question of whether the concept of communication difference extends to speech fluency and, if it does, to the related question of what a fluency difference would sound like. This issue has received little attention to date. In keeping with approaches used in the study of nonstandard dialects, a *fluency difference* might be defined as a fluency pattern that (a) varies in some identifiable way from that of typical fluent speakers and (b) the variation in fluency results from the effects of social or cultural factors and/or individualized stylistic preferences. One common scenario for a fluency difference would be the process of acquiring a second language. In this case, a speaker might exhibit certain forms of disfluency more often in his or her newly developing language than in the primary, established language. Other examples of speech patterns that could be considered as evidence of a fluency difference include the following:

Frequent use of the word "like." In some linguistic contexts, the word *like* functions as a verb (e.g., *I like cashews*); in other contexts, it functions as a comparative (e.g., *George was like a vulture, eating everything in sight*); and in other contexts, it functions as a qualifier, with a meaning similar to *about* or *approximately* (e.g., *The plant was like five feet tall*). Some speakers (e.g., certain subgroups of adolescent speakers in the United States) may use the word *like* frequently and in linguistic contexts that differ from those used by most speakers in the population. After reading Example 12–1 below, which contains multiple instances of the word *like,* one could argue that *like* functions similarly to the interjection *um* in many of its applications because it is audible, has a consistent phonetic form, and takes time to produce but does not add much meaning to the sentence other than, perhaps, a sense of uncertainty about how one feels regarding what just happened.

> Example 12–1: *Dude, I was <u>like</u> totally <u>like</u> into it when you were <u>like</u> doing that "eat like a vulture" thing. You know, <u>like</u>, that was <u>like</u> awesome.*

The term *sociolect* is used to refer to language forms or conventions that are used by certain social or demographic groups within a population (Wolfram, 2004). Typically, a speaker would use the sociolectal form, in this case *like*, most when interacting with peers from the social group. When interacting with people from other (mainstream) groups, however, the speaker would likely exhibit use of an alternate register (i.e., code switching), which would result in speech that features the much more conventional use of *like*. A speaker's nonstandard use of the word *like* raises questions about how it should be scored in a speech fluency analysis. If it is scored as disfluency, then the speaker may exhibit a frequency of total disfluency and a frequency of interjection that is greater than normal. If it is ignored, however, the client's disfluency frequency data would be expected to fall in the normal range. The disfluency data in Table 12–1 illustrate how disfluency frequency and speech rate would look under both scenarios. If the use of *like* and other similar words is attributed to sociolectal influences, the speaker should be regarded as exhibiting a fluency difference, rather than a fluency disorder.

Use of an exceptionally rapid speech rate.

Bakker and colleagues (Bakker, Myers, Raphael, & St. Louis, 2011) used the term *exceptionally rapid speech* to refer to a subgroup of speakers who demonstrate faster-than-typical speaking rates. In their research, Bakker et al. regarded the rate behavior as a variant of normal rate behavior rather than as a disorder, as the exceptionally rapid speech did not have a significant negative impact on the speakers' communicative competence, verbal participation, or self-concept as a competent speaker.

Use of nonstandard pause patterns.

Speakers sometimes manipulate pause duration and location in order to add emphasis, weight, or seriousness to what they are saying (O'Connell, Kowal, Sabin, Lamia, & Dannevik, 2010). Politicians often manipulate pause behavior when making public speeches. Poets sometimes also interject pauses at unexpected locations when reading their work aloud. Paul Harvey, a long-time radio commentator, was well known for his characteristic speaking style, which, at times, featured long and unusually placed pauses in speech. Interested readers can access recordings of politicians, poets, radio announcers, and other public presenters to gain a sense of the individual variation that exists in prosodic delivery patterns.

Developmental Disorders That Affect Fluency

Developmental Stuttering

In most cases, developmental stuttering is characterized by excessive disfluency in the form of repeating, prolonging, and/or blocking. Although people who stutter produce all types of repetition more often than typical speakers, the frequency of part-word repetitions usually is most aberrant in comparison to normal speakers. Findings from several studies show that, on average, children who stutter produce these disfluency types many times more often than children who do not stutter. Sound prolongations and fixed articulatory postures occur very infrequently among speakers who exhibit normal fluency; thus, the presence of these disfluency types—even at frequencies as low as 1 or 2 per 100 syllables—can indicate that a person stutters, especially when prolongations and fixed articulatory postures feature excessive physical tension. Children who stutter usually produce interjections and revisions at a frequency that is similar to children who do not stutter. Thus, the latter disfluency types usually are less reliable at differentiating the two groups. These characteristics are illustrated in Table 12–2, where hypothetical examples for subtypes of developmental fluency impairment are shown. As shown under developmental stuttering, total disfluency frequency is relatively high and repetitions, prolongations, and blocks constitute the majority of disfluency.

The repetitions, prolongations, and/or blocks that a person who stutters produces tend to cluster together on consecutive words or syllables much more often than those of speakers with typical fluency (Hubbard & Yairi, 1988; LaSalle & Conture, 1995), and the structure of speech disfluency is more apt to vary from the forms that typical speakers exhibit (Logan & LaSalle, 1999). Although the latter two characteristics are not required to make a diagnosis of developmental stuttering, their presence makes the diagnosis more certain. Speakers with developmental stuttering usually produce very few repetitions, prolongations, and/or blocks dur-ing contexts such as singing, unison reading, slowed/stretched speech, and speaking in time to a rhythmic stimulus such as the beat of a metronome. The presence of extensive stuttering in the later contexts would be quite unusual and perhaps a sign that the client's fluency problem is something other than developmental stuttering (Krishnan & Tiwari, 2013).

As noted, the presence of excessive or atypical repeating, prolonging, and blocking is usually essential to diagnosing developmental stuttering, and in most cases, the combined frequency for these three types of disfluency will be much greater than it is in a speaker with normal fluency functioning. For instance, Logan and LaSalle (1999) reported that the combined frequency for part-word repetitions, monosyllable word repetitions, and sound prolongations was 11.66 per 100 syllables for children who stuttered but only 1.27 per 100 syllables for children with typical fluency. Yairi (1997) reported a similar degree of discrepancy in a review of numerous studies published prior to the mid-1990s. Not all cases of developmental stuttering will show high frequencies of repeating, prolonging, and/or blocking, however. Consider, for example, the following fluency profile for a hypothetical case of stuttering in a 4-year-old child:

- The combined frequency of repetitions, prolongations, and blocks is 2.8 per 100 syllables;
- 80% of all disfluent segments include repeating, prolonging, or blocking;
- Sound prolongation is the most common type of disfluency, and most sound prolongations feature excessive physical tension;
- The mean duration during disfluent segments that include part-word repetition and sound prolongation is 1.67 s; and
- The child sometimes appears to be frustrated during disfluent speech.

Table 12–2. Fluency Profiles of Hypothetical Clients With Developmental Fluency Disorders

Variable	Developmental Subtype			
	Stuttering	Cluttering	Atypical Disfluency with Other Developmental Disorder[a]	Other Atypical Disfluency
Client age	12;0	12;0	12;0	12;0
Disfluency frequency (all types) per 100 syllables	12.00	12.00	24.00	5.00
RPBs per 100 syllables	10.00	2.00	20.00	3.00
IRs per 100 syllables	2.00	10.00	4.00	2.00
Percentage of total = RPBs	83%	17%	83%	60%
Most common disfluency type	Part-word repetition	Revision	Part-word repetition	Final sound repetition
Mean # of iterations per PWR/MWR	1.82	1.01	2.07	1.00
Articulation rate	WNL	Excessive	WNL	WNL
Speech rate	BNL	WNL	BNL	WNL
Repetition rhythm	Disrhythmic	Rhythmic	Disrhythmic	Rhythmic
M duration of RPBs	0.80 s	0.78 s	0.81 s	0.65 s
Speaking effort	Excessive	WNL	Excessive	WNL
Locations of fluency-based activity limitations	School, family settings	School, family settings	School, family settings	None
Fluency-based participation restrictions	Present	None	Present	None
Client's awareness of fluency difficulty	Often very aware	Minimally aware to unaware	Minimally aware to unaware	Minimally aware to unaware

Note: RPBs = repetitions, prolongations, and blocks; IRs = interjections and revisions; PWR = part-word repetition, MWR = monosyllable word repetition; WNL = within normal limits; BNL = below normal limits.

[a]The disfluency profile in this column illustrates what might be observed in some individuals with Down syndrome. In this case, the total disfluency frequency is relatively high, and the types of disfluency are consistent with those seen in developmental stuttering.

In this hypothetical case, the combined frequency of repetitions, prolongations, and blocks is not exceptionally high (2.8 per 100 syllables); however, all other fluency data are atypical. That is, with typically developing children, less than half of all disfluent segments will include repeating, prolonging, or blocking (Yairi, 1997). Sound prolongations usually will be among the least common types of disfluency, and most disfluent segments will not appear particularly effortful or trigger frustration (Yairi & Ambrose, 1999). The mean duration of disfluent segments featuring part-word repetition or sound prolongation usually is less than 1 s (Zebrowski, 1994). In this hypothetical case, the speech pattern still would be labeled as stuttering even though the observed frequency of repeating, prolonging, and blocking is not particularly high. This is because all other fluency measures are consistent with a diagnosis of developmental stuttering.

Occasionally, clients may be able to conceal anticipated repetitions, prolongations, and blocks effectively through the use of compensatory strategies such as word substitution or the purposeful use of stalling tactics such as interjection. In cases like these, the clinician must carefully analyze other dimensions of fluency (e.g., rate, effort, rhythm, naturalness) for signs of stuttering and/or ask the client whether compensatory strategies are being used to cope with impended stuttering-related disfluency. At other times, a client may report that he or she stutters in situations outside of the clinic; however, stuttered speech is not observed at all during the clinical evaluation, even after the clinician attempts to elicit stuttered speech through the introduction of various communicative stressors. Prior to making a diagnosis with such cases, the clinician must thoroughly validate the client's reports of stuttering. This can be done through the use of interview procedures like those from Cooper (1972) and Finn and colleagues (Finn, 1996, 1997; Finn et al., 2005), which were described in the previous section. There are a number of other stuttered-related questionnaires and inventories that can be used to elicit information about a person's stuttering experiences. These are described in Chapter 10. In addition, a clinician can ask the client to record samples of his or her speech from the settings when speech fluency is problematic. Activities such as these will enable the clinician to determine if the client is indeed stuttering.

With developmental stuttering, evidence of fluency difficulty usually is first noted during the preschool years, often between the ages of 2;6 and 4;0. Onset before age 2;0 is uncommon, but it can occur. As discussed in Chapter 6, the number of new cases of developmental stuttering diminishes greatly during the course of the elementary school years, and it generally is agreed that most of the risk for manifesting the disorder has passed by the age of 10 to 12 years. Some authors (e.g., Andrews, 1984) have questioned whether cases that feature stuttering onset after age 10 to 12 should even be classified as developmental stuttering (this issue is discussed further below under late-onset developmental stuttering). The precise etiology of developmental stuttering presently is unknown, but evidence points increasingly toward neurodevelopmental impairment. Such impairment is distinct from that which results from acquired conditions such as stroke, traumatic brain injury, neurodegenerative disease, and the use of certain drugs. The latter etiologies are nondevelopmental in nature and thus associated with acquired stuttering, which is described further below. Usually, a clinician will have access to information about the presence of developmental stuttering among a client's biological relatives. Although this information may be useful for certain aspects of treatment such as estimating prognosis or counseling the client about the nature and treatment of stuttering, it is not useful in arriving at a diagnosis of developmental stuttering. This is because having a family history is not a precondition for being diagnosed with stuttering. There is a substantial percentage of people who stutter—in some studies, it is estimated to be about 30%—who report that there is no one else in their family who stutters (Yairi & Ambrose, 2005).

With developmental stuttering, articulation rate usually is within normal limits. Speech rate, however, usually will be slower than normal because of the greater-than-normal amount of time spent in disfluency. Generally, the more disfluent a speaker is, the slower his or her speech rate will be (Logan, Byrd, Mazzocchi, & Gillam, 2011). The presence of abnormally long disfluencies can slow speech rate further. Stuttered speech typically is described as being "dysrhythmic." During the course of an utterance, normal speech rhythm is disrupted by excessive disfluency and/or excessively long disfluency, and the more disfluency a speaker produces, the more speech is likely to sound dysrhythmic. The disfluencies that a speaker produces also can sound dysrhythmic. This is particularly true during part- and whole-word repetition in speakers who stutter, wherein the editing phase of the repetitions (i.e., the silent period between iterations) often is briefer than it is in speakers with typical fluency, a pattern which makes the repetition sound dysrhythmic and "hurried" in relation to the surrounding fluent speech (Throneburg & Yairi, 1994).

Excessive physical effort may be present in some speakers, particularly speakers who are well past the onset of stuttering symptoms. With stuttering, excessive physical effort can be manifested in a variety of ways. For example, speakers who exhibit frequent or long disfluency may appear to struggle as they speak: Lip, tongue, or jaw muscles may show evidence of tremor, and speech breathing may appear dyssynchronous, sometimes to the extent that the speaker sounds as if he or she is running out of breath while speaking, talking with insufficient breath support, or straining to phonate. Excessive physical effort is not observed in all speakers who stutter; thus, unlike the scenario shown in Table 12–2, a client can be diagnosed with developmental stuttering without showing signs of excessive effort while talking. However, the presence of such behavior in combination with excessive repeating, prolonging, and blocking makes the diagnosis of developmental stuttering more straightforward than it otherwise would be.

Speakers may attempt to compensate for anticipated difficulty on upcoming words in any number of ways. Examples include the following: rearranging word order so that the anticipated word is repositioned to a later point in the utterance; substituting a synonym for a word that is expected to feature stuttering-related disfluency; and attempting to facilitate the production of articulatory movements by linking the onset of those movements in time either to the temporal patterning of a nonspeech movement (e.g., tapping a finger or foot, pounding a fist, taking a step) or to the tensing of a muscle (e.g., attempting to initiate voicing when muscles of the forearm become fully tensed). Compensatory behaviors such as these can add to the perception that the speaker is exerting excessive effort while talking. If the speaker routinely inserts unnecessary words into utterances in an attempt to circumvent certain words, the speaker's verbal expression may come across as rambling, unclear, or unfocused. At other times, the speaker may avoid initiating speech all together and instead will adopt a "speak if spoken to" mentality. The presence of compensatory behaviors such as these is not necessary for a diagnosis of stuttering, but if they are present, a diagnosis of stuttering becomes much more clear-cut.

Cluttering

Cluttering is a communication disorder that can affect speech fluency, rate, and intelligibility. Because fluency impairment often is not the only problem that the speaker has, it probably is more accurate to describe cluttering as a *developmental disorder that affects fluency* rather than as a fluency disorder. A host of symptoms have been ascribed to the disorder, but in recent years, it has been suggested that the essential symptoms of cluttered speech are the following: (1) a fast and/or irregular articulation rate; (2) reduced intelligibility of speech that results from coarticulatory imprecision; and (3) an atypically high frequency of revisions, interjections, and phrase repetitions (St. Louis, Raphael, Myers & Bakker, 2003). Other authorities note poor language organization, pausing irregularities, and poor self-awareness of communication deficits among the primary characteristics of the disorder (van Zaalen-op't Hof, Wijnen, & DeJonckere, 2009). Still others note deficits in language complexity, message cohesion, and topic maintenance (Myers, 1996). From this perspective, cluttering features elements of fluency dis-

order, articulation disorder, and language disorder. The disfluency pattern observed in cluttering is, in a general sense, the inverse of that seen in developmental stuttering (see Table 12–2). Although information about the onset of cluttering is sparse, it appears that the symptoms of the disorder are observable by late childhood to adolescence and are not attributable to nondevelopmental etiologies such as traumatic brain injury or illness.

Despite the seemingly clear-cut list of symptoms for cluttering, some researchers have questioned the reliability with which clinicians diagnose the disorder. For example, van Zaalen-op't Hof et al. (2009) asked two experienced speech-language pathologists (SLPs) to subjectively assign one of three diagnostic labels (i.e., stuttering, cluttering, or stuttering + cluttering) to 54 disfluent speakers after listening to several samples of their speech. Results showed that the SLPs assigned a common diagnostic label to only 27 of the 54 cases (50% of the total). In an additional analysis, however, the authors demonstrated that diagnostic agreement could be improved to about 80% when objective criteria pertaining to articulation rate, disfluency patterns, and articulatory accuracy were supplied.

In an additional analysis, van Zaalen-op't Hof et al. (2009) conducted objective, speech-based measures on only the stuttering and cluttering samples that the SLPs had rated consistently. Among these cases, the following characteristics were identified:

- The speakers who cluttered had a faster mean articulation rate (4.9 syll/s) than the speakers who stuttered (3.7 syll/s) but a comparable articulation rate to a control group of normally fluent speakers (5.9 syll/s) during a story-retelling task.

- More than half of the speakers who cluttered had an articulation rate that was more than 1 standard deviation above the group mean for all disfluent speakers during spontaneous speech. Fast articulation rate was not observed during either oral reading or story retelling, however.

- The articulation rates of speakers who cluttered were not more variable than those of speakers in the stuttering or control groups. Articulation rate was measured in spans of 10 to 20 consecutively fluent syllables, however. Measurement of shorter spans of fluent speech might have been a more sensitive measure of the "spurts" of rapid speech that often are ascribed to cluttering.

- On average, the combined frequency of revisions, interjections, and multiword repetitions for the speakers who cluttered was more than six times greater than the combined frequencies of their part-word repetitions, monosyllable word repetitions, and sound prolongations. Overall, 75% of speakers who cluttered fit this pattern. Conversely, 80% of the speakers who stuttered showed the inverse pattern of disfluency. So, most of the disfluencies that speakers who clutter produce tend to be revisions, interjections, and multiword repetitions.

- On average, speakers who cluttered produced about 10 times as many errors in articulatory accuracy as the speakers who stuttered and the speakers in the control group.

Overall, van Zaalen-op't Hof et al.'s (2009) findings were mostly consistent with the characteristics of cluttering presented by others (e.g., St. Louis et al., 2003). As with developmental stuttering, the more cluttering-related characteristics a client presents, the more a clinician can feel confident about a diagnosis of cluttering. The origins for the pattern of disfluency observed in cluttered speech are unclear; however, the occurrence of frequent revisions is consistent with difficulties in language formulation and organization (van Zaalen-op't Hof & DeJonckere, 2010), and the rate-based disturbances are consistent with impairment in the speech motor control system (Alm, 2011).

Stuttering-Cluttering

A third category under the heading of developmental fluency disorder is stuttering-cluttering (or cluttering-stuttering, depending on one's perspective). Whether this is a distinct disorder or a situation where two independent disorders coexist within the same individual is unclear. In either case, the key symptoms for this classification would be evidence of *both* stuttered speech (e.g., excessive production of repetitions, prolongations, and/or blocks) and cluttered speech (e.g., excessively fast articulation rate, bursts of rapidly articulated speech, a greater than normal frequency of reduced speech intelligibility resulting from poor coarticulation, excessive production of revision, interjections, and/or phase repetitions). Some anecdotal reports suggest that stuttering and cluttering co-occur often. For example, Daly (1993) stated that 40% of the children who attended a summer fluency camp presented symptoms of both disorders concurrently. Such reports should be viewed with caution, however, given the relatively poor agreement that SLPs have shown for differentiating cases of "pure cluttering," "pure stuttering," and "stuttering-cluttering" (van Zaalen-op't Hof et al., 2009). Further research is needed to specify the extent to which symptoms of stuttering and cluttering co-occur and to determine whether such co-occurrence is indicative of a distinct disorder.

Atypical Fluency in Conjunction With Other Developmental Disorders

This classification is used to describe atypical fluency patterns that may exist in speakers who exhibit developmental disorders other than stuttering and cluttering. Examples of such disorders include specific language impairment, autism spectrum disorder, intellectual impairment, and Down syndrome (see Table 12–2).

As explained in Chapter 9, the fluency patterns seen in children with specific language impairment do differ significantly, at least in a statistical sense, from the fluency patterns seen in normally developing children. The main pattern seems to be that children with specific language impairment tend to exhibit more total disfluency and, in some studies, more stutter-like disfluency than children with typical fluency (Guo, Tomblin, & Samelson, 2008; MacLachlan & Chapman, 1988). The absolute amount of disfluency and the magnitude of the difference between the two groups tend to be small, however. For example, in one study, the average frequency of stutter-like disfluency for children with specific language impairment was about 1 per 100 syllables (Boscolo, Bernstein Ratner, & Rescorla, 2002). Although this was greater than the observed frequency for the fluent control group, it still is well below the average frequencies seen in studies of speakers who are diagnosed with developmental stuttering. Thus, the production of 1 or 2 stutter-like disfluencies per 100 syllables, in the absence of other behavioral markers for stuttering, generally is not sufficient to warrant a diagnosis of developmental stuttering. For children with specific language impairment, the practical consequences of their atypical fluency patterns are likely to be minimal in comparison to the deficits that they exhibit in the area of language. Based on the research data thus far, the atypical fluency patterns seen in this population typically will not contribute substantially to whatever communication disability an individual has. In such cases, a child's language difficulties are likely to be assigned the highest priority in treatment, and fluency may not be targeted directly at all. To the extent that such disfluency stems from the language production difficulties that a child experiences, one would expect a child's fluency to improve over time as his or her language functioning improves through participation in language therapy activities.

The fluency anomalies that sometimes coincide with Asperger syndrome are likely to be more noticeable to casual listeners than those seen in conjunction with specific language impairment. Some children with Asperger syndrome have been observed to repeat word-final sounds. Repetition of this sort is very rare in speakers with typical fluency, speakers with developmental stuttering, speakers who clutter, and speakers with atypical fluency in conjunction with language impairment. It is even uncommon in speakers with acquired forms of stuttering. Unique forms of disfluency are likely to draw a listener's attention. Published reports to date suggest that when word-final repetition does occur, the frequency of occurrence is not particularly high. Thus, similar to specific language impairment, the practical consequences of the atypical fluency patterns are likely to be less in comparison to other communication-related challenges an individual with Asperger syndrome faces. The relative impact of fluency difficulty versus other communication difficulties has not, to our knowledge, been researched in populations other than developmental stuttering. Thus, these conclusions about the impact of the atypical disfluency seen in some individuals with Asperger syndrome and specific language impairment should be regarded as preliminary.

Other Forms of Atypical Disfluency

As noted in Chapter 9, there have been isolated reports of individuals who exhibit atypical disfluency patterns (e.g., final sound repetition) in the absence of any other identifiable causative or co-occurring condition such as language disorder, genetic syndrome, or acquired neurological dysfunction. In most case reports published to date, the reported atypical disfluency patterns do not appear to have resulted in marked communicative disability. The example in Table 12–2 shows a relatively mild case of atypical disfluency. In some cases, what appears to be disfluent speech may actually represent purposeful phonological behavior (Camarata, 1989).

Disfluent speech patterns, typical or atypical, always have a neurological basis. So, even in cases where an individual presents with an atypical form of disfluency and medical referrals have yielded negative findings, the clinician always should be mindful of the possibility that the disfluency is symptomatic of some more serious condition and be ready to make additional medical referrals should the client's functioning in fluency or general health undergo significant change.

This caution also applies to cases of late-onset stuttering that, on the surface, appear to be developmental in nature. There is no widely agreed-upon definition of late-onset stuttering, but if one uses the longitudinal data on stuttering-onset patterns from Andrews (1984) as a general guide, it might be defined as cases wherein the onset of excessive or atypical part-word repetitions, monosyllable word repetitions, sound prolongations, and blocks occur after age 12. Such cases simply may be a variant of developmental stuttering; however, in some instances, they may be the signal of some other underlying neuropathology (Lebrun, Retif, & Kaiser, 1983). To date, there are no common clinical practice guidelines for treating cases such as these, but as with cases of atypical disfluency, clinicians should at least be alert to the possibility that the disfluent speech is nondevelopmental in nature. If a nondevelopmental etiology is suspected, appropriate medical referrals are warranted.

Nondevelopmental Fluency Disorders

The third major classification category involves nondevelopmental or acquired forms of fluency impairment.

Acquired Stuttering

With acquired stuttering, the onset of fluency impairment can be linked to the occurrence of a specific event that impacts speech-language functioning in such a way that the speaker produces repetitions (particularly part-word repetitions), sound prolongations, and/or blocks more frequently than normal and more frequently than he or she had prior to the precipitating event. Examples of events that have been linked to acquired forms of stuttering include the following: stroke, traumatic brain injury, neurodegenerative disease, use of certain medications, migraine headaches, epilepsy, and acute psychological stress and/or mental illness (see Chapter 9 for a detailed review).

As explained in Chapter 9, each of these precipitating events affects neurological functioning in some way, through altering neuroanatomical structure and/or neurophysiological or neurochemical functioning. Thus, in a sense, each leads to a form of neurogenic stuttering. The use of neurogenic stuttering in the text differs from recent applications of the term in the fluency disorders literature, where it has been contrasted with psychogenic stuttering. As explained in Chapter 9, that distinction has several shortcomings, and in a general sense, all disfluency, even that produced by normally fluent speakers, is neurogenic. One approach to classifying acquired stuttering is to base subtypes on the type of neurologically related event that is linked to stuttering onset. Several examples of this approach follow:

- *Stuttering following traumatic brain injury*
- *Stuttering following stroke*
- *Stuttering following the introduction of medication*

These labels can be made more specific by identifying the location of the brain infarct, the type of stroke (hemorrhagic, ischemic), the type of neurodegenerative disease (e.g., dementia), the type of medication, and so forth.

Speakers with acquired forms of stuttering may show many of the same associated behaviors that occur with developmental stuttering. However, such behaviors do not need to be present in order to make a diagnosis of acquired stuttering. Excessive production of the signature stutter-like disfluency types is sufficient for diagnosis.

Acquired Cluttering

Is it possible for clutter-like speech to emerge in context of neurological injury or disease? This topic has received very little attention in the clinical research literature to date. Lebrun (1996) discussed the rate disturbance that accompanies extrapyramidal system diseases, such as Parkinson's disease, under the umbrella of acquired cluttering. Lebrun presented two cases with idiopathic Parkinson's disease, who displayed rapid rushes of speech along with poor speech intelligibility. He likened the speech patterns to the rate and intelligibility disturbances that are seen in the developmental form of cluttering.

Acquired Deficits in Verbal Fluency

Stuttering and cluttering are not the only types of fluency impairments that can result following neurological injury or disease. For example, several authors have described poor performance on verbal fluency tasks among patients with various forms of non-Alzheimer's dementia. As described in Chapter 10, The *Controlled Oral Word Association Test* (COWAT; Benton, Hamsher, & Sivan, 1994) and other similar, informal tasks have been used to examine phonemic, semantic, and generative action naming fluency in adult speakers. Other formal word generation tasks have been developed for use with children (see Chapter 10). With such tasks, speakers attempt to generate as many unique words as possible within a specified time frame, when given a categorical constraint (e.g., Tell me as many words as you can think of that start with "S"). Deficits in phonemic fluency have been described in patients with vascular dementia (Jones, Laukka, & Backman, 2006). Also, deficits in generative action naming fluency have been detected in patients with Parkinson's disease dementia (Henry & Crawford, 2004).

Rating Severity

After a clinician determines that a client presents a fluency disorder, it is customary to indicate the severity of the disorder. Severity ratings for fluency impairment usually focus on the degree of fluency-related impairment that is present. Instruments such as the *Stuttering Severity Instrument–Fourth Edition* (SSI-4; Riley, 2009) and the *Test of Childhood Stuttering* (TOCS, Gillam, Logan, & Pearson, 2009) feature norm-referenced metrics of severity. With the SSI-4, the client is compared against other people who stutter, and with the TOCS, the client is compared against both other people who stutter and speakers with normal fluency. Informal, Likert-style rating scales have been used with success to obtain holistic ratings of stuttering severity (Logan et al., 2011; O'Brian, Packman, & Onslow, 2004a; Yairi & Ambrose, 1999).

Statements of severity are most useful, however, when measures of fluency impairment such as those described in the preceding paragraph are supplemented with measures that capture the impact that stuttering has on the person's daily life. The latter kinds of measures capture the amount of disability that a person has. There are a number of instruments that capture the kinds of activity limitations and participation restrictions that a speaker exhibits, along with the kinds of environmental hindrances and personal feelings, beliefs, and attitudes that can hinder communication and negatively affect general quality of life. As described in Chapter 10, there are many published rating instruments that yield data on variables such as these. Several of these instruments are norm referenced and allow for comparisons against other people who stutter and/or speakers with normal fluency functioning (e.g., *Behavior Assessment Battery for School-Age Children Who Stutter* by Brutten and Vanryckeghem, 2007; *Overall Assessment of the Speaker's Experience of Stuttering (OASES)* by Yaruss and Quesal, 2008; *Test of Childhood Stuttering (TOCS)* by Gillam et al., 2009; and the *S-24 Scale* by Andrews and Cutler, 1974). When data from instruments like these are combined with quantitative measures of speech impairment severity and the client's own verbal reports of severity, it yields a better sense for the extent to which stuttering impacts a person's daily activities.

Making Recommendations

Upon completion of assessment activities and identification of the client's deficits or impairments, the clinician is poised to present the client with recommendations for what should happen next.

General Recommendations

Following an assessment, there are several possible recommendations that the clinician may present to the client. Each of the recommended actions is presented in the context of clinical counseling, wherein the clinician not only explains what he or she thinks should be done but also presents data that support the recommendation, describes how the recommended actions can be accomplished, provides the client with pertinent educational literature or resources, and solicits questions and comments from the client and/or the client's family members. The most common general recommendations to be presented following assessment are described below.

Dismissal

A recommendation for dismissal following an initial evaluation is most likely to occur when the assessment results indicate that the client is functioning within normal limits in all aspects of communicative functioning, and the client does not exhibit any speech-language behaviors that warrant reexamination.[2] A recommendation for dismissal also is likely to occur when re-evaluation results indicate that the client's fluency functioning has been within normal limits for a significant period of time (e.g., ~ one year) and all other aspects of speech-language performance are within normal limits as well. The latter scenario occurs in cases where speech fluency impairment has normal-

ized either through unassisted recovery or participation in speech-language treatment. In all cases, the clinician must explain to the client and/or the client's caregivers the evidence that supports a judgment of normal or normally developing fluency performance. In cases where a caregiver has expressed significant concern about a child's fluency development, yet the fluency assessment results clearly point toward normal performance, it usually is helpful to counsel caregivers with regard to what the symptoms of fluency impairment are and to encourage the caregiver to contact the clinician should these symptoms emerge in the future.

Re-evaluation

A recommendation for re-evaluation most often occurs when the clinician is uncertain about whether the client's fluency (or other aspects of speech-language performance) will remain within normal range in the months following the evaluation and thus should be monitored.[3] A decision to re-evaluate the client might come about in situations when the client currently functions in the normal range but has exhibited evidence of isolated fluency difficulty in the recent past or when some aspect of the client's current fluency performance is only marginally normal. A recommendation for re-evaluation implies that neither the client nor caregiver (when the client is a child) currently expresses or exhibits significant fluency-related distress and that other aspects of

---

[2]The discussion here is limited to recommendations involving speech-language performance in cases where only the speech-language pathologist (SLP) is involved in case management. It is assumed that swallowing functions are within normal limits and that there are no other indicators of behavioral impairment (e.g., hearing loss, attention deficit) that warrant referral to another professional.

[3]In this context, the term *re-evaluation* implies that the client will not be interacting with the client on a regular basis in the interval between the initial evaluation and the re-evaluation. Thus, the term does not include measures of posttreatment performance.

communicative functioning are within normal limits.

When a re-evaluation is recommended, the plan essentially involves monitoring the client's progress for the interval between the just-completed assessment and the future appointment when the re-evaluation takes place. As part of the monitoring plan, the clinician may engage in telephone consultations with the client (or the client's caregiver) on an as-needed basis should questions or concerns about fluency functioning arise. A typical time frame for re-evaluation is 1 to 6 months following the initial evaluation. Scheduling for the re-evaluation is driven by factors such as the extent to which the clinician and/or client are uncertain about the normalcy of the client's fluency, the amount of time that has elapsed since the client's past fluency difficulties, and the nature and severity of the client's past fluency difficulties. If the client's fluency performance remains in the normal range at the re-evaluation, the client then would be dismissed or scheduled for another (optional) re-evaluation. If the client's performance suggests the presence of fluency impairment at the time of re-evaluation, then the clinician most likely would recommend that the client enroll in treatment.

Treatment

A recommendation for treatment is made in situations where the client exhibits impaired fluency and wishes to address it. Usually, a recommendation for treatment involves regularly occurring appointments, which are held across a series of weeks (e.g., weekly 60-minute sessions across a 15-week period). At the end of the treatment period, fluency performance is re-evaluated and the clinician and cli-

ent then consider the need for additional treatment sessions. In certain work settings, other treatment scheduling options may be possible. For example, in a school setting, it may be possible to conduct semi-intensive treatment (e.g., 3-hour sessions for 5 consecutive days) during the week prior to the start of semester classes, and then follow that with weekly or biweekly appointments when the semester commences.

Referrals

A fourth type of recommendation involves referrals to other professionals. Referrals come about when the clinician suspects that the client presents additional areas of concern, and those areas are beyond the clinician's expertise or scope of practice. The nature of the referral will depend, of course, upon the nature of the areas of concern. Examples of professionals to whom referrals might be made include the following: a bilingual speech-language pathologist, a family practice physician, an otolaryngologist, a neurologist, a psychologist, a neuropsychologist, and an audiologist. Referrals can be presented in conjunction with recommendations for dismissal, re-evaluation, or treatment.

Other Considerations in Recommending Treatment

As indicated above, a clinician typically recommends treatment in situations where the client exhibits impaired fluency and the client (or the client's caregiver) expresses a desire for professional assistance in addressing the impairment and its associated effects on daily life. In most cases of disordered fluency, the decision to recommend treatment is straightforward. In fact, in many cases, clients come to the initial evaluation already knowing that they stutter or clutter and that they would like to establish a therapeutic relationship with the SLP. The decision about whether to recommend treatment is not always straightforward and clear-cut, however. Two scenarios in which a clinician may be uncertain about whether to commence treatment are discussed below.

Treating Developmental Stuttering in Preschool-Aged Children

Decisions about treatment with preschoolers who stutter can be complicated by the possibility that a child's stuttering might remit without formal treatment, a process that some (e.g., Martin & Lindamood, 1986) have termed "unassisted recovery." Findings from contemporary research suggest that roughly 75% of all preschoolers who stutter eventually normalize fluency in the absence of participation in formal speech therapy sessions (Yairi & Ambrose, 1999, 2005). At present, it is not possible to identify precisely which cases will resolve and which will persist. This creates the possibility that a clinician will provide treatment to a child who is on a path to recovery from stuttering, with or without therapy. The extent to which preschoolers' recovery or remission from developmental stuttering is truly "unassisted" has been questioned by researchers who argue that the informal, day-to-day comments and suggestions that parents make to a child's stuttering may constitute a form of treatment (e.g., Martin & Lindamood, 1986). In any case, the fact that preschoolers do indeed appear to recover from stuttering without participat-

ing in formalized speech therapy raises the question of which preschoolers who stutter should be recommended for treatment. This issue has generated considerable debate among experts and still is not completely settled.

Most experts agree that some form of active treatment is warranted in cases where a preschooler who stutters is distressed, frustrated, or concerned about his or her ability to communicate due to difficulties with speech fluency (Curlee & Yairi, 1997). Thus, even if a child has stuttered for a relatively short length of time, the presence of stuttering-related negative feelings, emotions, or communication experiences would outweigh whatever indicators of recovery a child might present and "tip the scales" in the direction of recommending treatment. The choice of whether to commence or defer treatment is less obvious when a child has been stuttering for a relatively short length of time, and the stuttered speech does not seem to result in significant communication disability or emotional distress. In such instances, the clinician may be inclined to monitor the child's fluency for some length of time, in the hope that the stuttered speech eventually will remit without treatment. A key question with this approach concerns the length of time a clinician should "wait and watch" before implementing treatment.

Several clinicians have noted that, with preschool-aged cases of stuttering, speech therapy can be aimed at parents as much as it can be aimed at children. In this view, the parent of a child who stutters can be counseled or can enroll in short-term training sessions that focus on increasing the parents' use of communicative behaviors that are likely to facilitate a child's fluency (Gregory, 2003;

Logan & Caruso, 1997; Richels & Conture, 2010; Starkweather, Gottwald, & Halfond, 1990). These prescriptive and preventative steps can be implemented on a routine basis in conjunction with a recommendation for actively monitoring a child's fluency. With this approach, the child's fluency then would be re-evalualated at some point in the future (e.g., after 3 to 6 months). Some clinicians (e.g., Martin & Lindamood, 1986; Starkweather et al., 1990) have argued that it is better to err on the side of caution in such circumstances and intervene, even if it is only indirectly, rather than wait passively to see if the stuttering resolves.

Several clinicians have developed guidelines for determining whether a preschooler who stutters should be enrolled in some form of active speech therapy or, instead, be assigned to some form of indirect intervention or, perhaps, a passive "wait-watch-monitor" strategy. With the latter strategy, the preschooler who stutters is on the clinician's "radar" but is not actively participating in regularly scheduled treatment sessions as he or she would be when enrolled in an active form of speech therapy. Curlee and Yairi (1997) suggested that direct (active) treatment of stuttering can be deferred for children who are between 2 to 5 years of age, provided that they are within 2 years of stuttering onset and there is no evidence of communicative distress, no evidence of concomitant communication disorders that require treatment, and the child's parents are not pressing for therapy. Yairi and colleagues' (see Yairi & Ambrose, 2005, for a summary) longitudinal research on stuttering outcomes in preschoolers who stutter has led to additional insights and guidelines about the factors that affect children's recovery from stuttering and, by

extension, factors that may affect which children are recommended for active participation in a treatment program. Yairi and Ambrose (2005) suggest several primary factors that clinicians should consider when deciding between whether to recommend treatment for a young child who stutters.

Family history of stuttering. Yairi and Ambrose (2005) stated that family history of stuttering is "one of the most powerful risk predictors" for persistent stuttering. The main pattern among preschoolers who stutter is that the child's risk for persistent stuttering increases if the child has other relatives who had or currently have persistent stuttering. Conversely, if the child's family includes other individuals who recovered from stuttering, the child is less likely to exhibit persistent stuttering. The latter cases nonetheless should be closely monitored, as the presence of recovered relatives does not ensure that the child also will recover.

Longitudinal trends in the frequency of stuttering-related disfluency. Yairi and Ambrose (2005) reported that most children who eventually met criteria for having recovered from stuttering showed a clear trend toward improved fluency in the weeks and months following stuttering onset. In their research, many children who eventually recovered from stuttering showed clear signs of recovery during the 12 months following symptom onset. Children who did not recover during the course of their project showed either a trend toward more frequent stuttering-related disfluency (i.e., the stuttering was becoming more severe over time) or a stable pattern of disfluency frequency in the months following onset (i.e., disfluency frequency neither markedly increased nor decreased). Interestingly, in their research, a child's frequency of stuttering-related disfluency near the time of stuttering onset did not seem to be a strong predictor of whether the child eventually recovered from stuttering. (Severity at later stages of the disorder [for example, 4 years post onset] was, however, viewed as a poor prognostic indicator for eventual recovery.) Children who recovered from stuttering also showed changes in the rhythmic structure of stuttering-related disfluency. That is, the duration of the "silent interval" (i.e., the editing phase) between iterations of a repetition became progressively longer over time in children who recovered. Children whose stuttering persisted, however, did not show such a pattern. In addition, the number of sound prolongations produced as a proportion of total disfluency gradually decreased in the children who were on a path toward recovery.

Amount of time elapsed since the onset of the child's stuttered speech. Yairi and Ambrose (2005) reported that, based on longitudinal data of stuttering recovery patterns, the longer the child exhibited stuttered speech, the less likely the child's stuttered speech was to resolve. For example, assuming all other factors were equal, a child who had been stuttering for 12 months had less likelihood of recovery than a child who had been stuttering for 3 months. In turn, a child who had been stuttering for 24 months had less likelihood of recovery than a child who had been stuttering for 12 months, and so on.

The current consensus is that if a child has been stuttering for 2 years or longer, that alone would be grounds for enrolling a child in treatment. This is true even in cases where the frequency of stuttering-related disfluency is not particularly high. For example, a child who has consistently produced between 4 to 5 stuttering-related disfluencies per 100 syllables during the course of 28 months would be seen as at risk for persistent stuttering (or, perhaps, even seen as already exhibiting persistent stuttering) and a candidate for enrollment in a treatment program. Regardless of a client's frequency of stuttering-related disfluency, a more conservative approach would be to recommend active treatment for any child who has stuttered for 1 year or more and has not exhibited signs of recovery such as a marked decrease in the frequency of stuttering-related disfluency. Given the potential negative effects that persistent stuttering can have on a speaker's attitudes toward communication and overall psychosocial well-being (Craig, Blumgart, & Tran, 2009; Vanryckeghem & Brutten, 1996, 2012; Yaruss & Quesal, 2006), a case can even be made for the use of a more conservative 6- to 9-month post onset window when evaluating the need for active treatment. As noted above, in cases where stuttering leads to marked communication disability or emotional distress, it is appropriate to commence some form of treatment even when the child is less than 6 months removed from the onset of stuttering symptoms.

As suggested in the preceding discussion, there is no fixed rule concerning to when intervention for stuttering should commence with young children. Given the many deleterious effects associated with stuttering, we are generally inclined to err on the side caution and intervene sooner rather than later.

Gender. Yairi and Ambrose (2005) reported that girls are more likely to exhibit recovery from stuttering than boys, and in girls, recovery takes place sooner in relation to stuttering onset than it does with boys. Thus, males have a greater risk for persistent stuttering, they are less likely to recover from stuttering than girls, and the total amount of time that they spend stuttering prior to recovery usually is more than it is with girls.

The child's age at the time of onset for stuttered speech. Yairi and Ambrose (2005) indicated that the effect of "age of stuttering onset" upon stuttering persistence was less clear than that of other variables. They did indicate, however, that the data suggested an increased risk for persistent stuttering as a child's age at time of stuttering onset increases. In this view, a child who first shows signs of stuttering at age 4 would be at greater risk of persistence then, say, a child who first shows signs of stuttering at age 2;6. Yairi and Ambrose speculated that self-awareness of stuttered speech, which tends to become more common past the age of 4 years, may play a role in the eventual outcome of the stuttering.

Other secondary factors. Yairi and Ambrose (2005) mentioned several other secondary factors that might be relevant to a child's recovery from stuttering. Examples of the latter factors include the following:

- Evidence of a *gradual decline in the number of extraneous head and neck movements* during the year following onset of stuttering. In their research, children who were on a path toward recovery from stuttering showed a gradual decline in the frequency of stuttering-related disfluency as well as "secondary" nonspeech movements.

- The presence of *poor phonological skills* at or near the time of stuttering onset. Children with this pattern were less likely to recover from stuttering than children who had normal or advanced phonological skills near the time of stuttering onset.

Addressing Differing Views on the Need for Treatment

Another situation in which the decision to recommend treatment may be unclear occurs when there is disagreement between parents and children regarding the need for fluency therapy. In our experience, differences of this sort are most likely to arise in the middle school and high school populations. Conflict sometimes arises when a parent expresses concern about the current or future impact of stuttering on the child's performance in school, work, or social development. The child, in contrast, indicates that he or she is not particularly concerned about the stuttering and expresses disinterest in attending fluency treatment sessions. Discrepancies like this sometimes are not easily resolved. It is best to commence a treatment plan only when all parties are receptive to participating. Potential responses to parent-child differences on the need for fluency therapy include the following: (a) defer treatment for 6- to 12-months, and then reintroduce the possibility of commencing fluency therapy at a time when, hopefully, the potential benefits of participation in treatment become more apparent to the child; and (b) implement treatment on a trial basis and, after completion of the trial period, revisit the child's willingness to participate.

Summary

The present chapter addressed issues related to the diagnosis of fluency impairment. Several categories of normal and disordered functioning were discussed. In clinical settings, clients often have a good sense for the type of disorder they have, even before they attend a fluency evaluation. In some cases, clients know that a fluency disorder exists, but they are uncertain about the nature of the disorder. For example, some clients will state that they stutter when in fact they clutter; others will say they stutter when, in fact, they exhibit disfluency that is associated with expressive language impairment. In treatment situations, it is useful for clients to have an accurate understanding of fluency impairment, as this will help them to interpret and troubleshoot the communication limitations that they present.

People in the general public and some health professionals may dismiss childhood stuttering as "normal" behavior and state that "everybody stutters." While it is true that many people produce isolated instances of stutter-like disfluency, only a small percentage of the population consistently exhibits the unique disfluency profile that characterizes the disorder known as developmental stuttering. Epidemiological data indicate that only about 5% of the population will exhibit this disorder during the course of their life span. Based on these data, it is clear that relatively few people stutter.

The diagnosis of stuttering sometimes is challenging with preschool-aged children. At this age, children generally are unable to describe their fluency experiences in detail. Thus, a clinician is unlikely to hear a preschooler report that, "I know what I want to say, but I can't say it" or "I want to say this word, but I feel stuck." Such verbal comments about fluency phenomenology are common in older children, adolescents, and adults, and they are useful in identifying stuttering in cases where speech symptoms alone may be insufficient to arrive at a diagnosis. In the absence of such information, clinicians may need to use qualified diagnostic labels such as "possible developmental stuttering" until the nature of the client's fluency functioning becomes more apparent after further observation.

Another area of potential uncertainty following a fluency evaluation concerns the issue of when to commence a treatment program with preschoolers who exhibit developmental stuttering. With this population, there is a possibility that the child might recover from stuttering in the absence of formal fluency intervention. Thus, to avoid treating children unnecessarily, it is important to identify those cases that are most likely to recover. Recent research has identified several behavioral indicators of recovery. Although these indicators offer some sense of whether a child's stuttering will persist, they are not close to being 100% predictive of a child's eventual outcome. The science of specifying the likelihood of recovery for specific individuals who stutter still is in its infancy. Ultimately, the existing speech-language indicators of recovery from stuttering will likely need to be supplemented or supplanted by biomarkers that relate more closely to the etiology of stuttering. Data from contemporary research indicate that certain genetic or neurodevelopmental measures may be suitable for this purpose.

SECTION
IV

Treatment Approaches

13

Treating Fluency Disorders: Goals and General Principles

It is customary in most textbooks on fluency disorders to review the treatment protocols that expert clinicians have developed at their particular clinics. There is, of course, value in seeing what experts do when they work with people who have impaired fluency. Prior to reviewing such information, however, it is first important to discuss the foundational aspects of clinical practice. The first foundational issue that warrants attention is *goal setting*. This is a critical component of treatment, because treatment goals essentially constitute the road map that the clinician and client will follow. If the treatment goals are misdirected or incomplete, then the treatment activities and associated outcomes will be misdirected or incomplete. The second foundational issue that warrants attention concerns the nature of the treatment approaches that clinicians use when helping clients to improve fluency functioning. Many of the evidence-based treatment programs for stuttering

have similar or overlapping components. This means that the evidence-based treatment protocol used at "Clinic A" is likely to be similar in some respects to the evidence-based treatment protocol used at "Clinic B." This situation suggests the need for clinicians to look beyond the particular "brand" of treatment that is being described in order to identify the essential *evidence-based principles* that characterize effective treatments (Bernstein Ratner, 2005). In essence, such principles constitute the common core of effective fluency intervention. These two issues—treatment goals and treatment principles—are discussed in detail in the present chapter.

Developing Treatment Goals

As indicated in the introductory comments above, the first step in intervention is to develop a treatment plan. The treatment plan is a statement of the general goals and specific objectives toward which the clinician and client will work.

Developing Comprehensive Goals

The effectiveness of a treatment plan is influenced in part by the extent to which the treatment plan addresses all aspects of a client's disability and functioning. Thus, it is essential to construct a treatment plan that is sufficiently comprehensive.

Working From Assessment Results

Assessment data are a main source of information for establishing treatment goals. Assuming that the assessment has addressed all relevant aspects of communicative functioning, the clinician should begin to get a sense for which aspects of communication are most in need of treatment. In most clinical settings, assessment data usually consist of both clinician-based observations and client-based reports. When developing treatment goals, it is essential that the clinician consider both perspectives. This reduces the likelihood that key problem areas will be overlooked in treatment. Client reports usually are a good source of information about communication disability and associated feelings, attitudes, and beliefs and, possibly, additional areas of impairment that are not detected via clinician-administered procedures during the assessment. Clinical assessment activities at the very least should screen for potential areas of communication impairment beyond fluency. It is not uncommon for children who are being treated for stuttering to exhibit concomitant disorders in speech sound pro-

duction and/or language comprehension and production. Similarly, many speakers who clutter present problems with both fluency (particularly rate) and speech intelligibility, and some clients also present evidence of additional impairment in areas such as language formulation and organization and cognitive functions such as attention.

Working From a Comprehensive Model of Fluency

Fluency is a multidimensional construct. The use of a multidimensional fluency model provides a clinician with a mechanism for ensuring that he or she addresses all aspects of a client's fluency functioning. As discussed later in the chapter, there is a long-standing practice in speech-language pathology of evaluating the success of stuttering treatment programs in terms of speech continuity. From this narrow perspective, cases that attain "0% syllables stuttered" or something close to that are seen as successful outcomes, and cases that exhibit higher posttreatment stuttering frequency scores are not. This practice is apparent even in the names of some intervention approaches (e.g., "stutter-free speech").

The main problem with evaluating treatment outcomes mainly in relation to stuttering frequency is that fluency is much more than the dimension of continuity. Indeed, many of the most effective and entertaining speakers in society are anything but "0% disfluent." Cooper (1986) referred to the overreliance on disfluency frequency data as the "frequency fallacy," and he argued that clinicians should utilize a variety of clinical measures when evaluating whether a treatment plan has been successful. The data on speakers' perceptions of fluency outcomes, with or without treatment, seem to support Cooper's argument. For example, the research literature for stuttering contains numerous reports of speakers who report feeling satisfied with their communication abilities even though their speech fluency has not entirely normalized (Anderson & Felsenfeld, 2003; Boberg & Kully, 1994; Cooper, 1986; Plexico, Manning, & DiLollo, 2005; Pollard, Ellis, Finan, & Ramig, 2009). As one of the participants in Plexico et al.'s (2005) study said, " . . . 95% of the time or more stuttering is not an issue... it's there and it's part of who I am, but it's not an issue in terms of decisions I make or . . . what I've achieved" (p. 15). The participant went on to comment that stuttering no longer dictated the day-to-day choices that the person made.

Thus, while normal speech continuity is worth striving for, clinicians and clients should remember that speech disfluency and effective communication are not mutually exclusive concepts.

In Chapter 1 of this text, a multidimensional model of fluency was described in detail. Components of the model include continuity, rate, rhythm, effort, naturalness, talkativeness, and stability. The scope of the model makes it easy to see that there are multiple measures available to document a client's changes in speech fluency. For example, one client might attain only a modest reduction in speech disfluency following a course of treatment and yet be pleased with his fluency outcome because of significant reductions in disfluency duration (an aspect of rhythm) and speech-related effort. Another client might show only modest reduction in disfluency frequency following a course of treatment yet still feel satisfied with the substantial increase in talkativeness that he has gained as a result of therapy. Although these clients may wish to con-

tinue to work at improving speech continuity and other dimensions of fluency, they and the clinician still can value the meaningful changes that have occurred. To summarize, when clinicians think of fluency as a multidimensional construct, it opens up an assortment of potential treatment goals and ways to measure treatment outcomes.

Working From a Comprehensive Model of Health Functioning

As noted above, treatment goals are derived from assessment data and a comprehensive model of fluency. After a clinician collects assessment data, it is helpful to organize the data in some conceptually valid manner. A useful tool for this purpose is the *International Classification of Functioning, Disability and Health* (ICF), an instrument that the World Health Organization (WHO, 2001) developed to provide health care workers with "a unified and standard language and framework for the description of health and health-related states" (p. 3). Several authors have described how the ICF framework can be applied to capturing the life experiences of people who stutter (e.g., American Speech-Language-Hearing Association [ASHA], 2004; Logan, 2005; Yaruss, 1998; Yaruss & Quesal, 2004). The ICF framework contains five primary components, three of which pertain to client functioning (i.e., *impairment, activity limitations, participation restrictions*) and two of which pertain to the context in which the client functions (i.e., *personal factors, environmental factors*). These five components offer an additional structure around which the clinician and client can generate treatment goals. Examples of the types of goals that follow from these components are shown in Table 13–1.

Table 13–1. Examples of Fluency-Related Goals Associated With Components of the ICF Instrument (World Health Organization, 2001)

ICF Component	Potential Goals to Target in Treatment
Impairment (and associated loss of function)	Remediate and/or compensate for fluency impairment: *Improve the client's capacity to speak fluently through the use of various fluency management skills.* • e.g., Improve/normalize speech continuity, rate, rhythm, effort, and naturalness.
Activity limitations	Reduce disability: *Reduce the number and severity of the client's activity limitations.* • Improve the client's fluency functioning in specific activities of daily living.
Participation restrictions	Reduce disability: *Increase the client's verbal participation within and across daily activities.* • Improve the extent to which the client participates verbally in specific situations. • Improve the number and variety of communicative tasks in which the client participates.
Personal factors	Reduce disability: *Reduce the impact of personal factors on the client's fluency functioning.* • Develop constructive, realistic, and/or accurate attitudes toward impairment and treatment. • Improve the accuracy with which the client interprets internal and external events that are associated with fluency impairment. • Develop strategies for managing feelings/emotions that disrupt speech fluency.
Environmental factors	Improve functioning: *Reduce the impact that environmental factors have on the client's fluency functioning.* • Develop supportive or facilitative listener reactions to the client's fluency impairment. • Reduce the occurrence of listener demands for rapid, fast-paced, or complex communication if such demands hinder fluency.

Note. ICF = International Classification of Disability, Functioning, and Health.

The most basic treatment goals deal with improving the client's *capacity* to manage his or her fluency impairment. In the ICF parlance, the term capacity refers to the client's optimal or maximal level of functioning as measured in a standard or controlled setting (which usually is the clinic meeting room). Included under the notion of managing fluency impairment are the various fluency management skills that form the core of a treatment program. These skills, when implemented, help the client reduce or lessen the symptoms of fluency impairment and any associated communication disability. Thus, it is standard for treatment plans to include goals that are aimed at building capacity. The reasoning is that if a client is unable to implement fluency management skills under optimal, controlled conditions, it is unlikely he or she will implement them under the often less-than-optimal conditions associated with real-world activities.

After a client develops the capacity to manage fluency in a controlled setting, he or she is set to transfer the newly developed capacity to beyond-clinic settings. When doing so, the client aims to lessen the various *activity limitations* that he or she presents. The activities that are targeted for intervention vary from person to person. For some clients, communication disability is present in virtually all daily activities. For others, it is present only in specific activities. After the clinician and client identify the problem activities, they can develop specific plans for how to change performance within them. As the client develops competence at managing fluency across various activities of daily living, the extent of his or her communication disability should diminish gradually. Thus, it is common for treatment plans to include goals that are aimed at reduced specific activity limitations that the client presents.

Participation restrictions are another aspect of disability that many speakers who stutter exhibit. This aspect of the ICF framework ties into the multidimensional fluency model that was discussed earlier in this section and in Chapter 1. People who stutter may expend considerable effort when talking and/or they may feel embarrassed about the way they talk. Effortful speech and negative feelings about how one talks will lead many speakers who stutter to talk less than they would like to talk. Thus, goals that

deal with participation often are aimed at increasing the *amount of talking* that a client does in specific situations as well as the *number* and *variety of situations* within which the client speaks. The long-term goal is not for a client to talk for the sake of talking but rather for a client to say as much as he or she would like to say within any given situation. Before pursing participation-related goals, it first may be necessary for a client to address his or her feelings, attitudes, and beliefs about communication and fluency impairment, if the feelings, attitudes, and beliefs are the primary source of the participation restriction.

Personal factors and *environmental factors* constitute the context within which the client functions. These contextual factors either can facilitate or hinder a client's fluency functioning. Overall, the main objective is to reduce or eliminate those personal and environmental factors that hinder the client's fluency functioning and to promote those personal and environmental factors that facilitate fluency functioning. Assessment activities (e.g., checklists, inventories, discussions) enable the clinician and client to identify the contextual factors that hinder and facilitate the client's fluency functioning most (see Chapter 10 for examples of pertinent assessment tools). This process leads naturally to the development of associated treatment goals.

Some treatment plans for speakers who stutter include goals that target personal factors; in particular, factors that pertain to a client's attitudes, feelings, and beliefs about his or her fluency impairment and the ways in which other people react to it. Many environmental factors can potentially hinder a client's fluency. Thus, treatment plans for speakers who stutter may include goals that target the ways in which the client's communication partners interact with the speaker and react to stuttered speech. For example, a treatment goal that is aimed at reducing the frequency with which a communication partner interrupts the client during disfluency is likely to facilitate fluency by providing the client with additional time to manage the disfluent segment. When treating children, clinicians typically first introduce treatment activities that pertain to parent or sibling communication behaviors in the clinic setting and then extend the activities to real-world settings. With adult clients who are seeking to change the behavior of friends, coworkers, and other such people, in-clinic activities are seldom possible. In these situations, clients may be called on to inform their communication partners of the kinds of changes they would like them to make (Schloss, Espin, Smith, & Suffolk, 1987). Many people, even those who do not stutter, find it difficult to engage in assertive behavior of this sort. With practice, however, clients can learn to assert their wishes by (a) telling the communication partner what he or she is doing (e.g., "I noticed that you interrupt me when I block on a word."), (b) informing the communication partner how this behavior affects the speaker (e.g., "This usually leads me to block longer and harder.), and (c) informing the communication partner what the speaker would like him or her to do instead (e.g., "I'd prefer it if you wait until I finish saying the word."). Schloss et al. (1987) examined the effects of a training program in which adults who stuttered learned to produce assertive behavior like that described above. The participants received more favorable interview ratings when using assertive behavior than they did when not making such comments.

Developing Appropriate Goals

The next issue to discuss concerns the need for establishing treatment goals that are consistent with the nature of the fluency disorder. Such a treatment plan will feature goals that deal directly with the types of speech production difficulties that clients present.

Working From an Accurate Model of Fluency Impairment

Views on the nature of stuttering have changed significantly during the past 60 years. Stuttering now is widely seen as a symptom of impairment or disfunction in the speech production system. Results from contemporary research studies point to an assortment of speech-related deficits in people who stutter when compared to nonstuttering speakers. Examples include the following:

- Evidence of impairment or inefficiency in speech motor learning (e.g., Bauerly & De Nil, 2011; Smits-Bandstra & De Nil, 2009; Smits-Bandstra, De Nil, & Saint-Cyr, 2006);
- Evidence of excessive variability in motor movements produced during tasks that require sequenced articulatory and manual movements (Kleinow & Smith, 2000; Olander, Smith, & Zelaznik, 2010);
- Evidence of slowness in the retrieval and/or assembly of the syntactic frames used in sentence production (e.g., Anderson & Conture, 2004);
- Evidence of neuroanatomical and neurophysiological deviations in regions of the brain involved with speech production (e.g., De Nil, Kroll, Lafaille, & Houle, 2003;

Foundas, Bollich, Corey, Hurley, & Heilman, 2001; Neumann et al., 2003); and

- Evidence that genetic factors play a role in determining a child's risk for developing stuttering (Dworzynski et al., 2007; van Beijsterveldt, Felsenfeld, & Boomsma, 2010).

Given the mounting evidence for motor system dysfunction in speakers who stutter, one might reasonably argue that stuttering should be classified as a type of *movement disorder*. This is in contrast to traditional practice, which is to assign stuttering into essentially its own "special" category (i.e., *fluency disorder*). The implications for how one classifies stuttering are not trivial, as views about the nature of a disorder are apt to influence the types of treatment goals and treatment techniques that one implements (Bernstein Ratner, 2005). For example, if a clinician regards stuttering as a movement disorder, then the primary treatment approaches for the disorder are likely to have more in common with treatments that are used with disorders such as dysarthria, apraxia, and speech sound disorder than they are, for example, with treatments that are used for personality disorders or anxiety disorders.

When writing about treatment outcomes, Rosenbek and LaPointe (1985) made the following observation about dysarthria:

> Only if a dysarthric patient's nervous system returns to normal will speech return too. The return to normal— either because of natural or physiologic recovery or because of medical treatment—is a rare circumstance indeed. Therefore the aim of all dysarthria treatment is compensated intelligibility. (p. 104)

Rosenbek and LaPointe's (1985) remarks about dysarthria seem apropos to persistent stuttering and most other fluency disorders. In other words, if stuttered speech is viewed as a symptom of neurologic impairment, then the initial aim for stuttering treatment will be *compensated fluency.* The notion of compensation implies that the speaker will attempt to speak as fluently as he or she is capable, in as many situations as possible, and for as long as possible, *given the limitations of his or her speech production system.* The concept of *effective compensation* is quite different from the concept of normalized fluency, in that it allows for the possibility that the client will continue to manifest impaired fluency, while normalized fluency does not. Given the mounting evidence to support a neurological basis for both stuttering and cluttering, it seems that "effective compensation" is a fundamental goal to aim toward in treatment and a fundamental variable to assess when evaluating treatment outcomes in speakers with disordered fluency, as well.

Incorporating Goals That Have Personal Significance

After identifying broad treatment goals such as those shown in Table 13–1, it is helpful to specify or personalize these goals in ways that reflect the client's unique circumstances. The process of personalizing treatment goals is illustrated in Figure 13–1. As shown, treatment goals can serve two broad functions. Some treatment goals deal with building the prerequisite skills for managing fluency impairment (i.e., *capacity-oriented goals*). Other treatment goals deal with functional outcomes, such as reducing disability in the activities of daily life (i.e., *performance-oriented goals*).

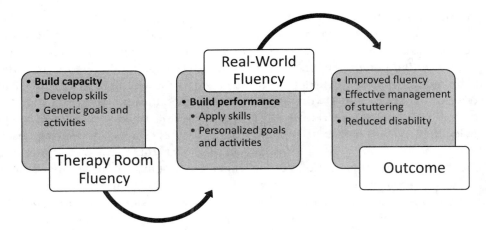

Figure 13–1. An illustration of the goal-setting process for the treatment of fluency disorders. Initial goals in treatment typically are aimed at building a speaker's capacity to speak with improved fluency under ideal conditions, such as in a therapy room setting. The activities involved in building capacity are generic in the sense that they consist of tasks most clients will do when developing basic competencies in fluency management skills. After the speaker establishes the capacity to use fluency management skills, the focus of treatment shifts toward goals that deal with fluency performance in real-world settings. The focus for these goals is on the specific activity limitations, participation restrictions, personal factors, and environmental factors the client faces. Thus, skills at this stage of treatment are personalized. In some cases, performance-based goals may be addressed concurrently with capacity-building activities. Attainment of these goals leads to an outcome. Given the nature of fluency disorders and the limitations of present treatments, it is suggested that an appropriate initial outcome for most clients with persistent stuttering is to develop the ability to manage the symptoms of fluency impairment so that fluency-related disability is markedly reduced or eliminated.

As stated earlier, the notion of capacity deals with a person's optimum level of functioning as measured in a standard setting such as the treatment room. Treatment goals that are oriented toward building the client's capacity are generic in nature, in that they pertain to the basic skills that many people with impaired fluency must master in order to reduce fluency-related disability in real-world activities. In contrast, treatment goals that are oriented toward reducing disability in real-world settings are individualized. That is, they pertain to the specific concerns that individual clients have about their fluency functioning in everyday situations.

Expressed fluency concerns can vary widely across clients. Examples of concerns that clients might express include the following:

- The impairment (e.g., "I often repeat sounds and words when I talk");
- Activity limitations that stem from the impairment (e.g., "It's really hard for me to introduce myself to customers at work.");
- Participation restrictions that stem from the impairment (e.g., "I really want to join the conversation when I'm attending my book club meeting, but I never do.");

- Personal factors associated with fluency impairment (e.g., "I feel very embarrassed when other people hear me stutter."); and
- Environmental factors associated with fluency impairment (e.g., "When I stutter, my boss always looks at me like he wants me to 'hurry up,' and then I stutter even more.").

The process of melding generic fluency management skills with individualized activities that are aimed at reducing the client's speech disability during real-world settings requires frequent and in-depth communication between the clinician and the client. Effective clinician-client communication is likely to increase the client's sense of "buy in" to the treatment process because it leads to treatment activities that are of personal significance to the client (Bothe & Richardson, 2011; Plexico, Manning, & DiLollo, 2010). As part of this collaborative relationship, the client can offer information about issues such as the specific fluency challenges that he or she faces in daily life, which challenges matter most, which aspects of a speaking activity are most concerning, and the extent to which he or she is willing to reveal the fluency impairment to others while attempting to attain the goal. The clinician can offer input on the types of treatment activities that are likely to help the client reduce communication disability in specific activities as well as insight into how the client can subdivide a goal (e.g., *improving fluency when placing an order at a restaurant*) into discrete, attainable steps. Through this process, the clinician and client can coauthor a treatment plan that is tailored to fit the client's unique experience of stuttering.

Defining Success

In his best-selling book on personal change, Stephen Covey (2013) identifies what he terms the "7 habits of highly effective people." One of the 7 habits on Covey's list is to "begin with the end in mind." In other words, people function most effectively when their daily activities are aligned with the goals or destinations that they hope to reach. This "habit" is applicable to people with fluency disorders, because their attempts to attain desired levels of fluency management may require considerable time, effort, struggle, and expense (Blumgart, Tran, & Craig, 2010b; Craig, Blumgart, & Tran, 2009; Plexico et al., 2005). In such cases, the long-range goal functions as a destination toward which one aspires and a reference point against which progress can be measured (Harackiewicz, Barron, Tauer, Carter, & Elliot, 2000). It is important that the clinician and client discuss the issue of long-range goals and, in doing so, learn how each other defines success. In our experience, the client's and the clinician's ideas of success often differ. If the discrepancy in viewpoints is not addressed, it can lead the clinician and client to work at cross-purposes during the course of a treatment program.

What Does the Client Want?

At the start of a treatment program, clients often have some sense of what they hope to accomplish. Four common outcomes that clients express at the start of treatment are discussed below. Clinicians should understand the basis and implications of each one.

"I want to be rid of stuttering." Clients who express a desire to be rid of stuttering essentially are striving to attain the sort of fluency that nonstuttering speakers experience. Guitar (2006) referred to this type of outcome as *spontaneous fluency,* which means that the client's fluency is within normal limits and the client accomplishes the fluency without needing to apply fluency management techniques consciously or with excessive effort. When a client who previously had stuttered maintains spontaneous fluency consistently across many consecutive months, the outcome is consistent with concepts such as *complete recovery* and *normalized fluency.* Over time, the client who is on this path becomes progressively less likely to self-identify as a person who stutters, and listeners become progressively more likely to identify the client as a typical speaker.

As noted elsewhere in this text, recovery from stuttering is most common during childhood. When normalized fluency results, it implies that the underlying impairment that caused the person to stutter either has fully resolved or has been fully compensated for (Neumann et al., 2005). The likelihood of attaining normalized fluency is age dependent, however. If a speaker stutters from childhood into adolescence or adulthood, normalization of speech fluency is less likely to occur. At present, the neurological mechanisms associated with recovery from stuttering are not well understood. The role of treatment in this process is not well understood either, as normalized fluency can occur in preschoolers who are not enrolled in formal treatment (Yairi & Ambrose, 1999). Results from neuroimaging data suggest that systematic practicing of rate-based stuttering management strategies results in changes in left-hemisphere neural activation, particularly in frontal and temporal lobe regions proximal to those that are involved in speech production within typical speakers (Boberg, Yeudall, Schop-flocher, & Bo-Lassen, 1983; De Nil et al., 2003; Neumann et al., 2005). Still, evidence of such changes is not equivalent to evidence of eliminating the fluency impairment. So, given the many uncertainties in determining which cases will recover from stuttering, clinicians should refrain from promising a client that fluency therapy will lead to full recovery from the disorder and normalized fluency. For the same reason, clinicians should not be overly enthusiastic about endorsing the client's desire to be rid of stuttering. That said, it also is not advisable for a clinician to tell a client that complete recovery from stuttering is an impossible outcome, for that too is unknown, and there are numerous documented cases where speakers reportedly attained normalized fluency long after the onset of stuttering symptoms (Wingate, 1964b).

So, how should a clinician respond when a client expresses the desire to be rid of stuttering? The first step is to validate the client's desire. Stuttering can result in significant communication disability and, over time, it can lead to significant emotional distress. It is understandable that a speaker would want to be rid of such a disorder. Given the lack of understanding about the role of fluency therapy in the attainment of normalized fluency, however, it is advisable to encourage the client first to strive toward intermediate outcomes that are realistic and attainable. These intermediate outcomes are, in a sense, destinations on the road to recovery. From this perspective, a client's success is defined in terms of developing the ability to realize significant reductions in communication disability. Such outcomes are consistent with current views on the etiology of stuttering and the notion of compensated fluency. Over time, the client may discover that the ability to manage stuttering effectively is a satisfying final destination. Data from a study by Plexico et al. (2005) exemplify this outcome. Plexico et al. analyzed the common experiences of adults who developed the ability to manage stuttering successfully over time and, from this analysis, they identified several common themes associated with successful stuttering management, including the following: an optimistic,positive view toward life; a sense of accomplishment, the sense that stuttering no longer played a primary factor in one's life choices; a reduction in stuttering-related anxiety, and a sense of being able to speak freely.

"I want to sound like a normal speaker." For other speakers who stutter, the primary long-range goal is to sound like a nonstuttering speaker. Clients who define success in this way aim for speech that is indistinguishable from that of nonstuttering speakers in terms of continuity, rate, rhythm, and naturalness. The speaker is not necessarily striving to resolve the impairment that causes stuttering but rather to compensate for it to such an extent that the effects of impairment are no longer apparent to the listener. Guitar (2006) used the term "controlled fluency" to refer to this type of speaking pattern.

A client who seeks to attain controlled fluency will continue to anticipate instances of stuttering-related disfluency and, thus, will continue to self-identify as a person who stutters. When the client is able to manage anticipated stuttering-related disfluency effectively through application of various stuttering management techniques, his or her speech will sound similar to that of typical speakers in terms of continuity. Controlled fluency implies a need to attend to speech production extensively in order to detect and then compensate for impending segments of disfluent speech. In our clinical

experience, many speakers who stutter find it effortful to implement controlled fluency for long periods of time. Some clients may aim for an outcome in which *all* instances of impending stuttering are managed effectively. Relatively few speakers who stutter are able to attain this lofty outcome, however, in part because of the difficulties associated with the need for continuous speech vigilance and in part because of the practical limitations associated with the use of treatments that are compensatory in nature.

The challenges associated with gaining complete control over fluency are reflected in the methods that contemporary researchers use to define "successful treatment outcomes." For instance, Bothe, Davidow, Bramlett, and Ingham (2006) considered a treatment outcome successful if the posttreatment stuttering frequency scores for research participants dropped below 5% syllables stuttered. Their standard for success is somewhat liberal when compared with past standards wherein the stated goal for some treatments was to "eliminate" the overt indicators of stuttering from posttreatment speech samples (e.g., Shames & Florance, 1980).

When a client expresses the desire to "sound like a normal speaker," it is important that the clinician clarify the client's expectations for success and his or her motivation for pursuing the goal. Ideally, the client's motivation for controlled fluency will stem from a desire to communicate more competently, compensate more effectively, or something similar. Motivations of this sort are consistent with the properties of present-day behavioral treatments. As noted above, most people who stutter—even adults—find it quite difficult to control fluency at all times. This means that symptoms of stuttered speech will be apparent at least some of the time that the person talks. Thus, when a client states the desire to implement controlled fluency on a "24/7" basis, it is advisable first to validate his or her push for excellence. Eventually, though, it is wise to counsel the client about the practical difficulties associated with that goal and to discuss alternate outcomes that are more feasible to attain. It also is worth encouraging the client to consider the possibility that one does not need to control fluency with 100% accuracy in order to communicate competently or eliminate stuttering-related communication disability.

"I want to hide my fluency impairment from listeners." For still other clients who stutter, the primary long-range goal is to conceal their fluency impairment from other people. As with clients who want to sound "normally fluent," clients who define success in terms of listener awareness aim for speech that is indistinguishable from that of nonstuttering speakers in terms of continuity, rate, rhythm, and naturalness. One way to accomplish this is through the use of controlled fluency. Speakers who yet have to learn formal strategies for how to control fluency or who realize only partial benefit from controlled fluency methods also may rely on potentially maladaptive compensations such as word avoidance, circumlocution, and attempting to time syllable initiation to rhythmic movements of nonspeech body parts such as a finger or hand. In short, the speaker may resort to whatever is necessary in order to conceal the overt symptoms of stuttering from listeners. A client who seeks to hide fluency impairment from others will continue to anticipate instances of stuttering-related disfluency and, thus, will continue to self-identify as a person who stutters.

When a client evaluates treatment success in terms of how well he or she can hide stuttering from others, it requires the clinician's immediate attention. In such cases, it is important for the clinician first to validate the client's concern about revealing fluency impairment to others. The desire to hide stuttering from listeners often is fueled by the speaker's expectation that listeners will have negative reactions toward the stuttered speech or people who stutter, as well as feelings of shame, embarrassment, frustration, and so forth, that the client may have developed over time in response to others' reactions and/or self-defined expectations for performance. Although the speaker's motivation for concealing fluency impairment through controlled fluency is understandable, it is not particularly constructive given the nature of the disorder and the limitations of contemporary treatments and self-devised compensatory strategies. That is, it is highly likely that others eventually will know that the client stutters. Consequently, the client ends up pursuing an unattainable goal.

The clinician's job in such cases is to help the client to alter his or her perspective on success. This likely will mean that the clinician introduces activities that are designed to promote the client's understanding of his or her fluency impairment and any disability that stems from it. The notion of understanding does not in any way imply that the client should feel resigned to a life of communication disability. Rather, it simply is intended to help the client develop a more accurate view of the current limits of his or her speech production system and to embrace the idea of learning to use the speech production system as effectively as possible. Clients can be very slow to shift from a "hide stuttering" perspective into a "communicate more competently" or a "reduce disability" perspective. Implicit within each of the latter perspectives is a willingness on the part of the client both to acknowledge that he or she has impaired fluency and to allow the symptoms of stuttering to be on display sometimes for others to see and hear. The latter outcome is discussed further in the next section.

"I want to stutter less severely." Some speakers who stutter recognize that they may not be able to control every instance of stuttering and simply want to stutter in a less severe way. Guitar (2006) referred to this outcome as "acceptable stuttering." With this pattern of speech, the speaker will continue to anticipate instances of stuttering and thus will continue to self-identify as a person who stutters. Rather than attempting to prevent or conceal impending disfluency, as was the case with the "controlled fluency" and "hide stuttering" outcomes described previously, the client instead attempts to minimize the severity or impact of disfluency as much as possible when it occurs. To do this most effectively, the client, of course, needs to feel comfortable with having other people hear the stuttered speech. The stuttering management strategies that commonly are used to reduce stuttering severity are quite similar to those that are used to control fluency. One main difference between them is that controlled fluency relies on the ability to *prevent* the effects of fluency impairment through active management of speech production at all times (i.e., both when fluency disruption is anticipated and when fluency disruption is not anticipated). In contrast, the notion of acceptable stuttering emphasizes the ability to *respond* to fluency disruption while it occurs, immediately after it occurs, and, eventually, immediately prior to when it occurs.

What Do Clinicians Expect?

Speech-language pathologists are likely to be in unanimous agreement that the success of a treatment program should not be defined in terms of a client's ability to hide stuttering from others. There also probably is widespread agreement among clinicians that the success of a treatment program for a speaker with an acquired fluency disorder should be defined in terms of the extent to which the speaker can compensate effectively for his or her fluency impairment. Curiously, however, when it comes to cases of developmental stuttering, there is less agreement with regard to what the long-term goal of fluency therapy should be and how clinical success should be defined. The main source of disagreement with regard to developmental stuttering seems to revolve around the extent to which clinicians feel that speakers who stutter should strive to attain controlled fluency and, with it, the ability to sound like a normally fluent speaker. The differing views on this matter are exemplified by statements that Cooper (1987) and Shames and Florance (1980) made about treatment outcomes. Cooper (1987, p. 381) stated that fluent speech is "an unrealistic goal" for many clients and that clinicians do clients a disservice when they pursue the "simplistic notion" that every client can develop fluent sounding speech. In contrast, Shames and Florance (1980, p. 19) stated that the primary goal of treatment is "to establish speech that is free of stuttering" and to help the speaker attain the self-perception of being "someone who no longer stutters." Although Cooper (1987) and Shames and Florance (1980) made their remarks years ago, differences in opinion about the long-term goal for therapy with speakers who stutter continue today. For instance, in an editorial column for the journal *Language, Speech, and Hearing Services in Schools,* Nippold (2011) decried what she perceived as a trend in the treatment literature toward encouraging children who stutter to accept stuttering and to focus on developing effective coping strategies for stuttering rather than on developing strategies that yield fluent sounding speech. The editorial prompted a vociferous response from Yaruss, Coleman, and Quesal (2012), who outlined the tenants of a broad-based approach to stuttering treatment that targeted both improved speech continuity *and* reduced stuttering-related disability, including disability that stems from feelings, attitudes, and emotions associated with fluency impairment.

Yaruss et al. (2012) maintained that helping clients gain acceptance of their fluency impairment does not preclude their ability to improve speech fluency and, if anything, is likely to increase those chances. The latter notion is consistent with the idea of compensated fluency, discussed earlier in this chapter. The speaker attempts to speak as fluently as possible, but accepts that, despite his or her best efforts, stuttering-related disfluency still may occur in some situations. When the disfluency does occur, the most constructive response is to accept that this is "part of the territory" that comes with persistent developmental stuttering. The speaker's goal at that point is to deal with the disfluency as effectively as possible through the use of whatever fluency management strategies he or she wishes to employ. An approach of this sort allows for the possibility of simultaneously striving toward both controlled fluency *and* acceptable stuttering, wherein speakers attempt to talk in a way that minimizes the occurrence of stuttering-related disfluency, and it allows for effective management or mod-

ification of stuttering-related disfluency if it should occur. The net result is that the speaker still may show signs of impairment but no longer shows additional signs of disability.

In a reply to Yaruss et al. (2012), Nippold (2012b) voiced general agreement with many points that Yaruss et al. raised, but reiterated the point stated in her 2011 editorial about the need for data on the efficacy of the assorted treatments used with school-aged children, and particularly those treatments that help children improve control over stuttering symptoms. The latter approach is not necessarily inconsistent with the idea of compensated fluency.

Staged Outcomes

Rather than defining success as an either/ or proposition, it may be more constructive to think of it as a staged construct. In this way, clients and clinicians can think of success in terms of near-, mid-, and long-term outcomes. With this approach, the outcome that a client works toward in the near term (e.g., 3 months from now) will differ from that for the mid-term (e.g., 1 year from now), which in turn will differ from that for the long term (e.g., 3 to 5 years from now). Thus, an adult client with moderately severe stuttering might aim to develop the capacity for controlled fluency and effective disfluency modification during the course of a semester, the ability to manage stuttering effectively in many daily activities during a 3-year period, and then aspire toward experiencing no stuttering-based disability during a 5-year period. An approach like this is consistent with Shapiro's (2011) idea that, for many clients with persistent fluency impairment, the successful management of stuttering is indeed a journey. Although clients often find that their speech motor patterns change relatively quickly, their stuttering-related emotions and attitudes change much more slowly. Thus, adoption of an extended time line for evaluating treatment outcomes helps clients to see that the journey toward successful stuttering management is progressing at a pace that is similar to that for other people who stutter.

General Treatment Principles

The focus for the remainder of the chapter shifts to general treatment principles that are embedded within many of the contemporary behavioral treatments for stuttering. Six principles are described; each is presented in Figure 13–2. As shown in

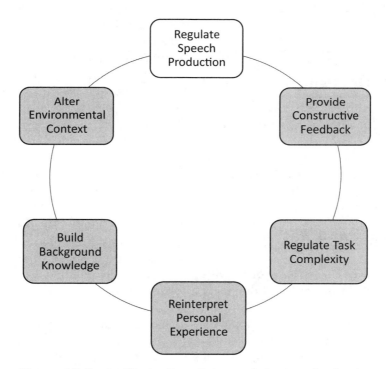

Figure 13–2. An illustration of six general principles for the treatment of stuttering and other fluency disorders. With the exception of regulated speech production, each of the principles pertains to the context within which the client talks. It is assumed that each of the principles connects with all of the other principles. For example, when a clinician or caregiver provides a client with constructive feedback about the client's fluency, the client may subsequently begin to regulate his or her speech production and may expand on background knowledge about the fluency disorder. Most of the treatment approaches described in the contemporary fluency disorders literature incorporate several of these principles; however, in most approaches, one or two of the principles are emphasized much more than the others.

the figure, five of the treatment principles deal with the context within which a client speaks. The remaining principle (regulation of speech production) deals directly with the act of speaking. In the remainder of the section, these principles are discussed in terms of their characteristics, rationale, and application. In clinical practice, a treatment plan might incorporate some or all of these principles, depending on the client's goals and the nature of his or her communication impairment.

Providing Clients With Feedback

Many treatment approaches incorporate the practice of providing clients with feedback about their speech fluency. The primary characteristics of this treatment principle are described in this section.

Overview and Rationale

Feedback involves the process of providing clients with information about their performance on a particular task. In the context of fluency therapy, the main focus is on providing clients with moment-to-moment feedback that relates to speech fluency. The rationale for providing feedback in a therapeutic setting is straightforward: it is difficult for a client to function in some new or different way if the client does not know how he or she currently functions. Feedback addresses this situation by helping the client become aware of what he or she is doing and, in some cases, how well he or she is doing it. Results from numerous studies indicate that the delivery of feedback immediately following stuttering-related disfluency

often leads to a decrease in the frequency and/or duration of the stuttering-related disfluency (Onslow, 1996; Prins & Hubbard, 1988).

Applications

Feedback has been used extensively in treatments for stuttering. In stuttering treatment programs, clinicians usually are the first to provide clients with systematic feedback about their performance. Over time, however, caregivers may do so, as well (Onslow, 1996). In some treatment approaches, the provision of systematic feedback constitutes the primary intervention strategy (e.g., Onslow, Packman, & Harrison, 2003). Over time, a clinician's feedback to a client can serve as a model for how to self-evaluate one's behavior. The ability to accurately self-evaluate one's performance is a critical component in the maintenance of treatment gains following the completion of a formal treatment session, as it leads directly to the identification of specific behaviors a client would need to change in order to get performance back on track. Table 13–2 contains several examples of ways in which speech-language pathologists have used feedback when treating clients who stutter. As shown in Table 13–2, the types of feedback that clinicians provide to clients vary in detail and purpose. Specific details about the various feedback types are described below.

Feedback as a Means of Highlighting Behavior

The most basic type of feedback is that which *highlights* the presence of a behavior. The clinician's aim is merely to signal to the client that a behavior of interest

Table 13–2. Types of Feedback Presented in Conjunction With Stuttering-Related Behavior

Type	Description	Feedback Examples	Presentation
Highlighting	Clinician informs client that client produced a behavior of interest (e.g., stuttering). Client is not asked to alter speech but may do so anyway.	• Mechanical signal (e.g., bell, light) • Gesture (e.g., hand raise, pointing, throat clear)	During or just after behavior of interest occurs
Evaluating	Clinician informs client about how client performed regarding predetermined criterion. Client is not asked to alter speech but may do so anyway.	• Verbal statements (e.g., "yes," "almost," "good," "not quite") • Gesture (e.g., a "slow down" gesture with arm movement)	During or just after behavior of interest occurs
Directing	Clinician informs client that client produced a particular behavior and, consequently, now should produce some other specified behavior.	• *Client:* Produces lip tremor on [p] in *pie* • *Clinician:* "Stop . . . " • *Client:* Stops saying [p], pauses for 5 s, restarts *pie* (hopefully without tremor)	During or just after behavior of interest occurs
Describing	After client produces a stuttering-related behavior, clinician tells client what client just did.	• *Client:* "G- g- g- get that out of here." • *Clinician:* "That sounded bumpy." • *Client:* "Put that over there." • *Clinician:* "That was smooth."	Just after behavior of interest occurs

has occurred. Feedback of this sort can be delivered in various ways (i.e., vocally, manual gestures, mechanical noises)—anything that is salient to the client. Examples of behaviors that a clinician or caregiver might attempt to highlight include stuttered or cluttered speech, fluent speech, and use of stuttering-related secondary behavior such as eye blinking. The clinician's main challenge when attempting to highlight client behavior is to present the feedback signal in close temporal proximity to the behavior of interest. The behavioral markers of stuttered speech

often are fleeting. For example, the part-word repetitions and sound prolongations of young children who stutter often last less than 1 second (Logan & Conture, 1997; Zebrowski, 1991, 1994). Thus, by the time the clinician presents the highlighting signal, the client may have already advanced the utterance by several syllables. At this point, the feedback is no longer precisely linked with the behavior that the clinician attempted to highlight, and the client may think that the clinician was highlighting a behavior other than the one the clinician intended to highlight.

Prins and Hubbard (1988) reviewed a number of experiments in which the effects of various response contingencies on stuttering frequency were examined. In experiments where aversive stimuli (i.e., electrical shock, loud tones, noise) were paired with stuttered speech, nine studies reported a decrease in stuttering frequency, three reported mixed results, and four reported no effect. In experiments where neutral stimuli (i.e., light, digital counter, pure tone) were paired with stuttered speech, one study reported a decrease in stuttering frequency, two reported mixed results, and two reported no effect. Fortunately, the use of aversive stimuli to highlight stuttering-related disfluency has fallen into disfavor since the 1980s. The findings from such studies did, however, demonstrate that speakers who stutter exhibit intrinsic resources for managing stuttering-related disfluency.

Feedback as a Means of Evaluating, Describing, or Directing Behavior

Another use of feedback is to *evaluate* what a client has done. With evaluative feedback, the clinician not only highlights a behavior that a client produces but also simultaneously comments on its accuracy, appropriateness, or desirability in relation to some predetermined standard. Evaluative feedback is, of course, a staple of learning in all sorts of domains. Teachers provide evaluative feedback to students on examinations; coaches provide evaluative feedback to athletes during practice drills; and parents provide evaluative feedback to their children during activities such as coloring and dressing.

Evaluative feedback can be simple in both form and content (e.g., "good," "not quite," "uh-oh"). In Prins and Hubbard's

(1988) review of response contingency research, there were two studies that reported significant reductions in stuttering frequency in conjunction with positive evaluative feedback (i.e., "good") and no studies with negative findings. In addition, among studies that utilized aversive forms of evaluative feedback (e.g., "no," "not good," "wrong," and laugher), nine reported a significant decrease in stuttering frequency, one reported mixed results, and one reported no effect. Interestingly, however, in two other studies, presentation of an ambiguous word (i.e., "tree") also resulted in a significant decrease in stuttering frequency (Cooper, Cady, & Robbins, 1970; Daly & Kimbarow, 1978). Thus, it may be that almost any type of verbal contingency that is linked with stuttered speech can prompt a client to recruit internal resources that reduce stuttering frequency.

In other cases, researchers have paired descriptive labels with speech production. Feedback of this sort constitutes a primary intervention strategy in the Lidcombe Program (Onslow et al., 2003), a well-researched treatment for preschoolers who stutter. Under the Lidcombe approach, clinicians and, eventually, caregivers deliver descriptive comments about a child's fluency during circumscribed intervention activities. The adults primarily make descriptive remarks about the child's fluent speech (e.g., "That sounded smooth"). Occasionally, however, they remark on the child's stuttered speech as well (e.g., "That sounded bumpy"). Although there is more to the Lidcombe treatment approach than these remarks, the descriptive feedback is a primary component of the approach. Implicit in the clinician's provision of the descriptive feedback is a request for the child to speak more fluently than he or she currently is.

The provision of such feedback to young children seems to be powerful, based on the many published accounts of positive treatment outcomes with the Lidcombe approach. It is interesting to note that, in the Lidcombe Program, clinicians devote little time to didactic instruction in speech production. Rather, the child essentially is left to figure out how to change "bumpy speech" into "smooth speech." To the extent that young children succeed at doing this, it again appears that people who stutter possess internal resources that enable them to compensate for the developmental impairment that causes them to stutter. Descriptive feedback is a mechanism that seems to prompt children to activate these resources. Clinicians and parents typically present the feedback on a predetermined schedule. Initially, feedback is provided often (in therapy activities, perhaps even continuously), but over time, it is faded and presented intermittently.

With older children, teens, and adults, clinicians also can, of course, present more detailed forms of evaluative feedback. Feedback of this sort typically would occur following the completion of a speaking task or following completion of speaking behaviors that are especially noteworthy. Detailed evaluative feedback provides clients with a critique of what they do during the course of an activity, as well as the clinician's assessment of what did and did not go well. Such information also provides clients with a model how they can self-evaluate their stuttering-related behavior.

Feedback also can be used in activities that are designed to direct or shape behavioral change more directly. When implementing feedback in this manner, the clinician administers a signal of some sort (e.g., a tone, a hand signal, a verbal remark such as "stop") that is contingent upon a stuttering-relevant behavior that the client has produced. The clinician attaches a contingency (e.g., stop talking for 5 seconds) to the client's stuttering-relevant behavior, which the client is to implement immediately after the clinician's presentation of the signal. The clinician delivers the feedback to the client in "real time;" that is, during or immediately after the behavior of interest. A number of single-subject experiments (e.g., James, 1981; James & Ingham, 1974; James, Ricciardelli, Rogers, & Hunter, 1989; Martin, Kuhl, & Haroldson, 1972) have demonstrated the effectiveness of this approach at reducing stuttering frequency, on both an immediate and a long-term basis.

Regulating Task Complexity

The next treatment principle pertains to the difficulty level associated with fluency intervention activities. Many treatment programs emphasize the importance of having clients develop fluency management strategies within the context of activities that are appropriately challenging.

Overview and Rationale

There are a host of variables that potentially can affect the likelihood that a speaker will stutter in a given utterance or situation. Some of the variables that affect speech fluency are intrinsic to the utterances a speaker produces (e.g., the number of syllables or syntactic units within an utterance, the stress patterns within a phrase, topic familiarity, the extent to which utterance form and content are rehearsed or formulaic). Other variables are associated with the behavior of the speaker's communication partner (e.g., the partner's speaking rate, interruption patterns, verbal and nonverbal reactions to stuttered speech). Still other variables are associated with characteristics of the communication environment (e.g., the presence of background noise, the number and nature of distracting stimuli, the amount of time the conversational participants have available to complete their conversation, the nature of the relationship between the speaker and the communication partner). Because variables such as these can impact stuttering-related behavior, speech-language pathologists usually attempt to control the extent to which they are present during treatment activities. One main reason for regulating task complexity is to create practice environments that are appropriately challenging in relation to a client's current level of fluency functioning. When the task demands of an activity are regulated in this way, the client is more likely to spend a relatively high percentage of the time during an activity engaged in successful fluency management than he or she would be if the task demands are not managed.

Applications

Regulation of task complexity is easiest to accomplish during in-clinic activities. In this setting, clinicians can design activities that help the speaker who stutters build his or her ability to apply specific fluency management skills in a controlled setting that is conducive to success. Because many fluency management skills are behavioral in nature, the activities are structured to promote opportunities for massed practice. In this regard, the activities have a structure that is similar to what an athlete

or musician would encounter during practice or a lesson.

It also is possible to regulate aspects of task complexity during real-world activities. Given the dynamic nature of events in real-world settings, however, it seldom is possible to control all relevant task complexity variables to the extent that it is possible within the clinic. Thus, activities that are conducted in beyond-clinic settings usually are less predictable and, hence, more challenging for fluency impaired speakers than activities that are conducted in within-clinic settings. Determination of appropriate levels of complexity for a particular task is essentially done on a trial and error basis. A clinician can identify the appropriate level for a particular activity through the use of informal assessment activities during a therapy session, wherein the key variable is presented to varying degrees and the client's fluency at each level is measured. In the treatment literature for fluency disorders, the aim generally is to determine the task level at which the client is able to perform with a high level of success, such as 90% or greater (e.g., Ingham, 1999; Ryan & Van Kirk Ryan, 1995; Shames & Florance, 1980). Over time, practice activities usually progress as follows: low task complexity → medium task complexity → high task complexity. When a client demonstrates satisfactory performance in the use of a particular fluency management skill at a particular task complexity level, subsequent practice activities are conducted at the next highest task complexity level. Thus, practice activities usually unfold over time in an "easiest to hardest" progression.

Speech-language pathologists often attempt to control the linguistic complexity of utterances that clients produce during in-clinic practice activities in the initial stages of treatment. Linguistic complexity can be defined in several ways. Examples of the most commonly manipulated linguistic variables during practice activities are shown in Table 13–3. As indicated in the table, phonological complexity is defined most often in terms of the number syllables per response. This variable is relatively easy to control at the word and phrase levels. However, as the number of syllables per utterance increases, it is likely that the number of words and syntactic constituents per utterance will increase as well. Thus, clinicians should be aware that the "syllable length" of an utterance may be confounded with these other variables.

The pragmatic function of an utterance also can be regulated in practice activities. For many years, it was thought that children stuttered more often when

Table 13–3. Variables That Clinicians Can Manipulate When Attempting to Control Task Complexity in Practice Activities

General	Specific	Examples
Phonologic	Number of syllables per word, phrase, or utterance	Word: *Ann* (1) vs. *Angelina* (4) Phrase: *In Denver* (3) vs. *In Philadelphia* (6) Utterance: *New York has the Knicks* (5) vs. *Oklahoma City has the Thunder* (10)
Syntactic	Number of syntactic units (constituents) per utterance	*John is hungry* (3) vs. *John ate pizza quickly today* (5)
	Phrasal elaboration	*Walter* vs. *Uncle Walter* vs. *My Uncle Walter*
	Developmental difficulty of syntactic form	*The boy is napping* vs. *After he eats lunch, the boy naps*
Pragmatic	Speech act type	*Assertive act* vs. *Responsive act* *Responding to request for information* vs. *Responding to request for clarification*
Temporal	Number of conversational turns per minute	*Few turns per minute* vs. *Many turns per minute*
	Time allotted for response production	*Open ended* vs. *Constrained*; *Short* vs. *Long*
Environment	Physical characteristics	*Quiet* vs. *Noisy*
	Audience characteristics	*Few audience members* vs. *Many audience members*; *Familiar* vs. *Unfamiliar*; *Patient* vs. *Impatient*
Clinician support	Feedback or cueing frequency	*Continuous* vs. *Intermittent*

Note. Numbers in parentheses indicate the number of linguistic units within a word, phrase, or utterance. Underlined text denotes syntactic constituents.

responding to questions than they did when making comments or statements. Subsequent research has demonstrated that this is not true, at least during conversational interactions between parents and children (Logan, 2003a; Weiss & Zebrowski, 1992). In this context, parents mainly tend to pose "close-ended requests" to their children. These are questions that can be answered in a word or a phrase (e.g., Parent: *What color is it?* Child: *Blue.*; Parent: *When are you leaving?* Child: *After lunch.*) Brief responses like these have a higher probability of being spoken fluently than responses that consist of fully developed sentences or several sentences in succession. The latter types of response are more likely to occur when a parent poses an "open-ended request" to a child (e.g., *Tell me about the movie.*) or when a child is making a comment or statement about an event. Certain request types do seem to be more challenging than others. For example, clients who stutter often report that it is more difficult to respond fluently to a request for clarification than it is to a request for information. Thus, in Example 13–1 below, the response to the request for clarification contains an instances of part-word repetition but the same target utterance, when produced as a response to a request for information is spoken fluently. The difference in fluency between the two versions of the utterance may occur because the speaker is expected to initiate the response to the request for clarification without the slightest bit of hesitation (since the speaker just said the sentence a few moments earlier).

Example 13–1:

Parent: Where are you going after school? (Request for Information)

Child: Over to Mario's house.

Parent: What did you say? Where are you going? (Request for Clarification)

Child: O- o- over to Mario's house.

Over time, as a client's capacity for managing stuttering-related disfluency improves, a clinician can systematically introduce fluency stressors like this during treatment activities so that the client can practice managing fluency in a range of discourse contexts.

Developing Background Knowledge

It is said that knowledge is power. The next treatment principle deals with helping fluency-impaired clients and their family members develop as much knowledge as possible about the nature of speech fluency and fluency disorders. Such knowledge most likely will prove to be useful during the course of a fluency intervention program.

Overview and Rationale

It is not uncommon for clients to enter into treatment having a limited and/or inaccurate understanding of their fluency disorder. This is potentially problematic because it can hinder communication between the clinician and client with regard to treatment activities, and it can lead to client to develop distorted or inaccurate concepts about the nature of his or her fluency impairment. Such misconceptions can contribute to the client's development of self-limiting thoughts and beliefs that relate to his or her communication skills and ability to benefit from therapy (Egan, 1998). In addition, it can limit a client's ability to self-evaluate his or her speech behavior in an objective manner. The latter skill is important in the modification of speech disfluency and also in the generalization and maintenance of fluency management skills. For these reasons, it is important that the clinician and client be "on the same page" with regard to their understanding of stuttering.

Application

It is not expected that clients will develop a professional-level understanding of fluency disorders (although some highly motivated clients do indeed develop this kind of understanding). Rather, the main objective is for clients to have a basic, age-appropriate understanding of what their fluency disorder is, how it affects their speech production and daily functioning, and what can be done to treat it. Background knowledge about stuttering can be presented at both "population" and "client" levels. Population-level information pertains to general facts about stuttering and people who stutter. Client-level information pertains to facts about the client's particular patterns of speech and associated experiences as a person who stutters.

There are a host of topics and issues that can be explored under the heading of stuttering knowledge. Examples of such topics are shown in Table 13–4. The client's age, development, and treatment needs will influence the depth with which topics like those in Table 13–4 are

Table 13–4. Examples of Topics to Explore When Building a Client's Understanding of Fluency Disorders

General Concepts	Specific Concepts
Nature of the fluency disorder	• Current views on etiology • Current epidemiological facts
Normal speech production	• Speech breathing, phonation, and articulation • Factors that contribute to disfluency
Common symptoms of fluency impairment	• Characteristics of stuttered speech (e.g., continuity, rate, rhythm, effort, naturalness, talkativeness, stability) • Common compensatory (secondary) behaviors • Factors that contribute to variations in stuttering severity • Characteristic activity limitations and participation restrictions • Fluency-enhancing conditions
Impact of the fluency disorder	• Common attitudes, feelings, and beliefs about speaking and stuttering • Characteristic strategies that speakers use to cope with stuttering • Listener reactions when interacting with people who stutter • Impact on quality of life (teasing, bullying, social aspects, employment effects, etc.)

Note. Similar topics can be explored to build knowledge of cluttering.

explored. Clients typically have a limited understanding of speech production. If self-evaluation strategies and speech regulation strategies are part of the treatment plan, there is value in reviewing concepts concerning the anatomy and physiology of speech production. Aspects of the various fluency dimensions are worth reviewing, as well, particularly those that are relevant to the client's stuttering pattern. With pre-teen-, teen-, and adult-aged clients, clinicians can delve further into details about certain concepts such as discussing speech disfluency patterns that are common in stuttering and those that occur most often in the client's speech. In some families, stuttering becomes a neglected or taboo topic of conversation. Consequently, the client rarely talks about his or her communication difficulties directly or at length (Logan & Yaruss, 1999; Rustin

& Cook, 1995). In such cases, the client may truly welcome the opportunities to talk about something that is such a central part of daily life and to discover that there are many other people who share the communication experiences that they encounter.

High-quality educational materials for stuttering are readily available through a variety of means. In addition to clinician-developed materials, there are print and video informational materials available for free or at nominal cost through a host of professional and consumer-oriented organizations (see Table 13–5 for examples). Most of these organizations also have well-developed websites that provide free, easy-to-access information. Several university and government sponsored websites provide information as well. Several people who stutter have started

Table 13–5. Examples of Sources Through Which Clients and Consumers Can Obtain Information About Stuttering

Associations and Organizations	Universities and Government Agencies
American Speech-Language-Hearing Association	The Stuttering Center of Western Pennsylvania
Australian Speak Easy Association	The Stuttering Homepage
Indian Stammering Association	The University College London Archive of Stuttered Speech
International Fluency Association	
International Stuttering Association	United States National Library of Medicine
Irish Stammering Association	United States National Institute on Deafness and Other Communication Disorders
The British Stammering Association	
The Canadian Stuttering Association	
The European League of Stuttering Associations	**Fiction and Nonfiction Books**
The National Stuttering Association	Autobiographical accounts of stuttering
The Stuttering Foundation	Fictional portrayals of stuttering in children's literature

Note. These sources are presented for illustrative purposes only. The associations, organizations, universities, and government agencies feature websites through which clients and consumers can access information. The list is not exhaustive, and the inclusion of a site in this table does not imply that the author endorses the website, its sponsor, or its associated content.

Web-based forums that are devoted to stuttering. Some of these websites provide opportunities for online chatting with other people who stutter and for viewing recorded lectures and discussions about various facets of stuttering. In the context of treatment, clinicians can screen such venues and, after deeming them appropriate, encourage or assign clients to review such information.

For older clients who enjoy books, there are a number of well-written autobiographies written by people who stutter. Lists of such books are available on websites such as *The Stuttering Homepage* or *The Stuttering Foundation* and through the search engines of commercial bookseller websites. For children and teens, there are a host of fictional accounts of stuttering. Logan, Mullins, and Jones (2008) reviewed 29 such books and discussed potential ways to use the books in the context of fluency therapy. Many of the books that they reviewed included accounts of how characters manage the social and emotional challenges that come with stuttering. Several books included vivid depictions of bullying. These fictional accounts provide an excellent starting point for discussions and problem-solving activities that deal with how children who stutter can manage similar challenges in their lives. In general, the introduction of informational materials into a treatment program provides opportunities for clients who stutter to discuss their speech experiences with other family members.

Altering Environmental Context

A person's functioning can be affected by surrounding events. Thus, when developing treatment plans for fluency-impaired speakers, clinicians should consider carefully the impact of environmental events on speech fluency.

Overview and Rationale

As indicated in the ICF framework (WHO, 2001), environmental factors either can facilitate or hinder an individual's functioning. For most clients who stutter, the severity of their stuttering will vary as a function of the environmental setting within which they speak. A host of environmental factors have been associated with the exacerbation of fluency difficulties in speakers who stutter (Bloodstein & Bernstein Ratner, 2008). Some of these factors are communicative in nature (e.g., the speech-language behaviors of a speaking partner). Others are socioemotional in nature (e.g., a speaking partner's verbal and nonverbal reactions to stuttered speech). And still others are societal or organizational in nature (e.g., a school district's policies for dealing with bullying behavior, the manner in which people who stutter are portrayed in film or media). Factors such as these can hinder a speaker's attempts at managing stuttering-related disfluency and thus are likely to warrant attention in many treatment plans.

Application

In the early stages of treatment, when a client is building the capacity for managing stuttering-related behaviors in the context of prescribed clinical and home-based activities, clinicians generally seek to control environmental stressors. The reasoning is that the fewer fluency stressors the client encounters during skill development, the more time the client will spend producing the newly developing fluency management skills successfully. During the performance-building phase of treatment, when the client begins to apply newly learned fluency management skills in real-world settings, environmental stressors are much more difficult to control. However, clinicians (and, sometimes, clients) can take steps to minimize their occurrence in family, classroom, and work settings by training key people in those environments to alter their communicative behaviors and emotional responses to stuttered speech in ways that are likely to facilitate fluency (Logan & Caruso, 1997; Starkweather, Gottwald, & Halfond, 1990; Gottwald, 2010). The specific behaviors to be altered or manipulated will vary across cases, but examples include the following:

- *Competition for obtaining a speaking turn* (conversational pace): Examples of relevant variables include the number of utterances produced by conversational participants per minute, the duration of pause times between conversational turns, and the number of conversational turns in which speakers talk simultaneously.
- *Competition for maintaining a speaking turn:* Examples of relevant variables include the frequency with which speaking partners interrupt the client's speech, and the frequency with which speaking partners attempt to fill in words when the client is in the midst of stuttering-related disfluency.
- *Partner's verbal and nonverbal responses when the client is speaking:* Examples of relevant variables include the frequency

with which the listener produces expressions or actions that suggest concern or impatience toward disfluent speech, the extent to which the listener makes remarks about the adequacy of the client's speech, and the frequency with which the listener offers speech-related advice to the client.

- *Communication setting:* Examples of relevant variables include audience size, audience composition (e.g., acquaintances vs. strangers), and physical settings (e.g., public space vs. private room).
- *The way in which the partner engages the client in conversation:* A partner's use of open-ended requests (e.g., *Tell me all about the movie.*) obligate the client to produce multiutterance responses, which may be challenging for clients who still are in the process of establishing the capacity for managing stuttering-related disfluency. In contrast, use of closed-ended requests (e.g., *What was the name of the movie? Was it very scary?*) obligate much shorter responses, and, in turn, increase the client's chances for successful management of stuttering in the situation (Logan & Caruso, 1997).

To summarize, the basic idea is that by minimizing the extent to which the client encounters environmental stressors when interacting with "communication allies" such as family members, friends, and coworkers, clinicians and clients can create semicontrolled practice contexts in real-world settings. Such contexts act as a bridge between the client's highly facilitative speaking environment in the clinic and the "rough-and-tumble" communicative situations that the client is certain to encounter when dealing with unrestrained communication partners who, in their enthusiasm to communicate, show little regard for the rules of communication etiquette or the challenges that people who stutter face in obtaining and maintaining conversational turns.

Teasing and bullying also come under the domain of environmental context. Children who stutter are more than four times as likely to be victims of bullying as children in the general population are, and children who have been bullied are more likely to exhibit lower levels of optimism and self-esteem than children who have not been bullied (Blood et al., 2011). When children are being bullied for disfluent speech or any other reason, it is essential for the clinician, parents, and other related professionals (e.g., teachers, school counselors, school administrators) to take steps to address it. In addition to coordinating efforts with school personnel, self-help organizations like *The National Stuttering Association* and *The Stuttering Foundation* publish resource materials and workbooks that clinicians can use to help children who stutter learn about bullying and develop strategies for responding to it.

Reinterpreting Personal Experience

Activities that come under this treatment principle pertain to the feelings, thoughts, and beliefs that clients have about issues such as fluency impairment and communication disability. One's feelings, thoughts,

and beliefs can influence how one behaves and, thus, these issues have relevance in many treatment plans.

Overview and Rationale

As noted elsewhere in this text, fluency impairment can lead to broad-based communication disability along with social- and speech-based anxiety, a reduced sense of self-efficacy, an assortment of negative attitudes toward speaking, and a reduction in the overall quality of life (Bray, Kehle, Lawless, & Theodore, 2003; Craig, 1990; Craig et al., 2009; Mulcahy, Hennessey, Beilby, & Byrnes, 2008; Vanryckeghem & Brutten, 1996; Yaruss, & Quesal, 2006). These psychosocial and cognitive effects can persist into adulthood, and remain even after having participated in treatment (Craig, Blumgart, & Tran, 2011). To the extent that these personal factors are present in specific clients, they have the potential to impact communicative functioning adversely, and thus they warrant attention during treatment.

According to the American Speech-Language-Hearing Association (2007), counseling activities that assist clients with issues related to acceptance, adaptation, and decision making about communicative functioning are included within the scope of the practice of speech-language pathology. Prior to providing services for any aspect of communicative functioning, including counseling, however, the practitioner must evaluate his or her experience and expertise to determine whether referral to another, more qualified speech-language pathologist is appropriate. If a client's emotional, mood, or personal adjustment difficulties go beyond the realm of communication-related events to adversely impact many areas of life, it is appropriate to refer the client to a qualified mental health professional for comprehensive assessment.

Application

Desensitization

One approach to helping clients reinterpret their stuttering-related experiences is by helping them change how they react when stuttering occurs or is expected to occur. The main goal is to help clients react to speech disfluency in an objective, problem-solving manner, rather than in an emotional manner (e.g., *"Okay, my speech is stuck. I can deal with it by _____"* vs. *"Oh no, I'm stuttering!"*). The use of desensitization in the treatment of stuttering is long-standing. For example, Van Riper (1973) devoted an entire chapter to desensitization in his text on treatment approaches for stuttering. Throughout the years, Van Riper and other clinicians (e.g., Guitar, 2006) have described an assortment of techniques that are aimed at reducing client sensitivity toward stuttering. Examples of several such techniques follow:

- *Analysis of disfluency.* The client describes the physical behaviors that characterize his or her current disfluency pattern (e.g., *"I pressed my tongue against the roof of my mouth, and I clenched my jaw."*) In some cases, the client might conduct this analysis by imitating the sorts of disfluency that he or she currently produces.
- *Deliberate manipulation of disfluency.* Guitar (2006) discusses the idea of "freezing" stuttering-related disfluency. As a client begins to repeat or prolong speech, the clinician instructs the client to hold (freeze) the disfluency

purposefully. The clinician may have the client voluntarily extend the disfluency for much longer than the client's typical disfluencies last, and eventually the duration of the disfluency becomes so long that any negative emotions that were present at the start of the disfluency have dissipated. In some cases the freezing may even evoke laughter—an emotional reaction that is not ordinarily part of stuttered speech. An extension of the freezing technique involves purposeful variation of speech during a held disfluency, wherein the client is coached to deliberately vary speech parameters such as repetition rate, muscle tension, vocal pitch, and so forth. Such behaviors are designed to foster a sense of control within the speaker over the way disfluency is expressed. The establishment of an internal *locus of control* (i.e., a belief such as, "I am in charge of this." or "I can do this.") has been associated with the extent to which adults who stutter favorably respond to the adversities that come with a lifetime of stuttering (Craig et al., 2011).

- *Voluntary stuttering.* With voluntary stuttering, the client purposefully introduces stutter-like disfluency into speech during conversation. The rationale behind the technique is that purposeful production of the feared behavior (in this case, stuttering) will lessen the fear of it over time. When a client is less fearful of stuttering in front of others, he or she will be Lbetter positioned to focus on employing fluency management skills.

In our experience, many speakers who stutter (not to mention, many clinicians) find voluntary stuttering very challenging to do, and many clients do not appreciate the rationale for the technique or its potential benefits, even after extensive explanation. For these reasons, it is not advisable to push voluntary stuttering on a client who is uncomfortable with the approach. Furthermore, much of the data to support the technique is anecdotal or case-based in nature. Despite some encouraging reports (e.g., Murphy, Yaruss, & Quesal, 2007), it seems that if the technique is to be used at all, it is most appropriate to implement it in conjunction with treatment strategies that are backed by stronger evidence, and the clinician should monitor the client's response to it carefully. Murphy et al. used such an approach when they combined traditional desensitization strategies with a cognitive restructuring treatment. The latter type of treatment is described in more detail in the following section.

Cognitive Behavioral Therapy

In recent years, a number of clinicians have incorporated elements of cognitive behavioral therapy (CBT) as a part of fluency treatment plans. This practice most commonly is implemented with adolescent and adults. CBT (e.g., Beck, 2011; Egan, 1998; Ellis & Harper, 1975; Nelson-Jones, 2002) is a multistep process in which the clinician and client analyze the way in which the client interprets life events, particularly those that relate to fluency impairment. It is organized around the identification of self-limiting beliefs that a client has, in this case, about his or her communication functioning (e.g., *I must be liked by everyone*; *I must perform excellently in everything I do*; *Things shouldn't go wrong in my life, and it's horrible when they do.*)

The following example, following principles described by Ellis and Harper (1975), illustrates how an activity might unfold in the context of a CBT activity:

A. *Antecedent event:* A client is talking with a salesperson. The client blocks on a word and, at that moment, the salesperson squints her eyes and looks at the client intently.
B. *Client's belief about event:* The salesperson thinks I'm weird. I can't let her hear me stutter again.
C. *Consequence of client's belief about event:* The client feels anxious and begins to avoid subsequent words that are about to be stuttered, which leaves the salesperson confused about what the client wants.

In this case, the focus of the treatment centers on the client's beliefs about the antecedent event (see point B above). Nelson-Jones (2002) offered a series of question types that clinicians can pose to clients in an effort to challenge and, ultimately, change their self-limiting beliefs. (In this context, the term *challenge* is not meant to suggest an adversarial or confrontational approach. Rather, the clinician first would establish that the questioning is done in the spirit of clinician-client collaboration to help the client function as effectively as possible.) After documenting the main facts of the event, the clinician and client then begin exploring the event, starting with the accuracy of the client's belief (part B in the example above). The clinician's first step might be to challenge the client's belief on empirical grounds (e.g., *Tell me how you know that the salesperson thinks you are weird. What proof do you have?*). Assuming that the client lacks such proof, the conversation then might shift toward the possibility that the salesperson squinted and stared for reasons other than what the client believed (e.g., *maybe the salesperson had never seen a person stutter before* or *maybe she thought you had a medical emergency*).

Also implied in the client's original belief is the notion that *the salesperson shouldn't be thinking that I'm weird* and that *other people shouldn't react at all when I stutter*. After identifying these underlying beliefs, the conversation might shift toward a time when the client entered into an unfamiliar situation with a person who had a disease or physical disability. (How did the client feel at that time? How did the client act? Did the client do anything that, in retrospect, he wished he hadn't done?) Eventually, this discussion then might lead to the creation of alternative interpretations of the interaction with the salesperson (e.g., *stuttering isn't very common, the salesperson is trying to figure it out*).

Finally, the clinician and client would explore the consequences of the client's current belief (i.e., *more severe stuttering, less effective communication*) and the way in which the client's thinking is (or isn't) helping the person attain the long-term goal of successful fluency management. The activity then might conclude with consideration of a worst-case scenario: What if the salesperson *was* thinking that you are weird? Ultimately, each of us only has limited influence on how we are regarded by others. So, the situation raises

the philosophical question of whether the client can be satisfied with how he or she spoke in a situation regardless of the salesperson's evaluation.

This approach can be extended to assist clients with developing a greater sense of openness about fluency impairment. Some people who stutter go to great lengths to hide their fluency impairment from others due to concern about how others may evaluate them. This leads to the use of assorted avoidance and postponement behaviors (e.g., word substitution, pretending to have forgotten what was to be said). Such strategies seldom are effective at hiding stuttering completely; they divert cognitive resources away from stuttering management; and they often have the counterproductive effect of diminishing communication (Blomgren, 2010). Thus, the goal is to nudge the client toward being more open about fluency impairment with others so that the client can devote more of his or her attentional resources toward fluency management. Blomgren notes that speakers can accomplish this goal by making simple, direct statements about their speech (e.g., *I stutter*), humorous remarks (e.g., *That's easy for you to say!*), or, less commonly, through use of voluntary stuttering.

Many clients, but particularly teenagers, find it quite difficult to acknowledge their stuttering to others (Blood, Blood, Tellis, & Gabel, 2003). We have found, when addressing this issue, it is important for clinicians to validate the client's concerns about self-disclosure of fluency impairment, and, if possible, provide opportunities for the client to interact with or read about other people who have had similar concerns. Clinicians also can model the act of self-disclosure during various activities, such as telephone conversations, in which they simulate stuttered speech. Empirical disputing (e.g., *Where is the proof that others will reject you if they know you stutter?*) and functional disputing (e.g., *How are you helping yourself manage stuttering more effectively by putting so much energy into hiding it from others?*), techniques described by Nelson-Jones (2002), can be used to open initial dialogue on this topic and to highlight the disadvantages of attempting to hide fluency impairment. We have found that it also is useful to have clients list the potential risks associated with being open about stuttering and then weigh the potential risks against the potential rewards. For many clients, the key question becomes: "Am I willing to risk the possibility that this listener will reject me in order to move closer to my goal of feeling in control of my speech fluency?" This is a question that only the client can answer, and the clinician should be prepared to support the client regardless of how he or she responds. Not every client will embrace the notion of taking communicative risks, however. Even if a client initially declines to confront potentially unpleasant listener reactions, the clinician can still play an important role in improving the client's communicative functioning by "planting the seeds" for how one can begin the process of performing activities that are challenging, uncomfortable, or threatening to do.

Regulating Speech Production

The last treatment principle to be discussed involves the regulation of speech production. Activities that come under this heading are aimed directly at changing how clients talk. As such, the concepts discussed in this section probably are most representative of what clients and laypeople think of when they hear the term "fluency intervention."

Overview and Rationale

Regulated speech production differs from the other fluency management principles discussed in this chapter. Whereas the other principles deal with the context in which the speaker talks, regulated speech production deals directly with how the speaker talks. The main objective is for the speaker to improve speech fluency through the deliberate regulation of one or more speech production parameters. In the context of stuttering treatment, the term *regulation* mainly refers to the practice of intentionally altering or controlling the motor movements that one makes while talking. Although regulated speech production can include slowed speech, the term is *not* synonymous with slow speech production. In other words, one can talk at a normal rate while consciously controlling or attending to aspects of articulation. Regulated speech is widely used as a strategy for the treatment of stuttering, particularly for clients in the pre-adolescent, adolescent, and adult years (Guitar & McCauley, 2010). Clients at these ages have the ability to conceptualize and attend to the mechanics of speech production more consistently than younger speakers do.

When regulated speech is used in connected discourse with speakers who stutter, it typically results in fewer continuity interruptions, as well as increased speech rate, improved rhythm, and the perception of less effortful and more natural-sounding speech (Logan, 2005). In many cases, the improvements in speech fluency are dramatic (e.g., Boberg & Kully, 1994). Similar improvements in fluency are noted with speakers who clutter when they regulate speech production (Myers, 2010). With more severe cases of stuttering, these improvements in fluency also may lead to improvements in the speaker's talkativeness. That is, the speaker's verbal output may increase during conversation, and the use of circumlocution and sentence reorganization as coping strategies may decrease to create a more succinct expression of ideas. The use of regulated speech often leads to fluency performance that is more stable over time, such that a fluency-impaired speaker develops the ability to talk with similar levels of fluency across many activities (Logan, 2005).

It is unclear exactly how regulated speech production results in improved fluency. The strategies discussed in this section typically require a speaker to attend to speech movements on a moment-to-moment basis. In speakers with impaired fluency, it is possible that added attention to aspects of speech production such as proprioception reduces the impact of the person's underlying impairment in speech motor control (Alm, 2011). It also is possible that the motor-based treatment strategies for stuttering are a type of *perturbation* within the speech production system. The term perturbation refers to a disturbance or change in how a movement is customarily executed. Researchers with an interest in speech-language pathology have conducted numerous studies on the effects of mechanical perturbation on articulatory movements. Guenther (2006) described the effects of a randomly introduced mechanical obstruction that altered the course of adults' customary jaw movements during a speaking task. Among other things, Guenther noted that

the mechanical perturbation resulted in increased neural activation within temporal and parietal lobe regions that are associated with sensory feedback. Results suggested that the perturbation required the speakers to generate novel syllable plans and that they no longer could rely on the syllable plans they had stored in memory. Because the novel plans were not well practiced, they obligated a greater-than-normal amount of sensory guidance to ensure that the speaker attained the articulatory goal. It is possible that a similar process exists when speakers who stutter attempt to consciously regulate the spatiotemporal characteristics of their articulatory movements.

According to a summary by Neumann and Euler (2010), findings from studies involving pre- and posttreatment comparisons of neural activation patterns in speakers who stutter indicate that the systematic use of motor-based therapy strategies tends to increase neural activity in key left-hemisphere brain regions that are inappropriately underactive in untreated speakers who stutter. The therapy techniques also seem to result in a "refunctionalization" of the basal ganglia and the cortico-striato-thalamico-cortical loop. Despite these positive effects, use of regulated speech motor patterns does not fully normalize neural functioning in speakers who stutter, even after extensive practice, as speakers who realize significant fluency improvement following therapy treatment continue to exhibit anomalies in neural activation (De Nil et al., 2003).

Applications

Most formalized therapies for stuttering include at least one skill that incorporates regulated speech production. As noted above, the act of regulating speech production implies that the client purposefully talks in a way that differs from his or her customary way of speaking. When talking in this mode, the speaker consciously attends to how he or she is speaking in order to produce a speech pattern that is different from his or her customary pattern. As such, the act of regulating speech production places both *physical* and *mental* demands on the speaker.

When it comes to regulating speech production, there are a limited number of variables that one can target. Three movement parameters that commonly are addressed in treatments for stuttering are:

- Timing, e.g., articulation rate, segment or syllable duration, pause duration and rhythmic patterns;
- Force, e.g., the manner in which one speech-related structure contacts another speech-related structure; and
- Spatial position, e.g., the location of one speech-related structure in relation to another speech-related structure.

Aerodynamic aspects of speech such as intraoral air pressure sometimes are targeted as well. Although these parameters may seem as if they are independent of one another, in reality, they are not. For example, when a person talks at a very fast articulation rate, the range of movement in the articulators is likely to decrease in order to meet the goal of getting from one vocal tract posture to another in a shorter-than-normal time frame. In the fluency disorders literature (e.g., Ramig & Bennett, 1997; Guitar, 2006), treatment strategies also are commonly organized in terms of the part of the speech production system that is being targeted. Con-

sequently, some strategies are aimed at the regulation of speech breathing, others at the regulation of phonation, and others at the regulation of articulation. This approach to differentiating fluency management strategies is somewhat artificial because respiratory, laryngeal, and supralaryngeal systems essentially function as a single coordinative structure during speech production (Hixon, Weismer, & Hoit, 2008). This means that changes in one part of the system are likely to lead to changes in other parts of the system. On this basis, it perhaps is better to think of the various regulated speech production strategies as differing in terms of where the speaker chooses to focus his or her attention when speaking (i.e., attending to speech breathing behavior, attending to laryngeal behavior, attending to supralaryngeal behavior).

Strategies That Emphasize Regulated Articulation

Regulation of articulation rate. One of the most common approaches to treating fluency disorders is to teach the speaker to regulate aspects of articulation. In most applications, the speaker first will practice speaking with a slower-than-normal articulation rate (e.g., 30 syllables per minute, which translates to 2 seconds per syllable). After the speaker meets predetermined criterion for mastery at that rate (e.g., in Shames and Florence's [1980] program, clients had to produce 30 minutes of talking with fewer than 1 stuttering-related disfluency per 100 syllables before moving to a faster articulation rate), the articulation rate target is progressively increased (e.g., very slow, slow, slightly slow) until eventually the speaker articulates at a normal rate. The speaker continuously monitors his or her articulatory behavior at each of these levels, even when using the normal articulation rate. Thus, this type of controlled fluency differs from the spontaneous fluency that an unimpaired speaker would use.

It is important that a speaker produces the regulated speech in as natural a manner as possible. Thus, even though the speaker may be using a slower-than-normal rate, the words and syllables still should be seamlessly connected. In addition, utterances still should exhibit normal intonational patterns, and syllable durations should be scaled so that the stress pattern of the utterance is proportionately equivalent to what it would be when the utterance is spoken at a normal speech rate. In other words, when using a slowed articulation rate, the speaker should refrain from pausing after every word, speaking in a monotone fashion, and making the duration of all syllables equivalent. Perhaps the best way to think of slow articulation rate is as "speaking in slow motion."

Regulation of phonetic transitions. Speakers who stutter often report that they can sense when instances of stuttering-related disfluency are about to occur. In such cases, the treatment strategy is to regulate articulatory movement in the syllable or syllables leading up to the place at which disfluency is anticipated. Consider Example 13–2 below, wherein a speaker anticipates stuttering on the words *Washington* and *Baltimore*.

Example 13–2:

Planned sentence: *We're going to Washington and Baltimore.*

Anticipated disfluency: *We're going to W̲- Washington and B̲- Baltimore.*

The speaker anticipates part-word repetitions during *Washington* (here the expected point of interruption is between the onset and the rime of the first syllable in *Washington*) and during *Baltimore* (here the expected point of interruption is between the onset and the rime of the first syllable in *Baltimore*). In a therapy setting, the strategy would be for the speaker to regulate the articulatory movements that lead up to the anticipated points of interruption. Van Riper (1973) referred to this strategy as *preparatory set*. Others have used terms such as *smooth transition* (Shames & Florance, 1980) and *easy, relaxed approach with smooth movements* (Gregory, 2003) to describe the adjustment. The speaker essentially has two choices for dealing with the anticipated disfluency in a way that differs from his or her customary (stuttered) method.

The first choice is to slow the rate of articulatory movement in the syllables that precede the expected points of interruption. So, for *Washington*, the speaker would increase the vowel duration in the word *to* along with the duration of the lip closure associated with the production of [w] in *Washington*. Thus, this portion of the utterance would be said seamlessly, as follows: *tooooWWWashington*. For *Baltimore*, the speaker would increase the duration of *and* (the [d] in that word would likely be lost to coarticulatory effects). The lip closure for the [b] in Baltimore also would be slowed, increasing its duration. Thus, this portion of the utterance would be said seamlessly, as follows: *aaannnBBBaltimore* (where the repeated "b's" indicate slow deliberate lip closure).

The second choice simply would be to attend to the articulatory movements that precede the onsets of both *Washington* and *Baltimore*. With this approach, the articulatory movements would not be noticeably slower than usual: The speaker would regulate the movements by devoting more attention than usual to movement velocity during vocal tract closure for the [w] and [b] in the two words. With the second approach, the listener would likely be unaware of the speaker's efforts to manage the anticipated disfluency. The speaker, in contrast, would be very aware of the management effort, since that is the essence of the therapy strategy. The second approach (management of anticipated disfluency in real time) is likely to be more challenging than the first for clients to execute successfully. Thus, it would likely follow extensive practice with use of the first approach (i.e., management of anticipated disfluency using slowed articulation). The regulated transition strategy described here essentially is nothing more than a microcosm of regulated articulation at a sentence level (described above). Slow transitions are progressively shaped into fast transitions, and through the process, the speaker monitors aspects of movement velocity, articulator location (proprioception), and, perhaps, movement force at the point of vocal tract constriction.

Other Forms of Regulated Speech Production

Although regulation of articulation rate seems to be the most common means of speech regulation in contemporary approaches to treating stuttering (Bothe et al., 2006), there are other ways that speakers can regulate speech production. Three of those approaches are discussed in this section.

Regulation of pauses. With pause regulation, a speaker aims to increase the frequency with which he or she pauses during the course of an utterance. Along with this, the speaker also can regulate (i.e., increase) the duration of pauses within and between utterances and conversational turns. The use of pausing as a treatment strategy with speakers who stutter has not been studied extensively. There are case reports of its application with both speakers who stutter and speakers who clutter, however (Daly, 2010).

Regulation of syllable-timing patterns. With the regulation of syllable-timing patterns, the speaker focuses on managing the rhythm of the syllables that comprise a spoken utterance. Syllable-timed speech typically is first established by asking a client to speak in time to a metronome. The beat may be relatively slow at first (e.g., 70 beats per minute) and, then, after the client establishes the ability to time syllables to the beat, the pace of the metronome is increased (e.g., 140 beats per minutes). When the skill is well established, the metronome is withdrawn and the speaker attempts to maintain the syllable-timed pattern independently. Andrews et al. (2012) reported favorable preliminary results in the use of this method for improving fluency with school-aged children who stutter. When provided with clinician feedback on speech naturalness, adult speakers who stutter can develop natural sounding speech while using this form of regulated speech, as well (Ingham, Sato, Finn, & Belknap, 2001).

Regulation of speech breathing. Other treatment approaches involve the regulation of speech breathing. The principles here are similar to those used in the regulation of articulation rate. A speaker can be taught to alter or monitor the duration of a breathing cycle or the duration of components within a breathing cycle (e.g., the amount of time spent on inspiration or expiration prior to and during the course of a spoken utterance, respectively). Speakers also can attempt to monitor changes in chest wall or abdominal wall positioning during the course of utterance production. The goal in the latter instance is to seek a steady, smooth return to resting level during the course of the utterance. There is some evidence of efficacy for treatments that involve regulated breathing (Bothe et al., 2006); however, some of these treatments (e.g., Azrin & Nunn, 1974) appear to incorporate fluency management strategies that go beyond breathing regulation, which makes it challenging to evaluate the contribution of the breathing component in the participants' fluency improvement.

Regulation of phonation. Some treatment approaches incorporate regulation of vowel duration as a means of improving fluency with speakers who stutter (Guitar, 2006). This approach relates closely to the regulation of articulation rate, described above. Another option is to regulate vocal fold contact. For words that begin with vowel sounds, speakers sometimes are taught to initiate phonation in a breathy manner. Such an approach is done presumably to counteract the effects of excessive vocal tension. The technique requires regulation of vocal fold positioning and tension and involves breathing regulation as well. The skill was a primary component in some older treatment approaches (e.g., Schwartz, 1977). To our knowledge, however, the evidence base for use of the technique as a primary treatment for stuttering is lacking. Further, there is little evidence to support the idea that speakers who stutter routinely present with unusually excessive tension in lip, jaw, or neck musculature or, necessarily, during all instances of stuttering-related disflu-

ency (Denny & Smith, 1992). Thus, regulated phonation is best supported when it results in increased vowel duration (Andrews, Howie, Dozsa, & Guitar, 1982).

Force. Speakers also are sometimes taught to regulate the force with which articulatory structures contact one another at specific places of articulation. This skill sometimes is termed *light (articulatory) contact*. The skill is particularly relevant to speech sounds that feature complete occlusion of the vocal tract (i.e., stops, affricates). When it is applied to laryngeal movement during vowel production, it seems to be consistent with the concept of *easy (vocal) onsets*. As Hixon et al. (2008) explain, force during speech production includes both passive and active components. Passive contributors to force include the natural recoil of muscles, cartilages, and connective tissues, the effects of gravity, and the surface tension that exists between approximated body structures. Hixon et al. indicate that active force is a more complex construct, as it reflects the effects of muscle contraction, the way in which muscles interact during simultaneous contraction, the mechanical status of the articulatory structures involved in a movement, and the nature of the activity. Although research into the biomechanical characteristics of regulated articulatory contact (as applied to the management of stuttering) is lacking, intuitively it would seem that movements of this sort would entail regulation of spatial aspects of movement; that is, the articulators may not approximate one another as completely as they ordinarily would do during unregulated speech and also the ability to dampen the movement velocity as an articulator approaches a place of articulation (Browman & Goldstein, 1990, 1992; Goldstein & Fowler, 2003). When a speaker deliberately attempts to make "light contact," the speaker presumably would need to control the deceleration of articulatory movements. The effects of this skill as a primary component in a treatment plan have not been well studied.

The Speaker's Experience of Speech Regulation

A speaker who stutters can apply regulated speech production in two ways. The first way is in a prevention fashion, which is consistent with the notion of controlled fluency. That is, the speaker enters a situation with a plan to regulate speech as much as possible during the course of the activity. To the extent that the speaker is able to implement the speech regulation strategies reliably, this approach should lead to less disfluency than the speaker would produce when not attempting to regulate speech. The second way is in a corrective fashion, which is consistent with the notion of acceptable stuttering. In other words, after saying a word disfluently, the speaker stops, and then repeats the word again while applying the principles of regulated speech. Corrections of this sort also can be done while the speaker is in the midst of stuttering-related disfluency. This notion of "re-doing" or "pulling out of" disfluent words is a principal component in the well-known treatment approach that Van Riper (1973) described. A similar version of the corrective application is implemented in the Lidcombe Program (Onslow et al., 2003), although in the latter application, the child is not explicitly asked to regulate aspects of speech production when reproducing the word. Onslow et al. speculated that the act of fluently reproducing a previously stuttered word may be more powerful than the other therapy components within the Lidcombe Program at bringing about improvement in young children's fluency.

To people who do not stutter, the act of regulating speech production may seem straightforward. This is reflected in the advice that well-meaning parents often dispense to children who stutter: *Just slow down.* For the speaker who stutters, however, the act of consistently monitoring speech, hour by hour, day after day, can be quite taxing. A rough analogy of the experience is to ask a person to suddenly begin walking about 10% slower than he or she normally does. This request may not be so difficult to fulfill in a quiet office with few distractions. However, it becomes much more difficult to do when the walker leaves the clinic and needs to maintain the slow-paced walking everywhere they go—when crossing busy streets, when attempting to catch buses that are about to leave, and when wanting to join neighbors for an evening stroll through the neighborhood. On top of this, the act of walking at a controlled pace feels unnatural. The challenges associated with "just walk slowly" are quite apparent in this example.

The process of regulating speech production is very similar to this—it is effortful, difficult to maintain in all situations, and can feel unnatural (Finn & Ingham, 1994). In cases of persistent stuttering, the need to continue regulation of speech production goes on across the life span (Anderson & Felsenfeld, 2003; Plexico et al., 2005). Thus, it is critical for clinicians, parents, and others who interact with people who stutter to understand the challenges associated with ongoing regulation of speech. Failure to grasp this concept can lead to unrealistic expectations of what a speaker should be able to accomplish after learning how to regulate speech production.

Summary

The present chapter dealt with foundational issues related to the treatment of fluency disorders. The issue of setting comprehensive and appropriate treatment goals was discussed at length. It was suggested that, to develop comprehensive treatment goals, clinicians first must conduct a comprehensive assessment of the client's communication functioning. When appropriate, the assessment should go beyond fluency to incorporate other aspects of communication, and both the clinician's and client's perspectives on communicative functioning should be explored. Treatment goals follow naturally from assessment results.

The use of a comprehensive fluency model can reduce the likelihood of developing a treatment plan that focuses exclusively on the number of disfluencies that a speaker produces. Although impairment in speech continuity is an important contributor to disability in disorders such as stuttering, consideration of other fluency dimensions will lead to a much broader perspective when evaluating treatment outcomes. Use of the ICF model or something similar provides a framework for developing a treatment plan that goes beyond the speaker's fluency impairment to consider issues such as how the client performs in real-world activities and how the client's feelings, attitudes, and beliefs and the actions of other people around the client may impact the client's fluency functioning.

The issue of developing appropriate goals was discussed at length, too. The main issue here is that the treatment strategies a clinician introduces should correspond to both the nature of the impairment that creates the fluency disorder and the consequences that follow the disorder. Developmental stuttering now is widely seen as a neurodevelopmental disorder that impacts motor system functioning. Thus, a treatment plan that consists solely of activities that are designed to relax a client is unlikely to have as much positive impact on the client's fluency performance as a treatment plan that is based on activities that directly target speech motor behavior. It also was suggested that an accurate understanding of the nature of stuttering will facilitate realistic views of treatment success. To date, none of the existing treatment methods for stuttering or cluttering reliably lead to a normalization of the underlying neurological conditions that cause the disorders. Until such a treatment is developed, the best course of action is to help clients attain compensated fluency. From this perspective, the client will strive to function as well as possible given the limitations of his or her speech production system. Clinicians can counsel clients with regard to issues related to developing realistic long-range goals for treatment and with setting meaningful interim goals, as well. When treatment does lead to normalized fluency, that outcome is, of course, to be celebrated. However, there are many other satisfactory treatment outcomes that clients can attain in which speech fluency is not entirely normalized, and these outcomes can be celebrated as well.

The second half of the chapter dealt with treatment principles. The characteristics and rationale of each principle was discussed, along with examples of how the principles are applied in contemporary treatment protocols. *Providing feedback* to clients is a principal component of all behavioral treatments for fluency impairment. As shown in the next chapter, feedback is a primary treatment agent in some evidence-based approaches for treating developmental stuttering. Most behavioral treatment approaches also incorporate the notion of *regulating task complexity*, at least during early stages of intervention when clients are establishing the capacity to produce basic fluency management skills. Eventually, of course, clients will need to deal with the complexities of real-world communication, and clinicians can help clients accomplish this by systematically introducing various "fluency stressors" into treatment activities. A third treatment principle—*developing background knowledge* about stuttering and stuttering-related disability—also was described at length. This principle is most relevant to older children, teens, and adults, as clients at these ages are more likely to engage in active self-management of impaired fluency than young children are. Still, young children can benefit from learning basic information about stuttering, particularly when they are feeling distressed at their difficulties in communicating fluently. Parents and clinicians can inform young children using age-appropriate language that some children experience "bumps" in speech when learning to talk and can label the emotions that children may experience as a result. Such an approach, when accompanied by reassurances of a parent's unconditional support and regard for the child, perhaps can prevent the development of more pervasive negative feelings and attitudes about stuttering in the future.

The fourth treatment principle dealt with the *regulation of environmental factors* that hinder fluency functioning. Some of these factors are communication based and can be addressed as needed by working with supportive communication partners on creating a speaking environment that is conducive to the application of fluency management skills. Bullying is another environmental stressor that some clients who stutter encounter, and it can have long-term negative effects on victims. Children who stutter are at greater risk than average to be bullied. Thus, clinicians must pay attention for evidence of bullying and be prepared to help clients respond to it if or when it occurs. Stuttering can have significant negative emotional and attitudinal impacts on affected speakers. Several approaches to helping client's *reinterpret stuttering-related experiences* were discussed. These included several methods of desensitization and basic principles of cognitive behavioral therapy (i.e., cognitive restructuring). Clinicians should be mindful that significant therapy-driven improvement in speech continuity is not always accompanied by comparable improvement in a client's self-concept, feelings about speech, and communication attitude. For many clients, negative feelings and attitudes about speech communication are as much a part of the disability that comes with fluency impairment as the disfluent speech and thus need to be monitored closely at all points in treatment, including the post-treatment "maintenance" phase.

The sixth module dealt with approaches to helping clients *regulate speech production*. This is a staple of most approaches to intervention for school-aged children and beyond, and there are basic elements of it in some treatment approaches for preschool-aged children. Most forms of speech regulation are targeted at speech articulation, particularly articulation rate. The use of slow articulation rate is a temporary strategy that is designed to introduce clients to the act of regulating speech movements. The long-range goal, however, is for clients to incorporate principles of regulated speech while using a normal rate of articulation and natural sounding speech. Principles of regulated speech often are applied with the goal of helping clients attain controlled fluency that sounds similar to that of typical speakers. Speakers who stutter also can apply the same speech strategies to modify instances of stuttering-related disfluency so that these interruptions in speech continuity have less of an impact on a speaker's communication. As the old saying goes, however, "there is no such thing as a free lunch." Speakers who stutter often find the act of regulating speech production to be effortful and unnatural. Although this may improve with time, clinicians, parents, and clients should take this into account when setting treatment goals and evaluating treatment outcomes. In clinical practice, clinicians can use the treatment principles outlined in this chapter as a starting point for designing treatment plans that meet the specific needs of individual clients.

14

Putting Treatment Principles Into Practice

In this chapter, the goal is to review some of the specific treatments that have been employed in the area of fluency disorders. The treatment literature for fluency disorders is extensive and largely oriented toward developmental stuttering. It includes authoritative accounts of how highly experienced clinicians conduct treatment, as well as a wide range of peer-reviewed articles in which the effects of various treatments have been evaluated scientifically.

There are three main categories of treatments for fluency disorders: *behavioral*, *assistive*, and *pharmacological*. Of the three, behavioral treatments by far are the most commonly used and the best researched; thus, they constitute the main focus of this chapter. Most behavioral treatments are aimed at altering aspects of speech production such as articulation rate, disfluency frequency, disfluency duration, and utterance length. Other behavioral treatments are aimed at altering the feelings, attitudes, and beliefs that

are associated with fluency impairment. Many contemporary interventions incorporate more than one type of behavioral treatment strategy. Rather than attempt to review all of the detailed behavioral treatment protocols that have been published throughout the years, the approach here, instead, is to examine a few representative treatments with regard to the underlying treatment principles upon which they are based. With this approach, the aim is to highlight both the similarities and the differences that exist among behavioral treatments for fluency disorders.

Assistive devices are tools or instruments that a speaker uses to enhance his or her communicative functioning. Devices that alter what a person hears while talking (e.g., masking devices, delayed auditory feedback devices, metronomes) have received the most attention with regard to their potential as treatments for stuttering. Pharmacological treatments also have been explored, mainly for their potential use in the treatment of developmental stuttering. Although pharmacological treatments remain largely experimental at present, they yield some interesting insights into the neural mechanisms that underlie speech fluency. Adult clients sometimes inquire about the possibility of drug-based treatments; thus, results from some experimental studies in this area are explored briefly, as well.

Initial Considerations

The Nature of Behavioral Treatments

Historically, behaviorally based interventions have been the treatment of choice for improving speech fluency in clients with fluency disorders. In some respects, contemporary treatment approaches for fluency disorders are not much different from those that were in vogue during the 1970s. The behavioral strategies that clinicians use to treat fluency disorders have been and continue to be regarded as *compensatory* in nature (De Nil, Kroll, Lafaille, & Houle, 2003; Neumann & Euler, 2010). In other words, the treatments are not purported to cure a person of the underlying impairment that causes a person to stutter or clutter. Rather, they primarily are intended to help a client use an impaired speech production system more effectively than he or she currently does. Despite this apparent limitation, behavioral treatments can be quite powerful. In fact, some speakers who stutter learn to compensate for their impaired fluency so well that they are able to eliminate or substantially reduce their overt symptoms of fluency impairment as well as their fluency-based communication disability.

Of course, not every client will compensate for fluency impairment so effectively. Thus, researchers and clinicians continue to search for treatments that are better than those that are used currently. Some of those treatments might include blended approaches, wherein behavioral treatments are combined with assistive devices and/or pharmacological interventions in an effort to maximize clients' communication performance. As Neumann and Euler (2010) discuss, data from recent neuroimaging studies indicate that some behavioral interventions—specifically those that entail intensive practice of regulated articulation rate—result in new patterns of neural activation that approximate those that are observed in normally fluent speakers. Neumann and Euler explain that these treatment-induced changes in neural activation provide evidence that certain types of behavioral interventions facilitate "repair" of an impaired speech production system in ways that enable speakers who stutter to communicate more fluently than they otherwise would do.

Treatment and Evidence-Based Practice

Perhaps the most significant change during the past 20 years with regard to the treatment of fluency disorders is the growing recognition that clinical practices need to be supported by evidence. That is, to the extent possible, clinicians should guide their decision-making during intervention by sound scientific, clinical, and patient-based evidence. The American Speech-Language-Hearing Association (ASHA, 2005) issued a position statement on this matter, which states that clinicians should "incorporate the principles of evidence-based practice in clinical decision making to provide high-quality clinical care." According to ASHA (2005), evidence-based practice "refers to an approach in which current, high-quality research evidence is integrated with practitioner expertise and client preferences and values into the process of making clinical decisions." Dollaghan (2007) described a three-part model of evidence-based practice that consists of *external evidence, internal evidence,* and *client/patient preferences.* The essential features of Dollaghan's model are described below.

External Evidence

Dollaghan (2007) states that *external evidence* refers to data that originate beyond a clinician's professional practice setting. External evidence typically is ranked in terms of quality. In such rankings, *randomized controlled trials* (RCTs) generally are regarded as being of higher quality than other types of research. RCTs are research studies that feature active manipulation of an independent variable (e.g., treatment versus no treatment) and random assignment of participants to the treatment groups. When implemented with sufficiently large samples, this process helps to control for the effect that extraneous variables might have on participant performance. The use of an untreated control group allows for groups to be compared on the basis of whether or not they received the treatment. A quasi-experimental design relies on precise matching of research participants to make the composition of the different treatment groups as similar as possible with regard to potentially confounding variables. Because of the difficulties inherent in matching participants on all potential confounding variables, it is regarded as a

weaker design than the RCT. Single-subject experimental research also is afforded less weight than the RCT in most rating systems. One limitation of the latter approach is that the results cannot be readily generalized to a broad population. Other sources of evidence, such as case studies and expert opinion are ranked as even lower types of evidence. Despite their limitations, single-subject experiments and case studies can play an important role in the evidence-building process. For example, these approaches are appropriate to use when examining the efficacy of a novel or previously untested treatment.

Internal Evidence

According to Dollaghan (2007), *internal evidence* involves data that a clinician amasses through systematic, empirical assessment of clients. As such, internal evidence helps a clinician identify the types of adjustments that might need to be made to externally supported treatments, in order to reflect the client's unique circumstances.

Patient Preferences

Dollaghan (2007) explains that *patient preferences* involve the choices that a fully informed patient makes with regard to treatment. According to Dollaghan, determination of patient preferences grows out of ongoing dialogue between the clinician, the patient, and, when appropriate, relevant family members. Such dialogue usually begins at the initial assessment, and it includes discussion about the patient's perceptions of his or her impairment and disability and the extent to which the patient wishes to participate actively in treatment decisions. Dollaghan notes that prior to commencing treatment, clinicians should present clients with potential approaches for treatment and their associated pros and cons. Included in this presentation should be information about the research base for each prospective treatment approach, its associated risks, estimates of the cost and time to treat, and the clinician's past experiences with the treatment. The overview concludes with the clinician's personal assessment of which approach seems best suited to the client's goals and current circumstances. After this, the client is invited to offer his or her thoughts on how treatment should proceed. Thus, discussion of client preferences helps to ensure that the treatment plan will reflect issues that are of primary importance to the client.

The inclusion of client preferences in the treatment process is not trivial. Findings from research with speakers who stutter indicate that clients' perceptions of treatment effectiveness are influenced not only by the fluency changes they make or their perceptions of clinicians' general knowledge about stuttering but also by their perceptions of how well clinicians understand the impact that fluency impairment has on the client (Plexico, Manning & DiLollo, 2010). Discussions with the client about treatment preferences can offer important insight into his or her experiences with stuttering.

Applying Evidence-Based Principles to Clinical Practice

Clinicians can access treatment research more easily today than at any time in the past due to the electronic storage of scholarly information and the rapid expansion of the Internet. Despite the advances that have been made in conceptualizing and promoting the use of evidence in clinical practice, a clinician's ability to implement evidence-based practice in a clinical context is limited by the amount and variety of high-quality research that is available. Clients often present complexities that participants in research studies do not present. Thus, a treatment protocol that was deemed efficacious for research participants who only stuttered may not be as effective for a patient who exhibits stuttering and some other concomitant impairment. Also, much of the research literature on stuttering pertains to "early-phase" research issues such as whether a particular treatment is more effective than no treatment at all. "Late-phase" research activities such as completion of multisite randomized clinical trials, assessment of long-term treatment outcomes, and comparisons of the cost effectiveness of specific treatments have received limited attention to date. As research efforts continue, more specific research questions undoubtedly will be examined (e.g., *Is "Treatment A" more effective than "Treatment B"? Is "Treatment A" more effective when used with preschoolers than it is when used with school-aged children?*). In the meantime, clinicians must be prepared for the possibility of having to adapt a particular type of treatment in ways that meet the needs of specific clients and to carefully evaluate the effects of such adaptations through the collection of "internal data" that capture how the client is responding to the treatment.

Overview of Behavioral Treatments for Stuttering

In the preceding chapter, six treatment principles for fluency disorders were discussed. The principles were derived from an analysis of the components that are present within contemporary treatment protocols that appear in the treatment literature. In this chapter, we revisit the principles to see how highly experienced clinical researchers have incorporated them into clinical practice with children, adolescents, and adults who stutter. These six principles are reviewed briefly below:

- *Provide clients with feedback:* Clinician and/or caregivers systematically introduce comments that serve to highlight, evaluate, or describe the client's stuttering-related behavior or that direct the client to change his or her behavior after producing a stuttering-related behavior.
- *Regulate task complexity:* Control the types of utterances that the client produces and/or the types of speaking tasks he or she participates in, particularly while the client is developing the capacity to produce fluency management skills.
- *Build the client's background knowledge:* Develop the client's understanding of the characteristics and consequences of fluency impairment; and assist the client with applying this knowledge toward self-management of fluency impairment and any related disability.
- *Alter the environmental context:* Reduce or eliminate factors that hinder the client's fluency, communication-related attitudes, and/or ability to practice fluency management skills.
- *Reinterpret personal experience*: Develop the client's ability to respond to fluency impairment, communication disability, and internal and external fluency stressors in ways that promote

effective fluency management and contribute positively to the client's quality of life.

- *Regulate speech production:* Help the client develop the ability to deliberately control and/or self-monitor speech-related movements (e.g., timing, spatial positioning, force).

A treatment plan for a particular client likely will incorporate concepts and strategies associated with more than one of these principles and, with some cases, the treatment plan will incorporate all of the principles.

One main area of difference among the many treatment approaches that are described in the clinical and research literature on stuttering concerns the degree to which specific treatment principles are emphasized. The treatment principle that a clinician emphasizes tends to be the mechanism that he or she relies on most to change the client's fluency functioning. For example, some clinicians have relied heavily on feedback (i.e., "response contingencies") as a mechanism for inducing change in the client's fluency. Other clinicians have relied heavily on the use of regulated speech production to induce the fluency change. Building background knowledge is not likely to be the sole basis for a treatment, but each of the other principles conceivably could be. The client's experiences in treatment will differ as a function of which treatment principles the clinician emphasizes most.

In many treatment approaches, clinicians use the treatment principles outlined in Chapter 13 (and described further below) as a starting point for designing multidimensional treatment protocols, in which the clinician may introduce the client to several of the behavioral strategies described in this section. Treatment protocols of this sort have been described in detail by many clinicians (e.g., Blomgren, 2010; Kully & Langevin, 1999; Kully, Langevin, & Lomheim, 2007; Logan, 2005).

Treatment Approaches That Emphasize Feedback About Speech Fluency

Treatments that are based on clinician-generated responses to the client's speech have a long history of use in speech-language pathology. Most applications of this treatment approach have occurred in the context of operant conditioning, which is a type of learning. Briefly, the learning paradigm in operant conditioning features three main components: a stimulus, a response, and a contingency that follows the response. Response contingencies either can increase the likelihood of the response occurring in the future (reinforcement) or decrease the likelihood of it occurring in the future (punishment)[1]. For example, imagine that a clinician presents a child with a stack of picture cards and then asks the child to name each of the pictures. When the clinician shows the child a picture of a ball (stimulus), the child is to respond by labeling the picture. If the child's response is compatible with the goal of the activity (e.g., to say words fluently), the clinician presents one type of response (e.g., *Good, that sounded very smooth!*), which is intended to increase the

likelihood of the fluent response occurring in the future. Depending on the structure of the activity, off-target responses (e.g., a stuttered response) might be met either with silence (i.e., no response) or a different form of feedback (e.g., *Oh, that one was a little bumpy.*) According to the theory, as the child is reinforced for fluent responses over time, the frequency of that behavior should increase, at least when the child is in the presence of the picture cards.

As noted in Chapter 13, a clinician can administer feedback in several ways, each subtly different from the others. Variations of feedback include the following: highlighting (i.e., *You did ___*); evaluating (i.e., *You did ___ correctly/incorrectly*); describing (i.e., *I will tell you about the positive and negative aspects of what you did*); and directing (i.e., *You did ___, therefore, I would like you to do ___ instead*).

With feedback-based interventions, the clinician acknowledges the client's stuttering directly. Depending on how the treatment is presented, the client, however, may or may not be directed explicitly to alter speech production. As noted earlier, in many applications, the use of clinician or caregiver feedback serves as the primary treatment agent. In other words, the treatment plan features little in the way of education about stuttering, little or no didactic instruction regarding how the client should modify his or her speech pattern, and relatively little attention to the complexity of the utterances that the client is attempting to produce. The clinician would, however, attend to

---

[1]The meaning of *punishment* in this context differs from the conventional sense of the word. That is, in the context of the original theory (e.g., Skinner, 1953), it is any response contingency that reduces the likelihood of a response occurring in the future. In some older studies of stuttering, the "punisher" was something clearly aversive (e.g., electric shock, a loud noise). In more recent applications, researchers downplay the reference to punishment and speak instead of "acknowledging" or "highlighting" stuttered speech (e.g., Onslow, Packman, & Harrison, 2003). In the present text, the term "evaluating" is used, as well. In any case, the clinician attempts to label, identify, or comment on what the client has done.

the physical setting within which treatment occurs—sessions in the early stages of treatment usually take place in controlled clinical settings.

Applications in Laboratory and Clinic Settings

Time-Out With Preschoolers During Conversational Interaction

Martin, Kuhl, and Haroldson (1972) reported on an intervention in which researchers conducted two single-subject experiments that involved highlighting children's stuttered speech in the context of a conversational interaction with a puppet. Martin et al. designed a lighted puppet theatre, which was set up so that the theatre lighting could be turned off remotely. The theatre was located behind a one-way mirror in a separate room from the preschool-aged participants. Each of the children was seen individually. A research assistant who was out of the children's view was charged with conversing with them through the puppet. After the researchers established baseline frequencies for stuttering, they implemented the experimental treatment, which involved a 10-second "time-out" from conversation after instances of stuttering. That is, when a child stuttered overtly, the puppet theatre went dark for 10 seconds and the puppet remained silent.

One of the children stuttered severely at baseline; thus, for the first 17 treatment sessions, the time-out procedure was applied only for stuttering-related disfluency that lasted 2 seconds or more. During the remaining 14 sessions, as the child's fluency improved, time-out was enacted following every instance of

stuttering-related disfluency. The second preschooler stuttered less severely. Thus, after completion of a five-session baseline phase, the time-out procedure was implemented following all instances of stuttering-related disfluency. This was done for 10 consecutive sessions. Martin et al. (1972) reported that both children responded quickly and positively to the time-out intervention, and at the end of the treatment phase, the percent of syllables stuttered had dropped to zero and remained that way during an "extinction phase" during which the children interacted with the puppet, but the time-out procedure was discontinued. Both children remained free of stuttered speech in the months following the treatment sessions. Martin et al. (1972) allowed for the possibility that the children's improvement could have resulted from recovery processes unrelated to the therapy; however, they considered this to be unlikely given the relatively stable stuttering frequency values both children exhibited during the baseline phase and the immediate improvements noted in their speech following introduction of the treatment.

Martin et al.'s (1972) research demonstrated that young children were capable of changing their speech fluency given nothing more than feedback that resulted in time-out from conversation. At the time Martin et al. published this study, some clinicians were reluctant to implement treatments that involved the act of making preschoolers aware of their stuttering. Martin et al. attributed this, in part, to the influence of Johnson's diagnosogenic theory, which centered on the claim that unwarranted parental concern over a child's fluency development was the root cause of the disorder. This claim led naturally to the idea that it was best to avoid acknowledging preschoolers' disfluent speech. Johnson (1949, p. 7) summarized his position succinctly in his *Open Letter to the Mother of a Stuttering Child*, when he urged that caregivers should do "absolutely nothing at any time, by word or deed or posture or facial expression" that would call a child's attention to a child's disfluent speech. Bluemel (1960), among others, also advocated against drawing attention to stuttered speech during early childhood. In his view, self-awareness of stuttering leads a child to produce various compensatory behaviors for it, and with it, a pattern of "secondary" stuttering. Based on findings from Martin et al. and other similar studies, it seems that these concerns were unwarranted.

Acknowledging Preschoolers' Stuttering

As the influence of the diagnosogenic theory waned during the 1970s and 1980s, a growing number of researchers began to examine the effects of treatments that directly targeted stuttering-related behaviors in preschoolers who stuttered. It was in this context that Onslow and colleagues (e.g., Onslow, 1992; Onslow, Andrews, & Lincoln, 1994; Onslow, Costa, & Rue, 1990) developed the *Lidcombe Program of Early Stuttering Invention*. The main component of the treatment involves having a clinician and, ultimately, a parent make evaluative comments about a child's fluency within the context of circumscribed daily activities. The program activities are designed to be a positive experience for children. Thus, most of the comments that the clinician and parent make about the child's fluency are done in conjunction with fluent speech (e.g., "That was smooth"). Comments about children's stuttered utterances (e.g., "That was bumpy") occur less often. After some stuttered

words, the clinician or parent prompts the child to retry words upon which they just have stuttered. The treatment primarily is parent-based. That is, clinicians train parents to recognize and respond to stuttered speech, and the parents use the training to implement the treatment. Clinicians then monitor the parents and children while the treatment is implemented. Since the early 1990s, Onslow and his colleagues at the Australian Stuttering Research Centre have published numerous studies that examine the effectiveness of the intervention. Among the findings to emerge from their research program include the following:

- Children who were treated successfully between the ages of 2 and 5 years using procedures from the Lidcombe Program maintained treatment gains of near-zero stuttering for 4 to 7 years after treatment. Data were collected from speech samples in home-based settings and from a parent questionnaire (Lincoln & Onslow, 1997; Onslow et al., 1994).

- Results from a randomized control trial showed that children who participated in the Lidcombe therapy exhibited significantly less stuttering than children in an untreated control group (Jones et al., 2005). A follow-up study showed that 84% of participants who could be contacted had maintained treatment gains of near-zero stuttering for, on average, 5 years (Jones et al., 2008). Children with no family history of stuttering showed more favorable treatment outcomes than children with a family history of recovery from stuttering (Jones et al., 2005).

- Children who were treated successfully using procedures from the Lidcombe Program did not show significant differences in pre- versus posttreatment speech timing measures (e.g., vowel duration, voice onset time, articulation rate) or maternal speech-language behaviors (Bonelli, Dixon, Bernstein Ratner, & Onslow, 2000; Onslow, Stocker, Packman, & McLeod, 2002). Thus, other than speaking more fluently, the child's speech patterns were not obviously different following treatment, and parents did not interact with the children in markedly different ways.
- Participation in the Lidcombe Program was a better predictor of a child's posttreatment fluency than the child's pretreatment severity was (Harrison, Onslow, & Menzies, 2004).
- Children's pretreatment stuttering severity and language development predicted 35% to 45% of the variance in the time it took children to complete the Lidcombe Program (Jones, Onslow, Harrison, & Packman, 2000); however, neither the child's age nor the elapsed time between stuttering onset and treatment onset predicted the amount of time needed to complete the program (Jones, Onslow, Harrison, & Packman, 2000). Thus, children who had stuttered for more than one year responded to the treatment as well as children who had stuttering for less than one year.
- Mothers reported a range of themes with regard to their experience in administering the program to their children. These themes included mention of challenges in fitting the treatment into daily routines and feelings of uncertainty over whether they were implementing the treatment correctly. Overall, however, they regarded the treatment as being effective and having an easy-to-follow theoretical basis (Goodhue, Onslow, Quine, O'Brian, & Hearne, 2010).
- Application of the Lidcombe treatment principles to school-aged children has been explored. Initial data suggest that the program results in significant reductions in stuttering frequency for school-aged children who stutter (Koushik, Shenker, & Onlow, 2009).

Feedback Applications With Adolescents and Adults Who Stutter

Several researchers have examined the effect of time-out on stuttering frequency with adolescents and adults who stutter. Costello (1975) reported data from three single-subject experiments that were conducted with 16- to 20-year-old males. All three participants responded positively to treatment, which took place in the context of reading, monologue, and conversation. When a participant stuttered, the clinician said, "stop," and then looked away from the client for 10 seconds, after which the clinician looked up at the participant, smiled, and instructed him to continue speaking. All three participants reduced stuttering frequency to near-zero levels during treatment, which was a noticeable improvement from baseline frequencies that ranged from approximately 6% to 12% syllables stuttered.

James (1976) compared the effect of various time-out intervals on fluency facilitation in adolescents and adults who stuttered during a monologue task. He found that intervals of 1, 5, 10, and 30 seconds yielded comparable outcomes, with stuttering frequency under time-out being reduced by approximately 50% to 66%. In another experiment (James & Ingham, 1974), it was shown that the participants' expectations about the effect of time-out on their fluency (i.e., being told it would help, being told it would hinder) had no impact on the amount of fluency improvement they attained: Fluency improved by 70% to 80% in each of the conditions. James, Ricciardelli, Rogers, and Hunter (1989) found that responsiveness to time-out in speakers who stutter could be improved through participation in intensive fluency intervention. On this basis, James et al. hypothesized that time-out leads to improved fluency because it prompts speakers who stutter to access fluency management capabilities that they otherwise may not fully utilize. The nature of these capabilities is unclear, however, as acoustic analysis of speech samples from school-aged children who exhibited improved fluency in the context of time-out do not exhibit any obvious changes in speech timing between the pre- and posttreatment conditions (Onslow, Packman, Stocker, van Doorn, & Siegel, 1997; Onslow et al., 2002).

Several researchers have examined the effect of self-imposed time-out on stuttering frequency. With this approach, speakers essentially attempt to stop their speech when stuttering-related disfluency occurs or is about to occur. In this way, a feedback-based form of treatment transforms into a type of self-regulated speech production. Hewat, Onslow, Packman, and O'Brian (2006) examined the effectiveness of a treatment program that fea-

tured self-regulated time-out and reported that the adolescents and adults in the study reduced stuttering frequency by an average of 54%. The treatment program involved individual sessions in which participants had to demonstrate more than 50% reduction in stuttering frequency and evidence of active application of the strategy for 60% of the time spent speaking during conversation. Overall, 77% of participants met this criterion, and more severe participants tended to realize more improvement in fluency than mild participants. Attainment of those goals led to additional individual activities that included application of self-imposed time-out in beyond-clinic settings and, for some participants, participation in group practice activities. Successful completion of those activities led to a maintenance phase that included continued clinician support. Participants' feedback for the program tended to be positive.

Findings from these studies generally are consistent with results reported by Bothe, Davidow, Bramlett, and Ingham (2006) in their systematic review of studies on behavioral treatments for stuttering that were published between 1970 and 2005. That is, all 11 of the studies that incorporated response contingencies resulted in posttreatment stuttering frequency scores of less than 5% syllables stuttered, and among the studies that examined long-term outcomes, results showed that participants were able to maintain the fluency improvement following treatment.

Improvements in fluency also have been reported in conjunction with treatments that incorporate certain types of biofeedback. For example, Craig et al. (1996) described results from a treatment program in which 9- to 14-year-old children used electromyographic (EMG) feedback to self-regulate stutter-like disfluency. The feedback was intended to increase the participants' awareness of and control over muscle tension and to help them maintain that control while conversing. All participants in the study were able to use this type of feedback to regulate speech production, as evidenced by posttreatment stuttering frequency that decreased to near-zero levels following the treatment phase. Participants demonstrated the ability to maintain a similar level of stuttering frequency following the termination of formal therapy. This approach illustrates another example of how speakers can use external feedback about their speech fluency to self-regulate aspects of their speech production.

Treatment Approaches That Emphasize Task Complexity

The regulation of task complexity (particularly *utterance complexity*) is a common component of many treatment programs for developmental stuttering. The principle is incorporated routinely within activities that are used to build a speaker's capacity to use fluency management skills. It also is incorporated within activities that are designed to help clients extend the use of fluency management skills from treatment room settings into real-world settings. The manipulation of task complexity as a primary treatment agent occurs less often, but it still is worth exploring in some detail in light of positive treatment outcomes reported to date.

Regulation of task complexity as a primary intervention strategy has been used mostly with children who stutter. As explained further below, the regulation of task complexity with adolescents and adults who stutter is more likely to be implemented as one of several intervention strategies in the context of a comprehensive, multidimensional treatment protocol. In the latter case, the effect of complexity regulation in treatment may be difficult to separate from that of other treatment components such as the provision of response contingent feedback and/or the speaker's use of a regulated speaking pattern.

Applications With Children Who Stutter

Ryan (1974) and Ingham (1999) provide detailed descriptions of treatments that are based on the regulation of task complexity. With Ryan's (1974) program, termed *Gradual Increase in Length and Complexity of Utterance* (GILCU), the clinician develops a series of practice activities in which task demands start out simply and become progressively more difficult with time, as the client progresses. Thus, the treatment essentially is a step-by-step approach to building a client's capacity for fluency management. In Ryan's description of the program within the 1974 text, treatment begins with reading at the one-word level. The client first is directed to read single words fluently. After mastering this level, the client progresses to reading two-word sequences fluently, and then three- to six-word sequences fluently, one- to four-sentence sequences fluently, and then eventually to reading fluently for progressively longer time intervals (e.g., 30 seconds, 1 minute, 2 minutes, etc.), up through 5 minutes of fluent reading. After attaining mastery within reading, the treatment cycles back to self-formulated words, from which the practice activities progress to monologue and, eventually, conversation. At all phases, the treatment follows a step-by-step structure.

If a child is unsuccessful at a particular step, the clinician is directed to model the correct (i.e., fluent) response for the client, which the client then imitates. If a child fails to meet outcome criteria at the end of a step sequence, the clinician then would restart the step sequence again at the beginning (e.g., at the one-word response level). When necessary, the GILCU framework easily can be combined with treatment strategies that emphasize regulated articulation rate or other forms of regulated speech. In this way, the client develops the ability to use regulated speech within the context of the step-by-step levels that characterize the GILCU approach. The principle of graduated complexity can be merged with other activities that a child might find appealing (e.g., producing a series of five target responses prior to taking a turn in a board game).

Ingham (1999) outlined a step-based treatment protocol for use with young children who stutter. The description of the program includes a highly detailed appendix that essentially constitutes a treatment manual. The program contains 21 steps, and for each step, Ingham specifies the treatment materials that are to be used (she termed them "discriminative stimuli"), the child's expected response to the materials (e.g., one stutter-free word), a description of the consequences that will follow desired (i.e., fluent) and undesired (i.e., stuttered) responses, and the criteria that the child must meet in order to proceed to the next step (e.g., 10 consecutive stutter-free responses). Step complexity within the program is similar to that in Ryan's GILCU approach, with target

responses increasing by the number of syllables per response and, eventually, by the time spent talking during monologue and conversation.

As noted earlier in this section, it is difficult to separate the contributions of the regulated complexity in these programs from those of the response contingent feedback that children receive. In both of the programs, the feedback is evaluative (e.g., "Great!," "Right!," "Not quite") and/or directive (e.g., "Stop!"). Interestingly, clients are given little to no explicit direction or instruction in how to talk fluently. As Ryan (1974, p. 54) stated, the program relies "heavily on the client's performance and the clinician's evaluation of the performance." If instructions are given, they are of a general nature (e.g., "Try to talk as smoothly as possible," "Try to talk with no stuttering"). In this respect, the treatment is similar to both the time-out and the Lidcombe approaches. That is, the client essentially is left to muster up internal resources for fluency management and implement those resources independently during the activities. As discussed in the next section, outcome data suggest that many clients are able to meet this challenge successfully.

Utterance Complexity Outcomes

Peer-reviewed treatment outcome data on the effects of regulated response complexity as a primary intervention strategy are not as extensive as those for the time-out and Lidcombe approaches. Ryan and Van Kirk Ryan (1995) compared treatment outcomes in children and teens who stuttered. Children in one group received a treatment that was based on GILCU principles, while children in another group received a treatment that used delayed auditory feedback (DAF) as a means of establishing regulated articulation rate. Overall, 96% of the children showed improvement in fluency, and the average time needed to establish the skills was 7.9 hours. In a transfer and maintenance phase that followed the active treatment phase, the children in the two groups again demonstrated a similar degree of fluency improvement. Among the children who completed all phases of study, mean stuttering frequency decreased from about eight stuttered words per minute during pretreatment to less than one stuttered word per minute 14 months later.

In a similarly designed study, Riley and Ingham (2000) compared treatment outcomes for a speech motor training therapy with those of an extended length of utterance therapy. For elementary-school-aged children, both treatments resulted in statistically significant reductions in stuttering frequency upon completion of 24 planned treatment sessions (for speech motor training, the median reduction was 36.5%, and for extended length of utterance, it was 63.5%). The speech motor training therapy resulted in significant increases in vowel duration and stop-gap duration between pre- and posttreatment measures. Children in the extended length of utterance treatment showed no changes in speech timing, and their speech timing resembled that of a control group of non-stuttering children.

Bothe, Davidow, Bramlett, and Ingham's (2006) systematic review of stuttering treatment research featured only two studies of regulated utterance complexity that met their inclusion criteria. One of the studies was the aforementioned study by Ryan and Van Kirk Ryan (1995). Both of these studies reported treatment outcomes in which stuttering frequency

was less than 5% syllables stuttered, and the participants were able to maintain the treatment gains at a 6-month follow-up.

Treatment Approaches That Emphasize Environmental Context

Another class of treatments for stuttering emphasizes the environmental context within which children speak. Treatments in which environmental context is a primary area of therapeutic focus typically are intended for young children who stutter. Treatments of this sort sometimes are characterized as a form of prevention, rather than as a form of remediation (Gottwald, 2010; Starkweather, Gottwald, & Halfond, 1990). In this context, prevention pertains to the goal of promoting normalized fluency in a young child or to the goal of preventing the consequences of a child's stuttering from developing into a significant disability.

Treatments of this sort usually are couched within a demands-capacities framework, and from that perspective, the goal essentially is to provide the child with as many speaking experiences as possible that promote fluent speech. In some ways, the approach involves a bit of transporting the ideal communication contexts that one finds in a therapy room into beyond-clinic settings, particularly settings within the child's home. Treatments that emphasize environmental context are broader in scope than treatments that emphasize regulation of task (utterance) complexity. For example, environment-oriented intervention approaches typically transpire in naturalistic settings and are aimed at altering aspects of parents' communication behavior in ways that minimize the extent to which a child is obligated to speak in situations that are likely to evoke or aggravate stuttering symptoms. As such, the treatment is less structured than the step-by-step approach that is used with approaches that emphasize graduated utterance complexity.

Parent Training Focus

As noted, the treatments that principally rely on altering environmental context typically are aimed more at *the parents of children who stutter* than they are at the children themselves (Botterill & Kelman, 2010). As such, environment-oriented treatments often are referred to as a form of *indirect intervention*. In other words, the intervention comes in the form of the communication environment that a parent creates. The parent attempts to develop a communication environment that "fits" with the child's current speech production functioning and, in doing so, minimizes the likelihood that the child will stutter.

Common goals in such treatments are to educate parents about the communication environments that tend to precipitate or aggravate stuttering symptoms in young children and to instruct them in recommended ways of responding to a child's stuttering or stuttering-related frustrations and concerns (Botterill & Kelman, 2010). Treatment programs often include parent-oriented training modules that are designed to help parents interact with children in ways that minimize the risk of precipitating or aggravating stuttering or that possibly may facilitate speech fluency (Gottwald, 2010). In this way, the treatment will seek to change some aspects of what parents currently do when interacting with their child and expand on other aspects of what they currently do (Botterill & Kelman, 2010).

Logan and Caruso (1997) summarized the sorts of communicative behaviors that parents typically strive for in environment-oriented treatments. These include the following:

- *Variables that effect conversational pace:* Included in this category are variables such as (a) the parent's speech rate; (b) the extent to which the parent's customary speech rate exceeds the child's customary speech rate; (c) the number and length of speaking turns that a parent produces in relation to the child; (d) the duration of pauses between the ends of the child's utterances and the beginnings of the parent's following utterances; (e) the percentage of the child's utterances that are marked by overlapping speech from the parent; and (f) the percentage of the child's utterances that are discontinued due to parent interruption. (These variables also can, of course, apply to other conversational partners such as siblings, friends, or grandparents.) The rationale is that fast-paced conversation is likely to increase the likelihood that a child will stutter and that parents can reduce this risk by regulating or slowing the pace of conversation.

- *Variables that affect conversational complexity:* Included in this category are parent-based behaviors that influence the linguistic or conceptual complexity of a child's utterances. Relevant variables include the following: (a) the frequency with which parents produce open-ended requests for information (e.g., Tell me about . . .); (b) the frequency with which parents make requests for clarification, repetition, or elaboration (e.g., "What was that? Huh, huh? Tell me more."); and (c) the extent to which parents introduce conceptually abstract or developmentally mismatched topics (e.g., "Tell grandma about the photosynthesis exhibit we saw at the museum today."). The rationale is that linguistically or conceptually complex conversation is likely to increase the likelihood that a child will stutter and that parents can reduce this risk by regulating or reducing conversational complexity.

As a rule, children who stutter are more likely to exhibit stuttered speech in discourse settings that are fast-paced and that promote or obligate the use of long, complicated utterances (Logan, 2003a; Logan & Caruso, 1997). Thus, the goal of an environment-oriented treatment is to minimize the occurrence of such events. As noted in the previous chapter, a host of other factors can come under the heading of environmental stressors. These include the ways in which speaking partners react to stuttered speech and the presence of bullying or unfriendly teasing. When such stressors are present, parents and clinicians can work to minimize or eliminate their occurrence, as well.

Outcomes for Parent-Oriented Interventions

It is easy to see how a supportive speaking environment would be advantageous to a child who stutters. The question becomes whether treatments that are oriented exclusively or primarily toward regulating environmental stressors are powerful enough to yield fluency improvements

that are comparable to those seen with other treatments for childhood stuttering. At present, research data are not available to answer this question unequivocally. Millard, Nicholas, and Cook (2008) reported on results of treatment for six preschool-aged children who stutter using a single-subject experimental design. The treatment featured six parent-training sessions and six home-based, parent-led sessions. The clinicians developed semi-individualized treatment programs for the children based on assessments of parent-child interaction patterns. Common features in all or most of the treatment plans included the provision of praise for target behaviors, directions for parents to follow the child's lead during play, and directions for parents to use comments more than questions when interacting with their child. Other directions that were applied to some cases included directions for parents to reduce their speech and alter or attend to family turn-taking behaviors. Millard et al. reported significant reductions in stuttering-related disfluency in four of the six cases. Additional data of this nature are needed for this type of intervention and to assess how treatment outcomes for parent-oriented interventions compare to those from other interventions such as feedback-oriented approaches like the Lidcombe Program.

Treatment Approaches That Emphasize Regulated Speech Production

In Chapter 13, the basic characteristics of regulated speech production were addressed. In this section of the present chapter, examples are provided to illustrate how these strategies are incorporated in treatment protocols. The literature on speech-based fluency management skills for the treatment of stuttering is quite large. Examples of sources that include descriptions of systematic treatment programs or protocols include the following: Boberg and Kully (1994); Craig et al. (1996); Hearne, Packman, Onslow, and O'Brian (2008); Logan (2005); Kully and Langevin (1999); Kully et al. (2007); Manning and DiLollo (2007), and Shames and Florance (1980). Given the similarities that exist among treatments that incorporate regulated speech, there are, of course, many other sources that could be cited as well. The goal here is not to review all possible approaches but rather to provide readers with a sense of the main issues that need to be considered when using these strategies in a treatment program. The focus in this section is on protocols that involve regulation of articulation rate. Similar protocols can be implemented for programs that seek to development fluency by some other means, such as through regulation of speech rhythm, phonation duration, or speech breathing.

Instructional Approaches

Published treatment protocols for regulated speech production usually are organized around either "top-down" instructional strategies or "bottom-up" instructional strategies. With the top-down approach, instruction of regulated speech begins with connected speech, typically either reading or narration, or, possibly, conversation and then highlights specific syllables or words as needed. With a bottom-up approach, practice activities begin with short target responses such as words or phrases and work progressively toward extended monologue and conversations. To our knowledge, there is no research to indicate whether one approach yields better outcomes than the other. Many of the treatment outcome studies for regulated articulation rate have used a top-down approach and reported successful outcomes. Because speech in a top-down approach (i.e., reading, narration) resembles real-world speaking more closely than speech in the bottom-up approach does, it seems like an appropriate place to initiate treatment. If the client struggles to manage fluency at these levels, the clinician simply can shift to the word or phrase levels associated with a bottom-up approach.

Initial Stages

Treatment of this sort usually is organized into stages or levels. Treatment begins with a skill-development stage (sometimes called "instatement"), wherein the client acquires the capacity to produce regulated speech. The skill-development stage typically is, itself, divided into substages. For example, when a client is learning to regulate articulation rate, treatment usually begins at a very slow articulation rate and then, as the client meets various performance criteria (which usually are defined in terms of speech continuity), articulation rate is increased in a step-by-step manner, until eventually, the client ends up speaking at a normal rate while continuing to monitor (self-regulate) speech. Training activities are relatively straightforward. In our practice, we have started with choral reading tasks, wherein the clinician and client read together aloud and the client follows the clinician model. The clinician model is withdrawn gradually over time so that the client speaks alone. A variation of this is to create audio recordings of various target rates and then have the client use the recording as a reference for the target rate. In some protocols, delayed auditory feedback is used as a tool for eliciting reduced articulation rate. Imitation of clinician models can be used as well. The latter approach works best in a bottom-up skill-training approach where the clinician produces a target rate while saying a word, phrase, or sentence about one picture, and the child generates a word, phrase, or sentence about another picture while attempting to match the rate of the clinician's modeled sentence. The Australian Stuttering Research Centre offers downloadable examples of slowed articulation rate on their website. In our experience, most clients learn the skill relatively quickly. Training sessions sometimes are done on an intensive basis but can be developed in more traditional weekly sessions as well.

Table 14–1 contains information about the relationship between various potential target rates for a treatment program and their equivalent values when converted to other rate measures. A normal articulation rate for adults would lie somewhere near the lower rows of the table (i.e., 240 to 300 syllables per minute). As shown, the slowest rate in the table (30 spm) is 10 times slower than the fastest rate in the table, and the second-slowest rate (60 spm) is five times slower. These very slow rates would be used only within the clinic during skill-building activities when the client is attempting to establish the capacity to produce connected speech that is free from disfluency. The client would not be asked to use these very slow rates in natural settings.

Not all programs utilize extremely slow articulation rates during the skill-building phase of treatment, and, in our experience, many speakers who stutter attain high levels of speech continuity when starting with a rate of 60 sps or more. So, a case could be made for targeting the least amount of rate reduction necessary in order to attain highly continuous speech. Research is needed to examine whether the use of extremely slow articulation rates during the skill-building phase offers any long-term advantage in terms of skill application in real-world settings or

Table 14–1. Conversions of Various Target Rates Into Other Rate-Based Measures

Target rate (in syllables per minute)	Converted Values		
	Seconds per syllable	Syllables per second	Time (in seconds) needed to say a 10-syllable utterance
30	2.00	0.5	20.0
60	1.00	1.0	10.0
90	0.67	1.5	6.7
120	0.50	2.0	5.0
180	0.33	3.0	3.3
240	0.25	4.0	2.5
300	0.20	5.0	2.0

in the client's ability to maintain fluency management skills after treatment ends. It also is important to note that the fastest rates in Table 14–1 may not be targeted as treatment goals either. For example, in Shames and Florence's (1980) protocol, the "top" speech rate falls somewhere in the mid-range of the values shown in Table 14–1. Most clients seem to be satisfied with using a "slow normal" articulation rate, as long as it results in minimal disfluency, sounds natural, and feels natural to produce.

As stated, the use of slow, prolonged speech patterns on the order of one to two syllables per second usually will enable clients who stutter to speak with high levels of speech continuity during connected speech, even when the spoken utterances are long and relatively complex. The client typically is encouraged to monitor articulation rate on a continual or near continual basis. Periodic presentation of prerecorded exemplars of model rates offers the client opportunities to self-evaluate the appropriateness of his or her rate. After the client establishes a pattern of smooth, continuous speech at a slow articulation rate, the clinician might, if necessary, address some finer points of regulated speech, such as the need for the client to blend word boundaries seamlessly, maintain a consistent articulation rate, and maintain natural-sounding inflectional or speech timing patterns. In some treatment protocols, the client learns to supplement regulated articulation rate with other forms of regulated speech behavior (e.g., regulated breathing). It is unclear whether the introduction of multiple regulatory strategies yields a better outcome than single-strategy approaches. That is another area that warrants investigation.

Introducing Strategies for Coping With Residual Stuttering-Related Disfluency

As noted earlier, many speakers who learn to produce controlled fluency through the use of regulated speech will continue to exhibit residual stuttering. This is not unexpected or a sign that the treatment "doesn't work." It merely underscores the limitations of current behavioral interventions in normalizing speech and the need to introduce strategies for managing residual disfluency. Many contemporary treatment protocols incorporate activities that are aimed at helping clients apply regulated speech production techniques during instances when stuttered speech occurs overtly. In this way, the client will learn how to manage stuttering-related disfluency in ways that limits its impact on communication. Van Riper (1973) described treatment strategies of this sort at length. Three main options for the speaker are:

1. *To re-do the stuttered word, trying to reproduce it with a greater amount of control than the initial disfluent version.* So, a word that is articulated initially with a physically tense, word-initial sound prolongation that lasted 4 seconds might be reproduced deliberately using slow, prolonged speech of the sort described earlier in this section. An example of a successful re-do would be a relatively effortless, 1-second sound prolongation of the sound that previously had stretched on tensely for more than 4 seconds. In Van Riper's (1973) terms, the speaker "cancelled" the old motor pattern and replaced it with a new pattern.

2. *To initiate regulation of speech fluency while in the midst of the disfluency.* With this approach, the client essentially decides to switch into "regulated speech mode" upon detection of a stuttering-related disfluency. At this point, the client begins to regulate the timing and/or tension of articulatory movements deliberately and, in doing so, begins to "pull out of" un-regulated disfluency and "slide in to" regulated speech. For example, during the midst of physically tense, word-initial sound prolongation, the client elects to actively manage speech timing and does so by deliberately prolonging the sound that is involved in the disfluency. This approach is intended to create a more controlled and orderly "exit" from the disfluency in comparison to what would have occurred if the speaker had made no attempt to regulate the disfluency. In this way, the speaker potentially reduces the impact of the disfluency on communication.

3. *To initiate regulation of speech a syllable or two in advance of anticipated stuttering.* As described in Chapter 13, a speaker can use regulated articulation rate on an as-needed basis within an utterance by electing to implement it in advance of points of anticipated stuttering-related disfluency. Of the three strategies listed for modifying stuttering-related disfluency, this approach typically results in the least disruption to the continuity, rate, rhythm, and naturalness of the ongoing utterance.

Later Stages

After the client demonstrates the ability to apply regulated articulation rate in conversation with minimal disfluency, an attempt is made to generalize the skill to real-world settings. The activities that are selected for initial application usually are chosen carefully with input from both the client and clinician. Usually, the aim is to select activities that offer the client a good chance of attaining goals. When formal treatment ends, the clinician and client establish a plan for helping the client maintain treatment gains. The plan might include suggestions for a regular practice routine in which the client reviews fluency management skills during periodic "refresher" visits and/or participates in a stuttering support group or some other group activity that offers consistent opportunities for skill application and maintenance of treatment gains.

Outcomes

Bothe, Davidow, Bramlett, and Ingham's (2006) systematic review of stuttering treatment research featured 14 studies that incorporated concepts consistent with regulated speech articulation (e.g., "prolonged speech," "smooth speech"). All of these studies reported posttreatment stuttering frequency scores of less than 5% syllables stuttered. Also, eight of the 14 studies featured follow-up measures of stuttering at least 6 months after treatment, and seven of the eight studies reported that participants were able to maintain treatment gains during that span. Relatively few studies assessed the impact of the treatment on social, emotional, and cognitive variables. Of those that did, four of four studies reported improvements in one or more of those variables, and three of four reported maintenance of those improvements at a 6-month follow-up. Langevin and colleagues (Langevin, Kully,

Teshima, Hagler, & Narasimha Prasad, 2010) reported on 18 participants who were reassessed five years after completing a broad-based intensive treatment that incorporated regulated speech. Overall, the participants had successfully maintained the treatment gains that were evidence immediately post treatment and they showed significantly improved in communication attitudes as well.

Addressing Social, Emotional, and Cognitive Factors

In contemporary clinical practice, social, emotional, and cognitive variables are not typically the main focus for treatment plans that are designed to treat stuttering. As has been demonstrated in previous chapters, stuttering is not fundamentally an emotional or psychological disorder. Nonetheless, social, emotional, and cognitive variables can contribute greatly to the communication-related disability that exists in specific clients, and as such, they can influence the client's perceptions of a treatment outcome and ability to maintain treatment gains over time. In such cases, social, emotional, and cognitive variables may indeed be a primary focus of treatment. Sheehan (1970) captured this scenario neatly by likening a speaker's experience of stuttering to that of an iceberg, wherein only a small portion of the total entity is on display to other people, and the large majority of it is hidden beneath the surface. In Sheehan's analogy, the speaker's speech disfluencies are on display, while the hidden components consist of feelings such as shame, guilt, and fear that arise as a result of accumulated negative experiences with disfluency,

along with the speaker's assorted tricks and false roles that are used to hide the speech impairment from other people.

The iceberg analogy reinforces a theme that is repeated in many places within this text: The sound of a person's speech is not always a good indicator of how a person feels about his skills as a speaker or, more broadly, about his value as a person. Still, a speaker's feelings of shame and self-consciousness often go hand-in-hand with his or her reports of experiencing speech-related struggle, avoidance, and expectancy to stutter (Ginsberg, 2000). Although improvements in speech fluency through participation in fluency therapy may help to improve some aspects of a speaker's social, emotional, or cognitive-behavioral functioning (Bothe, Davidow, Bramlett, & Ingham, 2006), clinicians still should be alert for the possibility that vestiges of stuttering-related disability remain below the surface.

In Chapter 13, several strategies for addressing the social, emotional, and cognitive consequences of stuttering were discussed. The strategies centered around three primary themes:

- Techniques that are designed to reduce a client's "sensitivity" or "reactivity" to stuttering-related behaviors while he or she is speaking;
- Techniques for interpreting stuttering-related experiences accurately and in a manner that is consistent with the notion of effective stuttering management; and
- Techniques for disclosing stuttered speech to others.

Research on the long-term effects of treatments that address these cognitive aspects of fluency functioning is limited.

Existing data suggest the treatments that directly target variables such as "unhelpful thoughts," hiding stuttering from others, and avoidance of words that are expected to be stuttered results in long-lasting improvements on measures of social anxiety and avoidance tendencies but, surprisingly, in some reports, do not seem to have long-lasting beneficial effects on speech fluency (Blomgren, Roy, Callister, & Merrill, 2005; Menzies et al., 2008). Thus, if long-lasting changes in speech fluency are sought, it likely will be necessary to target speech fluency directly and apart from a client's social and emotional concerns.

Murphy, Yaruss, and Quesal (2007) published a practical example of a treatment plan intended to promote desensitization. In this case, an 8-year-old male exhibited atypical performance on a scale of communicative attitudes, and he expressed a number of concerns verbally about his stuttering. Murphy et al. designed a treatment plan that included both speech management strategies and additional strategies that were designed to reduce the child's sensitivity to stuttering. The strategies included in the desensitization program were as follows:

- *Learning about stuttering and other people who stutter.* These activities were designed to help the client see that other people had learned to overcome the effects of stuttering. Part of the activity involved writing a letter to a famous person who stutters.
- *Interactions with other people who stutter* via a pen-pal activity and participation in a group that included other children who stutter. The pen-pal activity was part of a program run by The National Stuttering Association, a self-help

group for people who stutter. These activities provided the child with a sense of being part of a group of people who share many of the same concerns that he did about speaking.

- *Exploring stuttered disfluency and engaging in pseudostuttering.* With pseudostuttering, the child and clinician held contests to see who could produce the silliest disfluency. Exploration activities were oriented around "freezing" disfluencies purposefully and describing the resulting speech behaviors objectively. Activities such as these were designed to provide the child with a sense of control over disfluent speech.
- *Representing and exploring stuttering and stuttering-related emotions.* The child created models and drawings of stuttering-related experiences, and these were used as vehicles for prompting discussions about the feelings and emotions the child experienced with regard to stuttering.
- *Self-disclosure and changing unproductive self-talk.* Activities to promote self-disclosure included pseudostuttering, conducting surveys of people's knowledge about stuttering, and gaining experience with mentioning stuttering around people such as teachers and select friends. The self-talk activities were designed to provide the child with experiences at recognizing negative self-talk associated with stuttering (e.g., "I'm dumb.") and replacing such inaccurate and unproductive internal dialog with statements that provided a more accurate

assessment of the situation (e.g., "I stuttered. That has nothing to do with how smart I am.").

Posttreatment data showed positive changes in both the child's stuttering frequency and communication attitudes, and at a one-year follow-up assessment, he continued to participate regularly in class activities and reported feeling confident about his ability to manage stuttering successfully. This case example provides an illustration of the way in which clinicians can design a treatment program that targets aspects of speech production as well as communication-related attitudes and emotions. A number of the contemporary published treatment protocols for adolescents and adults who stutter are designed similarly. That is, they emphasize the attainment of (1) effective fluency management skills that are built around regulation of speech production, (2) effective attitudinal management skills that are built around desensitization to stuttering, and (3) the development of accurate and constructive interpretations of speech impairment and communicative disability.

Assistive Devices in the Treatment of Stuttering

As noted above, intervention programs for speakers who stutter typically are organized around speech-based behavioral techniques. Although there is evidence to support the efficacy of such techniques at reducing communicative disability, in cases of persistent stuttering the motor patterns associated with these interventions do not appear to become truly automatic (Armson & Kalinowski, 1994; Finn, 2008; Logan, 2005). Consequently, treated

speakers often must exert conscious effort after treatment to maintain the fluency improvements that were established during treatment. Given this limitation, some clinical researchers have explored the role of assistive devices in treatment. In some cases, the devices have been implemented as "stand-alone" treatments, and in other cases, they have been used to augment the speaker's development of regulated speech production skills.

Implementation in Treatment

With an assistive device, the speaker utilizes an external apparatus that—through processes that are not well understood—reduces the effect of the speaker's fluency impairment and results in improved speech fluency. One class of assistive devices for stuttering entails the altering of the auditory feedback that a speaker receives while talking (i.e., altered auditory feedback). There are two main forms of altered auditory feedback: *delayed auditory feedback* and *frequency altered feedback*.

Delayed Auditory Feedback

With delayed auditory feedback (DAF), a speaker hears his or her own voice at a slight delay while speaking. DAF devices have three main components: (1) a microphone that collects the person's speech signals as he or she speaks, (2) a signal processing system that gates the time at which the collected speech signals are released for playback, and (3) a speaker system that delivers the processed speech signals back to the person's ear canal. In most applications of DAF, vocal playback is delayed within a range of 50 to 250 ms. DAF devices traditionally have been used in the initial stages of fluency shaping protocols to help speakers who stutter develop precise control over articulation rate (Perkins, 1973; Perkins, Rudas, Johnson, Michael, & Curlee, 1974; Shames & Florence, 1980). With such approaches, speakers are taught to stretch or prolong speech sounds such that the effects of the delayed auditory feedback are negated. Long delay settings (e.g., 250 ms) yield very slow articulation rates (e.g., 30 words per minute) and, often, the elimination of all or most overt symptoms of stuttering. As the speaker reaches various performance criteria (e.g., 30 minutes of fluent speech at a specific rate), the delay of the playback signal is systematically moved closer to zero, at which point the speaker's articulation rate approaches that of a typical speaker. If the speaker can maintain fluent speech when the delay is reduced to near zero, the DAF device is removed, and the speaker then is charged with generalizing the budding fluent speech pattern to "real world" settings (Shames & Florence, 1980). In order to produce a "slow normal" articulation rate, the delay setting would be set at 50 to 75 ms.

Some researchers have speculated that speakers treat the delayed playback of their voice as a "second speech signal" and that DAF essentially is a special case of choral speech, another speech condition that has been found to yield marked reductions in stuttering symptoms. Kalinowski and colleagues (e.g., Kalinowski & Saltuklaroglu, 2003; Saltuklaroglu, Kalinowski, & Guntupalli, 2004) outlined a "mirror-neuron hypothesis," which, in very general terms, proposes that access to the so-called second speech signal leads to neural activation patterns that bypass the customary speech production pathways used by the speaker and, in doing so, result in more fluent speech production.

Frequency Altered Feedback

Frequency altered feedback (FAF) devices are similar to DAF devices, with the exception that, instead of delaying the playback of the auditory signal, the signal processing system shifts the frequency at which the collected speech signal is delivered to the person. The extent of frequency alteration is variable and may be shifted by as much as ± 1 octave. Thus, under FAF, a speaker hears his or her own voice at a higher or lower pitch than normal but without the obvious delay in auditory feedback that accompanies DAF (Stuart, Frazier, Kalinowski, & Vos, 2008). Figure 14–1 shows the relationship between DAF and FAF in terms of temporal and frequency characteristics.

Speaking under FAF has been found to enhance the speech fluency of speakers who stutter, and the effect is attained without requiring the speaker to make any obvious or deliberate changes in articulation rate (Natke, Grosser, & Kalveram, 2001). An important caveat to the above is that research into the effectiveness of FAF primarily has been conducted within laboratory settings during oral reading. During oral reading, exposure to FAF seems to reduce stuttering frequency by as much as 50% to 80%. However, stuttering reduction under FAF appears to be less than this during extended conversational tasks and some speakers seem to show relatively little fluency improvement during conversation or monologue under FAF (cf. Armson & Stuart, 1998; Howell, Sackin, & Williams, 1999; Ingham, Moglia, Frank, Ingham, & Cordes, 1997; Kalinowski, Stuart, Wamsley, & Rastatter, 1999).

For people who stutter, the extent of fluency improvement associated with DAF exposure seems comparable to—if not better than—that of FAF (Antipova,

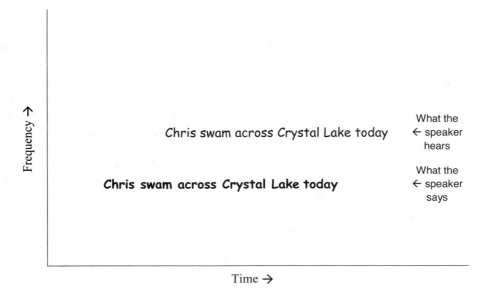

Figure 14–1. A diagram showing the relationship between normal auditory feedback (NAF) and altered auditory feedback (AAF) signals. The bottom sentence represents what the speaker hears when speaking normally (NAF). The top sentence represents how the speaker hears the normally spoken sentence when it is replayed under AAF through earphones. The *x*-axis captures the effect of DAF. In this example, the speaker has almost finished the word *swam* before hearing the onset of the sentence (*Chris*) through the earphones. The difference in the onset of articulation and the onset of hearing what was articulated equals the length of the delay in auditory feedback. The *y*-axis captures the effect of FAF. In this example, the FAF device is set so that the frequency of what the speaker says is shifted up (e.g., one-half octave), which would cause the speaker to perceive his or her voice at a higher pitch than normal. With some devices, DAF and FAF can be presented simultaneously. This would result in the speaker hearing the originally spoken utterance at a delay and at a higher pitch. Assuming an articulation rate of 5 syllables per second, the delay shown in this figure (i.e., approximately 200 ms for *Chris* and another 200 ms for *swam*) would be much longer than the delay settings that typically are used in fluency therapy (i.e., 50 to 250 ms).

Purdy, Blakeley, & Williams, 2008; Lincoln, Packman, & Onslow, 2006). Precise comparisons between DAF and FAF outcomes in speech fluency are difficult to make however, because, as noted above, DAF often has been used only as a tool for helping speakers who stutter develop "prolonged speech," a speech pattern that involves systematic regulation of articulation rate. As mentioned above, in such studies, DAF is withdrawn once a speaker demonstrates proficiency with the desired articulation rate patterns. The speaker then attempts to apply these newly developed articulation patterns independently in various real-world speaking situations. In contrast, research on FAF primarily has focused on basic "phase 1" and "phase 2" research issues such as establishing the extent to which frequency alterations facilitate fluency and identifying factors that are associated with the magnitude of its effect. Factors that have been examined in recent years include the effects that direction of frequency shift (i.e., upward or downward), magnitude of frequency shift (e.g., half octave or full octave), and feedback presentation mode (e.g., monaural or binaural) have on fluency. Research findings suggest that fluency enhancement does not vary substantially across the various types of feedback presentations (Antipova et al., 2008; Hargrave, Kalinowski, Stuart, Armson, & Jones, 1994; Lincoln et al., 2006; Stuart, Kalinowski, Armson, Stenstrom, & Jones, 1996).

Through the 1990s, *altered auditory feedback (*AAF) was delivered through relatively bulky devices that were highly conspicuous and/or cumbersome to use in real-world settings. In recent years, advances in electronics have led to the development of miniaturized AAF applications such as the SpeechEasy®, an assistive fluency device that is marketed and distributed by the Janus Development Group, Inc. Such devices resemble hearing aids. They can be worn in the ear canal or behind the ear and have the capability of delivering both DAF and FAF. Initial studies of speech fluency with adults who stutter suggest that the miniaturized devices facilitate fluency for speakers who stutter to the same extent as traditional "tabletop" or computer-based devices do. It remains to be determined whether concurrent presentation of DAF and FAF facilitates fluency in real-world settings to a greater extent than either DAF or FAF alone.

Thus far, most outcome data on AAF are from laboratory settings (Lincoln et al., 2006). Table 14–2 summarizes findings from several studies to illustrate the extent of change in stuttering frequency at a group level. The percent improvement scores in the table reflect the difference in stuttering frequency between normal auditory feedback and altered auditory feedback conditions. In all cases, mean stuttering frequencies were lower (better) in the AAF condition. Effect size differences are reported in terms of standard deviation units. The values in the table indicate moderate to very large effects for

Table 14–2. Examples of Fluency Improvements in Group Studies of Speakers Who Stutter While Using Altered Auditory Feedback (AAF)

Study	Study Characteristics				
	N	Task	Feedback	% SS Reduction	*d*
Armson et al. (2006)	13	C	D + F	36	0.40
Armson & Kiefte (2008)	31	M	D + F	63	0.99
Hargrave et al. (1994)	14	R	F	83	0.95
Howell, Sackin, & Williams (1999)	8	R	F	65	3.61
Stuart et al. (1996)	12	R	F	53	1.56

Note. *C* = conversational; *M* = monologue; *R* = reading; *D* = Delayed Auditory Feedback (DAF); *F* = Frequency Altered Feedback (FAF); SS = syllables stuttered.

device usage in the studies. The smallest effect size among the studies was reported for a conversational task, which is consistent with findings of AAF usage in real-world settings (see below).

AAF Effects in Real-World Contexts

Studies of AAF effects in real-world settings have become more common in recent years (e.g., O'Donnell, Armson, & Kiefte, 2008; Stuart, Kalinowski, Saltuklaroglu, & Guntupalli, 2006; Van Borsel, Reunes, & Van den Bergh, 2003). Van Borsel et al. (2003) examined long-term effects of DAF exposure in adults who stuttered severely. Stuttering frequency measures were conducted in a variety of tasks/settings across 3 months. Overall, most speakers showed significant improvement in speech fluency, and, importantly, improvements were noted during functional tasks such as conversational speech. More importantly, participants showed signs of generalizing the speech fluency gains made under DAF to normal auditory feedback (NAF) conditions. That is, after extended use of DAF, the participants tended to speak more fluently even when not wearing the portable DAF device. All of the participants in the study exhibited severe stuttering at the start of the study (about 30% to 40% of syllables were stuttered). Upon completion of the study, stuttering frequency had decreased to roughly 15% of syllables stuttered. Although that still is a significant amount of stuttering, a reduction of this magnitude is likely to be quite noticeable to both the speakers and listeners.

O'Donnell et al. (2008) examined the effects of SpeechEasy® usage over time during daily living situations with seven adults who stuttered. All participants showed a reduction in stuttering frequency of at least 30% when first exposed to the device; however, in subsequent laboratory sampling, three of seven participants exhibited somewhat more stuttering with the device than without it. Nonetheless, five of the seven participants exhibited fluency enhancement in at least some daily situations when wearing the device, along with more positive self-assessments of their communication-related attitudes, relative to baseline.

Lincoln and Walker (2007) surveyed 14 people who had used some type of AAF device to manage stuttering. Group data showed that 23% of the participants used the device "most of the time" and another 62% used it "some of the time." Overall, 64% of participants used the device on a daily basis. Participants reported that they were most apt to use the device in work-related activities, least apt to use the device during conversations with family, and the device generally was perceived as being effective at improving fluency in all of these situations. Indeed, 71% of the participants characterized the device as "very useful." There was some suggestion that a participant's level of self-consciousness about wearing the device affected the frequency with which the device was used.

Stuart et al. (2006) examined outcomes associated with AAF use during the course of a year. During reading and monologue tasks, the nine participants had maintained the significant reduction in stuttering frequency that they had demonstrated at their initial fitting. Overall, participants reported significant improvements in the severity of stuttering moments, the extent to which they avoided specific words and situations, and the extent to which they expected to stutter in various situations. A panel of listeners rated samples of the participants' speech that were elicited when wearing the device as sounding "more natural" than those that were elicited when the participants were not wearing the device.

Similarly, Pollard, Ellis, Finan, and Ramig (2009) examined the effects of SpeechEasy® usage across 4 months by analyzing biweekly speech samples from both clinic-based and beyond-clinic settings. Results showed variable outcomes across participants. Three of 11 participants showed improved scores on a quality of life measure, 6 of 11 reported improved fluency and increased confidence when talking, and 7 of 11 expressed interest in continuing with the device after treatment. At a group level, participants showed significantly better posttreatment scores on a self-rating measure of perceived stuttering severity.

Although existing research yields basic information about the effects of AAF devices on stuttered speech, many fundamental questions about the implementation, efficacy, and underlying mechanisms of AAF-based treatments remain unanswered or only partially understood. Some of the most salient clinical issues that require immediate study include: (1) the relative effectiveness of AAF-based intervention compared to behaviorally based fluency shaping interventions and (2) the extent to which use of behaviorally based fluency management skills are enhanced by concurrent access to AAF devices. In addition, much of the research on AAF devices has featured single-group pretest-posttest comparisons. This design is regarded as weak because of the inability to control for extraneous factors that might influence changes in participant performance such as maturation or familiarity with the research environment. Consequently, there is a need to conduct controlled studies that examine the effects of AAF usage in real-world settings.

Pharmacological Approaches to Treating Stuttering

Scientists have long been hopeful of finding effective drug-based treatments for stuttering. Saxon and Ludlow (2007) conducted a thorough review of the pre-2007 literature in this area. Part of their review focused on the strength of the research designs for studies in this area. They identified a total of 75 published reports that dealt with drug-based treatments for stuttering and found that none met criteria for Class I quality (i.e., randomized assignment to a control group, objective and blinded data collection and analysis, use of a large prospective design). According to Saxon and Ludlow, Class I studies yield information for determining whether a treatment is beneficial or not. Only 4 of the 75 studies met criteria for Class II quality (the design featured use of a matched control group as well as blinding and a small prospective design). Saxon and Ludlow explained that Class II studies allow readers to conclude whether a treatment is *probably* beneficial or not. The remaining studies were classified as either Class III (the design featured use of a control group, independent (but not blinded) data analysis, and a crossover designs) or Class IV (the study was uncontrolled and used patient reports as outcome measures, and a case series design). They stated that Class III studies only allow a reader to conclude whether a treatment is *possibly* beneficial, and Class IV studies do not allow for conclusions about the suitability of a drug for treatment.

Historically, researchers have been interested in evaluating the effects of drugs that target the neurotransmitter *dopamine* because of its actions in the basal ganglia, a region involved in the control of motor movements. After reviewing the results from these studies, Saxon and Ludlow (2007) concluded that pharmacological agents that directly affect the dopamine system (i.e., dopamine receptor blockers) are "probably beneficial" in treating stuttering. They noted that one drug in this category, haloperidol, which is used customarily in the treatment of psychosis, has the potential for very serious side effects (e.g., tardive dyskinesia) and, thus, can be excluded as a viable treatment option. They also noted that pimozide, another drug that acts as a dopamine receptor blocker, has been linked with side effects such as depression and the development of mild Parkinsonism in studies with speakers who stutter. Saxon and Ludlow reported that some other dopamine receptor blockers (i.e., tiapride, risperidone, clozapine) have fewer side effects and thus warrant further research.

Based on their review, Saxon and Ludlow (2007) concluded that norepinephrine reuptake inhibitors used in the treatment of depression (i.e., imipramine, desipramine) and calcium channel blockers (e.g., verapamil) are "possibly not beneficial." They also concluded that the study designs used to evaluate the use of selective serotonin reuptake inhibitors (SSRIs) such as clomipramine, paraxotine, and fluoxetine (typically used to treat depression) limited the conclusions one could make about their effects. They added that this might be a moot point because the reported side effects associated with certain SSRI drugs for some research participants (e.g., suicidal thoughts, depression) may be "prohibitive." Saxon and Ludlow also noted, that because most of the studies in their review took place across a relatively short time frame, more data are needed on the long-term effects of using medications to treat stuttering.

Bothe and colleagues (Bothe, Davidow, Bramlett, Franic, & Ingham, 2006) also evaluated the research literature for pharmacological approaches to treating stuttering. Their systematic review examined studies that were published between 1970 and 2005. The studies included in their systematic review were analyzed according to the extent to which they met predetermined criteria for methodology and treatment outcomes. Bothe et al. found that none of the 31 studies included in their review met more than three of the five methodological criteria they had specified (i.e., use of an experimental design, blinding during data collection, multiple data points for speech performance [including "before" and "after" measurements], data from beyond-clinic settings, and data on speech rate, speech naturalness, and observer agreement for these measures). In 4 of the 31 studies, stuttering frequency decreased by more than 50%, and only one study reported a posttreatment stuttering frequency of less than 5% syllables stuttered. In addition, evidence of short-term improvement in social, emotional, or cognitive variables was evident in only 4 of 31 studies. Among the studies with the strongest research design, none yielded unqualified evidence of favorable improvements in speech fluency or associated affective behaviors. Based on these findings, Bothe et al. questioned "the logic supporting the continued use of current pharmacological agents for stuttering."

More recently, Maguire et al. (2010) examined the effects of the drug pago-clone on stuttering-related behaviors in the context of a randomized, multisite clinical trial. As Maguire et al. explained, pagoclone is an agonist for GABA, which is a neurotransmitter that it is widely distributed in the brain and primarily acts to inhibit neuronal activity. GABA appears to modulate dopamine levels (e.g., higher concentrations of GABA are associated with lower concentrations of dopamine). In a previous paper, Wu et al. (1997) proposed that stuttered speech may be a symptom of excessive dopamine with resulting hyperexcitability in the speech motor system. Thus, pagoclone, a GABA-A selective receptor modulator, appeared to offer an approach toward reducing levels of dopamine without incurring the negative side effects of other dopaminergic drugs.

In their clinical trial, Maguire et al. (2010) treated 132 patients during an 8-week double blind, placebo-controlled, multicenter study. Overall, 88 participants received pagoclone and 44 received a placebo. Results showed that participants in the pagoclone group showed significantly better performance than those in the placebo-control group on a number of fluency-related measures. Fluency differences between the groups were apparent as early as 4 weeks after the introduction of pagoclone, where the experimental groups exhibited a 20% reduction in stuttering frequency versus a 5% reduction in the control group. Following the treatment phase of the study, participants could opt to enter an "open label" phase, during which they knew they were taking pago-clone. At 12-months post-baseline, participants who continued with pagoclone showed a 40% reduction in stuttering frequency relative to baseline and no serious or harmful side effects. Other measures indicated improvements in social anxiety and speech naturalness as well.

Although these results may sound promising, Ingham (2010) raised several limitations concerning the Maguire et al. (2010) study. Among his concerns were the following: (1) use of relatively short, in-clinic speech samples to assess treatment effects, (2) lack of evidence showing that the reported treatment effect for the drug exceeded natural variations in disfluency frequency associated with the disorder, (3) the magnitude of fluency improvement through the use of medication was substantially less than that reported for behavioral treatments of stuttering that emphasize regulated speech production, and (4) limited experience with stuttering measurement for data collectors at some research sites. Given these issues, Ingham concluded that trials such as this "contribute little" to the treatment of stuttering. Overall, it appears that considerably more research is needed with drug-based treatments before such an approach can be considered as a safe and viable alternative to behavioral treatments. Additional research also is needed to examine the role of drug-based treatments as an adjunct to traditional behavioral treatments.

Applying Fluency Management Strategies to Cluttering

Thus far, the discussion has focused primarily on approaches to improving speech fluency with speakers who stutter. The treatment literature in the area of cluttering is not nearly as well developed as it is in stuttering. That said, there is no a priori reason to think that some of the treatment strategies that lead to improved fluency management with people who stutter also might not do the same for people who clutter. Many of the treatment-oriented reports in the area of cluttering are case studies. The treatments described in the case studies are largely symptom-based and many of them incorporate rate regulation strategies. Examples of treatment outcomes in the area of cluttering included the following:

- Langevin and Boberg (1996) reported "substantial improvement" following an intensive rate-based treatment program in four participants who exhibited both cluttering and stuttering. The researchers noted, however, that the outcomes for these individuals were "less robust" than those for the participants who exhibited only stuttering.
- Craig (1996) reported on a client with cluttering and stuttering who improved fluency and articulation rate substantially following intensive rate-based treatment.
- St. Louis (1996) summarized findings from a series of case studies reported in a special issue of the *Journal of Fluency Disorders* and concluded that treatments emphasizing speech motor control were most common and that most case studies reported positive outcomes immediately following treatment; however, clients were much less consistent in their ability to maintain treatment gains during transfer and maintenance stages.

With stuttering, rate regulation is commonly accomplished by targeting a speaker's articulation rate. With cluttering, clinician's have also described the use of treatments that target pause behavior. For example, Daly (2010) reported anecdotal evidence on the usefulness of teaching people who clutter to increase pause frequency and pause duration as a means of improving communicative functioning. In the approach, development of target pause patterns is trained during oral reading, where pause locations are marked within printed passages. Daly stated that in addition to slowing rate, use of the pausing strategy also seems to facilitate language organization in speakers who clutter.

As with stuttering, clinicians who treat cluttering also have implemented multidimensional treatments that target the wide ranging deficits that can characterize the disorder. For example, Myers (2010, 2011) described a variety of practical strategies that are designed to help clients who clutter regulate articulation rate, monitor speech output consistently, and modulate syllable duration in ways that enhance the intelligibility of multisyllable words. The approach also includes strategies for building clients' "meta-awareness" of speech production components such as self-monitoring of speaking rate and listener comprehension as well as strategies for regulating speech timing in ways that normalize speaking rate and speech intelligibility. Bennett Lanouette (2011) also described a multidimensional approach to treating cluttering. The treatment strategies that she discussed are consistent with the treatment principles outlined in this chapter. Bennett Lanouette described intervention strategies that span five communication-related domains: cognition (e.g., self-awareness), language (e.g., language formulation and organization), pragmatics (e.g., topic maintenance, responding to listener cues regarding communication clarity), speech (e.g., fluency, rate, prosody, and articulation), and motor (e.g., movement coordination). The intervention strategies are designed to address the most common deficits that people who clutter exhibit. Reardon-Reeves (2010) reminded clinicians that people who clutter often present with several types of impairment, and she suggested that clinicians target a maximum of two problem behaviors per treatment activity. She explained that clients can work with the clinician to identify the two primary problem behaviors.

Evaluating Treatment Outcomes

In Figure 14–2, we present a framework for evaluating treatment outcomes. This framework follows an approach described by Yaruss and Quesal (2006), who argued for the importance of a broad-based view of client performance when assessing treatment outcomes. In the approach shown in Figure 14–2, performance is evaluated in terms of context or setting (clinic versus real-world) and the client's stage of treatment, including long-term follow-up. Clinic-based data capture the client's capacity for fluency management, while real-world data capture the application of that capacity in daily activities. Clinic and real-world data can be reported in terms

Setting/Stage		Fluency dimensions								Disability			
		Continuity	Rate	Rhythm	Effort	Naturalness	Talkativeness	Stability	Stuttering severity	Activity limitations	Participation restrictions	Personal factors	Environmental factors
Clinic	Pre-treatment												
	Post-treatment												
	Follow-up												
Real-world	Pre-treatment												
	Post-treatment												
	Follow-up												

Figure 14–2. Example of a framework for evaluating treatment outcomes. Client performance can be assessed in relation to setting, treatment stage, fluency dimension, and disability. Fluency-related measures consist largely of quantitative data such as the number of stuttered syllables per 100 syllables (continuity), duration and temporal structure of stuttering-related disfluency (rhythm), and performance variability (stability). Disability categories capture the impact of fluency performance on the client's functioning and the extent to which personal and environmental factors contribute to disability. In this framework, a client could demonstrate improvement in an aspect of fluency such as continuity in both clinic and real-world settings and yet continue to show evidence of disability such as participation restriction because of continuing embarrassment about being a person who stutters.

of fluency performance, which as shown in the figure, can be analyzed in relation to one or more fluency dimensions. These data then can be supplemented with data about disability, which primarily refers to the client's activity limitations and participation restrictions in communicative functioning but also encompasses aspects of personal functioning such as speech-related attitudes and emotions as well as environmental factors that might contribute to disability. Aspects of disability can be assessed by analyzing fluency data from real-world speech samples as well as client responses to oral interviews and the various stuttering-related rating instruments that are described in Chapter 10.

Use of a framework like this provides a means for capturing dissociations between quantitative measures of a client's fluency performance and the client's reports of lingering disability in real-world situations. For example, a client might demonstrate significant improvement in speech continuity within both clinic and real-world settings yet continue to experience disability in the form of participation restriction due to persisting embarrassment about being a person who stutters. The framework also provides a mechanism for capturing "positive outcomes" that are not reflected in continuity-based measures such as the percent of syllables stuttered. For example, a client might exhibit a posttreatment stuttering frequency of 7%, which could be taken as evidence of an unsuccessful outcome yet still report feeling quite satisfied with the outcome. Upon further assessment, the clinician might discover that the client's feeling of success stems from marked reductions in both disfluency duration and speech-related effort (i.e., "easier" stuttering), along with increased talkativeness, greater verbal participation, and evolving personal attitudes that result in growing acceptance of being identified as a "person who stutters." Quantitative data such as these can be supplemented with *qualitative data* in which clients describe their current speaking experiences (i.e., performance across various fluency dimensions, aspects of disability and functioning). The client's posttreatment content themes can be compared against those from the pretreatment assessment and used to document changes in communicative functioning.

Summary

This chapter explored methods of putting treatment principles into practice when working with people who stutter. Most treatments for stuttering are oriented toward changing the behavior of affected speakers and, as such, it is best to think of the treatments as providing speakers with a means of compensating for and/or coping with fluency impairment. Neuroimaging data suggest that motor-based behavioral treatments lead to changes in the neural systems involved in speech production, and these changes leave the impression that the speech production is, to some extent, "repaired" following treatment. With additional research, researchers should be able to determine whether the type of speech motor skill being practiced or the way in which practice is structured affects this process.

Ultimately, treatments for stuttering and other fluency disorders need to be based on evidence of their effectiveness. The process of evaluating the effectiveness for various treatments of stuttering is underway, and there is much work left for clinicians and researchers to do. In the meantime, the available treatment literature provides clinicians with a sense for the types of treatments that *should work* with a given client. From there, however, it is incumbent on the clinician to determine how specific treatments are likely to mesh with the unique performance profile of a particular client and the preferences that the client has with regard to how therapy should unfold. This process will likely result in individualized treatment protocols; that is, treatment delivery that differs somewhat from the "shelf version" of a published treatment protocol.

The bulk of the chapter dealt with various approaches to treating stuttering. Treatments were organized around general principles. Although the treatment principles identified here overlap to some degree, they nonetheless provide a useful framework for thinking about the concepts that receive the most emphasis in treatment. The effects of various "response contingencies" on stuttered speech have been studied extensively. This form of treatment is relatively simple in its structure—the clinician is providing a client with feedback about how he or she performs with regard to speech fluency. The fact that simple response contingencies such as, "That was smooth" or "That was bumpy" affect the expression of stuttering is somewhat remarkable. It was suggested here, as it has been elsewhere, that such treatments "work" by nudging clients to access fluency control mechanisms that they may not have accessed ordinarily. The fact that treatments such as these sometimes are associated with a speaker eventually recovering from stuttering also is intriguing and raises additional questions about the nature of the relationship between behavioral treatments and the underlying impairment that causes children to stutter.

Response contingencies sometimes are presented in the context of treatment activities that feature carefully structured practice stimuli. The most common form of such treatments involves gradual increases in utterance length and complexity. Such treatments have not been researched as extensively as some of the other treatments that emphasize response feedback. The effect of treatments that are oriented toward creating a fluency-friendly speaking environment for children also warrants additional research. Expansion of research efforts in these areas will allow clinicians to determine whether some treatment principles are more powerful than others at ameliorating the effects of stuttering and which kinds of environmental variables stress fluency most.

Treatments that emphasize the use of regulated speech production are widely used, particularly with older children, adolescents, and adults who stutter. Fluency management strategies often focus on the regulation of articulation rate; however, other aspects of speech production have been targeted as well. Data are most plentiful for rate-based treatments, but data on the effects of other forms of speech regulation (e.g., speech rhythm) are emerging as well. Many studies evaluate treatment outcomes in terms of stuttering frequency, which is to be expected; however, given the limitations of current behavioral treatments, a case can be made for evaluating other aspects of fluency and for tying fluency-based measures into broader notions of the client's communication disability and quality of life. Several of the contemporary stuttering treatment protocols include modules that target social, emotion, and/or cognitive aspects of functioning. Additional research is warranted to contrast the outcomes associated with treatments that target both speech and affective functioning against those treatments that target only speech functioning.

The limitations associated with behavioral treatments have led researchers to explore alternate modes of treatment. Devices that alter the speaker's auditory feedback during speech have been studied with increasing frequency in recent years, in part, because advances in electronics have led to the development of portable devices that can be used in real-world situations. Although research findings suggest that such devices help speakers improve fluency during certain laboratory tasks, the effect of such devices on fluency performance in real-world settings requires additional study.

Various types of drug-based treatments for stuttering have been examined, as well. The side effects associated with some medications seem to rule out their use as a general treatment for stuttering. Newer drugs that modulate the functioning of specific systems within the nervous system, particularly systems that are involved in the regulation of speech motor movements, seem to have potential for ameliorating the effects of stuttering. The use of assistive devices and pharmacological treatments with stuttering is, of course, not an either/or proposition. Several researchers have discussed the need for studies that examine the extent to which the effects of traditional behavioral treatments might be enhanced by combining them with other types of treatment.

The take-home message is this: Although existing treatments for fluency disorders have limitations, they still can have powerful facilitative effects on a client's ability to communicate effectively. Of course, effective treatment depends on more than only treatment strategies. The clinician plays a critical part in the process too. During the course of treatment, the clinician is likely to assume many roles —therapist, teacher, coach, guide, role model, facilitator, advisor, taskmaster, and unwavering supporter. Each of these roles may be necessary, as the path toward successful fluency management sometimes is lengthy and challenging for the client to traverse. However, for both the client and the clinician, it is a path that is well worth traveling, because even though the ability to speak fluently may seem quite ordinary to most people, it is anything but ordinary for the person with impaired fluency. And for the clinician and client who are working together to address this issue, the attainment of effective fluency management can indeed be truly extraordinary.

References

Abe, K., Yokoyama, R., & Yorifuji, S. (1993). Repetitive speech disorders resulting from infarcts in the paramedian thalami and midbrain. *Journal of Neurology, Neurosurgery, and Psychiatry, 56*, 1024–1026.

Ackermann, H., & Riecker, A. (2010). Cerebral control of motor aspects of speech production: Neurophysiological and functional imaging data. In B. Maassen & P. van Lieshout (Eds.), *Speech motor control: New developments in basic and applied research* (pp. 117–134). Oxford, UK: Oxford University Press.

Adams, M. R. (1977). A clinical strategy for differentiating the normally nonfluent child and the incipient stutterer. *Journal of Fluency Disorders, 2*, 141–148.

Adams, M. R. (1990). The demands and capacities model: Theoretical elaborations. *Journal of Fluency Disorders, 15*, 135–141.

Adams, M. R., & Hayden, P. (1976). The ability of stutterers and nonstutterers to initiate and terminate phonation during production of an isolated vowel. *Journal of Speech and Hearing Research, 19*, 290–296.

Adams, M. R., Lewis, J. I., & Besozzi, T. E. (1973). The effect of reduced reading rate on stuttering frequency. *Journal of Speech and Hearing Research, 16*, 671–675.

Al-Ghamedei, A., & Logan, K. J. (2012, November). *A survey of contemporary fluency assessment practices.* Poster presented at the annual meeting of the American Speech-Language-Hearing Association, Atlanta, GA.

Alm, P. A. (2011). Cluttering: A neurological perspective. In D. Ward & K. Scaler Scott (Eds.), *Cluttering: A handbook of research, intervention and education* (pp. 3–28). New York, NY: Psychology Press.

Ambrose, N. G., & Yairi, E. (1994). The development of awareness of stuttering in preschool children. *Journal of Fluency Disorders, 19*, 229–245.

Ambrose, N. G., & Yairi, E. (1999). Normative disfluency data for early childhood stuttering. *Journal of Speech, Language, and Hearing Research, 42*, 895–909.

American Association on Intellectual and Developmental Disabilities (AAIDD). (2013). *Definition of intellectual disability.* Author. Retrieved January 3, 2014, from http://aaidd.org/intellectual-disability/definition

American Psychological Association (APA). (2014). *Bullying.* Author. Retrieved February 10, 2014, from https://www.apa.org/topics/bullying/index.aspx

American Speech-Language-Hearing Association (ASHA). (1995). *Guidelines for practice in stuttering treatment* [Guidelines]. Retrieved from http://www.asha.org/policy

American Speech-Language-Hearing Association. (2004). *Preferred practice patterns for the profession of speech-language pathology* [Preferred practice patterns]. Retrieved from http://www.asha.org/policy

American Speech-Language-Hearing Association. (2005). Evidence-based practice in communication disorders [Position statement]. Retrieved from http://www.asha.org/policy

American Speech-Language-Hearing Association. (2007). *Scope of practice in speech-language pathology* [Scope of practice]. Retrieved from http://www.asha.org/policy

Anderson, J. D. (2007). Phonological neighborhood and word frequency effects in the stuttered disfluencies of children who stutter. *Journal of Speech, Language, and Hearing Research, 50,* 229–247.

Anderson, J. D., & Byrd, C. T. (2008). Phonotactic probability effects in children who stutter. *Journal of Speech, Language, and Hearing Research, 51,* 851–866.

Anderson, J. D., & Conture, E. G. (2004) Sentence structure priming in children who do and do not stutter. *Journal of Speech, Language, and Hearing Research, 47,* 552–571.

Anderson, J. D., Pellowski, M. W., Conture, E. G., & Kelly, E. M. (2003). Temperamental characteristics of young children who stutter. *Journal of Speech, Language, and Hearing Research, 46,* 1221–1233.

Anderson, J. D., & Wagovich, S. A. (2010). Relationships among linguistic processing speed, phonological working memory, and attention in children who stutter. *Journal of Fluency Disorders, 35,* 216–234.

Anderson, J. D., Wagovich, S. A., & Hall, N. E. (2006). Nonword repetition skills in young children who do and do not stutter. *Journal of Fluency Disorders, 31,* 177–199.

Anderson, T. K., & Felsenfeld, S. (2003). A thematic analysis of late recovery from stuttering. *American Journal of Speech-Language Pathology, 12,* 243–253.

Andrews, C., O'Brian, S., Harrison, E., Onslow, M., Packman, A., & Menzies, R. (2012). Syllable-timed speech treatment for school-age children who stutter: A phase I trial. *Language, Speech, and Hearing Services in Schools, 43,* 359–369.

Andrews, G. (1984). The epidemiology of stuttering. In R. F. Curlee & W. H. Perkins (Eds.), *Nature and treatment of stuttering: New directions* (pp. 1–12). Boston, MA: College-Hill Press.

Andrews, G., Craig, A., Feyer, A. M., Hoddinott, S., Howie, P., & Neilson, M. (1983). Stuttering: A review of research findings and theories circa 1982. *Journal of Speech and Hearing Disorders, 48,* 226–246.

Andrews, G., & Cutler, J. (1974). Stuttering therapy: The relation between changes in symptom level and attitudes. *Journal of Speech and Hearing Disorders, 39,* 312–319.

Andrews, G., & Harris, M. (with Garside, R. & Kay, D.). (1964). *The syndrome of stuttering.* Clinics in Developmental Medicine, No. 17. London, England: The Spastics Society Medical Education and Information Unit in association with Heinemann Medical Books.

Andrews, G., & Harvey, R. (1981). Regression to the mean in pretreatment measures of stuttering. *Journal of Speech and Hearing Disorders, 46,* 204–207.

Andrews, G., Howie, P. M., Dozsa, M., & Guitar, B. (1982). Stuttering: Speech pattern characteristics under fluency-inducing conditions. *Journal of Speech and Hearing Research, 25,* 208–216.

Andrews, G., Morris-Yates, A., Howie, P., & Martin, N. (1991). Genetic factors in stuttering confirmed (Letter). *Archives of General Psychiatry, 48,* 1034–1035.

Antipova, E. A., Purdy, S. C., Blakeley, M., & Williams, S. (2008). Effects of altered auditory feedback (AAF) on stuttering frequency during monologue speech production. *Journal of Fluency Disorders, 33,* 274–290.

Apple, W., Streeter, L. A., & Krauss, R. M. (1979). Effects of pitch and speech rate on personal attributions. *Journal of Personality and Social Psychology, 37,* 715–727.

Aram, D. M., Meyers, S. C., & Ekelman, B. L. (1990). Fluency of conversational speech in children with unilateral brain lesions. *Brain and Language, 38,* 105–121.

Ardila, A., & Lopez, M. V. (1986). Severe stuttering associated with right hemisphere lesion. *Brain and Language, 27,* 239–246.

Armson, J., Jenson, S., Gallant, D., Kalinowski, J., & Fee, E. J. (1997). The relationship between degree of audible struggle and judgments of childhood disfluencies as stuttered or not stuttered. *American Journal of Speech-Language Pathology, 6,* 42–50.

Armson, J., & Kalinowski, J. (1994). Interpreting results of the fluent speech paradigm in stuttering research: Dificulties in separting cause from effect. *Journal of Speech and Hearing Research, 37,* 69–82.

Armson, J., & Kiefte, M. (2008). The effect of SpeechEasy® on stuttering frequency, speech rate, and speech naturalness. *Journal of Fluency Disorders, 33,* 120–134.

Armson, J., Kiefte, M., Mason, J., & De Croos, D. (2006). The effect of SpeechEasy® on stuttering frequency in laboratory conditions. *Journal of Fluency Disorders, 31,* 137–152.

Armson, J., & Stuart, A. (1998). Effect of extended exposure to frequency-altered feedback on stuttering during reading and monologue. *Journal of Speech, Language, and Hearing Research, 41,* 479–490.

Arndt, J., & Healey, E. C. (2001). Concomitant disorders in school-age children who stutter. *Language, Speech, and Hearing Services in Schools, 32,* 68–78.

Arnold, H. S., Conture, E. G., Key, A. F., & Walden, T. (2011). Emotional reactivity, regulation, and childhood stuttering: A behavioral and electrophysiological study. *Journal of Communication Disorders, 44,* 276–293.

Arnold, H. S., Conture, E. G., & Ohde, R. N. (2005). Phonological neighborhood density in the picture naming of young children who stutter: Preliminary study. *Journal of Fluency Disorders, 30,* 125–148.

Au-Yeung, J., Howell, P., & Pilgrim, L. (1998). Phonological words and stuttering on function words. *Journal of Speech, Language, and Hearing Research, 41,* 1019–1030.

Azrin, N. H., & Nunn, R. G. (1974). A rapid method of eliminating stuttering by a regulated breathing approach. *Behaviour Research and Therapy, 12,* 279–286.

Baddeley, A. D. (1992). Working memory. *Science, 255,* 556–559.

Bakker, K. (2010). The measurement of cluttering severity. In K. Bakker, F. L. Myers, & L. J. Raphael (Eds.), *Proceedings of the First World Conference on Cluttering* (pp. 211–219). International Cluttering Association. Retrieved November 2, 2013, from http://associations.missouristate.edu/ICA/

Bakker, K., Brutten, G. J., Janssen, P., & van der Meulen, S. (1991). An eyemarking study of anticipation and dysfluency among elementary school stutterers. *Journal of Fluency Disorders, 16,* 25–33.

Bakker, K., Myers, F. L., Raphael, L. J., & St. Louis, K. O. (2011). A preliminary comparison of speech rate, self-evaluation, and disfluency of people who speak exceptionally fast, clutter, or speak normally. In D. Ward & K. Scaler Scott (Eds.), *Cluttering: A handbook of research, intervention and education* (pp. 45–65). New York, NY: Psychology Press.

Bakker, K., & Riley, G. D. (2009). *Computerized scoring of stuttering severity (CSSS-2.0).* Austin, TX: Pro-Ed.

Balasubramanian, V., Cronin, K. L., & Max, L. (2010). Dysfluency levels during repeated readings, choral readings, and readings with altered auditory feedback in two cases of acquired neurogenic stuttering. *Journal of Neurolinguistics, 23,* 488–500.

Balasubramanian, V., Max, L., Van Borsel, J., Rayca, K. O., & Richardson, D. (2003). Acquired stuttering following right frontal and bilateral pontine lesion: A case study. *Brain and Cognition, 53,* 185–189.

Ball, M. J., Müller, N., & Rutter, B. (2010). *Phonology for communication disorders.* New York, NY: Psychology Press.

Barch, D. M., & Berenbaum, H. (1997). Language generation in schizophrenia and mania: The relationships among verbosity. *Journal of Psycholinguistic Research, 26,* 401–412.

Bauerly, K. R., & De Nil, L. F. (2011). Speech sequence skill learning in adults who stutter. *Journal of Fluency Disorders, 36,* 349–360.

Bauman-Waengler, J. A. (2012). *Articulatory and phonological impairments: A clinical focus* (4th ed.). Upper Saddle River, NJ: Pearson Education.

Beck, J. S. (2011). *Cognitive behavior therapy: Basics and beyond* (2nd ed.). New York: NY: Guilford Press.

Behrman, A. (2007). *Speech and voice science.* San Diego, CA: Plural.

Bella, S. D., & Berkowska, M. (2009). Singing and its neuronal substrates: Evidence from the general population. *Contemporary Music Review, 28,* 279–291.

Bennett Lanouette, E. B. (2011). Intervention strategies for cluttering disorders. In D.

Ward & K. Scaler Scott (Eds.), *Cluttering: A handbook of research, intervention and education* (pp. 175–197). New York, NY: Psychology Press.

Benton, A. L. (1967). Problems of test construction in the field of aphasia. *Cortex, 3*, 32–58.

Benton, A. L., Hamsher, K., & Sivan, A. B. (1994). *Multilingual Aphasia Examination.* Iowa City, IA: AJA Associates.

Berg, T. (1998). *Linguistic structures and change.* New York, NY: Oxford University Press.

Berg, T., & Abd-El-Jawad, H. (1996). The unfolding of suprasegmental representations: A cross-linguistic perspective. *Journal of Linguistics, 32*, 291–324.

Bernstein Ratner, N. (1988). Response to Quesal: Terminology in stuttering research [Letter to the editor]. *Journal of Speech and Hearing Disorders, 53*, 350.

Bernstein Ratner, N. (2005). Evidence-based practice in stuttering: Some questions to consider. *Journal of Fluency Disorders, 30*, 163–188.

Bernstein Ratner, N., Rooney, B., & MacWhinney, B. (1996). Analysis of stuttering using CHILDES and CLAN. *Clinical Linguistics and Phonetics, 10*, 169–187.

Bernstein Ratner, N., & Sih, C. C. (1987). Effects of gradual increases in sentence length and complexity on children's dysfluency. *Journal of Speech and Hearing Disorders, 52*, 278–287.

Bernstein Ratner, N., & Silverman, S. (2000). Parental perceptions of children's communicative development at stuttering onset. *Journal of Speech, Language, and Hearing Research, 43*, 1252–1263.

Berry, M. F. (1937). Twinning in stuttering families. *Human Biology, 9*, 329–346.

Berry, M. F. (1938). A common denominator in twinning and stuttering. *Journal of Speech and Hearing Disorders, 3*, 51–57.

Berry, R. C., & Silverman, F. H. (1972). Equality of intervals on the Lewis-Sherman scale of stuttering severity. *Journal of Speech and Hearing Research, 15*, 185–188.

Bhatnagar, S., & Andy, O. J. (1989). Alleviation of acquired stuttering with human centre-median thalamic stimulation. *Journal of Neurology, Neurosurgery, and Psychiatry, 52*, 1182–1184.

Bishop, J. H., Williams, H. G., & Cooper, W. A. (1991). Age and task complexity variables in motor performance of children with articulation-disordered, stuttering, and normal speech. *Journal of Fluency Disorders, 16*, 219–228.

Bleumel, C. S. (1932). Primary and secondary stammering. *Quarterly Journal of Speech, 18*, 187–200.

Bleumel, C. S. (1960). Concepts of stammering: A century in review. *Journal of Speech and Hearing Disorders, 25*, 24–32.

Bliss, L. S., & McCabe, A. (2008). Patterns of discourse coherence: Variations in genre performance in children with language impairment. *Imagination, Cognition, and Personality, 28*, 137–154.

Bliss, L. S., McCabe, A., & Miranda, A. E. (1998). Narrative assessment profile: Discourse analysis for school-age children. *Journal of Communication Disorders, 31*, 347–363.

Blomgren, M. (2010). Stuttering treatment for adults: An update on contemporary approaches. *Seminars in Speech and Language, 31*, 272–282.

Blomgren, M., Nagarajan, S. S., Lee, J. N., Li, T., & Alvord, L. (2003). Preliminary results of a functional MRI study of brain activation patterns in stuttering and nonstuttering speakers during a lexical access task. *Journal of Fluency Disorders, 28*, 337–356.

Blomgren, M., Roy, N., Callister, T., & Merrill, R. M. (2005). Intensive stuttering modification therapy: A multidimensional assessment of treatment outcomes. *Journal of Speech, Language, and Hearing Research, 48*, 509–523.

Blood, G. W., Blood, I. M., Bennett, S., Simpson, K. C., & Susman, E. J. (1994). Subjective anxiety measurements and cortisol responses in adults who stutter. *Journal of Speech and Hearing Research, 37*, 760–768.

Blood, G. W., Blood, I. M., Maloney, K., Meyer, C. D., & Qualls, C. (2007). Anxiety levels in adolescents who stutter. *Journal of Communication Disorders, 40*, 452–469.

Blood, G. W., Blood, I. M., Tellis, G. M., & Gabel, R. M. (2003). A preliminary study of self-esteem, stigma, and disclosure in adolescents who stutter. *Journal of Fluency Disorders, 28,* 143–159.

Blood, G. W., Blood, I. M., Tramontana, M. G., Sylvia, A. J., Boyle, M. P., & Motzko, G. R. (2011). Self-reported experience of bullying of students who stutter: Relations with life satisfaction, life orientation, and self-esteem. *Perceptual and Motor Skills, 113,* 353–364.

Blood, G. W., Ridenour, V., Jr., Qualls, C., & Hammer, C. (2003). Co-occurring disorders in children who stutter. *Journal of Communication Disorders, 36,* 427–448.

Blood, G. W., & Seider, R. (1981). The concomitant problems of young stutterers. *Journal of Speech and Hearing Disorders, 46,* 31–33.

Blood, I. M., Wertz, H., Blood, G. W., Bennett, S., & Simpson, K. C., (1997). The effects of life stressor and daily stressors on stuttering. *Journal of Speech, Language, and Hearing Research, 40,* 134–143.

Bloodstein, O. (1958). Stuttering as an anticipatory struggle reaction. In J. Eisenson (Ed.), *Stuttering: A symposium* (pp. 1–70). New York, NY: Harper & Row.

Bloodstein, O. (1960a). The development of stuttering: I. Changes in nine basic features. *Journal of Speech and Hearing Disorders, 25,* 219–237.

Bloodstein, O. (1960b). The development of stuttering: II. Development phases. *Journal of Speech and Hearing Disorders, 25,* 366–376.

Bloodstein, O., & Bernstein Ratner, N. (2008). *A handbook on stuttering* (6th ed.). Clifton Park, NY: Thomson Delmar Learning.

Bloodstein, O., & Gantwerk, B. F. (1967). Grammatical function in relation to stuttering in young children. *Journal of Speech and Hearing Research, 10,* 786–789.

Bloodstein, O., & Grossman, M. (1981). Early stutterings: Some aspects of their form and distribution. *Journal of Speech and Hearing Research, 24,* 298–302.

Bloom, L., & Lahey, M. (1978). *Language development and language disorders.* New York, NY: John Wiley & Sons.

Blumgart, E., Tran, Y., & Craig, A. (2010a). Social anxiety disorder in adults who stutter. *Depression and Anxiety, 27,* 687–692.

Blumgart, E., Tran, Y., & Craig, A. (2010b). An investigation into the personal financial costs associated with stuttering. *Journal of Fluency Disorders, 35,* 203–215.

Boberg, E., & Kully, D. (1994). Long-term results of an intensive treatment program for adults and adolescents who stutter. *Journal of Speech and Hearing Research, 37,* 1050–1059.

Boberg, E., Yeudall, L. T., Schopflocher, D., & Bo-Lassen, P. (1983). The effect of an intensive behavioral program on the distribution of EEG alpha power in stutterers during the processing of verbal and visuospatial information. *Journal of Fluency Disorders, 8,* 245–263.

Bock, K., & Levelt, W. J. M. (1994). Language production: Grammatical encoding. In M. A. Gernsbacher (Ed.), *Handbook of psycholinguistics* (pp. 741–779). New York, NY: Academic Press.

Boey, R. A., Van de Heyning, P. H., Wuyts, F. L., Heylen, L., Stoop, R., & De Bodt, M. S. (2009). Awareness and reactions of young stuttering children aged 2–7 years old towards their speech disfluency. *Journal of Communication Disorders, 42,* 334–346.

Bohland, J. W., Bullock, D., & Guenther, F. H. (2009). Neural representations and mechanisms for the performance of simple speech sequences. *Journal of Cognitive Neuroscience, 22,* 1504–1529.

Boller, F., Boller, M., Denes, G., Timberlake, W. H., Zieper, I., & Albert M. (1973). Familial palilalia. *Neurology, 23,* 1117–1125.

Bonelli, P., Dixon, M., Bernstein Ratner, N., & Onslow, M. (2000). Child and parent speech and language following the Lidcombe Programme of early stuttering intervention. *Clinical Linguistics and Phonetics, 14,* 427–446.

Bonfanti, B. H., & Culatta, R. (1977). An analysis of the fluency patterns of institutionalized retarded adults. *Journal of Fluency Disorders, 2,* 117–128.

Boomer, D. S., & Laver, J. D. (1973). Slips of the tongue. In V. Fromkin (Ed.), *Speech errors as linguistic evidence.* (pp. 120–131). The Hague, Netherlands: Mouton.

Borden, G. J., & Harris, K. S. (1984). *Speech science primer: Physiology, acoustics, and perception of speech* (2nd ed.). Baltimore, MD: Lippincott Williams & Wilkins.

Bortfeld, H., Leon, S. D., Bloom, J. E., Schober, M. F., & Brennan, S. E. (2001). Disfluency rates in conversation: Effects of age, relationship, topic, role, and gender. *Language and Speech, 44,* 123–147.

Boscolo, B., Bernstein Ratner, N., & Rescorla, L. (2002). Fluency of school-aged children with a history of specific expressive language impairment: An exploratory study. *American Journal of Speech-Language Pathology, 11,* 41–49.

Bosshardt, H. (1999). Effects of concurrent mental calculation on stuttering, inhalation, and speech timing. *Journal of Fluency Disorders, 24,* 43–72.

Bosshardt, H. (2002). Effects of congruent cognitive processing on the fluency of word repetition: Comparison between persons who do and do not stutter. *Journal of Fluency Disorders, 27,* 93–114.

Bothe, A. K., Davidow, J. H., Bramlett, R. E., Franic, D. M., & Ingham, R. J. (2006). Stuttering treatment research 1970–2005: II. Systematic review incorporating trial quality assessment of pharmacological approaches. *American Journal of Speech-Language Pathology, 15,* 342–352.

Bothe, A. K., Davidow, J. H., Bramlett, R. E., & Ingham, R. J. (2006). Stuttering treatment research 1970–2005: I. Systematic review incorporating trial quality assessment of behavioral, cognitive, and related approaches. *American Journal of Speech-Language Pathology, 15,* 321–341.

Bothe, A. K., & Richardson, J. D. (2011). Statistical, practical, clinical, and personal significance: Definitions and applications in speech-language pathology. *American Journal of Speech-Language Pathology, 20,* 233–242.

Botterill, W., & Kelman, E. (2010). Palin parent-child interaction. In B. Guitar & R. McCauley (Eds.), *Treatment of stuttering: Established and emerging interventions* (pp. 63–90). Baltimore, MD: Lippincott Williams & Wilkins.

Brady, W. A., & Hall, D. E. (1976). The prevalence of stuttering among school-age children. *Language, Speech, and Hearing Services in Schools, 7,* 75–81.

Bray, M., Kehle, T. J., Lawless, K. A., & Theodore, L. A. (2003). The relationship of self-efficacy and depression to stuttering. *American Journal of Speech-Language Pathology, 12,* 425–431.

Brazell, T. R., & Logan, K. J. (2001, November). *Stuttering children with concomitant problems: A survey of treatment practices.* Poster presented at the annual convention of the American Speech-Language-Hearing Association, New Orleans, LA.

Breznitz, Z. (2006). *Fluency in reading: Synchronization of processes.* Mahwah, NJ: Lawrence Erlbaum Associates.

Bricker-Katz, G., Lincoln, M., & McCabe, P. (2009). A life-time of stuttering: How emotional reactions to stuttering impact activities and participation in older people. *Disability and Rehabilitation: An International, Multidisciplinary Journal, 31,* 1742–1752.

Brookshire, R. H., & Nicholas, L. E. (1995). Performance deviations in the connected speech of adults with no brain damage and adults with aphasia. *American Journal of Speech-Language Pathology, 4,* 118–123.

Brosch, S., Häge, A., & Johansen, H. S. (2002). Prognostic indicators for stuttering: The value of computer-based speech analysis. *Brain and Language, 82,* 75–86.

Browman, C. P., & Goldstein, L. (1990). Gestural specification using dynamically-defined articulatory structures. *Journal of Phonetics, 18,* 299–320.

Browman, C. P., & Goldstein, L. (1992). Articulatory phonology: An overview. *Phonetica, 49,* 155–180.

Brown, B. L., Giles, H., & Thakerar, J. N. (1985). Speaker evaluations as a function of speech rate, accent, and context. *Language & Communication, 5,* 207–220.

Brown, R. (1973). *A first language*. Cambridge, MA: Harvard University Press.

Brown, S. F. (1937). The influence of grammatical function on the incidence of stuttering. *Journal of Speech and Hearing Disorders, 2*, 207–215.

Brown, S. F. (1938). A further study of stuttering in relation to various speech sounds. *Quarterly Journal of Speech, 24*, 390–397.

Brown, S. F. (1945). The loci of stuttering in the speech sequence. *Journal of Speech and Hearing Disorders, 10*, 181–192.

Brown, S. F., Ingham, R. J., Ingham, J. C., Laird, A. R., & Fox, P. T. (2005). Stuttered and fluent speech production: An ALE meta-analysis of functional neuroimaging studies. *Human Brain Mapping, 25*, 105–117.

Brundage, S. B., Bothe, A. K., Lengeling, A. N., & Evans, J. J. (2006). Comparing judgments of stuttering made by students, clinicians, and highly experienced judges. *Journal of Fluency Disorders, 31*, 271–283.

Brutten, E. J., & Shoemaker, D. J. (1967). *The modification of stuttering*. Englewood Cliffs, NJ: Prentice Hall.

Brutten, G. J. (1975). Stuttering: Topography, assessment and behavior change strategies. In J. Eisenson (Ed.), *Stuttering: A second symposium* (pp. 199–262). New York, NY: Harper & Row.

Brutten G. J., & Vanryckeghem, M. (2007). *Behavior Assessment Battery for School-Age Children Who Stutter.* San Diego, CA: Plural.

Buhr, A., & Zebrowski, P. (2009). Sentence position and syntactic complexity of stuttering in early childhood: A longitudinal study. *Journal of Fluency Disorders, 34*, 155–172.

Bunton, K. (2008). Speech versus nonspeech: Different tasks, different neural organization. *Seminars in Speech and Language, 29*, 267–275.

Burch, J. M., Kiernan, T. E. J., & Demaer-schalk, B. M. (2013). Neurogenic stuttering with right hemisphere stroke: A case presentation. *Journal of Neurolinguistics, 26*, 207–213.

Burger, R., & Wijnen, F. (1999). Phonological encoding and word stress in stuttering and nonstuttering subjects. *Journal of Fluency Disorders, 24*, 91–106.

Byrd, C. T., Conture, E. G., & Ohde, R. N. (2007). Phonological priming in young children who stutter: Holistic versus incremental processing. *American Journal of Speech-Language Pathology, 16*, 43–53.

Byrd, C. T., Logan, K. J., & Gillam, R. B. (2012). Speech disfluency in school-age children's conversational and narrative discourse. *Language, Speech, and Hearing Services in Schools, 43*, 153–163.

Byrd, D. (1993). 54,000 American stops. *UCLA Working Paper in Phonetics, 83*, 97–116.

Camarata, S. T. (1989). Final consonant repetition: A linguistic perspective. *Journal of Speech and Hearing Disorders, 54*, 159–162.

Canter, G. J. (1971). Observations of neurogenic stuttering: A contribution to differential diagnosis. *British Journal of Disorders of Communication, 6*, 139–143.

Carey, W. B., & McDevitt, S. C. (1995). *The Carey Temperament Scales*. Scottsdale, AZ: Behavioral-Developmental Initiatives.

Caruso, A. J., Abbs, J. H., & Gracco, V. L. (1988). Kinematic analysis of multiple movement coordination during speech in stutterers. *Brain, 111*, 439–456.

Caruso, A. J., Chodzko-Zajko, W. J., Bidinger, D. A., & Sommers, R. K. (1994). Adults who stutter: Responses to cognitive stress. *Journal of Speech and Hearing Research, 37*, 746–754.

Caruso, A. J., Conture, E. G., & Colton, R. H. (1988). Selected temporal parameters of coordination associated with stuttering in children. *Journal of Fluency Disorders, 13*, 57–82.

Cerhan, J., Folsom, A., Mortimer, J., Shahar, E., Knopman, D., McGovern, P., . . . Heiss, G. (1998). Correlates of cognitive function in middle-aged adults. *Gerontology, 44*, 95–105.

Chakraborty, N., & Logan, K. J. (2013, November) *Factors that contribute to listeners' judgments of naturalness in children's speech*. Poster presented at the annual convention of the American Speech-Language-Hearing Association, Chicago, IL.

Chall, D. (1983). *Stages of reading development*. New York, NY: McGraw-Hill.

Chang, S. E., Erickson, K. I., Ambrose, N. G., Hasegawa-Johnson, M. A., & Ludlow, C. L. (2008). Brain anatomy differences in childhood stuttering. *Neuroimage, 39*, 1333–1344.

Chang, S. E., Horwitz, B., Ostuni, J., Reynolds, R., & Ludlow, C. L. (2011). Evidence of left inferior frontal-premotor structural and functional connectivity deficits in adults who stutter. *Cerebral Cortex, 21*(11), 2507–2518.

Chang, S. E., Kenney, M. K., Loucks, T. M., & Ludlow, C. L. (2009). Brain activation abnormalities during speech and non-speech in stuttering speakers. *Neuroimage, 46*, 201–212.

Chapman, A. H., & Cooper, E. B. (1973). Nature of stuttering in a mentally retarded population. *American Journal of Mental Deficiency, 38*, 153–157.

Chard, D. J., Pikulski, J. J., & McDonagh, S. H. (2006). Fluency: The link between decoding and comprehension for struggling readers. In T. Rasinski, C. Blachowicz, & K. Lems (Eds.), *Fluency instruction: Research-based best practices* (pp. 39–61). New York, NY: Guilford Press.

Chertkow, H., & Bub, D. (1990). Semantic memory loss in Alzheimer-type dementia. In M. F. Schwartz (Ed.), *Modular deficits in Alzheimer-type dementia* (pp. 207–244). Cambridge, MA: MIT Press.

Chmela, K. A., & Reardon, N. (2001). *The school-aged child who stutters: Working effectively with attitudes and emotions*. Memphis, TN: Stuttering Foundation of America.

Cholin, J. (2008). The mental syllabary in speech production: An integration of different approaches and domains. *Aphasiology, 22*, 1127–1141.

Cholin, J., & Levelt, W. J. M. (2009). Effects of syllable preparation and syllable frequency in speech production: Further evidence for syllabic units at a post-lexical level. *Language and Cognitive Processes, 24*, 662–684.

Cholin, J., Schiller, N. O., & Levelt, W. M. (2004). The preparation of syllables in speech production. *Journal of Memory and Language, 50*, 47–61.

Choo, A., Kraft, S., Olivero, W., Ambrose, N. G., Sharma, H., Chang, S., & Loucks, T. M. (2011). Corpus callosum differences associated with persistent stuttering in adults. *Journal of Communication Disorders, 44*, 470–477.

Cipolotti, L., Bisiacchi, P.S., Denes, G., & Gallo, A. (1988). Acquired stuttering: A motor programming disorder? *European Neurology, 28*, 321–325.

Cloutman, L., Newhart, M., Davis, C., Heidler-Gary, J., & Hillis, A. (2009). Acute recovery of oral word production following stroke: Patterns of performance as predictors of recovery. *Behavioural Neurology, 21*, 145–153.

Coggon, D., Rose, G., & Barker, D. J. P. (1997) *Epidemiology for the uninitiated*. London, UK: BMJ.

Cohen, J. (1988). *Statistical power analysis for the behavioral sciences* (2nd ed.). Hillsdale, NJ: Lawrence Erlbaum Associates.

Colburn, N., & Mysak, E. D. (1982a). Developmental disfluency and emerging grammar: I. Disfluency characteristics in early syntactic utterances. *Journal of Speech and Hearing Research, 25*, 414–420.

Colburn, N., & Mysak, E. D. (1982b). Developmental disfluency and emerging grammar: II. Co-occurrence of disfluency with specified semantic-syntactic structures. *Journal of Speech and Hearing Research, 25*, 421–427.

Collins, A. M., & Loftus, E. F. (1975). A spreading activation theory of semantic processing. *Psychological Review, 82*, 407–428.

Collins, C. R., & Blood, G. W. (1990). Acknowledgment and severity of stuttering as factors influencing nonstutterers' perceptions of stutterers. *Journal of Speech and Hearing Disorders, 55*, 75–81.

Conture, E. G. (1990). *Stuttering* (2nd ed.). Englewood Cliffs, NJ: Prentice Hall.

Conture, E. G. (2001). *Stuttering: Its nature, diagnosis, and treatment*. Boston, MA: Allyn & Bacon.

Conture, E. G., Colton, R. H., & Gleason, J. R. (1988). Selected temporal aspects of coordination during fluent speech of young stutterers. *Journal of Speech and Hearing Research, 31*, 640–653.

Conture, E. G., & Kelly, E. M. (1991). Young stutterers' nonspeech behaviors during stuttering. *Journal of Speech and Hearing Research, 34*, 1041–1056.

Conture, E. G., Schwartz, H. D., & Brewer, D. W. (1985). Laryngeal behavior during stuttering: A further study. *Journal of Speech and Hearing Research, 28*, 233–240.

Conture, E. G., Walden, T. A., Arnold, H. S., Graham, C. G., Hartfield, K. N., & Karrass, J. (2006). Communication-emotional model of stuttering. In N. Bernstein & J. Tetnowski (Eds.), *Current issues in stuttering research and practice* (pp. 17–46). Mahwah, NJ: Lawrence Erlbaum Associates.

Cooper, E. B. (1972). Recovery from stuttering in a junior and senior high school population. *Journal of Speech and Hearing Research, 15*, 632–638.

Cooper, E. B. (1986). The mentally retarded stutterer. In K. O. St. Louis (Ed.), *The atypical stutterer: Principles and practices of rehabilitation* (pp. 123–154). Orlando, FL: Academic Press.

Cooper, E. B. (1987). The chronic perseverative stuttering syndrome: Incurable stuttering. *Journal of Fluency Disorders, 12*, 381–388.

Cooper, E. B., Cady, B. B., & Robbins, C. J. (1970). The effect of the verbal stimulus words, "wrong," "right," and "tree" on the disfluency rates of stutterers and nonstutterers. *Journal of Speech and Hearing Research, 13*, 239–244.

Cooper, G. M. (2000). *The cell: A molecular approach* (2nd ed.) [Lysosomes]. Sunderland, MA: Sinauer Associates. Retrieved from http://www.ncbi.nlm.nih.gov/books/NBK9953/

Corcoran, J., & Stewart, M. (1998). Stories of stuttering: A qualitative analysis of interview narratives. *Journal of Fluency Disorders, 23*, 247–264.

Cordes, A. K. (2000). Individual and consensus judgments of disfluency types in the speech of persons who stutter. *Journal of Speech, Language, and Hearing Research, 43*, 951–964.

Cordes, A. K., & Ingham, R. J. (1994). The reliability of observational data: II. Issues in the identification and measurement of stuttering events. *Journal of Speech and Hearing Research, 37*, 279–294.

Coriat, I. H. (1943). Theory. In E. F. Hahn (Ed.), *Stuttering: Significant theories and therapies* (pp. 27–29). Stanford University, CA: Stanford University Press.

Costello, J. (1975). The establishment of fluency with time-out procedures: Three case studies. *Journal of Speech and Hearing Disorders, 40*, 216–231.

Cosyns, M., Mortier, G., Janssens, S., Saharan, N., Stevens, E., & Van Borsel, J. (2010). Speech fluency in neurofibromatosis type 1. *Journal of Fluency Disorders, 35*, 59–69.

Covey, S. (2013). *The 7 habits of highly effective people.* New York, NY: Simon & Schuster.

Cox, N. J., Seider, R. A., & Kidd, K. K. (1984). Some environmental factors and hypotheses for stuttering in families with several stutterers. *Journal of Speech and Hearing Research, 27*, 543–548.

Craig, A. (1990). An investigation into the relationship between anxiety and stuttering. *Journal of Speech and Hearing Disorders, 55*, 290–294.

Craig, A. (1996). Long-term effects of intensive treatment for a client with both a cluttering and stuttering disorder. *Journal of Fluency Disorders, 21*, 329–335.

Craig, A. (1998). Relapse following treatment for stuttering: A critical review and correlative data. *Journal of Fluency Disorders, 23*, 1–30.

Craig, A. (2010). The importance of conducting controlled clinical trial in the fluency disorders with emphasis on cluttering. In K. Bakker, F. L. Myers, & L. J. Raphael (Eds.), *Proceedings of the First World Conference on Cluttering* (pp. 220–229). International Cluttering Association. Retrieved November 2, 2013, from http://associations.missouristate.edu/ICA/

Craig, A., & Andrews, G. (1985). The prediction and prevention of relapse in stuttering: The value of self-control techniques and locus of control measures. *Behavior Modification, 9,* 427–442.

Craig, A., Blumgart, E., & Tran, Y. (2009). The impact of stuttering on the quality of life in adults who stutter. *Journal of Fluency Disorders, 34,* 61–71.

Craig, A., Blumgart, E., & Tran, Y. (2011). Resilience and stuttering: Factors that protect people from the adversity of chronic stuttering. *Journal of Speech, Language, and Hearing Research, 54,* 1485–1496.

Craig, A., Hancock, K., Chang, E., McCready, C., Shepley, A., McCaul, A., . . . Reilly, K. (1996). A controlled clinical trial for stuttering in persons aged 9 to 14 years. *Journal of Speech and Hearing Research, 39,* 808–826.

Craig, A., Hancock, K., Tran, Y., Craig, M., & Peters, K. (2002). Epidemiology of stuttering in the community across the entire life span. *Journal of Speech, Language, and Hearing Research, 45,* 1097–1105.

Craig, A. R., & Cleary, P. J. (1982). Reduction of stuttering by young male stutterers using EMG feedback. *Biofeedback and Self-Regulation, 7,* 241–255.

Craig, A. R., Franklin, J. A., & Andrews, G. (1984). A scale to measure locus of control of behaviour. *British Journal of Medical Psychology, 57,* 173–180.

Craig, H. K., & Washington, J. A. (2004). Grade-related changes in the production of African American English. *Journal of Speech, Language, and Hearing Research, 47,* 450–463.

Cross, D. E., & Luper, H. L. (1979). Voice reaction time of stuttering and nonstuttering children and adults. *Journal of Fluency Disorders, 4,* 59–77.

Cross, D. E., & Olson, P. (1987). Interaction between jaw kinematics and voice onset for stutterers and nonstutterers in a VRT task. *Journal of Fluency Disorders, 12,* 367–380.

Crystal, D., & Varley, R. (1998). *Introduction to language pathology.* Baltimore, MD: Paul H. Brookes.

Crystal, T., & House, A. (1990). Articulation rate and the duration of syllables and stress groups in connected speech. *Journal of the Acoustical Society of America, 88,* 101–112.

Cuadrado, E. M., & Weber-Fox, C. M. (2003). Atypical syntactic processing in individuals who stutter: Evidence from event-related brain potentials and behavioral measures. *Journal of Speech and Hearing Research, 46,* 960–976.

Cuetos, F., Gonzalez-Nosti, M., & Martínez, C. (2005). The picture-naming task in the analysis of cognitive deterioration in Alzheimer's disease. *Aphasiology, 19,* 545–557.

Culatta, R., & Sloan, A. (1977). The acquisition of the label "stuttering" by primary level schoolchildren. *Journal of Fluency Disorders, 2,* 29–34.

Cullinan, W. L., & Springer, M. T. (1980). Voice initiation and termination times in stuttering and nonstuttering children. *Journal of Speech and Hearing Research, 23,* 344–360.

Curlee, R. F. (1981). Observer agreement on disfluency and stuttering. *Journal of Speech and Hearing Research, 24,* 595–600.

Curlee, R. F. (1996). Cluttering: Data in search of understanding. *Journal of Fluency Disorders, 21,* 367–371.

Curlee, R. F., & Yairi, E. (1997). Early intervention with early childhood stuttering: A critical examination of the data. *American Journal of Speech-Language Pathology, 6,* 8–18.

Curry, F. K., & Gregory, H. H. (1969). The performance of stutterers on dichotic listening tasks thought to reflect cerebral dominance. *Journal of Speech and Hearing Research, 12,* 73–82.

Cykowski, M. D., Fox, P. T., Ingham, R. J., Ingham, J. C., & Robin, D. A. (2010). A study of the reproducibility and etiology of diffusion anisotropy differences in developmental stuttering: A potential role for impaired myelination. *Neuroimage, 52,* 1495–1504.

Cykowski, M. D., Kochunov, P. V., Ingham, R. J., Ingham, J. C., Mangin, J. F., Riviere, D., . . . Fox, P. T. (2008). Perisylvian sulcal morphology and cerebral asymmetry patterns in adults who stutter. *Cerebral Cortex, 18,* 571–583.

Dabul, B. L. (2000). *Apraxia Battery for Adults–Second Edition [ABA–2].* Austin, TX: Pro-Ed.

Daly, D. (1986). The clutterer. In K. O. St. Louis (Ed.), *The atypical stutterer: Principles and practices of rehabilitation* (pp. 155–192). Orlando, FL: Academic Press.

Daly, D. (1992). Helping the clutterer: Therapy considerations. In F. L. Myers & K. O. St. Louis (Eds.), *Cluttering: A clinical perspective*. Leicester, UK: Far Communications.

Daly, D. (1993). Cluttering: The orphan of speech-language pathology. *American Journal of Speech-Language Pathology, 2*, 6–8.

Daly, D. (2010). Treating cluttering: The power of the pause. In J. Kuster (Ed.), *Proceedings of the International Cluttering Online Conference, 2010*. Retrieved October 28, 2013, from http://www.mnsu.edu/comdis/ica1/icacon1.html

Daly, D., & Cantrell, R. (2006, July). *Cluttering: Characteristics identified as diagnostically significant by 60 fluency experts*. Paper presented at the 5th World Congress on Fluency Disorders, Dublin, Ireland.

Daly, D. A., & Burnett, M. L. (1996). Cluttering: Assessment, treatment planning, and case study illustration. *Journal of Fluency Disorders, 21*, 239–248.

Daly, D. A., & Burnett, M. L. (1999). Cluttering: Traditional views and new perspectives. In R. F. Curlee (Ed.), *Stuttering and related disorders of fluency* (pp. 222–254). New York, NY: Thieme Medical.

Daly, D. A., & Kimbarow, M. L. (1978). Stuttering as operant behavior: Effects of the verbal stimuli wrong, right, and tree on the disfluency rates of school-age stutterers and nonstutterers. *Journal of Speech and Hearing Research, 21*, 589–597.

Daniels, D. E., Gabel, R. M., & Hughes, S. (2012). Recounting the K–12 school experiences of adults who stutter: A qualitative analysis. *Journal of Fluency Disorders, 37*, 71–82.

Davis, S., Howell, P., & Cooke, F. (2002). Sociodynamic relationships between children who stutter and their non-stuttering classmates. *Journal of Child Psychology and Psychiatry and Allied Disciplines, 43*, 939–947.

Defloor, T., Van Borsel, J., & Curts, L. (2000). Speech fluency in Prader-Willi syndrome. *Journal of Fluency Disorders, 25*, 85–98.

DeJoy, D. A., & Gregory, H. H. (1985). The relationship between age and frequency of disfluency in preschool children. *Journal of Fluency Disorders, 10*, 107–122.

Dell, G. S. (1986). A spreading activation theory of retrieval in sentence production. *Psychological Review, 93*, 288–331.

Dell, G. S., Juliano, C., & Govindjee, J. (1993). Structure and content in language production: A theory of frames constraints in phonological speech errors. *Cognitive Science, 17*, 149–195.

Dell, G. S., & Warker, J. A. (2007). Using slips to study phonotactic learning in the laboratory. In C. T. Schütze & V. S. Ferreira (Eds.), *MIT working papers in linguistics: Vol. 53. The state of the art in speech error research: Proceedings of the LSA Institute Workshop* (pp. 75–94). Cambridge, MA: MITWPL.

Dembowski, J., & Watson, B. C. (1991). Preparation time and response complexity effects on stutterers' and nonstutterers' acoustic LRT. *Journal of Speech and Hearing Research, 34*, 49–59.

De Nil, L. F., & Brutten, G. J. (1991). Speech-associated attitudes of stuttering and nonstuttering children. *Journal of Speech, Language, and Hearing Research, 34*, 60–66.

De Nil, L. F., Jokel, R., & Rochon, E. (2007). Etiology, symptomatology, and treatment of neurogenic stuttering. In E. G. Conture & R. F. Curlee (Eds.), *Stuttering and related disorders of fluency* (pp. 326–343). New York, NY: Thieme Medical.

De Nil, L. F., & Kroll, R. M. (1995). The relationship between locus of control and long-term stuttering treatment outcome in adult stutterers. *Journal of Fluency Disorders, 20*, 345–364.

De Nil, L. F., Kroll, R. M., Lafaille, S. J., & Houle, S. (2003). A positron emission tomography study of short- and long-term treatment effects on functional brain activation in adults who stutter. *Journal of Fluency Disorders, 28*, 357–380.

De Nil, L. F., Sasisekaran, J., van Lieshout, P. H. H. M., & Sandor, P. (2005). Speech disfluencies in individuals with Tourette syndrome. *Journal of Psychosomatic Research, 58*, 97–102.

Denny, M., & Smith, A. (1992). Gradations in a pattern of neuromuscular activity associated with stuttering. *Journal of Speech and Hearing Research, 35,* 1216–1229.

Deputy, P. N., Nakasone, H., & Tosi, O. (1982). Analysis of pauses occurring in the speech of children with consistent misarticulations. *Journal of Communication Disorders, 15,* 43–54.

Dewey, J. (2010). My experiences with cluttering. In J. Kuster (Ed.), *Proceedings of the International Cluttering Online Conference,* 2010. Retrieved from http://www.mnsu.edu/comdis/ica1/icacon1.html

Dickson, S. (1971). Incipient stuttering and spontaneous remission of stuttered speech. *Journal of Communication Disorders, 4,* 99–110.

Diedrich, W. M. (1984). Cluttering: Its diagnosis. In H. Winitz (Ed.), *Treating articulation disorders: For clinicians by clinicians* (pp. 307–323). Baltimore, MD: University Park Press.

Dijkstra, K., Bourgeois, M. S., Allen, R. S., & Burgio, L. D. (2004). Conversational coherence: Discourse analysis of older adults with and without dementia. *Journal of Neurolinguistics, 17,* 263.

Dollaghan, C. A. (2007). *The handbook for evidence-based practice in communication disorders.* Baltimore, MD: Paul H. Brookes.

Dollaghan, C. A., & Campbell, T. (1992). A procedure for classifying disruptions in spontaneous language samples. *Topics in Language Disorders, 12,* 56–68.

Dore, J. (1974). A pragmatic description of early language development. *Journal of Psycholinguistic Research, 3,* 343–350.

Douglas, J. M. (2010). Relation of executive functioning to pragmatic outcome following severe traumatic brain injury. *Journal of Speech, Language, and Hearing Research, 53,* 365–382.

Drayna, D. (2011). Possible genetic factors in cluttering. In D. Ward & K. Scaler Scott (Eds.), *Cluttering: A handbook of research, intervention and education* (pp. 29–33). New York, NY: Psychology Press.

Duffy, J. (1995). *Motor speech disorders.* Baltimore, MD: Mosby.

Dworzynski, K., Remington, A., Rijsdijk, F., Howell, P., & Plomin, R. (2007). Genetic etiology in cases of recovered and persistent stuttering in an unselected, longitudinal sample of young twins. *American Journal of Speech-Language Pathology, 16,* 169–178.

Dyson, A. T. (1988). Phonetic inventories of 2- and 3-year-old children. *Journal of Speech and Hearing Disorders, 53,* 89–93.

Egan, G. (1998). *The skilled helper: A problem-management approach to helping* (6th ed.). Pacific Grove, CA: Brooks/Cole.

Eggers, K., De Nil, L. F., & Van den Bergh, B. H. (2009). Factorial temperament structure in stuttering, voice-disordered, and typically developing children. *Journal of Speech, Language, and Hearing Research, 52,* 1610–1622.

Ehri, L. C. (1995). Phases of development in learning to read words by sight. *Journal of Research in Reading, 18,* 116–125.

Einarsdóttir, J., & Ingham, R. J. (2005). Have disfluency-type measures contributed to the understanding and treatment of developmental stuttering? *American Journal of Speech-Language Pathology, 14,* 260–273.

Ellis, A., & Harper, R. A. (1975). *A new guide to rational living.* Englewood Cliffs, NJ: Prentice Hall.

Endler, N. S., Edwards, J. M., Vitelli, R., & Parker, J. D. A. (1989). Assessment of state and trait anxiety: Endler Multidimensional Anxiety Scales. *Anxiety Research, 2,* 1–14.

Ezrati-Vinacour, R., & Levin, I. (2004). The relationship between anxiety and stuttering: A multidimensional approach. *Journal of Fluency Disorders, 29,* 135–148.

Ezrati-Vinacour, R., Platzky, R., & Yairi, E. (2001). The young child's awareness of stuttering-like disfluency. *Journal of Speech, Language, and Hearing Research, 44,* 368–380.

Felsenfeld, S., Kirk, K. M., Zhu, G., Statham, D. J., Neale, M. C., & Martin, N. G. (2000). A study of the genetic and environmental etiology of stuttering in a selected twin sample. *Behavior Genetics, 30,* 359–366.

Ferreira, F. (1993). The creation of prosody during sentence processing. *Psychological Review, 100*, 233–253.

Ferreira, F. (2007). Prosody and performance in language production. *Language and Cognitive Processes, 22*, 1151–1177.

Fey, M. E. (1986). *Language intervention with young children*. San Diego, CA: College-Hill Press.

Fillmore, C. J. (1979). On fluency. In C. J. Fillmore, D. Kempler, & W. S. Y. Wang (Eds.), *Individual differences in language ability and language behavior* (pp. 85–101). New York, NY: Academic Press.

Finn, P. (1996). Establishing the validity of recovery from stuttering without formal treatment. *Journal of Speech and Hearing Research, 39*, 1171–1181.

Finn, P. (1997) Adults recovered from stuttering without formal treatment: Perceptual assessment of speech normalcy. *Journal of Speech, Language, and Hearing Research, 40*, 821–831.

Finn, P. (2008). Self-control and the treatment of stuttering. In E. G. Conture & R. F. Curlee (Eds.), *Stuttering and related disorders of fluency* (3rd ed., pp. 344–360). New York, NY: Thieme Medical.

Finn, P., Howard, R., & Kubala, R. (2005). Unassisted recovery from stuttering: Self-perceptions of current speech behavior, attitudes, and feelings. *Journal of Fluency Disorders, 30*, 281–305.

Finn, P., & Ingham, R. J. (1994). Stutterer's self-ratings of how natural speech sounds and feels. *Journal of Speech and Hearing Research, 37*, 326–340.

Finn, P., Ingham, R. J., Ambrose, N. G., & Yairi, E. (1997). Children recovered from stuttering without formal treatment: Perceptual assessment of speech normalcy. *Journal of Speech, Language, and Hearing Research, 40*, 867–876.

Fisher, S. E. (2010). Genetic susceptibility to stuttering [Comment on mutations in the lysosomal enzyme-targeting pathway and persistent stuttering]. *New England Journal of Medicine, 362*, 750–752.

Fletcher, J. M. (1914) An experimental study of stuttering. *American Journal of Psychology, 25*, 201–255.

Fletcher, S. G. (1972). Time-by-count measurement of diadochokinetic syllable rate. *Journal of Speech and Hearing Research, 15*, 763–770.

Flipsen, P., Jr. (2006). Syllables per word in typical and delayed speech acquisition. *Clinical Linguistics and Phonetics, 20*, 293–301.

Fon, J., Johnson, K., & Chen, S. (2011). Durational patterning at syntactic and discourse boundaries in Mandarin spontaneous speech. *Language and Speech, 54*, 5–32.

Forrest, K. & Iuzzini, J. (2008). A comparison of oral motor and production training for children with speech sound disorders. *Seminars in Speech and Language, 29*, 304–311.

Foundas, A. L., Bollich, A. M., Corey, D. M., Hurley, M., & Heilman, K. M. (2001). Anomalous anatomy of speech-language areas in adults with persistent developmental stuttering. *Neurology, 57*, 207–215.

Foundas, A. L., Bollich, A. M., Feldman, J. J., Corey, D. M., Hurley, M. M., Lemen, L. C., & Heilman, K. M. (2004). Aberrant auditory processing and atypical planum temporale in developmental stuttering. *Neurology, 63*, 1640–1646.

Foundas, A. L., Corey, D. M., Angeles, V. V., Bollich, A. M., Crabtree-Hartman, E. E., & Heilman, K. M. (2003). Atypical cerebral laterality in adults with persistent developmental stuttering. *Neurology, 61*, 1378–1385.

Fowler, C. A. (2003). Speech production and perception. In A. F. Healy & R. W. Proctor (Eds.), *Handbook of psychology: Experimental psychology* (Vol. 4, pp. 237–266). Hoboken, NJ: John Wiley & Sons.

Fowler, C. A. (2007). Speech production. In M. G. Gaskell (Ed.), *The Oxford handbook of psycholinguistics* (pp. 489–501). Oxford, UK: Oxford University Press.

Fowler, C. A., & Housum, J. (1987). Talkers' signaling of "new" and "old" words in speech and listeners' perception and use of the distinction. *Journal of Memory and Language, 26*, 489–504.

Fowler, C. A., & Turvey, M. T. (1980). Immediate compensation in bite-block speech. *Phonetica, 37*, 306–325.

Francis D., Clark N., & Humphreys, G. (2002). Circumlocution-induced naming (CIN): A treatment for effecting generalisation in anomia? *Aphasiology, 16*, 243–259.

Franic, D. M., & Bothe, A. K. (2008). Psychometric evaluation of condition-specific instruments used to assess health-related quality of life, attitudes, and related constructs in stuttering. *American Journal of Speech-Language Pathology, 17*, 60–80.

Frank, A., & Bloodstein, O. (1971). Frequency of stuttering following repeated unison readings. *Journal of Speech and Hearing Research, 14*, 519–524.

Franz, E. A., Zelaznik, H. N., & Smith, A. (1992). Evidence of common timing processes in the control of manual, orofacial, and speech movements. *Journal of Motor Behavior, 24*, 281–287.

Freeman, F. J., & Ushijima, T. (1978). Laryngeal muscle activity during stuttering. *Journal of Speech and Hearing Research, 21*, 538–562.

Freund, H. (1952). Studies in the interrelationship between stuttering and cluttering. *Folia Phoniatrica, 4*, 146–168.

Friel-Patti, S. (1994). Commitment to theory. *American Journal of Speech-Language Pathology, 3*, 30–34.

Fromkin, V. A. (1971). The non-anomalous nature of anomalous utterances. *Language, 47*, 27–52.

Gabel, R. M., Blood, G. W., Tellis, G. M., & Althouse, M. T. (2004). Measuring role entrapment of people who stutter. *Journal of Fluency Disorders, 29*, 27–49.

Gaines, N. D., Runyan, C. M., & Meyers, S. C. (1991). A comparison of young stutterers' fluent versus stuttered utterances on measures of length and complexity. *Journal of Speech, Language, and Hearing Research, 34*, 37–42.

Garrett, M. F. (1975). The analysis of sentence production. In G. Bower (Ed.), *Psychology of learning and motivation: Advances in research and theory* (Vol. 9, pp. 133–177). New York, NY: Academic Press.

Garrett, M. F. (1984). Disorders of lexical selection. *Cognition, 42*, 143–180.

Gay, T. (1978). Effect of speaking rate on vowel formant movements. *Journal of the Acoustical Society of America, 63*, 223–230.

Gay, T., Ushijima, T., Hirose, H., & Cooper, F. S. (1974). Effect of speaking rate on labial consonant-vowel articulation. *Journal of Phonetics, 2*, 47–63.

Gertner, B. L., Rice, M. L., & Hadley, P. A. (1994). Influence of communicative competence on peer preferences in a preschool classroom. *Journal of Speech and Hearing Research, 37*, 913–923.

Ghosh, S. S., Tourville, J. A., & Guenther, F. H. (2008). A neuroimaging study of premotor lateralization and cerebellar involvement in the production of phonemes and syllables. *Journal of Speech, Language, and Hearing Research, 51*, 1183–1202.

Gickling, E. E., & Armstrong, D. L. (1978). Levels of instructional difficulty as related to on-task behavior, task completion, and comprehension. *Journal of Learning Disabilities, 11*, 559–566.

Giddan, J. J., Ross, G. J., Sechler, L. L., & Becker, B. R. (1997). Selective mutism in elementary school: Multidisciplinary interventions. *Language, Speech, and Hearing Services in Schools, 28*, 127–133.

Gierut, J. A. (1999). Syllable onsets: Clusters and adjuncts in acquisition. *Journal of Speech, Language, and Hearing Research, 42*, 708–726.

Gillam, R. B., Logan, K. J., & Pearson, N. A. (2009). *Test of Childhood Stuttering (TOCS)*. Austin, TX: Pro-Ed.

Gillam, R. B., & Pearson, N. A. (2004). *Test of Narrative Language*. Austin, TX: Pro-Ed.

Gillespie, S. K., & Cooper, E. B. (1973). Prevalence of speech problems in junior and senior high schools. *Journal of Speech and Hearing Research, 16*, 739–743.

Ginsberg, A. (2000). Shame, self-consciousness, and locus of control in people who stutter. *The Journal of Genetic Psychology: Research and Theory on Human Development*, *161*, 389–399.

Ginther, A., Dimova, S., & Yang, R. (2010). Conceptual and empirical relationships between temporal measures of fluency and oral English proficiency with implications for automated scoring. *Language Testing*, *27*, 379–399.

Gleason, J. B. (2013). The development of language. In J. B. Gleason & N. Bernstein Ratner (Eds.), *The development of language* (8th ed., pp. 1–29). Boston, MA: Pearson Education.

Glosser, G., & Deser, T. (1990). Patterns of discourse production among neurological patients with fluent language disorders. *Brain and Language*, *40*, 67–88.

Goberman, A. L., Hughes, S., & Haydock, T. (2011). Acoustic characteristics of public speaking: Anxiety and practice effects. *Speech Communication*, *53*, 867–876.

Goldman, R., & Fristoe, M. (2000). *Goldman-Fristoe Test of Articulation-2*. Circle Pines, MN: American Guidance Services.

Goldsmith (1990). *Autosegmental and metrical phonology*. Oxford, UK: Blackwell.

Goldstein, L., & Fowler, C.A. (2003). A phonology for public language use. In N. O. Schiller & A. S. Meyer (Eds.), *Phonetics and phonology in language comprehension and production: Differences and similarities* (pp. 159–207). Berlin, Germany: Mouton de Gruyter.

Goodglass, H., Kaplan, E., & Barresi, B. (2000). *Boston Diagnostic Aphasia Examination* (3rd ed.). San Antonio, TX: PsychCorp.

Goodhue, R., Onslow, M., Quine, S., O'Brian, S., & Hearne, A. (2010). The Lidcombe Program of early stuttering intervention: Mothers' experiences. *Journal of Fluency Disorders*, *35*, 70–84.

Gordon, P. A., & Luper, H. L. (1989). Speech disfluencies in nonstutterers: Syntactic complexity and production task effects. *Journal of Fluency Disorders*, *14*, 429–445.

Gordon, P. A., Luper, H. L., & Peterson, H. A. (1986). The effects of syntactic complexity on the occurrence of disfluencies in 5-year-old nonstutterers. *Journal of Fluency Disorders*, *11*, 151–164.

Gottsleben, R. H. (1955). The incidence of stuttering in a group of mongoloids. *Training School Bulletin*, *51*, 209–218.

Gottwald, S. R. (2010). Stuttering prevention and early intervention: A multidimensional approach. In B. Guitar & R. McCauley (Eds.), *Treatment of stuttering: Established and emerging interventions* (pp. 91–117). Baltimore, MD: Lippincott Williams & Wilkins.

Gracco, V. L. (1990). Characteristics of speech as a motor control system. In. G. R. Hammond (Ed.), *Cerebral control of speech and limb movements* (pp. 3–28). Amsterdam: North-Holland.

Gracco, V. L., & Abbs, J. H. (1985). Dynamic control of the perioral system during speech: Kinematic analyses of autogenic and non-autogenic sensorimotor processes. *Journal of Neurophysiology*, *54*, 418–432.

Graf, O. (1955). Incidence of stuttering among twins. In W. J. Johnson & R. R. Leutenegger (Eds.), *Stuttering in children and adults*. Minneapolis, MN: University of Minnesota Press.

Grant, A. C., Biousse, V., Cook, A. A., & Newman, N. J. (1999). Stroke-associated stuttering. *Archives of Neurology*, *56*, 624–627.

Gregory, H. H. (with Campbell, J. H., Gregory, C. B., & Hill, D. G.) (2003). *Stuttering therapy: Rationale and procedures*. Boston, MA: Allyn & Bacon.

Grice, H. P. (1975). Logic and conversation. In P. Cole & J. L. Morgan (Eds.), *Speech acts* (pp. 41–58). New York, NY: Academic Press.

Guenther, F. H. (1995). Speech sound acquisition, coarticulation, and rate effects in a neural network model of speech production. *Psychological Review*, *102*, 594–621.

Guenther, F. H. (2003). Neural control of speech movements. In N. O. Schiller & A. S. Meyer (Eds.), *Phonetics and phonology in language comprehension and production: Differences and similarities* (pp. 209–239). Berlin, Germany: Mouton de Gruyter.

Guenther, F. H. (2006). Cortical interactions underlying the production of speech sounds. *Journal of Communication Disorders, 39,* 350–365.

Guitar, B. (1975). Reduction of stuttering frequency using analog electromyographic feedback. *Journal of Speech and Hearing Research, 18,* 672–685.

Guitar, B. (2006). *Stuttering: An integrated approach to its nature and treatment* (3rd ed.). Philadelphia, PA: Lippincott Williams & Wilkins.

Guitar, B., Guitar, C., Neilson, P., O'Dwyer, N., & Andrews, G. (1988). Onset sequencing of selected lip muscles in stutterers and nonstutterers. *Journal of Speech and Hearing Research, 31,* 28–35.

Guitar, B., & McCauley, R. J. (2010). An overview of treatments for preschool stuttering. In B. Guitar & R. J. McCauley (Eds.), *Treatment of stuttering: Established and emerging interventions* (pp. 56–62). Baltimore, MD: Lippincott Williams & Wilkins.

Guo, L., Tomblin, J. B., & Samelson, V. (2008). Speech disruptions in the narratives of English-speaking children with specific language impairment. *Journal of Speech, Language, and Hearing Research, 51,* 722–738.

Hakim, H. B., & Bernstein Ratner, N. (2004). Nonword repetition abilities of children who stutter: An exploratory study. *Journal of Fluency Disorders, 29,* 179–199.

Hall, K., Amir, O., & Yairi, E. (1999). A longitudinal investigation of speaking rate in preschool children who stutter. *Journal of Speech, Language, and Hearing Research, 42,* 1367–1377.

Hall, N. E. (1999). Speech disruptions in preschool children with specific language impairment and phonological impairment. *Clinical Linguistics & Phonetics, 13,* 295–307.

Hall, N. E., Yamashita, T. S., & Aram, D. M. (1993). Relationship between language and fluency in children with developmental language disorders. *Journal of Speech and Hearing Research, 23,* 568–579.

Hancock, K., Craig, A., McCready, C., McCaul, A., Costello, D., Campbell, K., & Gilmore, G. (1998). Two- to six-year controlled-trial stuttering outcomes for children and adolescents. *Journal of Speech, Language, and Hearing Research, 41,* 1242–1252.

Hand, C. R., & Haynes, W. O. (1983). Linguistic processing and reaction time differences in stutterers and nonstutterers. *Journal of Speech and Hearing Research, 26,* 181–185.

Hanna, R., Wilfling, F., & McNeill, B. (1975). A biofeedback treatment for stuttering. *Journal of Speech and Hearing Disorders, 40,* 270–273.

Hanson, B. R., Gronhovd, D., & Rice, P. L. (1981). A shortened version of the Southern Illinois University Speech Situation Checklist for the identification of speech related anxiety. *Journal of Fluency Disorders, 6,* 351–360.

Harackiewicz, J. M., Barron, K. E., Tauer, J. M., Carter, S. M., & Elliot, A. J. (2000). Short-term and long-term consequences of achievement goals: Predicting interest and performance over time. *Journal of Educational Psychology, 92,* 316–300.

Hargrave, S., Kalinowski, J., Stuart, A., Armson, J., & Jones, K. (1994). Effect of frequency-altered feedback on stuttering frequency at normal and fast speech rates. *Journal of Speech and Hearing Research, 37,* 1313–1319.

Harris, H. F. (1996). Elective mutism: A tutorial. *Language, Speech, and Hearing Services in Schools, 27,* 10–15.

Harris, T., & Hodges, R. (1995) *The literacy dictionary.* Newark, DE: International Reading Association.

Harrison, E., Onslow, M., & Menzies, R. (2004). Dismantling the Lidcombe Program of early stuttering intervention: Verbal contingencies for stuttering and clinical measurement. *International Journal of Language & Communication Disorders, 39,* 257–267.

Hartinger, M., & Moosehammer, C. (2009). Investigation of speech motor skills in cluttering by means of EMMA. In K. Bakker, F. L. Myers, & L. J. Raphael (Eds.), *Proceedings of the First World Conference on Cluttering* (pp. 153–161). International Cluttering Association. Retrieved from http://associations.missouristate.edu/ICA/

Hasbrouck, J., & Tindal, G. A. (2006). Oral reading fluency norms: A valuable assessment tool for reading teachers. *The Reading Teacher, 59*, 636–644.

Hayhow, R., Cray, A. M., & Enderby, P. (2002). Stammering and therapy views of people who stammer. *Journal of Fluency Disorders, 27*, 1–17.

Hearne, A., Packman, A., Onslow, M., & O'Brian, S. (2008). Developing treatment for adolescents who stutter: A phase I trial of the Camperdown Program. *Language, Speech, and Hearing Services in Schools, 39*, 487–497.

Heath, S. B. (1982). What no bedtime story means: Narrative skills at home and school. *Language in Society, 11*, 49–76.

Helm, N., Butler, R., & Canter, G. (1980). Neurogenic acquired stuttering. *Journal of Fluency Disorders, 5*, 269–279.

Helm-Estabrooks, N. (1986). Diagnosis and management of neurogenic stuttering in adults. In K. O. St. Louis (Ed.), *The atypical stutterer: Principles and practices of rehabilitation* (pp. 193–217). Orlando, FL: Academic Press.

Helm-Estabrooks, N., Yeo, R., Geschwind, N., Freedman, M., & Weinstein, C. (1986). Stuttering: Disappearance and reappearance with acquired brain lesions. *Neurology, 36*, 1109–1112.

Henry, J. D., & Crawford, J. R. (2004). Verbal fluency deficits in Parkinson's disease: A meta-analysis. *Journal of the International Neuropsychological Society, 10*, 608–622.

Hewat, S., Onslow, M., Packman, A., & O'Brian, S. (2006). A Phase II clinical trial of self-imposed time-out treatment for stuttering in adults and adolescents. *Disability and Rehabilitation: An International, Multidisciplinary Journal, 28*, 33–42.

Hieke, A. E. (1981). A content-processing view of hesitation phenomena. *Language and Speech, 24*, 147–160.

Hieke, A. E., Kowal, S., & O'Connell, D. C. (1983). The trouble with "articulatory" pauses. *Language and Speech, 26*, 203–214.

Higuchi, T. (2000). Disruption of kinematic coordination in throwing under stress. *Japanese Psychological Research, 42*, 168–177.

Hixon, T. J. (1973). Respiratory function in speech. In F. D. Minifie, T. J. Hixon, & F. Williams (Eds.), *Normal aspects of speech, hearing, and language* (pp. 82–101). Englewood Cliffs, NJ: Prentice Hall.

Hixon, T. J., Weismer, G., & Hoit, J. D. (2008) *Preclinical speech science.* San Diego, CA: Plural.

Hodgman, H., & Logan, K. J. (2013, November). *A comparison on naturalness and effort ratings in stuttered and fluent speech samples.* Poster presented at the annual convention of the American Speech-Language-Hearing Association, Chicago, IL.

Hoit, J. D., Lansing, R. W., & Perona, K. E. (2007). Speaking-related dyspnea in healthy adults. *Journal of Speech, Language, and Hearing Research, 50*, 361–374.

Howell, P. (2011). *Recovery from stuttering.* New York, NY: Psychology Press.

Howell, P., & Au-Yeung, J. (1995). The association between stuttering, Brown's factors, and phonological categories in child stutterers ranging in age between 2 and 12 years. *Journal of Fluency Disorders, 20*, 331–344.

Howell, P., Au-Yeung, J., & Sackin, S. S. (1999). Exchange of stuttering from function words to content words with age. *Journal of Speech, Language, and Hearing Research, 42*, 345–354.

Howell, P., & Davis, S. (2011). The epidemiology of cluttering with stuttering. In D. Ward & K. Scaler Scott (Eds.), *Cluttering: A handbook of research, intervention and education* (pp. 69–89). New York, NY: Psychology Press.

Howell, P., Sackin, S. S., & Rustin, L. L. (1995). Comparison of speech motor development in stutterers and fluent speakers between 7 and 12 years old. *Journal of Fluency Disorders, 20*, 243–255.

Howell, P., Sackin, S. S., & Williams, R. (1999). Differential effects of frequency-shifted feedback between child and adult stutterers. *Journal of Fluency Disorders, 24*, 127–136.

Howie, P. M. (1981). Concordance for stuttering in monozygotic and dizygotic twin pairs. *Journal of Speech and Hearing Research, 24*, 317–321.

Hubbard, C. P., & Prins, D. (1994). Word familiarity, syllabic stress pattern, and stuttering. *Journal of Speech and Hearing Research, 37*, 564–571.

Hubbard, C. P., & Yairi, E. (1988). Clustering of disfluencies in the speech of stuttering and nonstuttering preschool children. *Journal of Speech and Hearing Research, 31*, 228–233.

Huggins, A. W. (1972). Just noticeable differences for segment duration in natural speech. *Journal of the Acoustical Society of America, 51*, 1270–1278.

Hugh-Jones, S., & Smith, P. K. (1999). Self-reports of short- and long-term effects of bullying on children who stammer. *British Journal of Educational Psychology, 69*, 141–158.

Hulstijn, W., Summers, J. J., van Lieshout, P. H., & Peters, H. F. (1992). Timing in finger tapping and speech: A comparison between stutterers and fluent speakers. *Human Movement Science, 11*, 113–124.

Indefrey, P. (2007). Brain imaging studies of language production. In G. Gaskell (Ed.), *The Oxford handbook of psycholinguistics* (pp. 547–564). Oxford, UK: Oxford University Press.

Indefrey, P., & Levelt, W. J. M. (2004). The spatial and temporal signatures of word production components. *Cognition, 92*, 101–144.

Ingham, J. C. (1999). Behavioral treatment of young children who stutter: An extended length of utterance method. In R. F. Curlee (Ed.), *Stuttering and related disorders of fluency* (2nd ed., pp. 80–109). New York, NY: Thieme Medical.

Ingham, J. C., & Ingham, R. J. (2011). *The Stuttering Measurement System (SMS) training manual (Student's manual)*. Santa Barbara, CA: University of California.

Ingham, J. C., & Riley, G. (1998). Guidelines for documentation of treatment efficacy for young children who stutter. *Journal of*

Speech, Language, and Hearing Research, 41, 753–770.

Ingham, R. J. (2010). Comments on article by Maguire et al.: Pagoclone trial: Questionable findings for stuttering treatment. *Journal of Clinical Psychopharmacology, 30*, 649–650.

Ingham, R. J., Bothe, A. K., Jang, E., Yates, L., Cotton, J., & Seybold, I. (2009). Measurement of speech effort during fluency-inducing conditions in adults who do and do not stutter. *Journal of Speech, Language, and Hearing Research, 52*, 1286–1301.

Ingham, R. J., & Cordes, A. K. (1992) Interclinic differences in stuttering-event counts. *Journal of Fluency Disorders, 17*, 171–176.

Ingham, R. J., Cordes, A. K., & Gow, M. L. (1993) Time-interval measurement of stuttering: Modifying interjudge agreement. *Journal of Speech and Hearing Research, 36*, 503–515.

Ingham, R. J., Fox, P. T., Ingham, J. C., Xiong, J., Zamarripa, F., Hardies, L. J., & Lancaster, J. L. (2004). Brain correlates of stuttering and syllable production: Gender comparison and replication. *Journal of Speech, Language, and Hearing Research, 47*, 321–341.

Ingham, R. J., Gow, M., & Costello, J. M. (1985). Stuttering and speech naturalness: Some additional data. *Journal of Speech and Hearing Disorders, 50*, 217–219.

Ingham, R. J., Grafton, S. T., Bothe, A. K., & Ingham, J. C. (2012). Brain activity in adults who stutter: Similarities across speaking tasks and correlations with stuttering frequency and speaking rate. *Brain and Language, 122*, 11–24.

Ingham, R. J., Ingham, J. C., Moglia, R., & Kilgo, M. (n.d). *SMS: Stuttering Measurement System* [Software and training manual and practice materials.]. Retrieved from http://sms.id.ucsb.edu/#

Ingham, R. J., Martin, R. R., Haroldson, S. K., Onslow, M., & Leney, M. (1985). Modification of listener-judged naturalness in the speech of stutterers. *Journal of Speech and Hearing Research, 28*, 495–504.

Ingham, R. J., Martin, R. R., & Kuhl, P. (1974). Modification and control of rate of speaking by stutterers. *Journal of Speech and Hearing Research, 17,* 489–496.

Ingham, R. J., Moglia, R. A., Frank, P., Ingham, J. C., & Cordes, A. K. (1997). Experimental investigation of the effects of frequency-altered auditory feedback on the speech of adults who stutter. *Journal of Speech, Language, and Hearing Research, 40,* 361–372.

Ingham, R. J., & Packman, A. C. (1978). Perceptual assessment of normalcy of speech following stuttering therapy. *Journal of Speech and Hearing Research, 21,* 63–73.

Ingham, R. J., Sato, W., Finn, P., & Belknap, H. (2001). The modification of speech naturalness during rhythmic stimulation treatment of stuttering. *Journal of Speech, Language, and Hearing Research, 44,* 841–852.

Ingham, R. J., Warner, A., Byrd, A., & Cotton, J. (2006). Speech effort measurement and stuttering: Investigating the chorus reading effect. *Journal of Speech and Hearing Research, 49,* 660–670.

Iverach, L., Jones, M., O'Brian, S., Block, S., Lincoln, M., Harrison, E., . . . Onslow, M. (2010a). Mood and substance use disorders among adults seeking speech treatment for stuttering. *Journal of Speech, Language, and Hearing Research, 53,* 1178–1190.

Iverach, L., O'Brian, S., Jones, M., Block, S., Lincoln, M., Harrison, E., . . . Onslow, M. (2009). Prevalence of anxiety disorders among adults seeking speech therapy for stuttering. *Journal of Anxiety Disorders, 23,* 928–934.

Iverach, L., O'Brian, S., Jones, M., Block, S., Lincoln, M., Harrison, E., . . . Onslow, M. (2010b). The five factor model of personality applied to adults who stutter. *Journal of Communication Disorders, 43,* 120–132.

James, J. E. (1976). The influence of duration of the effects of time-out from speaking. *Journal of Speech and Hearing Research, 19,* 206–215.

James, J. E. (1981). Behavioral self-control of stuttering using time-out from speaking. *Journal of Applied Behavior Analysis, 14,* 25–37.

James, J. E., & Ingham, R. J. (1974). The influence of stutterer's expectancies of improvement upon response to time-out. *Journal of Speech and Hearing Research, 17,* 86–93.

James, J. E., Ricciardelli, L. A., Rogers, P., & Hunter, C. E. (1989). A preliminary analysis of the ameliorative effects of time-out from speaking on stuttering. *Journal of Speech and Hearing Research, 32,* 604–610.

Jayaram, M. (1984). Distribution of stuttering in sentences: Relationship to sentence length and clause position. *Journal of Speech and Hearing Research, 27,* 329–338.

Jeffries, K. J., Fritz, J. B., & Braun, A. R. (2003). Words in melody: An $H_2{}^{15}O$ PET study of brain activation during singing and speaking. *Neuroreport: For Rapid Communication of Neuroscience Research, 14,* 749–754.

Johnson, K. N., Karrass, J., Conture, E. G., & Walden, T. (2009). Influence of stuttering variation on talker group classification in preschool children: Preliminary findings. *Journal of Communication Disorders, 42,* 195–210.

Johnson, K. N., Walden, T. A., Conture, E. G., & Karrass, J. (2010). Spontaneous regulation of emotions in preschool children who stutter: Preliminary findings. *Journal of Speech, Language, and Hearing Research, 53,* 1478–1495.

Johnson, W. (1942). A study of the onset and development of stuttering. *Journal of Speech and Hearing Disorders, 7,* 251–257.

Johnson, W. (1949). An open letter to the mother of a stuttering child. *Journal of Speech and Hearing Disorders, 14,* 3–8.

Johnson, W. (1961). Measurements of oral reading and speaking rate and disfluency of adult male and female stutterers and nonstutterers [Monograph Supplement No. 7]. *Journal of Speech and Hearing Disorders, 26,* 1–20.

Johnson, W., & Associates. (1959). *The onset of stuttering: Research findings and implications.* Minneapolis, MN: University of Minneapolis Press.

Johnson, W., Boehmler, R. M., Dahlstrom, W. G., Darley, F. L., Goodstein, L. D., Kools, J. A., . . . Young, M. A. (1959). *The onset of stuttering.* Minneapolis, MN: University of Minnesota Press.

Johnson, W., & Colley, W. H. (1945). The relationship between frequency and duration of stuttering. *Journal of Speech and Hearing Disorders, 10,* 35–38.

Johnson, W., & Rosen, P. (1937). Studies in the psychology of stuttering: VII. Effect of certain changes in speech pattern upon stuttering frequency, *Journal of Speech and Hearing Disorders, 2,* 105–109.

Johnson, W., Van Riper, C., Davis, D., Scarbrough, H., Hunsley, Y., Bakes, F., . . . Dwyer, S. (1942). A study of the onset and development of stuttering. *Journal of Speech Disorders, 7,* 251–257.

Jokel, R., De Nil, L. F., & Sharpe, A. K. (2007). Speech disfluencies in adults with neurogenic stuttering associated with stroke and traumatic brain injury. *Journal of Medical Speech-Language Pathology, 15,* 243–261.

Jones, K. M., Logan, K. J., & Shrivastav, R. (2005, November). *Duration, rate, and phoneme-type effects on listeners' judgments of prolongations.* Poster presented at the annual convention of the American Speech-Language-Hearing Association, San Diego, CA.

Jones, M., Onslow, M., Harrison, E., & Packman, A. (2000). Treating stuttering in young children: Predicting treatment time in the Lidcombe Program. *Journal of Speech, Language, and Hearing Research, 43,* 1440.

Jones, M., Onslow, M., Packman, A., O'Brian, S., Hearne, A., Williams, S., . . . Schwarz, I. (2008). Extended follow-up of a randomized controlled trial of the Lidcombe Program of early stuttering intervention. *International Journal of Language & Communication Disorders, 43,* 649–661.

Jones, M., Onslow, M., Packman, A., Williams, S., Ormond, T., Schwarz, I., & Gebski, V. (2005). Randomised controlled trial of the Lidcombe Programme of early stuttering intervention. *British Medical Journal, 331,* 659.

Jones, R. K. (1966). Observations on stammering after localized cerebral injury. *Journal of Neurology, Neurosurgery and Psychiatry, 29,* 192–195.

Jones, R. M., Fox, R. A., & Jacewicz, E. (2012). The effects of concurrent cognitive load on phonological processing in adults who stutter. *Journal of Speech, Language, and Hearing Research, 55,* 1862–1875.

Jones, S., Laukka, E. J., & Backman, L. (2006). Differential verbal fluency deficits in the preclinical stages of Alzheimer's disease and vascular dementia. *Cortex, 42,* 347–355.

Jourdain, S. (2000). A native-like ability to circumlocute. *Modern Language Journal, 84,* 185–195.

Kalinowski, J., Armson, J., & Stuart, A. (1995). Effect of normal and fast articulatory rates on stuttering frequency. *Journal of Fluency Disorders, 20,* 293–302.

Kalinowski, J., & Saltuklaroglu, T. (2003). Choral speech: The amelioration of stuttering via imitation and the mirror neuronal system. *Neuroscience & Biobehavioral Reviews, 27,* 339–347.

Kalinowski, J., Stuart, A., Wamsley, L., & Rastatter, M. P. (1999). Effects of monitoring condition and frequency-altered feedback on stuttering frequency. *Journal of Speech, Language, and Hearing Research, 42,* 1347–1354.

Kang, C., Riazuddin, S., Mundorff, J., Krasnewich, D., Friedman, P., Mullikin, J. C., & Drayna, D. (2010). Mutations in the lysosomal enzyme-targeting pathway and persistent stuttering. *New England Journal of Medicine, 362,* 677–685.

Karrass, J., Walden, T. A., Conture, E. G., Graham, C. G., Arnold, H. S., Hartfield, K. N., & Schwenk, K. A. (2006). Relation of emotional reactivity and regulation to childhood stuttering. *Journal of Communication Disorders, 39,* 402–423.

Kefalianos, E., Onslow, M., Ukoumunne, O., Block, S., & Reilly, S. (2014). Stuttering, temperament and anxiety: Data from a community cohort aged 2–4 years. *Journal of Speech, Language, and Hearing Research.* Advance online publication. doi:10.1044/2014_JSLHR-S-13-0069

Kell, C. A., Neumann, K., von Kriegstein, K., Posenenske, C., von Gudenberg, A. W., Euler, H., & Giraud, A. (2009). How the brain repairs stuttering. *Brain: A Journal of Neurology, 132,* 2747–2760.

Kelly, E. M. (1994). Speech rates and turn-taking behaviors of children who stutter and their fathers. *Journal of Speech and Hearing Research, 37,* 1284–1294.

Kelly, E. M., & Conture, E. G. (1992). Speaking rates, response time latencies, and interrupting behaviors of young stutterers, nonstutterers, and their mothers. *Journal of Speech and Hearing Research, 35,* 1256–1267.

Kelly, E. M., Smith, A., & Goffman, L. (1995). Orofacial muscle activity of children who stutter: A preliminary study. *Journal of Speech and Hearing Research, 38,* 1025–1036.

Kempen, G. (1977). Conceptualizing and formulating in sentence production. In S. Rosenberg (Ed.), *Sentence production: Developments in research and theory* (pp. 259–274). Hillsdale, NJ: Lawrence Erlbaum Associates.

Kempen, G. (1978). Sentence construction by a psychologically plausible formulator. In R. Campbell & P. Smith (Eds.), *Recent advances in the psychology of language: Vol. 2. Formal and experimental approaches* (pp. 103–123). New York, NY: Plenum Press.

Kent, R. D. (1984). Stuttering as a temporal programming disorder. In R. Curlee & W. Perkins (Eds.), *Nature and treatment of stuttering: New directions* (pp. 283–301). San Diego, CA: College-Hill Press.

Kent, R. D. (2004). The uniqueness of speech among motor systems. *Clinical Linguistics and Phonetics, 18,* 495–505.

Kent, R. D., & LaPointe, L. (1982) Acoustic properties of pathologic reiterative utterances: A case study of palilalia. *Journal of Speech and Hearing Research, 25,* 95–99.

Kent, R. D., & Read, C. (1992). *The acoustic analysis of speech.* San Diego, CA: Singular.

Kent, R. D., & Vorperian, H. K. (2013). Speech impairment in Down syndrome: A review. *Journal of Speech, Language, and Hearing Research, 56,* 178–210.

Kenyon, E. (1943). The etiology of stammering: The psychophysiologic facts which concern the production of speech sounds and of stammering. *Journal of Speech and Hearing Disorders, 8,* 347–348.

Kertesz, A. (2006). *Western Aphasia Battery–Revised.* San Antonio, TX: PsychCorp.

Ketelaars, M. P., Hermans, S. I. A., Cuperus, J., Jansonius, K., & Verhoeven, L. (2011). Semantic abilities in children with pragmatic language impairment: The case of picture naming skills. *Journal of Speech, Language, and Hearing Research, 54,* 87–98.

Kidd, K. K. (1984). Stuttering as a genetic disorder. In R. F. Curlee & W. H. Perkins (Eds.), *Nature and treatment of stuttering: New directions* (pp. 149–170). Boston, MA: College-Hill Press.

Kidd, K. K., Kidd, J. R., & Records, M. A. (1978). The possible causes of the sex ratio in stuttering and its implications. *Journal of Fluency Disorders, 3,* 13–23.

Kimura, D. (1961). Cerebral dominance and the perception of verbal stimuli. *Canadian Journal of Psychology, 14,* 166–177.

Klatt, D. (1974). The duration of [s] in English words. *Journal of Speech and Hearing Research, 17,* 51–63.

Klatt, D. (1975) Vowel lengthening is syntactically determined in a connected discourse. *Journal of Phonetics, 3,* 129–140.

Kleinow, J., & Smith, A. (2000). Influences of length and syntactic complexity on the speech motor stability of the fluent speech of adults who stutter. *Journal of Speech, Language, and Hearing Research, 43,* 548–559.

Klompas, M., & Ross, E. (2004). Life experiences of people who stutter, and the perceived impact of stuttering on quality of life: Personal accounts of South African individuals. *Journal of Fluency Disorders, 29,* 275–305.

Kloth, S. A. M., Janssen, P., Kraaimaat, F. W., & Brutten, G. J. (1995). Communicative behavior of mothers of stuttering and nonstuttering high-risk children prior to the onset of stuttering. *Journal of Fluency Disorders, 20,* 365–377.

Kloth, S. A. M., Janssen, P., Kraaimaat, F. W., & Brutten, G. J. (1998). Child and mother variables in the development of stuttering among high-risk children: A longitudinal study. *Journal of Fluency Disorders, 23,* 217–230.

Kloth, S. A. M., Kraaimaat, F. W., & Brutten, G. J. (1995). Speech-motor and linguistic skills of young stutterers prior to onset. *Journal of Fluency Disorders, 20*, 157–170.

Kloth, S. A. M., Kraaimaat, F. W., Janssen, P., & Brutten, G. J. (1999). Persistence and remission of incipient stuttering among high-risk children. *Journal of Fluency Disorders, 24*, 253–265.

Klouda, G. V., & Cooper, W. E. (1988). Contrastive stress, intonation, and stuttering frequency. *Language and Speech, 31*, 3–20.

Knott, J. R., Johnson, W., & Webster, M. J. (1937). Studies in the psychology of stuttering: II: A quantitative evaluation of expectation of stuttering in relation to the occurrence of stuttering. *Journal of Speech and Hearing Disorders, 2*, 20–22.

Koushik, S., Shenker, R., & Onslow, M. (2009). Follow-up of 6–10-year-old stuttering children after Lidcombe Program treatment: A phase I trial. *Journal of Fluency Disorders, 34*, 279–290.

Kowal, S., O'Connell, D. C., & Sabin, E. J. (1975). Development of temporal patterning and vocal hesitations in spontaneous narratives. *Journal of Psycholinguistic Research, 4*, 195–207.

Kraft, S. J., & Yairi, E. (2012). The genetic bases of stuttering: The state of the art, 2011. *Folia Phoniatrica et Logopaedica, 64*, 34–47.

Krishnan, G., & Tiwari, S. (2013). Differential diagnosis in developmental and acquired neurogenic stuttering: Do fluency-enhancing conditions dissociate the two? *Journal of Neurolinguistics, 26*, 252–257.

Kröger, B. J., Birkholz, P., Lowit, A., & Neuschaefer-Rube, C. (2010). Phonemic, sensory, and motor representations in an action-based neurocomputational model of speech production (ACT). In B. Maassen & P. van Lieshout (Eds.), *Speech motor control: New developments in basic and applied research* (pp. 23–36). New York, NY: Oxford University Press.

Kully, D., & Boberg, E. (1988). An investigation of inter-clinic agreement in the identification of fluent and stuttered syllables. *Journal of Fluency Disorders, 13*, 309–318.

Kully, D., & Langevin, M. (1999). Intensive treatment for stuttering adolescents. In R. F. Curlee (Ed.), *Stuttering and related disorders of fluency* (2nd ed., pp. 139–159). New York, NY: Thieme Medical.

Kully, D., Langevin, M., & Lomheim, H. (2007). Intensive treatment of stuttering in adolescents and adults. In E. G. Conture & R. F. Curlee (Eds.), *Stuttering and related disorders of fluency* (pp. 213–232). New York, NY: Thieme Medical.

Lange, P. G. (2008). An implicature for *um*: Signaling relative expertise. *Discourse Studies, 10*, 191–204.

Langevin, M. (2009). The peer attitudes toward children who stutter scale: Reliability, known groups validity, and negativity of elementary school-age children's attitudes. *Journal of Fluency Disorders, 34*, 72–86.

Langevin, M., & Boberg, E. (1996). Results of intensive stuttering therapy with adults who clutter and stutter. *Journal of Fluency Disorders, 21*, 315–327.

Langevin, M., Kully, D., Teshima, S., Hagler, P., & Narasimha Prasad, N. G. (2010). Five-year longitudinal treatment outcomes of the ISTAR comprehensive stuttering program. *Journal of Fluency Disorders, 35*, 123–140.

Lankford, S. D., & Cooper, E. B. (1974). Recovery from stuttering as viewed by parents of self-diagnosed recovered stutterers. *Journal of Communication Disorders, 7*, 171–180.

LaPointe, L. L., & Horner, J. (1981). Palilalia: A descriptive study of pathological reiterative utterances. *Journal of Speech and Hearing Disorders, 46*, 34–38.

LaSalle, L. R., & Conture, E. G. (1995). Disfluency clusters of children who stutter: Relation of stutterings to self-repairs. *Journal of Speech and Hearing Research, 38*, 965–977.

Lattermann, C., Shenker, R. C., & Thordardottir, E. (2005). Progression of language complexity during treatment with the Lidcombe Program for early stuttering intervention. *American Journal Speech-Language Pathology, 14*, 242–253.

Leaper, C., & Ayres, M. M. (2007). A meta-analytic review of gender variations in adults' language use: Talkativeness, affiliative speech, and assertive speech. *Personality and Social Psychology Review, 11,* 328–363.

Leaper, C., & Smith, T. E. (2004). A meta-analytic review of gender variations in children's language use: Talkativeness, affiliative speech, and assertive speech. *Developmental Psychology, 40,* 993–1027.

Lebrun, Y. (1996). Cluttering after brain damage. *Journal of Fluency Disorders, 3–4,* 289–295.

Lebrun, Y., & Leleux, C. (1985). Acquired stuttering following right brain damage in dextrals. *Journal of Fluency Disorders, 10,* 137–141.

Lebrun, Y., Leleux, C., Rousseau, J., & Devreux, F. (1983). Acquired stuttering. *Journal of Fluency Disorders, 8,* 323–330.

Lebrun, Y., Retif, J., & Kaiser, G. (1983). Acquired stuttering as a forerunner of motorneuron disease. *Journal of Fluency Disorders, 8,* 161–167.

Lebrun, Y., & Van Borsel, J. (1990). Final sound repetitions. *Journal of Fluency Disorders, 15,* 107–113.

Lee, L. L. (1974). *Developmental sentence analysis.* Evanston, IL: Northwestern University Press.

Lees, R. M., Boyle, B. E., & Woolfson, L. (1996). Is cluttering a motor disorder? *Journal of Fluency Disorders, 21,* 281–288.

Lehiste, I. (1973). Rhythmic units and syntactic units in production and perception. *Journal of the Acoustical Society of America, 54,* 1228–1234.

Levelt, W. J. M. (1983). Monitoring and self-repair in speech. *Cognition, 14,* 41–104.

Levelt, W. J. M. (1989). *Speaking: From intention to articulation.* Cambridge, MA: MIT Press.

Levelt, W. J. M. (2001). Spoken word production: A theory of lexical access. *Proceedings of the National Academy of Sciences, 98,* 13464–13471.

Levelt, W. J. M., Roelofs, A., & Meyer, A. S. (1999). A theory of lexical access in speech production. *Behavioral and Brain Sciences, 22,* 1–75.

Liberman, A. M., Cooper, F. S., Shankweiler, D. P., & Studdert-Kennedy, M. M. (1967). Perception of the speech code. *Psychological Review, 74,* 431–461.

Liberman, M., & Prince, A. (1977). On stress and linguistic rhythm. *Linguistic Inquiry, 8,* 249–336.

Lickley, R. J., Hartsuiker, R. J., Corley, M., Russell, M., & Nelson, R. (2005). Judgment of disfluency in people who stutter and people who do not stutter: Results from magnitude estimation. *Language and Speech, 48,* 299–312.

Liles, B. Z. (1993). Narrative discourse in children with language disorders and children with normal language: A critical review of the literature. *Journal of Speech and Hearing Research, 36,* 868–882.

Lincoln, M., & Onslow, M. (1997). Long-term outcome of early intervention for stuttering. *American Journal of Speech-Language Pathology, 6,* 51–58.

Lincoln, M., Packman, A., & Onslow, M. (2006). Altered auditory feedback and the treatment of stuttering: A review. *Journal of Fluency Disorders, 31,* 71–89.

Lincoln, M., & Walker, C. (2007). A survey of Australian adult users of altered auditory feedback devices for stuttering: Use patterns, perceived effectiveness, and satisfaction. *Disability and Rehabilitation, 29,* 1510–1517.

Loban, W. (1976). *Language development: Kindergarten through grade twelve.* Urbana, IL: National Council of Teachers of English.

Logan, K. J. (2001). The effect of syntactic complexity upon the speech fluency of adolescents and adults who stutter. *Journal of Fluency Disorders, 26,* 85–106.

Logan, K. J. (2003a). Language and fluency characteristics of preschoolers' multiple-utterance conversational turns. *Journal of Speech, Language, and Hearing Research, 46,* 178–188.

Logan, K. J. (2003b). The effect of syntactic structure upon speech initiation times of stuttering and nonstuttering speakers. *Journal of Fluency Disorders, 28,* 17–35.

Logan, K. J. (2005). Improving communicative functioning with school-aged children who stutter. In R. Lees & C. Stark (Eds.), *The treatment of stuttering in the young school-aged child* (pp. 108–139). London, UK: Whurr.

Logan, K. J. (2009) Supplemental clinical assessment activities. In R. B. Gillam, K. J. Logan, & N. A. Pearson (Eds.), *Test of Childhood Stuttering* [Examiner's manual] (pp. 77–104). Austin, TX: Pro-Ed.

Logan, K. J. (2010). Helping clients who clutter regulate speaking rate. In J. Kuster (Ed.), *Proceedings of the International Cluttering Online Conference, 2010.* Retrieved October 28, 2013, from http://www.mnsu.edu/comdis/ica1/icacon1.html

Logan, K. J. (2011). Stuttering (developmental). In J. Kreutzer, J. DeLuca, & B. Kaplan (Eds.), *Encyclopedia of clinical neuropsychology* (pp. 2420–2422). New York, NY: Springer Reference.

Logan, K. J., Byrd, C. T., Mazzocchi, E. M., & Gillam, R. B. (2011). Speaking rate characteristics of elementary-school-aged children who do and do not stutter. *Journal of Communication Disorders, 44,* 130–147.

Logan, K. J., & Caruso, A. J. (1997). Parents as partners in the treatment of childhood stuttering. *Seminars in Speech and Language, 18,* 309–326, 2420–2422

Logan, K. J., & Conture, E. G. (1995). Length, grammatical complexity, and rate differences in stuttered and fluent conversational utterances of children who stutter. *Journal of Fluency Disorders, 20,* 35–61.

Logan, K. J., & Conture, E. G. (1997). Selected temporal, grammatical, and phonological characteristics of conversational utterances. *Journal of Speech, Language, and Hearing Research, 40,* 107.

Logan, K. J., & Gillam, R. B. (2006, November). *A comparison of two sampling approaches in fluency analysis.* Poster presented at the annual convention of the American Speech-Language-Hearing Association, Miami, FL.

Logan, K. J., & Haj Tas, M. A. (2007). Effect of sample size on the measurement of stutter-like disfluencies. *Perspectives on Fluency and Fluency Disorders, 17,* 3–6.

Logan, K. J., & LaSalle, L. R. (1999). Grammatical characteristics of children's conversational utterances that contain disfluency clusters. *Journal of Speech, Language, and Hearing Research, 42,* 80–91.

Logan, K. J., Louko, L. J., Edwards, M. L., & Conture, E. G. (1995, December). *Differences in young children's phonological skills across stuttering severity levels.* Poster presented at the annual convention of the American Speech-Language-Hearing Association, Orlando, FL.

Logan, K. J., & Maren, S. M. (1998, November*). Palilalic-like speech in a school-aged child who stutters.* Poster presented at the annual convention of the American Speech-Language-Hearing Association, San Antonio, TX.

Logan, K. J., Mullins, M. S., & Jones, K. M. (2008). The depiction of stuttering in contemporary juvenile fiction: Implications for clinical practice. *Psychology in the Schools, 45,* 609–626.

Logan, K. J., & O'Connor, E. M. (2012). Factors affecting occupational advice for speakers who do and do not stutter. *Journal of Fluency Disorders, 37,* 25–41.

Logan, K. J., Roberts, R. R., Pretto, A. P., & Morey, M. J. (2002). Speaking slowly: Effects of four self-guided training approaches on adults' speech rate and naturalness. *American Journal of Speech-Language Pathology, 11,* 163–174.

Logan, K. J., & Willis, J. R. (2011). The accuracy with which adults who do not stutter predict stuttering-related communication attitudes. *Journal of Fluency Disorders, 36,* 334–348.

Logan, K. J., & Yaruss, J. S. (1999). Helping parents address attitudinal and emotional factors with young children who stutter. *Contemporary Issues in Communication Science and Disorders, 26,* 69–81.

Loonstra, A., Tarlow, A., & Sellers, A. (2001). COWAT metanorms across age, gender, and education. *Applied Neuropsychology, 8,* 161–166.

Louis, E. D., Winfield, L., Fahn, S., & Ford, B. (2001). Speech dysfluency exacerbated by levodopa in Parkinson's disease. *Movement Disorders, 16,* 562–581.

Louko, L. J., Edwards, M. L., & Conture, E. G. (1990). Phonological characteristics of young stutterers and their normally fluent peers: Preliminary observations. *Journal of Fluency Disorders, 15,* 191–210.

Ludlow, C., Rosenberg, J., Salazar, A., Grafman, J., & Smutok, M. (1987). Site of penetrating brain lesions causing chronic acquired stuttering. *Annals of Neurology, 22,* 60–66.

MacDonald, J. D., & Martin, R. R. (1973). Stuttering and disfluency as two reliable and unambiguous response classes. *Journal of Speech and Hearing Research, 16,* 691–699.

MacFarlane, W. B., Hanson, M., Walton, W., & Mellon, C. D. (1991). Stuttering in five generations of a single family: A preliminary report including evidence supporting a sex-modified mode of transmission. *Journal of Fluency Disorders, 16,* 117–123.

MacKay, D. G., & MacDonald, M. C. (1984). Stuttering as a sequencing and timing disorder. In R. F. Curlee & W. H. Perkins (Eds.), *Nature and treatment of stuttering: New directions* (pp. 261–282). Boston, MA: College-Hill Press.

Mackenzie, C. (2000). Adult spoken discourse: The influences of age and education. *International Journal of Language and Communication Disorders, 35,* 269–285.

MacLachlan, B. G., & Chapman, R. S. (1988). Communication breakdowns in normal and language learning-disabled children's conversation and narration. *Journal of Speech and Hearing Disorders, 53,* 2–7.

MacNeilage, P. F. (1970) Motor control of serial ordering of speech. *Psychological Review, 77,* 182–196.

MacWhinney, B. (1995). The CHILDES Project: Computational tools for analyzing talk (2nd ed.). Hillsdale, NJ: Lawrence Erlbaum Associates.

MacWhinney, B., & Osser, H. (1977). Verbal planning functions in children's speech. *Child Development, 48,* 978–985.

Maguire, G., Franklin, D., Vatakis, N. G., Morgenshtern, E., Denko, T., Yaruss, J. S., . . . Riley, G. (2010). Exploratory randomized clinical study of pagoclone in persistent developmental stuttering: The examining pagoclone for persistent developmental stuttering study. *Journal of Clinical Psychopharmacology, 30,* 48–56.

Mahr, G. C., & Torosian, T. (1999). Anxiety and social phobia in stuttering. *Journal of Fluency Disorders, 24,* 119–126.

Mahurin-Smith, J., & Ambrose, N. G., (2013). Breastfeeding may protect against persistent stuttering. *Journal of Communication Disorders, 46,* 351–360.

Makela, E. H., Sullivan, P., & Taylor, M. (1994). Sertraline and speech blockage. *Journal of Clinical Psychopharmacology, 14,* 432–433.

Makeun, G. H. (1909). A brief history of the treatment of stammering with some suggestions as to modern methods. *Medical Record, 76,* 1015–1017.

Malecot, A. (1955) An experimental study of force of articulation. *Studia Linguistica, 9,* 35.

Manning, W. H. (1994). *The SEA Scale: Self-efficacy scaling for adolescents who stutter.* Presentation to the annual meeting of American Speech-Language-Hearing Association, New Orleans, LA.

Manning, W. H. (2010). *Clinical decision making in fluency disorders* (3rd ed.). Clifton Park, NY: Delmar Cengage Learning.

Manning, W. H., & Beck, J. G. (2013). Personality dysfunction in adults who stutter: Another look. *Journal of Fluency Disorders, 38,* 184–192.

Manning, W. H., Dailey, D., & Wallace, S. (1984). Attitude and personality characteristics of older stutterers. *Journal of Fluency Disorders, 9,* 207–215.

Manning, W. H., & DiLollo, A. (2007). Management of stuttering for adolescents and adults: Traditional approaches. In E. Conture & R. F. Curlee (Eds.), *Stuttering and related disorders of fluency* (pp. 233–255). New York, NY: Thieme Medical.

Månsson, H. (2000). Childhood stuttering: Incidence and development. *Journal of Fluency Disorders, 25,* 47–57.

Market, K. E., Montague, J. C., Buffalo, M. D., & Drummond, S. S. (1990). Acquired stuttering: Descriptive data and treatment outcome. *Journal of Fluency Disorders, 15,* 21–33.

Marshall, R. C., & Neuburger, S. I. (1987). Effects of delayed auditory feedback on acquired stuttering following head injury. *Journal of Fluency Disorders, 12,* 355–365.

Martin, R. R., & Haroldson, S. K. (1981). Stuttering identification: Standard definition and the moment of stuttering. *Journal of Speech and Hearing Research, 24,* 59–63.

Martin, R. R., & Haroldson, S. K. (1992). Stuttering and speech naturalness: Audio and audiovisual judgments. *Journal of Speech and Hearing Research, 35,* 521–528.

Martin, R. R., Haroldson, S. K., & Triden, K. A. (1984). Stuttering and speech naturalness. *Journal of Speech and Hearing Disorders, 49,* 53–58.

Martin, R. R., Kuhl, P., & Haroldson, S. K. (1972). An experimental treatment with two preschool stuttering children. *Journal of Speech and Hearing Research, 15,* 743–752.

Martin, R. R., & Lindamood, L. P. (1986). Stuttering and spontaneous recovery: Implications for the speech-language pathologist. *Language, Speech, and Hearing Services in Schools, 17,* 207–218.

Martin, R. R., & Siegel, G. M. (1966). The effects of response contingent shock on stuttering. *Journal of Speech and Hearing Research, 9,* 340–352.

Martin, R. R., St. Louis, K., Haroldson, S., & Hasbrouck, J. (1975). Punishment and negative reinforcement of stuttering using electric shock. *Journal of Speech and Hearing Research, 18,* 478–490.

Maske-Cash, W. S., & Curlee, R. F. (1995). Effect of utterance length and meaningfulness on the speech initiation times of children who stutter and children who do not stutter. *Journal of Speech and Hearing Research, 38,* 18–25.

Mathews, J. (1986). Historical prologue. In G. H. Shames & H. Rubin (Eds.), *Stuttering then and now* (pp. 5–18). Columbus, OH: Charles E. Merrill.

Max, L., & Baldwin, C. J. (2010). The role of motor learning in stuttering adaptation: Repeated versus novel utterances in a practice–retention paradigm. *Journal of Fluency Disorders, 35,* 33–43.

Max, L., Caruso, A., & Vandevenne, A. (1997). Decreased stuttering frequency during repeated readings: A motor learning perspective. *Journal of Fluency Disorders, 22,* 17–34.

Max, L., & Caruso, A. J. (1998). Adaptation of stuttering frequency during repeated readings: Associated changes in acoustic parameters of perceptually fluent speech. *Journal of Speech, Language, and Hearing Research, 41,* 1265–1281.

Max, L., Guenther, F. H., Gracco, V. L., Ghosh, S. S., & Wallace, M. E. (2004). Unstable or insufficiently activated internal models and feedback-biased motor control as sources of dysfluency: A theoretical model of stuttering. *Contemporary Issues in Communication Science and Disorders, 31,* 105–122.

Maxwell, D. L., & Satake, E. (2006). *Research and statistical methods in communication sciences and disorders.* Clifton Park, NY: Thomson Delmar Learning

McAllister, J., & Kingston, M. (2005). Final part-word repetitions in school-age children: Two case studies. *Journal of Fluency Disorders, 30,* 255–267.

McClean, M. D., Goldsmith, H., & Cerf, A. (1984). Lower-lip EMG and displacement during bilabial disfluencies in adult stutterers. *Journal of Speech and Hearing Research, 27,* 342–349.

McClean, M. D., & McLean, A., Jr. (1985). Case report of stuttering acquired in association with phenytoin use for post-head-injury seizures. *Journal of Fluency Disorders, 10,* 241–255.

McClean, M. D., & Runyan, C. M. (2000). Variations in the relative speeds of orofacial structures with stuttering severity. *Journal of Speech, Language, and Hearing Research, 43,* 1524–1531.

McClean, M. D., & Tasko, S. M. (2002). Association of orofacial with laryngeal and respiratory motor output during speech. *Experimental Brain Research, 146,* 481–489.

McDevitt, S. C., & Carey, W. B. (1978). The measurement of temperament in 3–7 year old children. *Journal of Child Psychology & Psychiatry, 19,* 245–253.

McGraw-Hill Education. (2014). *First performances–Fox in a Box.* Monterrey, CA: CTB/McGraw-Hill.

McKeehan, A. B. (1994). Student experiences with fluency facilitating speech strategies. *Journal of Fluency Disorders, 19,* 113–123.

McKinnon, D. H., McLeod, S., & Reilly, S. (2007). The prevalence of stuttering, voice, and speech-sound disorders in primary school students in Australia. *Language, Speech, and Hearing Services in Schools, 38,* 5–15.

McKnight, R. C., & Cullinan, W. L. (1987). Subgroups of stuttering children: Speech and voice reaction times, segmental durations, and naming latencies. *Journal of Fluency Disorders, 12,* 217–233.

Meilijson, S. R., Kasher, A., & Elizur, A. (2004). Language performance in chronic schizophrenia: A pragmatic approach. *Journal of Speech, Language, and Hearing Research, 47,* 695–713.

Menzies, R. G., O'Brian, S., Onslow, M., Packman, A., St. Clare, T., & Block, S. (2008). An experimental clinical trial of a cognitive-behavior therapy package for chronic stuttering. *Journal of Speech, Language, and Hearing Research, 51,* 1451–1464.

Merits-Patterson, R., & Reed, C. G. (1981). Disfluencies in the speech of language-delayed children. *Journal of Speech and Hearing Research, 24,* 55–58.

Merritt, D. D., & Liles, B. Z. (1989). Narrative analysis: Clinical applications of story generation and story retelling. *Journal of Speech and Hearing Disorders, 54,* 429–438.

Messenger, M., Onslow, M., Packman, A., & Menzies, R. (2004). Social anxiety in stuttering: Measuring negative social expectancies. *Journal of Fluency Disorders, 29,* 201–212.

Meyers, S. C., & Freeman, F. J. (1985). Mother and child speech rates as a variable in stuttering and disfluency. *Journal of Speech and Hearing Research, 28,* 436–444.

Meyers, S. C., Hall, N. E., & Aram, D. M. (1990). Fluency and language recovery in a child with a left hemisphere lesion. *Journal of Fluency Disorders, 15,* 159–173.

Miles, S., & Bernstein Ratner, N. (2001). Parental language input to children at stuttering onset. *Journal of Speech, Language, and Hearing Research, 44,* 1116–1130.

Millard, S. K., Nicholas, A., & Cook, F. M. (2008). Is parent-child interaction therapy effective in reducing stuttering? *Journal of Speech, Language, and Hearing Research, 51,* 636–650.

Miller, J. F. (1981). *Assessing language production in children: Experimental procedures.* Baltimore, MD: University Park Press.

Miller, J. F., Chapman, R. S., & Nockerts, A. (1998). *Systematic analysis of language transcripts: Basic SALT programs for Windows®.* Madison, WI: Waisman Research Center, University of Wisconsin.

Miller, S., & Watson, B. C. (1992). The relationship between communication attitude, anxiety, and depression in stutterers and nonstutterers. *Journal of Speech and Hearing Research, 35,* 789–798.

Minifie, F. D., & Cooker, H. S. (1964). A disfluency index. *Journal of Speech and Hearing Disorders, 29,* 189–192.

Molt, L. (1996). An examination of various aspects of auditory processing in clutterers. *Journal of Fluency Disorders, 21,* 215–225.

Montgomery, B. M., & Fitch, J. L. (1988). The prevalence of stuttering in the hearing-impaired school age population. *Journal of Speech and Hearing Disorders, 53,* 131–135.

Moore, W. H. (1976). Bilateral tachistoscopic word perception of stutterers and normal subjects. *Brain and Language, 3,* 434–442.

Moore, W. H. (1984). Central nervous system characteristics of stutterers. In R. F. Curlee & W. H. Perkins (Eds.), *Nature and treatment of stuttering: New directions* (pp. 49–72). Boston, MA: College-Hill Press.

Morley, M. E. (1957). *The development and disorders of speech in childhood.* Edinburgh, UK: Livingstone.

Mowrer, D. E. (1987). Repetition of final consonants in the speech of a young child.

Journal of Speech and Hearing Disorders, 52, 174–178.

Mulcahy, K., Hennessey, N., Beilby, J., & Byrnes, M. (2008). Social anxiety and the severity and typography of stuttering in adolescents. *Journal of Fluency Disorders, 33,* 306–319.

Munson, B., & Solomon, N. (2004). The effect of phonological neighborhood density on vowel articulation. *Journal of Speech, Language, and Hearing Research, 47,* 1048–1058.

Murphy, W. P., Yaruss, J., & Quesal, R. W. (2007). Enhancing treatment for school-age children who stutter I. Reducing negative reactions through desensitization and cognitive restructuring. *Journal of Fluency Disorders, 32,* 121–138.

Myers, F. L. (1996). Cluttering: A matter of perspective. *Journal of Fluency Disorders, 21,* 175–185.

Myers, F. L. (2010) Primacy of self-awareness and the modulation of rate in the treatment of cluttering. In K. Bakker, F. L. Myers, & L. J. Raphael (Eds.), *Proceedings of the First World Conference on Cluttering* (pp. 108–114). International Cluttering Association. Retrieved November 2, 2013, from http://associations.missouristate.edu/ICA/

Myers, F. L. (2011). Treatment of cluttering: A cognitive-behavioral approach centered on rate control. In D. Ward & K. Scaler Scott (Eds.), *Cluttering: A handbook of research, intervention and education* (pp. 152–174). New York, NY: Psychology Press.

Myers, F. L., & St. Louis, K. O. (1992). *Cluttering: A clinical perspective.* Leicester, UK: Far Communications.

Myers, F. L., & St. Louis, K. O. (1996). Two youths who clutter, but is that the only similarity? *Journal of Fluency Disorders, 21,* 297–304.

Namasivayam, A. K., & van Lieshout, P. (2008). Investigating speech motor practice and learning in people who stutter. *Journal of Fluency Disorders, 33,* 32–51.

Naremore, R. C., & Dever, R. B. (1975). Language performance of educable mentally retarded and normal children at five age levels. *Journal of Speech and Hearing Research, 18,* 82–95.

Nathan, R., & Stanovich, K. (1991). The causes and consequences of differences in reading fluency. *Theory Into Practice, 30,* 177–184.

Nathani, S., Oller, D. K., & Cobo-Lewis, A. (2003). Final syllable lengthening (FSL) in infant vocalizations. *Journal of Child Language, 30,* 3–25.

National Center for Education Statistics (NCES). (2002). *National assessment of educational progress (NAEP) oral reading fluency scale, Grade 4, 2002.* Author. Retrieved from http://nces.ed.gov/nationsreportcard/studies/ors/scale.asp

National Center for Learning Disabilities (NCLD). (2014). *What are learning disabilities?* Author. Retrieved from http://ncld.org/types-learning-disabilities/what-is-ld/what-are-learning-disabilities

National Institute of Mental Health. (2014). *Attention deficit hyperactivity disorder.* Author. Retrieved from http://www.nimh.nih.gov/health/topics/attention-deficit-hyperactivity-disorder-adhd/index.shtml

National Institute of Neurological Disorders and Stroke (NINDS). (2014). *Tourette syndrome information page.* Author. Retrieved from http://www.ninds.nih.gov/disorders/tourette/tourette.htm

Natke, U., Grosser, K., & Kalveram, T. (2001). Fluency, fundamental frequency, and speech rate under frequency-shifted feedback in stuttering and nonstuttering persons. *Journal of Fluency Disorders, 26,* 227–241.

Natke, U., Sandrieser, P., Pietrowsky, R., & Kalveram, K. (2006). Disfluency data of German preschool children who stutter and comparison children. *Journal of Fluency Disorders, 31,* 165–176.

Navarro-Ruiz, M., & Rallo-Fabra, L. (2001). Characteristics of mazes produced by SLI children. *Clinical Linguistics & Phonetics, 15,* 63–66.

Navon, D. (1984). Resources—A theoretical soup stone. *Psychological Review, 91,* 216–234.

Neath, I., & Surprenant, A. M. (2003) *Human memory* (2nd ed.). Belmont, CA: Wadsworth/Thomson Learning.

Neel, A. T., & Palmer, P. M. (2012). Is tongue strength an important influence on rate of articulation in diadochokinetic and reading tasks? *Journal of Speech, Language, and Hearing Research, 55,* 235–246.

Neilson, M. D., & Neilson, P. D. (1987). Speech motor control and stuttering: A computational model of adaptive sensory-motor processing. *Speech Communication, 6,* 325–333.

Nelson, S. E., Hunter, N., & Walter, M. (1945). Stuttering in twin types. *Journal of Speech and Hearing Disorders, 10,* 335–343.

Nelson-Jones, R. (2002). *Essential counseling and therapy skills: The skilled client model.* London, UK: Sage.

Nespor, M., & Vogel, I., (1986). *Prosodic phonology.* Dordrecht: Foris.

Neumann, K., & Euler, H. (2010). Neuroimaging and stuttering. In B. Guitar & R. McCauley (Eds.), *Treatment of stuttering: Established and emerging interventions* (pp. 355–377). Baltimore, MD: Lippincott Williams & Wilkins.

Neumann, K., Euler, H. A., von Gudenberg, A., Giraud, A., Lanfermann, H., Gall, V., & Preibisch, C. (2003). The nature and treatment of stuttering as revealed by fMRI: A within- and between-group comparison. *Journal of Fluency Disorders, 28,* 381–410.

Neumann, K., Preibisch, C., Euler, H. A., von Gudenberg, A., Lanfermann, H., Gall, V., & Giraud, A. (2005). Cortical plasticity associated with stuttering therapy. *Journal of Fluency Disorders, 30,* 23–39.

Newcomer, P. L., & Hammill, D. D. (2008) *Test of Language Development: Primary*–4th Edition [TOLD:P:4]. Austin, TX: Pro-Ed.

Nichols, A. C. (1966). Audience ratings of the "naturalness" of spoken and written sentences. *Speech Monographs, 33,* 156–159.

Nicolosi, L., Harryman, E., & Kresheck, J. (1989). *Terminology of communication disorders.* (3rd ed.). Baltimore, MD: Lippincott Williams & Wilkins.

Nippold, M. A. (2011). Stuttering in school-age children: A call for treatment research. *Language, Speech, and Hearing Services in Schools, 42,* 99–101.

Nippold, M. A. (2012a). Stuttering and language ability in children: Questioning the connection. *American Journal of Speech-Language Pathology, 21,* 183–196.

Nippold, M. A. (2012b). When a school-aged child stutters, let's focus on the primary problem. *Language, Speech, and Hearing Services in Schools, 43,* 549–551.

Nippold, M. A., & Rudzinski, M. (1995). Parents' speech and children's stuttering: A critique of the literature. *Journal of Speech and Hearing Research, 38,* 978–989.

Nippold, M. A., Schwarz, I. E., & Jescheniak, J. (1991). Narrative ability in school-age stuttering boys: A preliminary investigation. *Journal of Fluency Disorders, 16,* 289–308.

Norrick, N. R. (2008). Using large corpora of conversation to investigate narrative: The case of interjections in conversational storytelling performance. *International Journal of Corpus Linguistics, 13,* 438–464.

Norrick, N. R. (2009). Interjections as pragmatic markers. *Journal of Pragmatics, 41,* 866–891.

Norris, J. (1995). Expanding language norms for school-age children and adolescents: Is it pragmatic? *Language, Speech, and Hearing Services in Schools, 26,* 342–352.

Nowack, W. J., & Stone, R. (1987). Acquired stuttering and bilateral cerebral disease. *Journal of Fluency Disorders, 12,* 141–146.

Ntourou, K., Conture, E. G., & Lipsey, M. W. (2011). Language abilities of children who stutter: A meta-analytical review. *American Journal of Speech-Language Pathology, 20,* 163–179.

O'Brian, S., Packman, A., & Onslow, M. (2004a). Self-rating of stuttering severity as a clinical tool. *American Journal of Speech-Language Pathology, 13,* 219–226.

O'Brian, S., Packman, A., Onslow, M., & O'Brian, N. (2004b). Measurement of stuttering in adults: Comparison of stuttering-rate and severity-scaling methods. *Journal of Speech, Language, and Hearing Research, 47,* 1081–1087.

O'Connell, D. C., Kowal, S., Sabin, E. J., Lamia, J. F., & Dannevik, M. (2010). Start-up rhetoric in eight speeches of Barack Obama. *Journal of Psycholinguistic Research, 39,* 393–409.

O'Donnell, J. J., Armson, J., & Kiefte, M. (2008). The effectiveness of SpeechEasy during situations of daily living. *Journal of Fluency Disorders, 33,* 99–119.

Okalidou, A., & Kampanaros, M. (2001). Teacher perceptions of communication impairment at screening stage in preschool children living in Patras, Greece. *International Journal of Language & Communication Disorders, 36,* 489–502.

Olander, L., Smith, A., & Zelaznik, H. N. (2010). Evidence that a motor timing deficit is a factor in the development of stuttering. *Journal of Speech, Language, and Hearing Research, 53,* 876–886.

Oller, D. K. (1973). The effect of position in utterance on speech segment duration in English. *Journal of the Acoustical Society of America, 54,* 1235–1247.

Onslow, M. (1992). Choosing a treatment procedure for early stuttering: Issues and future directions. *Journal of Speech and Hearing Research, 35,* 983–993.

Onslow, M. (1996). *Behavioral management of stuttering.* San Diego, CA: Singular.

Onslow, M., Andrews, C., & Lincoln, M. (1994). A control/experimental trial of an operant treatment for early stuttering. *Journal of Speech and Hearing Research, 37,* 1244–1259.

Onslow, M., Costa, L., & Rue, S. (1990). Direct early intervention with stuttering: Some preliminary data. *Journal of Speech and Hearing Disorders, 55,* 405–416.

Onslow, M., Gardner, K., Bryant, K. M., Stuckings, C. L., & Knight, T. (1992). Stuttered and normal speech events in early childhood: The validity of a behavioral data language. *Journal of Speech and Hearing Research, 35,* 79–87.

Onslow, M., & Ingham, R. J. (1987). Speech quality measurement and the management of stuttering. *Journal of Speech and Hearing Disorders, 52,* 2–17.

Onslow, M., Packman, A., & Harrison, E. (2003). *The Lidcombe Program of early stuttering intervention: A clinician's guide.* Austin, TX: Pro-Ed.

Onslow, M., Packman, A., Stocker, S., van Doorn, J., & Siegel, G. M. (1997). Control of children's stuttering with response-contingent time-out: Behavioral, perceptual, and acoustic data. *Journal of Speech, Language, and Hearing Research, 40,* 121–133.

Onslow, M., Stocker, S., Packman, A., & McLeod, S. (2002). Speech timing in children after the Lidcombe Program of early stuttering intervention. *Clinical Linguistics & Phonetics, 16,* 21–33.

Orlikoff, R. F., & Baken, R. J. (1993). *Clinical speech and voice measurement.* San Diego, CA: Singular.

Ornstein, A. F., & Manning, W. H. (1985). Self-efficacy scaling by adult stutterers. *Journal of Communication Disorders, 18,* 313–320.

Osawa, A., Maeshima, S., & Yoshimora, T. (2006). Acquired stuttering in a patient with Wernicke's aphasia. *Journal of Clinical Neuroscience, 13,* 1066–1069.

Otto, F. M., & Yairi, E. (1974). An analysis of the speech disfluencies in Down's syndrome and in normally intelligent subjects. *Journal of Fluency Disorders, 1,* 26–32.

Özdemir, E., Norton, A., & Schlaug, G. (2006). Shared and distinct neural correlates of singing and speaking. *Neuroimage, 33,* 628–635.

Packman, A., Onslow, M., Richard, F., & Van Doorn, J. (1996). Syllabic stress and variability: A model of stuttering. *Clinical Linguistics and Phonetics, 10,* 235–263.

Paden, E., Yairi, E., & Ambrose, N. G. (1999). Early childhood stuttering II: Initial status of phonological abilities. *Journal of Speech, Language, and Hearing Research, 42,* 1113–1124.

Paden, E. P., Yairi, E., & Ambrose, N. G. (2002). Phonological progress during the first 2 years of stuttering. *Journal of Speech, Language, and Hearing Research, 45,* 256–267.

Panico, J., & Healey, E. C. (2009). Influence of text type, topic familiarity, and stuttering frequency on listener recall, comprehension, and mental effort. *Journal of Speech, Language, and Hearing Research, 52,* 534–546.

Parnell, M., & Amerman, J. D. (1977). Subjective evaluation of articulatory effort. *Journal of Speech and Hearing Research, 20,* 644–652.

Parrish, W. M. (1951). The concept of "naturalness." *Quarterly Journal of Speech, 37,* 448–450.

Paul, R., & Smith, R. L. (1993). Narrative skills in 4-year-olds with normal, impaired, and late-developing language, *Journal of Speech and Hearing Research, 36,* 592–598.

Pearl, S. Z., & Bernthal, J. E. (1980). The effect of grammatical complexity upon disfluency behavior of nonstuttering preschool children. *Journal of Fluency Disorders, 5,* 55–68.

Pellowski, M. W., & Conture, E. G. (2002). Characteristics of speech disfluency and stuttering behaviors in 3- and 4-year-old children. *Journal of Speech, Language, and Hearing Research, 45,* 20–34.

Perfetti, C. A. (1985). *Reading ability.* New York, NY: Oxford University Press.

Perkins, W. H. (1973). Replacement of stuttering with normal speech: I. Rationale. *Journal of Speech and Hearing Disorders, 38,* 283–294.

Perkins, W. H., Bell, J., Johnson, L., & Stochs, J. (1979). Phone rate and the effective planning time hypothesis of stuttering. *Journal of Speech and Hearing Research, 22,* 747–755.

Perkins, W. H., Kent, R. D., & Curlee, R. F. (1991). A theory of neuropsycholinguistic function in stuttering. *Journal of Speech and Hearing Research, 34,* 734–752.

Perkins, W. H., Rudas, J., Johnson, L., Michael, W. B., & Curlee, R. F. (1974). Replacement of stuttering with normal speech: III. Clinical effectiveness. *Journal of Speech and Hearing Disorders, 39,* 416–428.

Philofsky, A., Fidler, D. J., & Hepburn, S. (2007). Pragmatic language profiles of school-age children with autism spectrum disorders and Williams syndrome. *American Journal of Speech-Language Pathology, 16,* 368–380.

Pikulski, J. J., & Chard, D. J. (2005). Fluency: Bridge between decoding and reading comprehension. *The Reading Teacher, 58,* 510–519.

Pindzola, R. H., Jenkins, M. M., & Lokken, K. J. (1989). Speaking rates of young children. *Language, Speech, and Hearing Services in Schools, 20,* 133–138.

Pindzola, R. H., & White, D. T. (1986). A protocol for differentiating the incipient stutterer. *Language, Speech, and Hearing Services in Schools, 17,* 2–15.

Plexico, L. W., Cleary, J. E., McAlpine, A., & Plumb, A. M. (2010). Disfluency characteristics observed in young children with autism spectrum disorders: A preliminary report. *Perspectives on Fluency and Fluency Disorders, 20,* 42–50.

Plexico, L. W., Manning, W. H., & DiLollo, A. (2005). A phenomenological understanding of successful stuttering management. *Journal of Fluency Disorders, 30,* 1–22.

Plexico, L. W., Manning, W. H., & DiLollo, A. (2010). Client perceptions of effective and ineffective therapeutic alliances during treatment for stuttering. *Journal of Fluency Disorders, 35,* 333–354.

Pollard, R., Ellis, J. B., Finan, D., & Ramig, P. R. (2009). Effects of the SpeechEasy on objective and perceived aspects of stuttering: A 6-month, Phase I clinical trial in naturalistic environments. *Journal of Speech, Language, and Hearing Research, 52,* 516–533.

Porfert, A. R., & Rosenfield, D. B. (1978). Prevalence of stuttering. *Journal of Neurology, Neurosurgery & Psychiatry, 41,* 954–956.

Porter, H. V. K. (1939). Studies in the psychology of stuttering: XIV. Stuttering phenomena in relation to size and personnel of audience. *Journal of Speech and Hearing Disorders, 4,* 323–333.

Porter, J. N., Collins, P. F., Muetzel, R. L., Lim, K. O., & Luciana, M. (2011). Associations between cortical thickness and verbal fluency in childhood, adolescence, and young adulthood. *Neuroimage, 55,* 1865–1877.

Postma, A., & Kolk, H. (1990). Speech errors, disfluencies, and self-repairs of stutterers in two accuracy conditions. *Journal of Fluency Disorders, 15,* 291–303.

Postma, A., & Kolk, H. (1991). Manual reaction times and error rates in stutterers. *Perceptual and Motor Skills, 72,* 627–630.

Postma, A., & Kolk, H. (1993). The covert repair hypothesis: Prearticulatory repair processes in normal and stuttered disfluencies. *Journal of Speech and Hearing Research, 36,* 472–487.

Postma, A., Kolk, H., & Povel, D. (1990). Speech planning and execution in stutterers. *Journal of Fluency Disorders, 15,* 49–59.

Prelock, P. A., & Panagos, J. M. (1989). The influence of processing mode on the sentence productions of language-disordered and normal children. *Clinical Linguistics and Phonetics, 3,* 251–263.

Preus, A. (1990). Treatment of mentally retarded stutterers. *Journal of Fluency Disorders, 15,* 223–233.

Preus, A. (1992). Cluttering and stuttering: Related, different, or antagonistic disorders? In F. L. Myers & K. O. St. Louis (Eds.), *Cluttering: A clinical perspective* (pp. 55–70). Leicester, UK: Far Communications.

Preus, A. (1996). Stuttering upgraded. *Journal of Fluency Disorders, 21,* 349–357.

Prins, D., & Hubbard, C. P. (1988). Response contingent stimuli and stuttering: Issues and implications. *Journal of Speech and Hearing Research, 31,* 696–709.

Prins, D., Hubbard, C. P., & Krause, M. (1991). Syllabic stress and the occurrence of stuttering. *Journal of Speech and Hearing Research, 34,* 1011–1016.

Prins, D., & Lohr, F. (1972). Behavioral dimensions of stuttered speech. *Journal of Speech and Hearing Research, 15,* 61–71.

Proctor, A., Yairi, E., Duff, M. C., & Zhang, J. (2008). Prevalence of stuttering in African American preschoolers. *Journal of Speech, Language, and Hearing Research, 51,* 1465–1479.

Prosek, R. A., & House, A. S. (1975). Intraoral air pressure as a feedback cue in consonant production. *Journal of Speech and Hearing Research, 18,* 133–147.

Prosek, R. A., Walden, B. E., Montgomery, A. A., & Schwartz, D. M. (1979). Some correlates of stuttering severity judgments. *Journal of Fluency Disorders, 4,* 215–222.

Quesal, R. W. (1988). Inexact use of "disfluency" and "disfluency" in stuttering research [Letter to the editor]. *Journal of Speech and Hearing Disorders, 53,* 349–350.

Quillian, M. R. (1967). Word concepts: A theory and simulation of some basic semantic capabilities. *Behavioral Science, 12,* 410–430.

Rami, M. K., Kalinowski, J., Stuart, A., & Rastatter, M. P. (2003). Self-perceptions of speech language pathologists-in-training before and after pseudostuttering experiences on the telephone. *Disability and Rehabilitation, 25,* 491–496.

Ramig, P., & Bennett, E. M. (1997). Clinical management of children: Direct management strategies. In R. F. Curlee & G. M. Siegel (Eds.), *Nature and treatment of stuttering: New directions* (pp. 292–313). Needham Heights, MA: Allyn & Bacon.

Ramig, P. R., & Dodge, D. M. (2005). *The child and adolescent stuttering treatment and activity resource guide.* Clifton Park, NY: Thomson Delmar Learning.

Ramig, P. R., Krieger, S. M., & Adams, M. R. (1982). Vocal changes in stutterers and non-stutterers when talking to children. *Journal of Fluency Disorders, 7,* 369–384.

Rasinski, T. V. (2012). Why reading fluency should be hot! *The Reading Teacher, 65,* 516–522.

Rathvon, N. (2004). *Early reading assessment: A practitioner's handbook.* New York, NY: Guilford Press.

Reardon, N. A., & Yaruss, J. S. (2004). *The source for stuttering: Ages 7–18.* East Moline, IL: LinguiSystems.

Reardon-Reeves, N. (2010). Two thumbs up! In J. Kuster (Ed.), *Proceedings of the International Cluttering Online Conference, 2010.* Retrieved from http://www.mnsu.edu/comdis/ica1/icacon1.html

Reichel, I. (2010). Treating the person who clutters and stutters. In K. Bakker, F. L. Myers, & L. J. Raphael (Eds.), *Proceedings of the First World Conference on Cluttering* (pp. 99–107). International Cluttering Association. Retrieved from http://associations.missouristate.edu/ICA/

Reilly, J., Rodriguez, A. D., Lamy, M., & Neils-Strunjas, J. (2010). Cognition, language, and clinical pathological features of non-

Alzheimer's dementias: An overview. *Journal of Communication Disorders, 43*, 438–452.

Reilly, S., Onslow, M., Packman, A., Cini, E., Conway, L., Ukoumunne, O. C., . . . Wake, M. (2013). Natural history of stuttering to 4 years of age: A prospective community-based study. *Pediatrics, 132*, 460–467.

Rentschler, G. J., Driver, L. E., & Callaway, E. A. (1984). The onset of stuttering following drug overdose. *Journal of Fluency Disorders, 9*, 265–284.

Reynolds, C. R., & Richmond, B. O. (1985). *Revised Children's Manifest Anxiety Scale (RCMAS) manual*. Los Angeles, CA: Western Psychological Services.

Riaz, N., Steinberg, S., Ahmad, J., Pluzhnikov, A., Riazuddin, S., Cox, N. J., & Drayna, D. (2005). Genomewide significant linkage to stuttering on chromosome 12. *American Journal of Human Genetics, 76*(4), 647–651.

Richels, C., & Conture, E. G. (2010). Indirect treatment of childhood stuttering: Diagnostic predictors of treatment outcome. In B. Guitar & R. McCauley (Eds.), *Treatment of stuttering: Established and emerging interventions* (pp. 18–55). Baltimore, MD: Lippincott Williams & Wilkins.

Riecker, A., Mathiak, K., Wildgruber, D., Erb, M., Hertrich, I., Grodd, W., & Ackermann, H. (2005). fMRI reveals two distinct cerebral networks subserving speech motor control. *Neurology, 64*, 700–706.

Riley, G. D. (1994). *Stuttering severity instrument* (3rd ed.). Austin, TX: Pro-Ed.

Riley, G. D. (2009). *Stuttering severity instrument* (4th ed.). Austin, TX: Pro-Ed.

Riley, G. D., & Ingham, J. C. (2000). Acoustic duration changes associated with two types of treatment for children who stutter. *Journal of Speech, Language, and Hearing Research, 43*, 965–978.

Riley, J., Riley, G., & Maguire, G. (2004). Subjective screening of stuttering severity, locus of control, and avoidance: Research edition. *Journal of Fluency Disorders, 29*, 51–62.

Rispoli, M. (2003). Changes in the nature of sentence production during the period of grammatical development. *Journal of Speech, Language, and Hearing Research, 46*, 818–830.

Robb, M., Maclagan, M., & Chen, Y. (2004). Speaking rates of American and New Zealand varieties of English. *Clinical Linguistics and Phonetics, 18*, 1–15.

Robbins, J., & Klee, T. (1987). Clinical assessment of oropharyngeal motor development in young children. *Journal of Speech and Hearing Disorders, 52*, 271–277.

Rochester, S. (1973). The significance of pauses in spontaneous speech. *Journal of Psycholinguistic Research, 2*, 51–81.

Rodríguez-Aranda, C., & Martinussen, M. (2006). Age-related differences in performance of phonemic verbal fluency measured by Controlled Oral Word Association Task (COWAT): A meta-analytic study. *Developmental Neuropsychology, 30*, 697–717.

Roelofs, A. (1997). The WEAVER model of word-form encoding in speech production. *Cognition, 64*, 249–84.

Roelofs, A. (2000). WEAVER++ and other computational models of lemma retrieval and word-form encoding. In L. Wheeldon (Ed.), *Aspects of language production* (pp. 71–114). Philadelphia, PA: Taylor & Francis.

Roelofs, A. (2003). Modeling the relation between the production and recognition of spoken word forms. In N. O. Schiller & A. S. Meyer (Eds.), *Phonetics and phonology in language comprehension and production: Differences and similarities* (pp. 115–158). Berlin, Germany: Mouton de Gruyter.

Roelofs, A., & Meyer, A. S. (1998). Metrical structure in planning the production of spoken words. *Journal of Experimental Psychology: Learning, Memory, & Cognition, 24*, 922–939.

Rogalski, Y., Altmann, L. J. P., Plummer-D'Amato, P., Behrman, A. L., & Marsiske, M. (2010). Discourse coherence and cognition after stroke: A dual task study. *Journal of Communication Disorders, 43*, 212–224.

Rosenbek, J., Messert, B., Collins, M., & Wertz, R. (1978). Stuttering following brain damage. *Brain and Language, 6*, 82–96.

Rosenbek, J. C. (1984). Stuttering secondary to nervous system damage. In R. F. Curlee & W. H. Perkins (Eds.), *Nature and treatment of stuttering: New directions* (pp. 31–48). Boston, MA: College-Hill Press.

Rosenbek, J. C., & LaPointe, L. L. (1985). The dysarthrias: Description, diagnosis, and treatment. In D. F. Johns (Ed.), *Clinical management of neurogenic communicative disorders* (2nd ed., pp. 97–152). Boston, MA: Little, Brown and Company.

Rosenfield, D., & Jerger, J. (1984). Stuttering and auditory function. In R. F. Curlee & G. M. Siegel (Eds.), *Nature and treatment of stuttering: New directions* (pp. 73–88). Needham Heights, MA: Allyn & Bacon.

Ross, T. P., Weinberg, M., Furr, A. E., Carter, S. E., Evans-Blake, L., & Parham, S. (2005). The temporal stability of cluster and switch scores using a modified COWAT procedure. *Archives of Clinical Neuropsychology, 20,* 983–996.

Rothbart, M. K., & Bates, J. E. (1998). Temperament. In N. Eisenberg (Ed.), *Handbook of child psychology, 5th ed.: Vol 3. Social, emotional, and personality development* (pp. 105–176). Hoboken, NJ: John Wiley & Sons.

Rousey, C. G., Arjunan, K. N., & Rousey, C. L. (1986). Successful treatment of stuttering following closed head injury. *Journal of Fluency Disorders, 11,* 257–261.

Rudmin, F. (1984). Parent's reports of stress and articulation oscillation as factors in a preschooler's disfluencies. *Journal of Fluency Disorders, 9,* 85–87.

Ruff, R. M., Light, R. H., Parker, S. B., & Levin, H. S. (1996). Benton Controlled Oral Word Association Test: Reliability and updated norms. *Archives of Clinical Neuropsychology, 11,* 329–338.

Runyan, C. M., Bell, J. N., & Prosek, R. A. (1990). Speech naturalness ratings of treated stutterers. *Journal of Speech and Hearing Disorders, 55,* 434–438.

Rustin, L., & Cook, F. (1995). Parental involvement in the treatment of stuttering. *Language, Speech, and Hearing Services in Schools, 26,* 127–137.

Ryan, B. (1974). *Programmed therapy for stuttering in children and adults.* Springfield, IL: Charles C. Thomas.

Ryan, B. (1992). Articulation, rate, and fluency characteristics of stuttering and nonstuttering preschool children. *Journal of Speech and Hearing Research, 35,* 333–342.

Ryan, B. P., & Van Kirk Ryan, B. (1995). Programmed stuttering treatment for children: Comparison of two establishment programs through transfer, maintenance, and follow-up. *Journal of Speech and Hearing Research, 38,* 61–75.

Saltuklaroglu, T., & Kalinowski, J., (2005). How effective is therapy for childhood stuttering? Dissecting and reinterpreting the evidence in light of spontaneous recovery rates. *International Journal of Language and Communication Disorders, 40,* 359–374.

Saltuklaroglu, T., Kalinowski, J., & Guntupalli, V. K. (2004). Towards a common neural substrate in the immediate and effective inhibition of stuttering. *International Journal of Neuroscience, 114,* 435–450.

Samuels, S. J. (1979). The method of repeated readings. *The Reading Teacher, 32,* 403–408.

Sander, E. K. (1963). Frequency of syllable repetition and 'stutterer' judgments. *Journal of Speech and Hearing Disorders, 28,* 19–30.

Sapienza, C., & Ruddy, B. H. (2009). *Voice disorders.* San Diego, CA: Plural.

Sawyer, J., Chon, H., & Ambrose, N. G. (2008). Influences of rate, length, and complexity on speech disfluency in a single-speech sample in preschool children who stutter. *Journal of Fluency Disorders, 33,* 220–240.

Sawyer, J., & Yairi, E. (2006). The effect of sample size on the assessment of stuttering severity. *American Journal of Speech-Language Pathology, 15,* 36–44.

Saxon, K. G., & Ludlow, C. L. (2007). A critical review of the effect of drugs on stuttering. In E. G. Conture & R. F. Curlee (Eds.), *Stuttering and related disorders of fluency* (pp. 277–294). New York, NY: Thieme Medical.

Scaler Scott, K. (2011) Cluttering and autism spectrum disorders. In D. Ward & K. Scaler Scott (Eds.), *Cluttering: A handbook of research, intervention and education* (pp. 115–134). New York, NY: Psychology Press.

Scaler Scott, K., Grossman, H. L., & Tetnowski, J. A. (2010). A survey of cluttering instruction in fluency courses. In K. Bakker, F. L. Myers, & L. J. Raphael (Eds.), *Proceedings of the First World Conference on Cluttering* (pp. 171–179). International Cluttering Association. Retrieved November 2, 2013, from http://associations.missouristate.edu/ICA/

Schiavetti, N., Sacco, P. R., Metz, D. E., & Sitler, R. W. (1983). Direct magnitude estimation and interval scaling of stuttering events. *Journal of Speech and Hearing Research*, *26*, 568–573.

Schiller, N. O., Meyer, A. S., Baayen, R. H., & Levelt, W. J. M. (1996). A comparison of lexeme and speech syllables in Dutch. *Journal of Quantitative Linguistics*, *3*, 8–28.

Schlanger, B. B., & Gottsleben, R. H. (1957). Analysis of speech defects among the institutional mentally retarded. *Journal of Speech and Hearing Disorders*, *22*, 98–103.

Schloss, P. J., Espin, C. A., Smith, M. A., & Suffolk, D. R. (1987). Developing assertiveness during employment interviews with young adults who stutter. *Journal of Speech and Hearing Disorders*, *52*, 30–36.

Schmidt, L., Lebreton, M., Cléry-Melin, M., Daunizeau, J., & Pessiglione, M. (2012). Neural mechanisms underlying motivation of mental versus physical effort. *PLoS Biology*, *10*, 1–13.

Schönpflug, U. (2008). Pauses in elementary school children's verbatim and gist free recall of a story. *Cognitive Development*, *23*, 385–394.

Schriefers, H., Meyer, A. S., & Levelt, W. J. M. (1990). Exploring the time course of lexical access in production: Picture-word interference studies. *Journal of Memory and Language*, *29*, 86–102.

Schuell, H., Jenkins, J. J., & Jiminez-Pabon, E. (1964). *Aphasia in adults: Diagnosis, prognosis, and treatment*. New York, NY: Harper & Row.

Schulte, K. (2009). *Communication and communication disorders: Empirical examination of characteristics and coexisting disorders on cluttering* (Doctoral dissertation). University of Technology, Dortmund, Germany.

Schwartz, M. F. (1977). *Stutter no more*. New York, NY: Simon & Schuster.

Schwenk, K. A., Conture, E. G., & Walden, T. A. (2007). Reaction to background stimulation of preschool children who do and do not stutter. *Journal of Communication Disorders*, *40*, 129–141.

Scott, C. M., & Windsor, J. (2000). General spoken language performance measures in spoken and written narrative and expository discourse of school-aged children with language learning disabilities. *Journal of Speech, Language, and Hearing Research*, *43*, 324–339.

Searle, J. R. (1975). A taxonomy of illocutionary acts. In K. Gunderson (Ed.), *Language, mind, and knowledge: Minnesota studies in the philosophy of science* (Vol. 7, pp. 344–369). Minneapolis: University of Minnesota Press.

Seery, C. H. (2005). Differential diagnosis of stuttering for forensic purposes. *American Journal of Speech-Language Pathology*, *14*, 284–294.

Seery, C. H., Watkins, R. V., Mangelsdorf, S. C., & Shigeto, A. (2007). Subtyping stuttering II: Contributions from language and temperament. *Journal of Fluency Disorders*, *32*, 197–217.

Seider, R. A., Gladstien, K. L., & Kidd, K. K. (1983). Recovery and persistence of stuttering among relatives of stutterers. *Journal of Speech and Hearing Disorders*, *48*, 402–409.

Selkirk, E. O. (1984). *Phonology and syntax: The relation between sound and structure*. Cambridge, MA: MIT Press.

Semel, E., Wiig, E. H., & Secord, W. A. (2003). *Clinical Evaluation of Language Fundamentals®–Fourth Edition [CELF–4]*. San Antonio, TX: Pearson.

Shames, G. H., & Florance, C. L. (1980) *Stutter-free speech: A goal for therapy*. Columbus, OH: Charles E. Merrill.

Shapiro, D. A. (2011) *Stuttering intervention: A collaborative journey to fluency freedom*. Austin, TX: Pro-Ed.

Shattuck-Hufnagel, S. (1979). Speech errors as evidence for a serial order mechanism in sentence production. In W. E. Cooper & E. C. T. Walker (Eds.), *Sentence processing* (pp. 295–342). Hillsdale, NJ: Lawrence Erlbaum Associates.

Shearer, W. M., & Williams, J. (1965). Self-recovery from stuttering. *Journal of Speech and Hearing Disorders, 30,* 288–290.

Sheehan, J. G. (1958). Conflict theory of stuttering. In J. Eisenson (Ed.), *Stuttering: A symposium* (pp. 121–166). New York, NY: Harper & Row.

Sheehan, J. G. (1970). *Stuttering: Research and therapy.* New York, NY: Harper & Row.

Sheehan, J. G., & Martyn, M. M. (1966). Spontaneous recovery from stuttering. *Journal of Speech and Hearing Research, 9,* 121–135.

Sheehan, J. G., & Martyn, M. M. (1970). Stuttering and its disappearance. *Journal of Speech and Hearing Research, 13,* 279–289.

Sheehan, J. G., Martyn, M. M., & Kilburn, K. L. (1968). Speech disorders in retardation. *American Journal of Mental Deficiency, 73,* 251–256.

Shriberg, L. D., Aram, D. M., & Kwiatkowski, J. (1997a). Developmental apraxia of speech: I. Descriptive and theoretical perspectives. *Journal of Speech, Language, and Hearing Research, 40,* 273–285.

Shriberg, L. D., Aram, D. M., & Kwiatkowski, J. (1997b). Developmental apraxia of speech: II. Towards a diagnostic marker. *Journal of Speech, Language, and Hearing Research, 40,* 286–312.

Shriberg, L. D., Aram, D. M., & Kwiatkowski, J. (1997c). Developmental apraxia of speech: III. A subtype marked by inappropriate stress. *Journal of Speech, Language, and Hearing Research, 40,* 313–337.

Shriberg, L. D., Austin, D., Lewis, B. A., Mc-Sweeny, J. L., & Wilson, D. L. (1997). The Speech Disorders Classification System (SDCS): Extensions and lifespan reference data. *Journal of Speech, Language, and Hearing Research, 40,* 723–740.

Shriberg, L. D., & Kwiatkowski, J. (1982). Phonological disorders: I. A diagnostic classification system. *Journal of Speech and Hearing Disorders, 47,* 226–241.

Shriberg, L. D., Paul, R., McSweeney, J., Klin, A., Cohen, D., & Volkmar, F. (2001). Speech and prosody characteristics of adolescents and adults with high-functioning autism and Asperger syndrome. *Journal of Speech, Language, and Hearing Research, 44,* 1097–1115.

Shugart, Y. Y., Mundorff, J., Kilshaw, J., Doheny, K., Doan, B., Wanyee, J., . . . Drayna, D. (2004). Results of a genome-wide linkage scan for stuttering. *American Journal of Medical Genetics A, 124,* 133–135.

Shumak, I. C. (1955). A speech rating sheet for stutterers. In W. Johnson & R. R. Leutenegger (Eds.), *Stuttering in children and adults* (pp. 341–347). Minneapolis, MN: University of Minnesota Press.

Silbergleit, A. K., Feit, H., & Silbergleit, R. (2009). Neurogenic stuttering in corticobasal ganglionic degeneration: A case report. *Journal of Neurolinguistics, 22,* 83–90.

Silverman, E.-M., & Williams, D. E. (1967b). A comparison of stuttering and nonstuttering children in terms of five measures of oral language development. *Journal of Communication Disorders, 1,* 305–309.

Silverman, F. H., & Williams, D. E. (1967a). Loci of disfluencies in the speech of nonstutterers during oral reading. *Journal of Speech and Hearing Research, 10,* 790–794.

Silverman, S. W., & Bernstein Ratner, N. (1997). Syntactic complexity, fluency, and accuracy of sentence imitation in adolescents. *Journal of Speech, Language, and Hearing Research, 40,* 95–106.

Sisskin, V. (2006). Speech disfluency in Asperger's syndrome: Two cases of interest. *Perspectives on Fluency and Fluency Disorders, 16,* 12–14.

Sjölander, K., & Beskow, J. (2006). *Wavesurfer* [Computer software and manual]. Retrieved from http://speech.kth.se/wavesurfer/index.html

Skinner, B. F. (1953). *Science and human behavior.* New York, NY: Macmillan.

Smith, A. (1989). Neural drive to muscles in stuttering. *Journal of Speech and Hearing Research, 32,* 252–264.

Smith, A. (1992). 'A theory of neuropsycholinguistic function in stuttering': Commentary. *Journal of Speech and Hearing Research, 35,* 805–809.

Smith, A., Denny, M., Shaffer, L. A., Kelly, E. M., & Hirano, M. (1996). Activity of intrinsic laryngeal muscles in fluent and disfluent speech. *Journal of Speech and Hearing Research, 39*, 329–348.

Smith, A., & Goffman, L. (1998). Stability and patterning of speech movement sequences in children and adults. *Journal of Speech, Language, and Hearing Research, 41*, 18–30.

Smith, A., Goffman, L., Sasisekaran, J., & Weber-Fox, C. (2012). Language and motor abilities of preschool children who stutter: Evidence from behavioral and kinematic indices of nonword repetition performance. *Journal of Fluency Disorders, 37*, 344–358.

Smith, A., & Kelly, E. (1997). Stuttering: A dynamic multifactorial model. In R. F. Curlee & G. M. Siegel (Eds.), *Nature and treatment of stuttering: New directions* (pp. 204–217). Needham Heights, MA: Allyn & Bacon.

Smith, A., & Kleinow, J. (2000). Kinematic correlates of speaking rate changes in stuttering and normally fluent adults. *Journal of Speech, Language, and Hearing Research, 43*, 521–536.

Smith, A., Luschei, E., Denny, M., Wood, J. L., Hirano, M., & Badylak, S. (1993). Spectral analyses of activity of laryngeal and orofacial muscles in stutterers. *Journal of Neurology, Neurosurgery, and Psychiatry, 56*, 1303–1311.

Smith, A., Sadagopan, N., Walsh, B., & Weber-Fox (2010). Increasing phonological complexity reveals heightened instability in inter-articulatory coordination in adults who stutter. *Journal of Fluency Disorders, 35*, 1–18.

Smith, A., & Weber, C. M. (1988, April). The need for an integrated perspective on stuttering. *ASHA, 30*, 30–32.

Smith, B. L., Brown, B. L., Strong, W. J., & Rencher, A. C. (1975). Effects of speech rate on personality perception. *Language and Speech, 18*, 145–152.

Smits-Bandstra, S. & De Nil, L. F. (2006). *Sequency skill learning and the transition to automaticity in adults who stutter.* Dissertation Abstracts International, DAI-B 68/01, 288 (AAT NR22037).

Smits-Bandstra, S., & De Nil, L. F. (2007). Sequence skill learning in persons who stutter: Implications for cortico-striato-thalamo-cortical dysfunction. *Journal of Fluency Disorders, 32*, 251–278.

Smits-Bandstra, S., & De Nil, L. F. (2009). Speech skill learning of persons who stutter and fluent speakers under single and dual task conditions. *Clinical Linguistics & Phonetics, 23*, 38–57.

Smits-Bandstra, S., De Nil, L. F., & Rochon, E. (2006). The transition to increased automaticity during finger sequence learning in adult males who stutter. *Journal of Fluency Disorders, 31*, 22–42.

Smits-Bandstra, S., De Nil, L. F., & Saint-Cyr, J. A. (2006) Speech and nonspeech sequence skill learning in adults who stutter. *Journal of Fluency Disorders, 31*, 116–131.

Snow, D. (1994). Phrase–final syllable lengthening and intonation in early child speech. *Journal of Speech and Hearing Research, 37*, 831–840.

Snow, D. (1997). Children's acquisition of speech timing in English: A comparative study of voice onset time and final syllable vowel lengthening. *Journal of Child Language, 24*, 35–56.

Soderberg, G. A. (1966). The relations of stuttering to word length and word frequency. *Journal of Speech and Hearing Research, 9*, 584–589.

Soderberg, G. A. (1967). Linguistic factors in stuttering. *Journal of Speech and Hearing Research, 10*, 801–810.

Sommer, M., Koch, M. A., Paulus, W., Weiller, C., & Büchel, C. (2002). Disconnection of speech-relevant brain areas in persistent developmental stuttering. *The Lancet, 360*(9330), 380–383.

Sommers, R. K., Brady, W. A., & Moore, W. H. (1975). Dichotic ear preferences of stuttering children and adults. *Perceptual and Motor Skills, 41*, 931–938.

Spielberger, C. D., Gorsuch, R. L., Lushene, R. E., & Vagg, P. R. (1983). *Manual for the State-Trait Anxiety Inventory.* Palo Alto, CA: Consulting Psychologists Press.

St. Louis, K. O. (1992). On defining stuttering. In F. L. Myers & K. O. St. Louis (Eds.), *Clut-*

tering: A clinical perspective (pp. 37–53). Leicester, UK: Far Communications.

St. Louis, K. O. (1996). A tabular summary of cluttering subjects in the special edition. *Journal of Fluency Disorders, 21,* 337–344.

St. Louis, K. O. (2010). A ten-year agenda for cluttering: Excerpts featuring seven key guidelines. In K. Bakker, F. L. Myers, & L. J. Raphael (Eds.), *Proceedings of the First World Conference on Cluttering* (pp. 20–30). International Cluttering Association. Retrieved November 2, 2013, from http://associations.missouristate.edu/ICA/

St. Louis, K. O., Coskun, M., Ozdemir, S., Topbas, S., Goranova, E., & Filatova, Y. (2010a). Public attitudes toward cluttering and stuttering: USA, Bulgaria, Turkey, and Russia. In K. Bakker, F. L. Myers, & L. J. Raphael (Eds.), *Proceedings of the First World Conference on Cluttering* (pp. 190–198). International Cluttering Association. Retrieved November 2, 2013, from http://associations.missouristate.edu/ICA/

St. Louis, K. O., Goranova, E., Georgieva, D., Coskun, M., Filatova, Y., & McCaffrey, E. (2010b). Public awareness of cluttering: USA, Bulgaria, Turkey, and Russia. In K. Bakker, F. L. Myers, & L. J. Raphael (Eds.), *Proceedings of the First World Conference on Cluttering* (pp. 180–189). International Cluttering Association. Retrieved November 2, 2013, from http://associations.missouristate.edu/ICA/

St. Louis, K. O., & Hinzman, A. R. (1986). Studies of cluttering: Perceptions of cluttering by speech-language pathologists and educators. *Journal of Fluency Disorders, 11,* 131–149.

St. Louis, K. O., Hinzman, A. R., & Hull, F. M. (1985). Studies of cluttering: Disfluency and language measures in young possible clutterers and stutterers. *Journal of Fluency Disorders, 10,* 151–172.

St. Louis, K. O., Murray, C. D., & Ashworth, M. S. (1991). Coexisting communication disorders in a random sample of school-aged stutterers. *Journal of Fluency Disorders, 16,* 13–23

St. Louis, K. O., Myers, F. L., Bakker, K., & Raphael, L. J. (2007). Understanding and treating of cluttering. In E. G. Conture &

R. F. Curlee (Eds.), *Stuttering and related disorders of fluency* (3rd ed., pp. 297–325). New York, NY: Thieme Medical.

St. Louis, K. O., Myers, F. L., Cassidy, L. J., & Michael, A. J. (1996). Efficacy of delayed auditory feedback for treating cluttering: Two case studies. *Journal of Fluency Disorders, 21,* 305–314.

St. Louis, K. O., Myers, F. L., Faragasso, K., Townsend, P. S., & Gallaher, A. J. (2004). Perceptual aspects of cluttered speech. *Journal of Fluency Disorders, 29,* 213–235.

St. Louis, K. O., Raphael, L. J., Myers, F. L., & Bakker, K. (2003, November) Cluttering updated. *The ASHA Leader.* Retrieved from http://www.asha.org/Publications/leader/2003/031118/f031118a.htm

St. Louis, K. O., & Rustin, L. (1986). Professional awareness of cluttering. In F. L. Myers & K. O. St. Louis (Eds.), *Cluttering: A clinical perspective* (pp. 23–35). Leicester, UK: Far Communications.

St. Louis, K. O., & Schulte, K. (2011). Defining cluttering: The lowest common denominator. In D. Ward & K. Scaler Scott (Eds.), *Cluttering: A handbook of research, intervention and education* (pp. 233–253). New York, NY: Psychology Press.

Stager, S. V., Jeffries, K. J., & Braun, A. R. (2003). Common features of fluency-evoking conditions studied in stuttering subjects and controls: An $H_2^{15}O$ PET study. *Journal of Fluency Disorders, 28,* 319–336.

Stager, S. V., & Ludlow, C. L. (1998). The effects of fluency-evoking conditions on voicing onset types in persons who do and do not stutter. *Journal of Communication Disorders, 31,* 33–52.

Stansfield, J. (1995). Word-final disfluencies in adults with learning difficulties. *Journal of Fluency Disorders, 20,* 1–10.

Starkweather, C. W. (1987). *Fluency and stuttering.* Englewood Cliffs, NJ: Prentice Hall.

Starkweather, C. W., Franklin, S., & Smigo, T. M. (1984). Vocal and finger reaction times in stutterers and nonstutterers: Differences and correlations. *Journal of Speech and Hearing Research, 27,* 193–196.

Starkweather, C. W., Gottwald, S. R., & Halfond, M. M. (1990). *Stuttering prevention: A clini-*

cal method. Englewood Cliffs, NJ: Prentice Hall.

Stathopoulos, E. T., & Weismer, G. (1983). Closure duration of stop consonants. *Journal of Phonetics, 11,* 395–400.

Stein, N. L., & Glenn, C. G. (1979). An analysis of story comprehension in elementary school children. In R. O. Freedle (Ed.), *Discourse processing: Multidisciplinary perspectives.* Norwood, NJ: Ablex.

Steinberg, M. E., Bernstein Ratner, N., Gaillard, W., & Berl, M. (2013). Fluency patterns in narratives from children with localization related epilepsy. *Journal of Fluency Disorders, 38,* 193–205.

Stemberger, J. P. (1982). Syntactic errors in speech. *Journal of Pyscholingusitc Research, 11,* 313–345.

Stemberger, J. P. (1989). Speech errors in early child language production. *Journal of Memory and Language, 28,* 164–188.

Stevens, K. N. (1972). The quantal nature of speech: Evidence from articulatory-acoustic data. In P. B. Denes & E. E. David, Jr. (Eds.), *Human communication: A unified view* (pp. 51–66). New York, NY: McGraw-Hill.

Stevens, S. S. (1975). Partition scales and paradoxes. In G. Stevens (Ed.), *Psychophysics* (pp. 134–171). New York, NY: John Wiley & Sons.

Stribling, P., Rae, J., & Dickerson, P. (2007). Two forms of spoken repetition in a girl with autism. *International Journal of Language & Communication Disorders, 42,* 427–444.

Stuart, A., Frazier, C. L., Kalinowski, J., & Vos, P. W. (2008). The effect of frequency altered feedback on stuttering duration and type. *Journal of Speech, Language, and Hearing Research, 51,* 889–897.

Stuart, A., Kalinowski, J., Armson, J., Stenstrom, R., & Jones, K. (1996). Fluency effect of frequency alterations of plus/minus one-half and one-quarter octave shifts in auditory feedback of people who stutter. *Journal of Speech and Hearing Research, 39,* 396–401.

Stuart, A., Kalinowski, J., Saltuklaroglu, T., & Guntupalli, V. K. (2006). Investigations of the impact of altered auditory feedback in-the-ear devices on the speech of people who stutter: One-year follow-up. *Disability and Rehabilitation: An International, Multidisciplinary Journal, 28,* 757–765.

Sturm, J. A., & Seery, C. H. (2007). Speech and articulatory rates of school-age children in conversation and narrative contexts. *Language, Speech, and Hearing Services in Schools, 38,* 47–59.

Subramanian, A., Yairi, E., & Amir, O. (2003). Second formant transitions in fluent speech of persistent and recovered preschool children who stutter. *Journal of Communication Disorders, 36,* 59–75.

Subtelny, J. D., Worth, J. H., & Sakuda, M. (1966). Intraoral pressure and rate of flow during speech. *Journal of Speech and Hearing Research, 9,* 498–518.

Suresh, R., Ambrose, N. G., Roe, C., Pluzhnikov, A., Wittke-Thompson, J., Ng, M. C., . . . Cox, N. J. (2006). New complexities in the genetics of stuttering: Significant sex-specific linkage signals. *American Journal of Human Genetics, 78,* 554–563.

Susca, M., & Healey, E. C. (2001). Perceptions of simulated stuttering and fluency. *Journal of Speech, Language, and Hearing Research, 44,* 61–72.

Tani, T., & Sakai, Y. (2011). Stuttering after right cerebellar infarction: A case study. *Journal of Fluency Disorders, 35,* 141–145.

Taylor, I. K. (1966). What words are stuttered? *Psychological Bulletin, 65,* 233–242.

Taylor, R. M., & Morrison, L. P. (1996). *Taylor–Johnson temperament analysis manual.* Thousand Oaks, CA: Psychological Publications.

Teesson, K., Packman, A., & Onslow, M. (2003). The Lidcombe behavioral data language of stuttering. *Journal of Speech, Language, and Hearing Research, 46,* 1009–1015.

Teigland, A. (1996). A study of pragmatic skills of clutterers and normal speakers. *Journal of Fluency Disorders, 21,* 201–214.

Teshima, S., Langevin, M., Hagler, P., & Kully, D. (2010). Post-treatment speech naturalness of comprehensive stuttering program clients and differences in ratings among listener groups. *Journal of Fluency Disorders, 35,* 44–58.

Theys, C., van Wieringen, A., & De Nil, L. F. (2008). A clinician survey of speech and non-speech characteristics of neurogenic stuttering. *Journal of Fluency Disorders, 33*, 1–23.

Theys, C., van Wieringen, A., Sunaert, S. S., Thijs, V. V., & De Nil, L. F. (2011). A one-year prospective study of neurogenic stuttering following stroke: Incidence and co-occurring disorders. *Journal of Communication Disorders, 44*, 678–687.

Theys, C., van Wieringen, A., Tuyls, L., & De Nil, L. F. (2009). Acquired stuttering in a 16-year-old boy. *Journal of Neurolinguistics, 22*, 427–435.

Throneburg, R. N., & Yairi, E. (1994). Temporal dynamics of repetitions during the early stage of childhood stuttering: An acoustic study. *Journal of Speech and Hearing Research, 37*, 1067–1075.

Throneburg, R. N., & Yairi, E. (2001). Durational, proportionate, and absolute frequency characteristics of disfluencies: A longitudinal study regarding persistence and recovery. *Journal of Speech, Language, and Hearing Research, 44*, 38–51.

Throneburg, R. N., Yairi, E., & Paden, E. P. (1994). Relation between phonologic difficulty and the occurrence of disfluencies in the early stage of stuttering. *Journal of Speech and Hearing Research, 37*, 504–509.

Tiffany, W. R. (1980). The effect of syllable structure on diadochokinetic and reading rates. *Journal of Speech and Hearing Disorders, 23*, 894–908.

Trautman, L., Healey, E., Brown, T. A., Brown, P., & Jermano, S. (1999). A further analysis of narrative skills of children who stutter. *Journal of Communication Disorders, 32*, 297–315.

Trautman, L., Healey, E., & Norris, J. A. (2001). The effects of contextualization on fluency in three groups of children. *Journal of Speech, Language, and Hearing Research, 44*, 564–576

Travis, L. E. (1927). Dysintegration of the breathing movements during stuttering. *Archives of Neurology and Psychiatry, 18*, 673–690.

Travis, L. E. (1931). *Speech pathology.* New York, NY: Appleton-Century.

Travis, L. E. (1934). Disassociation of the homologous muscle function in stuttering. *Archives of Neurology and Psychiatry, 31*, 127–133.

Travis, L. E. (1971). The unspeakable feelings of people with special reference to stuttering. In L. E. Travis (Ed.), *Handbook of speech pathology and audiology* (pp. 1009–1033). Englewood Cliffs, NJ: Prentice Hall.

Treptow, M. A., Burns, M. K., & McComas, J. J. (2007). Reading at the frustration, instructional, and independent levels: The effects on students' reading comprehension and time on task. *School Psychology Review, 36*, 159–166.

Tsao, Y., & Weismer, G. (1997). Interspeaker variation in habitual speaking rate: Evidence for a neuromuscular component. *Journal of Speech, Language, and Hearing Research, 40*, 858–866.

Tsao, Y., Weismer, G., & Iqbal, K. (2006). Interspeaker variation in habitual speaking rate: Additional evidence. *Journal of Speech, Language, and Hearing Research, 49*, 1156–1164.

Tsiamtsiouris, J., & Cairns, H. S. (2013). Effects of sentence-structure complexity on speech initiation time and disfluency. *Journal of Fluency Disorders, 38*, 30–44.

Tulving, E. (1983) *Elements of episodic memory.* New York, NY: Oxford University Press.

Tulviste, T., Mizera, L., & De Geer, B. (2006). Teenagers' contribution to family mealtime conversations in Estonia, Sweden, and the U.S.: A comparative study. In A. Columbus (Ed.), *Advances in psychology research* (Vol. 45, pp. 159–180). Hauppauge, NY: Nova Science.

Tulviste, T., Mizera, L., De Geer, B., & Tryggvason, M. (2003). A silent Finn, a silent Finno-Ugric, or a silent Nordic? A comparative study of Estonian, Finnish, and Swedish mother-adolescent interactions. *Applied Psycholinguistics, 24*, 249–265.

Turget, N., Utku, U., & Balci, K. (2002). A case of acquired stuttering resulting from left parietal infarction. *Acta Neurologica Scandinavica, 105*, 408–410.

Umeda, N. (1977). Consonant duration in American English. *Journal of the Acoustical Society of America, 61,* 846–858.

van Beijsterveldt, C., Felsenfeld, S., & Boomsma, D. (2010). Bivariate genetic analyses of stuttering and nonfluency in a large sample of 5-year-old twins. *Journal of Speech, Language, and Hearing Research, 53,* 609–619.

Van Borsel, J., & Medeiros de Britto Pereira, M. M. (2005). Assessment of stuttering in a familiar versus an unfamiliar language. *Journal of Fluency Disorders, 30,* 109–124.

Van Borsel, J., Goethals, L., & Vanryckeghem, M. (2004). Disfluency in Tourette syndrome: Observational study in three cases. *Folia Phoniatrica et Logopaedica, 56,* 358–366.

Van Borsel, J., Moeyaert, J., Mostaert, C., Rosseel, R., Van Loo, E., & Van Renterghem, T. (2006). Prevalence of stuttering in regular and special school populations in Belgium based on teacher perceptions. *Folia Phoniatrica et Logopaedica, 58,* 289–302.

Van Borsel, J., Reunes, G., & Van den Bergh, N. (2003). Delayed auditory feedback in the treatment of stuttering: Clients as consumers. *International Journal of Language and Communication Disorders, 38,* 119–129.

Van Borsel, J., & Taillieu, C. (2001). Neurogenic stuttering versus developmental stuttering: An observer judgment study. *Journal of Communication Disorders, 34,* 1–11.

Van Borsel, J., & Tetnowski, J. A. (2007). Fluency disorders in genetic syndromes. *Journal of Fluency Disorders, 32,* 279–296.

Van Borsel, J., & Vandermuelen, A. (2008) Cluttering in Down syndrome. *Folia Phoniatrica et Logopaedica, 60,* 312–317.

Van Borsel, J., Van Lierde, K., Van Cauwenberge, P., Guldemont, I., & Van Orshoven, M. (1998). Severe acquired stuttering following injury of the left supplementary motor region: A case report. *Journal of Fluency Disorders, 23,* 49–58.

Van Borsel, J., & Vanryckeghem, M. (2000). Dysfluency and phonic tics in Tourette syndrome: A case report. *Journal of Communication Disorders, 33,* 227–240.

van Lieshout, P. H. H. M., Starkweather, C. W., Hulstijn, W., & Peters, H. F. M. (1995). Effects of linguistic correlates of stuttering on EMG activity in nonstuttering speakers. *Journal of Speech and Hearing Research, 38,* 360–372.

Van Riper, C. (1971). *The nature of stuttering.* Englewood Cliffs, NJ: Prentice Hall.

Van Riper, C. (1973). *The treatment of stuttering.* Englewood Cliffs, NJ: Prentice Hall.

Van Riper, C. (1982). *The nature of stuttering* (2nd ed.). Englewood Cliffs, NJ: Prentice Hall.

van Zaalen-op't Hof, Y., & DeJonckere, P. H. (2010). Cluttering: A language-based fluency disorder. In J. Kuster (Ed.), *Proceedings of the International Cluttering Online Conference, 2010.* Retrieved October 28, 2013, from http://www.mnsu.edu/comdis/ica1/icacon1.html

van Zaalen-op't Hof, Y., Wijnen, F., & DeJonckere, P. H. (2009). Differential diagnostic characteristics between cluttering and stuttering—Part one. *Journal of Fluency Disorders, 34,* 137–154.

Vanryckeghem, M., & Brutten, G. J. (1996). The relationship between communication attitude and fluency failure of stuttering and nonstuttering children. *Journal of Fluency Disorders, 21,* 109–118.

Vanryckeghem, M., & Brutten, G. J. (2012). A comparative investigation of the BigCat and Erickson S-24 measures of speech-associated attitude. *Journal of Communication Disorders, 45,* 340–347.

Wada, J. (1949). A new method for the determination of the side of cerebral speech dominance. *Medical Biology, 14,* 221–222.

Walker, B. J., Mokhtari, K., & Sargent, S. (2006). In T. Rasinski, C. Blachowicz, & K. Lems (Eds.), *Fluency instruction: Research-based best practices* (pp. 86–105). New York, NY: Guilford Press.

Walker, J. F., & Archibald, L. M. D. (2006). Articulation rates in preschool children: A 3-year longitudinal study. *International Journal of Language and Communication Disorders, 41,* 541–565.

Walker, J. F., Archibald, L. M. D., Cherniak, S. R., & Fish, V. G. (1992). Articulation rate in 3- and 5-year-old children. *Journal of Speech and Hearing Research, 35,* 4–13.

Wall, M. J., Starkweather, C. W., & Cairns, H. S. (1981). Syntactic influences on stuttering in young child stutterers. *Journal of Fluency Disorders, 6,* 283–298.

Walsh, B., & Smith, A. (2013). Oral electromyographic activation patterns for speech are similar in preschoolers who do and do not stutter. *Journal of Speech, Language, and Hearing Research, 56,* 1441–1454.

Ward, D. (2006). *Stuttering and cluttering: Frameworks for understanding and treatment.* New York, NY: Psychology Press.

Ward, D. (2011). Scope and constraint in the diagnosis of cluttering: Combining two perspectives. In D. Ward & K. Scaler Scott (Eds.), *Cluttering: A handbook of research, intervention and education* (pp. 254–262). New York, NY: Psychology Press.

Ward, D., & Scaler Scott, K. (2011). *Cluttering: A handbook of research, intervention and education.* New York, NY: Psychology Press.

Wardle, M., Cederbaum, K., & de Wit, H. (2011). Quantifying talk: Developing reliable measures of verbal productivity. *Behavior Research Methods, 43,* 168–178.

Watkins, K. E., Smith, S. M., Davis, S., & Howell, P. (2008). Structural and functional abnormalities of the motor system in developmental stuttering. *Brain: A Journal of Neurology, 131,* 50–59.

Watkins, R. V., & Yairi, E. (1997). Language production abilities of children whose stuttering persisted or recovered. *Journal of Speech, Language, and Hearing Research, 40,* 385–399.

Watkins, R. V., Yairi, E., & Ambrose, N. G. (1999). Early childhood stuttering III: Initial status of expressive language abilities. *Journal Speech, Language, and Hearing Research, 42,* 1125–1135.

Watson, B. C., Pool, K. D., Devous, M. D., Sr., Freeman, F. J., & Finitzo, T. (1992). Brain blood flow related to acoustic laryngeal reaction time in adult developmental stutterers. *Journal of Speech and Hearing Research, 35,* 555–561.

Weber, C. M., & Smith, A. (1990). Autonomic correlates of stuttering and speech assessed in a range of experimental tasks. *Journal of Speech and Hearing Research, 33,* 690–706.

Weber-Fox, C., & Hampton, A. (2008). Stuttering and natural speech processing of semantic and syntactic constraints on verbs. *Journal of Speech and Hearing Research, 51,* 1058–1071.

Weber-Fox, C., Spencer, R. M. C., Spruill, J. E., III, & Smith, A. (2004). Phonologic processing in adults who stutter: Electrophysiological and behavioral evidence. *Journal of Speech and Hearing Research, 47,* 1244–1258.

Weber-Fox, C., Wray, A., & Arnold, H. (2013). Early childhood stuttering and electrophysiological indices of language processing. *Journal of Fluency Disorders, 38,* 206–221.

Webster, W. G. (1986). Sequence reproduction deficits in stutterers tested under nonspeeded conditions. *Journal of Fluency Disorders, 14,* 79–86.

Webster, W. G. (1989). Sequence initiation performance by stutterers under conditions of response competition. *Brain and Language, 36,* 286–300.

Webster, W. G. (1990). Evidence in bimanual finger tapping of an attentional component to stuttering. *Behavioral Brain Research, 37,* 93–100.

Weiss, A. L., & Zebrowski, P. M. (1991). Patterns of assertiveness and responsiveness in parental interactions with stuttering and fluent children. *Journal of Fluency Disorders, 16,* 125–141.

Weiss, A. L., & Zebrowski, P. M. (1992). Disfluencies in the conversations of young children who stutter: Some answers about questions. *Journal of Speech and Hearing Research, 35,* 1230–1238.

Weiss, A. L., & Zebrowski, P. M. (1994). The narrative productions of children who stutter: A preliminary view. *Journal of Fluency Disorders, 19,* 39–63.

Weiss, D. (1964). *Cluttering.* Englewood Cliffs, NJ: Prentice Hall.

West, R. (1958). An agnostic's speculations about stuttering. In J. Eisenson (Ed.), *Stuttering: A symposium* (pp. 167–222). New York, NY: Harper & Row.

Westby, C. E. (1974). Language performance of stuttering and nonstuttering children. *Journal of Communication Disorders, 12,* 133–145.

Wexler, K. B. (1982). Developmental disfluency in 2-, 4-, and 6-year-old boys in neutral and stress situations. *Journal of Speech and Hearing Research, 25,* 229–234.

Wheeldon, L. (2000). Generating prosodic structure. In L. Wheeldon (Ed.), *Aspects of language production* (pp. 249–274). Philadelphia, PA: Taylor & Francis.

Wiederholt, J. L., & Bryant, B. R. (2012). *Gray Oral Reading Tests-5* (GORT-5), Austin, TX: Pro-Ed.

Wijnen, F. (1990). The development of sentence planning. *Journal of Child Language, 17,* 651–675.

Wijnen, F., & Boers, I. (1994). Phonological priming effects in stutterers. *Journal of Fluency Disorders, 19,* 1–20.

Williams, D. E. (1978). Differential diagnosis of disorders of fluency. In F. L. Darley & D. C. Spriestersbach (Eds.), *Diagnostic methods in speech pathology* (2nd ed., pp. 409–438). New York, NY: Harper & Row.

Williams, D. E., Darley, F. L., & Spriestersbach, D. C. (1978). Appraisal of rate and fluency. In F. L. Darley & D. C. Spriestersbach (Eds.), *Diagnostic methods in speech pathology* (pp. 256–283). New York, NY: Harper & Row.

Williams, D. E., & Kent, L. R. (1958). Listener evaluations of speech interruptions. *Journal of Speech and Hearing Research, 1,* 124–131.

Williams, D. E., Silverman, F. H., & Kools, J. A. (1968). Disfluency behavior of elementary school stutterers and non-stutterers: The adaptation effect. *Journal of Speech and Hearing Research, 11,* 622–630.

Williams, D. F., & Wener, D. L. (1996). Cluttering and stuttering exhibited in a young professional. *Journal of Fluency Disorders, 21,* 261–269.

Wilson, E. M., Green, J. R., Yunusova, Y., & Moore, C. (2008). Task specificity in early oral motor development. *Seminars in Speech and Language, 29,* 257–266.

Wingate, M. E. (1964a). A standard definition of stuttering. *Journal of Speech and Hearing Disorders, 29,* 484–489.

Wingate, M. E. (1964b). Recovery from stuttering. *Journal of Speech and Hearing Disorders, 29,* 312–321.

Wingate, M. E. (1967). Stuttering and word length. *Journal of Speech and Hearing Research, 10,* 146–152.

Wingate, M. E. (1984a). Pause loci in stuttered and normal speech. *Journal of Fluency Disorders, 9,* 227–235.

Wingate, M. E. (1984b). Stutter events and linguistic stress. *Journal of Fluency Disorders, 9,* 295–300.

Wingate, M. E. (1988). *The structure of stuttering: A psycholinguistic analysis.* New York, NY: Springer-Verlag.

Wittke-Thompson, J. K., Ambrose, N. G., Yairi, E., Roe, C., Cook, E. H., Ober, C., & Cox, N. J. (2007). Genetic studies of stuttering in a founder population. *Journal of Fluency Disorders, 32,* 33–50.

Wolfram, W. (2004). Social varieties of American English. In E. Finegan & J. R. Rickford (Eds.), *Language in the USA: Themes for the twenty-first century.* New York, NY: Cambridge University Press.

Wolk, L., Edwards, M., & Conture, E. G. (1993). Coexistence of stuttering and disordered phonology in young children. *Journal of Speech and Hearing Research, 36,* 906–917.

Wong, J. (2010). Cluttering—A parent's perspective. In J. Kuster (Ed.), *Proceedings of the International Cluttering Online Conference, 2010.* Retrieved October 28, 2013, from http://www.mnsu.edu/comdis/ica1/icacon1.html

Woolf, G. (1967). The assessment of stuttering as struggle, avoidance, and expectancy. *British Journal of Disorders of Communication, 2,* 158–171.

Workplace Bullying Institute (WBI). (2014). *The WBI definition of workplace bullying.* Author. Retrieved March 22, 2014, from http://www.workplacebullying.org/individuals/problem/definition/

World Health Organization (WHO). (2001). *International classification of function-*

ing, disability, and health: Short version. Geneva, Switzerland: Author.

World Health Organization (WHO). (2010). Stuttering. In Author: *ICD-10 Classification of Mental and Behavioral Disorders.* Retrieved from http://www.who.int/classifications/icd/en/bluebook.pdf

Wright, A., & Ayre, A. (2000). *Wright & Ayre Stuttering Self-Rating Profile* (WASSP). Bicester, UK: Speechmark.

Wright, C. E., (1979). Duration differences between rare and common words and their implications for the interpretation of word frequency effects. *Memory & Cognition, 7,* 411–419.

Wu, J. C., Maguire, G., Riley, G., Lee, A., Keator, D., Tang, C., . . . Najafi, A. (1997). Increased dopamine activity associated with stuttering. *Neuroreport: An International Journal for the Rapid Communication of Research in Neuroscience, 8,* 767–770.

Yairi, E. (1981). Disfluencies of normally speaking two-year-old children. *Journal of Speech and Hearing Research, 24,* 490–495.

Yairi, E. (1982). Longitudinal studies of disfluencies in two-year-old children. *Journal of Speech and Hearing Research, 25,* 155–160.

Yairi, E. (1997). Disfluency characteristics of childhood stuttering. In R. F. Curlee & G. M. Siegel (Eds.), *Nature and treatment of stuttering: New directions* (pp. 49–78). Needham Heights, MA: Allyn & Bacon.

Yairi, E. (2007). Subtyping stuttering I: A review. *Journal of Fluency Disorders, 32,* 165–196.

Yairi, E., & Ambrose, N. G. (1992a). A longitudinal study of stuttering in children: A preliminary report. *Journal of Speech and Hearing Research, 35,* 755–760.

Yairi, E., & Ambrose, N. G. (1992b). Onset of stuttering in preschool children: Selected factors. *Journal of Speech and Hearing Research, 35,* 782–788.

Yairi, E. & Ambrose, N. G. (1999). Early childhood stuttering I: Persistency and recovery rates. *Journal of Speech, Language, and Hearing Research, 42,* 1097–1112.

Yairi, E., & Ambrose, N. G. (2005). *Early childhood stuttering: For clinicians by clinicians.* Austin, TX: Pro-Ed.

Yairi, E., Ambrose, N., & Cox, N. (1996). Genetics of stuttering: A critical review. *Journal of Speech and Hearing Research, 39,* 771–784.

Yairi, E., Ambrose, N. G., & Niermann, R. (1993). The early months of stuttering: A developmental study. *Journal of Speech and Hearing Research, 36,* 521–528.

Yairi, E., Ambrose, N. G., Paden, E. P., & Throneburg, R. N. (1996). Predictive factors of persistence and recovery: Pathways of childhood stuttering. *Journal of Communication Disorders, 29,* 51–77.

Yairi, E., & Clifton, N. (1972). The disfluent speech behavior of preschool children, high school seniors, and geriatric persons. *Journal of Speech and Hearing Research, 15,* 714–719.

Yairi, E., & Hall, K. D. (1993). Temporal relations within repetitions of preschool children near the onset of stuttering: A preliminary report. *Journal of Communication Disorders, 26,* 231–244.

Yairi, E., & Seery, C. (2011). *Stuttering: Foundations and clinical applications.* Boston, MA: Pearson.

Yaruss, J. S. (1997). Clinical implications of situational variability in preschool children who stutter. *Journal of Fluency Disorders, 22,* 187–203.

Yaruss, J. S. (1998). Describing the consequences of disorders: Stuttering and the international classification of impairments, disabilities, and handicaps. *Journal of Speech, Language, and Hearing Research, 49,* 249–257.

Yaruss, J. S. (1999). Utterance length, syntactic complexity, and childhood stuttering. *Journal of Speech, Language, and Hearing Research, 42,* 329–344.

Yaruss, J. S. (2000). Converting between word and syllable counts in children's conversational speech samples. *Journal of Fluency Disorders, 25,* 305–316.

Yaruss, J. S., Coleman, C. E., & Quesal, R. W. (2012). Stuttering in school-age children: A comprehensive approach to treatment. *Language, Speech, and Hearing Services in Schools, 43,* 536–548.

Yaruss, J. S., LaSalle, L. R., & Conture, E. G. (1998) Evaluating stuttering in young children: Diagnostic data. *American Journal of Speech-Language Pathology, 7*, 62–76.

Yaruss, J. S., & Logan, K. J. (2002). Evaluating rate, accuracy, and fluency of young children's diadochokinetic productions: A preliminary investigation. *Journal of Fluency Disorders, 27*, 65–86.

Yaruss, J. S., Max, M. S., Newman, R., & Campbell, J. H. (1998). Comparing real-time and transcript-based techniques for measuring stuttering. *Journal of Fluency Disorders, 23*, 137–151.

Yaruss, J. S., & Quesal, R. W. (2004). Stuttering and the International Classification of Functioning, Disability, and Health: An update. *Journal of Communication Disorders, 37*, 35–52.

Yaruss, J. S., & Quesal, R. W. (2006). Overall Assessment of the Speaker's Experience of Stuttering (OASES): Documenting multiple outcomes in stuttering treatment. *Journal of Fluency Disorders, 31*, 90–115.

Yaruss, J. S., & Quesal, R. W. (2008). *Overall Assessment of the Speaker's Experience of Stuttering (OASES)*. Minneapolis, MN: Pearson.

Young, M. A. (1961). Predicting ratings of severity of stuttering. *Journal of Speech and Hearing Disorders, Monograph Supplement 7*, 31–54.

Young, M. A. (1975). Onset, prevalence, and recovery from stuttering. *Journal of Speech and Hearing Disorders, 40*, 49–58.

Young, M. A. (1981). Articulation effort: Transitivity and observer agreement. *Journal of Speech and Hearing Research, 24*, 224–232.

Zackheim, C. T., & Conture, E. G. (2003). Childhood stuttering and speech disfluencies in relation to children's mean length of utter-ance: A preliminary study. *Journal of Fluency Disorders, 28*, 115–142.

Zarate, J. (2013). The neural control of singing. *Frontiers in Human Neuroscience, 7*, 237. doi:10.3389/fnhum.2013.00237

Zebrowski, P. M. (1991). Duration of the speech disfluencies of beginning stutterers. *Journal of Speech and Hearing Research, 34*, 483–491.

Zebrowski, P. M. (1994). Duration of sound prolongation and sound/syllable repetition in children who stutter: Preliminary observations. *Journal of Speech and Hearing Research, 37*, 254–263.

Zebrowski, P. M., & Conture, E. G. (1989). Judgments of disfluency by mothers of stuttering and normally fluent children. *Journal of Speech and Hearing Research, 32*, 625–634.

Zebrowski, P. M., Conture, E. G., & Cudahy, E. A. (1985). Acoustic analysis of young stutterers' fluency: Preliminary observations. *Journal of Fluency Disorders, 10*, 173–192.

Zelaznik, H. N., Smith, A., Franz, E. A., & Ho, M. (1997). Differences in bimanual coordination associated with stuttering. *Acta Psychologica, 96*, 229–243.

Zimmermann, G. (1980). Stuttering: A disorder of movement. *Journal of Speech and Hearing Research, 23*, 122–136.

Zukowski, A. (2013). Putting words together. In J. B. Gleason & N. Bernstein Ratner (Eds.), *The development of language* (8th ed., pp. 120–162). Boston, MA: Pearson Education.

Zutell, J., & Rasinski, T. V. (1991). Training teachers to attend to their students' oral reading fluency. *Theory Into Practice, 30*, 211–217.

Index